# MASTER TECHNIQUES IN ORTHOPAEDIC SURGERY

■

# THE FOOT AND ANKLE

*Second Edition*

# MASTER TECHNIQUES IN ORTHOPAEDIC SURGERY

## Series Editor
## Roby C. Thompson, Jr., M.D.

### THE FOOT AND ANKLE
Second Edition: Harold B. Kitaoka, M.D.

First Edition: Kenneth A. Johnson, M.D.

### RECONSTRUCTIVE KNEE SURGERY
Douglas W. Jackson, M.D.

### KNEE ARTHROPLASTY
Second Edition: Paul A. Lotke, M.D. and Jess H. Lonner, M.D.

First Edition: Paul A. Lotke, M.D.

### THE HIP
Clement B. Sledge, M.D.

### THE SPINE
Second Edition: David S. Bradford, M.D. and Thomas A. Zdeblick, M.D.

First Edition: David S. Bradford, M.D.

### THE SHOULDER
Edward V. Craig, M.D.

### THE ELBOW
Bernard F. Morrey, M.D.

### THE WRIST
Richard H. Gelberman, M.D.

### THE HAND
Second Edition: James W. Strickland, M.D. and Thomas J. Graham, M.D.

First Edition: James W. Strickland, M.D.

### FRACTURES
Donald A. Wiss, M.D.

# THE FOOT AND ANKLE

## Second Edition

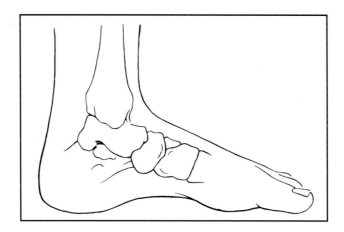

## Editor

### HAROLD B. KITAOKA, M.D.
**Head, Foot and Ankle Section
Department of Orthopaedics
Mayo Clinic and Mayo Foundation
Professor of Orthopaedics
Mayo School of Medicine
Rochester, Minnesota**

## Illustrator

### Deborah Ravin
**Phoenix, Arizona**

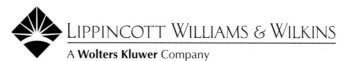

# LIPPINCOTT WILLIAMS & WILKINS
A **Wolters Kluwer** Company

Philadelphia · Baltimore · New York · London
Buenos Aires · Hong Kong · Sydney · Tokyo

*Acquisitions Editor:* James Merritt
*Developmental Editor:* Julia Seto
*Production Editor:* Elaine Verriest McClusky
*Manufacturing Manager:* Tim Reynolds
*Cover Designer:* Karen Quigley
*Compositor:* Maryland Composition

**© 2002 by LIPPINCOTT WILLIAMS & WILKINS**
**530 Walnut Street**
**Philadelphia, PA 19106 USA**
**LWW.com**

Printed in China

---

**Library of Congress Cataloging-in-Publication Data**

The foot and ankle / editor, Harold B. Kitaoka ; illustrator, Deborah Ravin.—2nd ed.
    p. ; cm.—(Master techniques in orthopaedic surgery)
  Includes bibliographical references and index.
  ISBN-13: 978-0-7817-3363-2
  ISBN-l0: 0-7817-3363-4
    1. Foot—Surgery. 2. Ankle—Surgery. I. Kitaoka, Harold B. II. Master techniques in orthopaedic surgery (2nd ed.) ·
  [DNLM: 1. Ankle—surgery. 2. Foot—surgery. 3. Orthopedics. WE 880 F6859 2002]
  RD781 .F572 2002
  617.5′85059—dc21

                                              2002016192

---

10 9 8 7 6 5 4 3

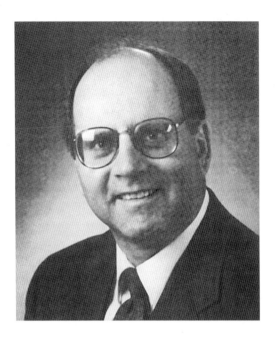

To Kenneth A. Johnson, colleague, friend, and pioneer in the foot and ankle specialty. Dr. Johnson was a consultant at the Mayo Clinic Scottsdale, past president of the American Orthopaedic Foot and Ankle Society, and editor of the first edition of the *Master Techniques in Orthopaedic Surgery: The Foot and Ankle.*

To the contributors—superb surgeons and educators—who gave up their personal time in order to share their expertise.

To our families, who strongly supported the efforts required to bring this book to fruition.

To the memory of my late mother, Shizu Kitaoka, and to my father Hiroo Kitaoka.

■

# CONTENTS

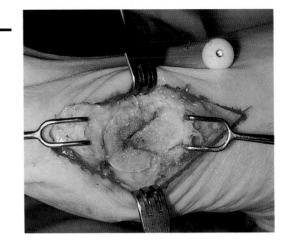

# PART IV   HINDFOOT

# CONTRIBUTORS

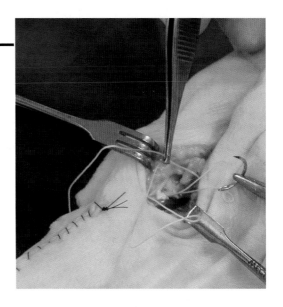

**Ian J. Alexander, M.D.**
*Department of Orthopaedic Surgery, Northeastern Ohio Universities College of Medicine, Rootstown, Ohio*

**James A. Amis, M.D.**
*Director of Foot/Ankle Service, Clinical Instructor, Department of Orthopaedic Surgery, University of Cincinnati; and Active Staff, Department of Orthopaedic Surgery, Good Samaritan Hospital, Cincinnati, Ohio*

**Robert B. Anderson, M.D.**
*Chief, Foot and Ankle Service, Department of Orthopaedics and Vice-Chairman, Department of Orthopaedic Surgery, Carolinas Medical Center; and Private Practice, Miller Orthopaedic Clinic, Charlotte, North Carolina*

**Donald E. Baxter, M.D.**
*Fondren, Houston, Texas*

**Irwin L. Bliss, M.D.**
*Assistant Clinical Professor, Department of Orthopaedic Surgery, University of California Los Angeles Medical Center; and Attending Surgeon, Department of Orthopaedic Surgery, Cedars Sinai Medical Center, Los Angeles, California*

**W. Grant Braly, M.D.**
*Clinical Assistant Professor, Department of Orthopaedic Surgery, University of Texas Health Science Center-Houston; and Associate, Fondren Orthopedic Group, Foot and Ankle Section, Texas Orthopedic Hospital, Houston, Texas*

**Timothy J. Bray, M.D.**
*Clinical Professor Orthopaedic Surgery, University of California-Davis Medical Center, Sacramento, California; and Reno Orthopaedic Clinic, Reno, Nevada*

**James W. Brodsky, M.D.**
*Clinical Professor, Department of Orthopaedic Surgery, University of Texas Southwestern Medical School; and Director, Foot and Ankle Surgery Fellowship, Baylor University Medical Center and University of Texas Southwestern Medical School, Dallas, Texas*

**Jason H. Calhoun, M.D.**
*Professor and Chairman, Department of Orthopaedics and Rehabilitation, University of Texas Medical Branch, Galveston, Texas*

**Laurette Chang, M.D.**
*Fellow, The Center for Orthopaedic Care, Inc., Cincinnati, Ohio*

**Stephen F. Conti, M.D.**
*Associate Professor, Department of Orthopaedic Surgery, University of Pittsburgh School of Medicine; and Chief, Division of Foot and Ankle Surgery, University of Pittsburgh Physicians, Pittsburgh, Pennsylvania*

**Michael J. Coughlin, M.D.**
*Clinical Professor, Department of Orthopaedic Surgery, Oregon Health Sciences University, Portland, Oregon; and Private Practice, Boise, Idaho*

**Diane L. Dahm, M.D.**
*Assistant Professor, Department of Orthopaedic Surgery, Mayo Clinic, Rochester, Minnesota*

**W. Hodges Davis, M.D.**
*Chief, Foot and Ankle Service, Department of Orthopaedic Surgery, Carolinas Medical Center; and Private Practice, Miller Orthopaedic Clinic, Charlotte, North Carolina*

**David J. Dixon, M.D.**
*Private Practice, Foot and Ankle Surgery, Northeast Orthopaedics; and Attending, Albany Medical Center, Albany, New York*

**Carol Frey, M.D.**
*Assistant Clinical Professor, Department of Orthopaedic Surgery, University of California Los Angeles; and Chief, Foot and Ankle Surgery, West Coast Sports Performance, Manhattan Beach, California*

**Richard E. Gellman, M.D., P.C.**
*Orthopaedic Surgeon, Portland Orthopaedic Specialists, Portland, Oregon*

**Gregory P. Guyton, M.D.**
*Assistant Professor, Department of Orthopaedic Surgery; and Foot and Ankle Service, Department of Orthopaedics, University of North Carolina at Chapel Hill, Chapel Hill, North Carolina*

**William G. Hamilton, M.D.**
*Clinical Professor, Department of Orthopaedic Surgery, Columbia University College of Physicians and Surgeons; Senior Attending, St. Luke's-Roosevelt Hospital Center; and Orthopedic Associates of New York, New York, New York*

**Sigvard T. Hansen, Jr., M.D.**
*Professor, Department of Orthopaedics and Sports Medicine, University of Washington; and Harborview Medical Center, Seattle, Washington*

**Carl T. Hasselman, M.D.**
*Clinical Instructor, Department of Orthopaedic Surgery, University of Pittsburgh; and Surgeon, Three Rivers Orthopaedic Associates, Pittsburgh, Pennsylvania*

**Steven A. Herbst, M.D.**
*Foot and Ankle Division, Central Indiana Orthopaedics, Muncie, Indiana*

**Christopher B. Hirose, M.D.**
*Resident in Orthopaedic Surgery, Department of Orthopaedic Surgery, Washington University School of Medicine; and Barnes-Jewish Hospital, St. Louis, Missouri*

**Jeffrey E. Johnson, M.D.**
*Associate Professor, Department of Orthopaedic Surgery, Washington University School of Medicine; and Associate Professor, Department of Orthopaedic Surgery, Barnes-Jewish Hospital, St. Louis, Missouri*

**Steven J. Kavros, D.P.M.**
*Assistant Professor, Department of Orthopaedic Surgery, Mayo Clinic, Rochester, Minnesota*

**Todd A. Kile, M.D.**
*Assistant Professor Orthopaedic Surgery, Mayo Graduate School of Medicine, Mayo Clinic, Rochester, Minnesota; and Consultant and Chair, Foot and Ankle Surgery, Department of Orthopaedic Surgery, Mayo Clinic Scottsdale and Hospital, Scottsdale, Arizona*

**Gary Kish, M.D.**
*Department of Orthopaedics, Portsmouth Regional Hospital, Portsmouth, New Hampshire*

**Harold B. Kitaoka, M.D.**
*Head, Foot and Ankle Section, Department of Orthopaedics, Mayo Clinic and Mayo Foundation; and Professor of Orthopaedics, Mayo School of Medicine, Rochester, Minnesota*

**Roger A. Mann, M.D.**
*Director, Foot Fellowship Program, Private Practice, Oakland, California*

**Arthur Manoli II, M.D.**
*Director, Michigan International Foot & Ankle Center, Pontiac, Michigan*

**James Michelson, M.D.**
*Professor, Orthopaedic Surgery and Director of Clinical Informatics, The George Washington University School of Medicine and Health Sciences, Washington, DC*

**Mark S. Myerson, M.D.**
*Attending Surgeon, Department of Orthopaedics, Union Memorial Hospital, Baltimore, Maryland*

**Javad Parvizi, M.D.**
*Chief Resident, Department of Orthopaedic Surgery, Mayo Clinic, Rochester, Minnesota*

**Glenn B. Pfeffer, M.D.**
*Assistant Clinical Professor, Department of Orthopaedics, University of California, San Francisco; and California Pacific Medical Center, San Francisco, California*

**E. Greer Richardson, M.D.**
*Professor, Orthopedic Surgery, Campbell Clinic-University of Tennessee, Germantown; and Director, Foot and Ankle Service and Fellowship, Department of Orthopaedic Surgery, University of Tennessee Teaching Hospital, Memphis, Tennessee*

**Michael M. Romash, M.D., COL. M.C., USA (RET.)**
*Clinical Assistant Professor, Department of Surgery, Uniformed Services University of Health Sciences, Bethesda, Maryland; and Orthopaedic Surgeon, Orthopaedic Foot and Ankle Center of Hampton Roads, Chesapeake General Hospital, Chesapeake, Virginia*

**Charles L. Saltzman, M.D.**
*Professor, Departments of Orthopaedic Surgery, and Biomedical Engineering, University of Iowa, Iowa City, Iowa*

**G. James Sammarco, M.D.**
*Volunteer Professor, Department of Orthopaedic Surgery, University of Cincinnati School of Medicine; and Director, Foot and Ankle Fellowship, The Center for Orthopaedic Care, Inc., Cincinnati, Ohio*

**Melanie Sanders, M.D.**
*Private Practice, OrthoIndy, Indianapolis, Indiana*

**Roy Sanders, M.D.**
*Clinical Professor, Division of Orthopaedic Surgery, University of South Florida; and Chief, Department of Orthopaedics, Tampa General Hospital, Tampa, Florida*

**Bruce J. Sangeorzan, M.D.**
*Professor, Department of Orthopaedics and Sports Medicine, University of Washington; and Chief of Service, Department of Orthopaedics and Sports Medicine, Harborview Medical Center, Seattle, Washington*

**Lew C. Schon, M.D.**
*Attending Surgeon, Department of Orthopaedics, Union Memorial Hospital, Baltimore, Maryland*

**Michael J. Shereff, M.D.**
*Clinical Professor, Department of Orthopaedic Surgery, Medical University of South Carolina; and Director, Foot and Ankle Center, Orthopaedic Specialists of Charleston, Charleston, South Carolina*

**Lex A. Simpson, M.D.**
*Chief, Department of Orthopaedic Surgery, Cleveland
Clinic Florida, Weston, Florida*

**Ronald W. Smith, M.D.**
*Associate Clinical Professor, Department of Orthopaedic
Surgery, University of California at Los Angeles, Los Angeles; and Chief, Foot and Ankle Service, Department of Orthopaedic Surgery, Harbor-UCLA Medical Center, Torrance, California*

**Joel D. Stewart, M.D.**
*Instructor in Surgery, Department of Surgery, Uniformed
Services University of the Health Sciences, Bethesda,
Maryland; and Staff, Foot and Ankle, Department of Or-
thopaedics, Naval Medical Center Portsmouth,
Portsmouth, Virginia*

**James W. Stone, M.D.**
*Assistant Clinical Professor, Department of Orthopaedic
Surgery, Medical College of Wisconsin, Milwaukee, Wis-
consin*

**David B. Thordarson, M.D.**
*Associate Professor and Chief, Foot and Ankle Trauma and
Reconstructive Surgery, Department of Orthopaedic
Surgery, Keck School of Medicine, University of Southern
California, Los Angeles, California*

**Norman S. Turner, M.D.**
*Consultant, Department of Orthopaedic Surgery, Mayo
Clinic, Rochester, Minnesota*

**Keith L. Wapner, M.D.**
*Clinical Professor, Department of Orthopaedic Surgery,
University of Pennsylvania; Professor, Department of Or-
thopaedic Surgery, MCP Hahnemann University; and Fel-
lowship Director, Orthopaedic Foot & Ankle Surgery,
Pennsylvania Hospital, Philadelphia, Pennsylvania*

**Bernhardt Weber, M.D.**
*Titular-Professor, Department of Orthopaedic Surgery,
University of Bern, Bern; and Staff Member, Department of
Orthopedic Surgery, Orthopedics at Rosenberg, St. Gallen,
Switzerland*

**Yue Shuen Wong, M.B., B.S., F.R.C.S. (EDIN)**
*Consultant, Department of Orthopaedic Surgery, Alexan-
dra Hospital, Singapore*

# ACKNOWLEDGMENTS

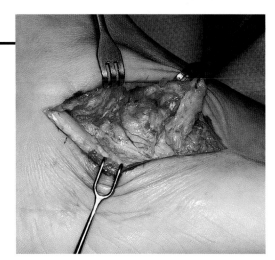

Our understanding of problems affecting the foot and ankle has greatly advanced in the past two decades, because of the contributions of many experts. There are a number of "giants" in the field, who paved the way for improved operative techniques, clinical investigations, and basic science research. The international and interdisciplinary efforts of the orthopaedic community have resulted in advances which have been applied to the clinical practice of orthopaedics. My gratitude and appreciation are extended to mentors in orthopaedics, foot and ankle surgery, and research, including Andrea Cracchiolo III, Kenneth A. Johnson, Melvin H. Jahss, Edward O. Leventen, Kai-Nan An, J. Patrick Flanagan, John Sellman, and Irwin Bliss. I recognize my colleagues at the Mayo Clinic and elsewhere who have fostered my interest in the foot and ankle specialty. I wish to acknowledge the secretarial support of Diane Wurst and Donna Riemersa. I recognize the contribution of the supremely talented medical illustrator, Deborah Ravin, and the editorial work at Lippincott Williams & Wilkins by James Merritt and Julia Seto.

The effort and time required to prepare this volume came at the expense of personal life. I acknowledge the patience and support of my wife Linda, and my sons Robert and John.

# SERIES PREFACE

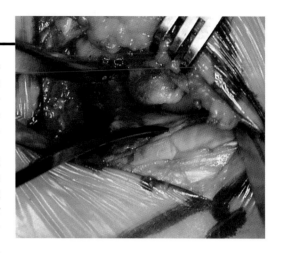

The first volume of the series *Master Techniques in Orthopaedic Surgery* was published in 1994. Our goal in assembling the series was to create easy-to-follow descriptions of operative techniques that would help orthopaedists through the challenges of daily practice. The books were intended to be more than just technical manuals, they were designed to impart the personal experience of the "master orthopaedic surgeons."

*Master Techniques in Orthopaedic Surgery* has become precisely what we hoped for—books that are used again and again, and are found at home and in the offices of practicing orthopaedists and residents in training. Most importantly, they are recommended by orthopaedists who look to them for practical advice and suggestions concerning the difficult but common problems they encounter.

The series is now entering its second edition phase. You will again find recognized leaders as volume editors, known for their contributions to research, education, and the advancement of the surgical state of the art. Chapter authors have been selected for their experience, operative skills, and recognized expertise with a particular technique. The classic procedures are still included; some techniques have changed as new technology has been incorporated; and new procedures that have been popularized during the last several years have been added.

We are maintaining the same user-friendly format that was so well-received when the series was first introduced—a standardized presentation of information replete with tips and pearls gained through years of experience, with abundant color photographs and drawings to guide you step-by-step through the procedures.

With these new editions, we again invite you into the operating room to peer over the shoulder of the surgeon at work. It is our goal to offer the orthopaedic surgeon seeking an improved proficiency in practice access to the maximum confidence in selecting and executing the appropriate surgery for the individual patient.

*Roby C. Thompson, Jr., M.D.*
*Series Editor*

# PREFACE

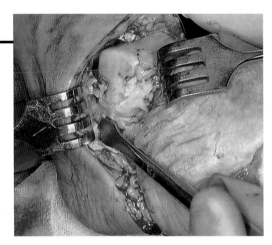

This volume is an advanced surgical technique book, describing more than 50 of the most important operations related to trauma and reconstruction of the foot and ankle. The specialty has changed considerably since the first edition of the book over eight years ago, and the procedures selected for the present volume have been revised accordingly. The chapters from the first edition have been completely rewritten or updated, with newly added procedures such as the Weil osteotomy, fibular grooving operation, subtalar distraction arthrodesis, popliteal block anesthesia, and ankle block anesthesia. New chapters are included on topics such as total ankle arthroplasty, mosaicplasty for osteochondral lesions of the talus, tendon transfer for foot drop, medial displacement calcaneal osteotomy, talus fracture open reduction and fixation, tibial periarticular fracture reduction and fixation, arthroscopic ankle arthrodesis, ankle arthroscopy for osteochondral lesions, phalangeal osteotomy with cheilectomy, lesser toe reconstruction, and tibiotalocalcaneal arthrodesis with intramedullary nail fixation. Each chapter was prepared by one or more experts, with the specific operation described in a step-by-step fashion with intraoperative photographs, clinical photographs, and drawings. It is our hope that this volume will be valuable to surgeons worldwide and ultimately result in the improved quality of patient care.

*Harold B. Kitaoka, M.D.*

# PART I

## Phalanges

# 1

# Marginal Toenail Ablation

## Melanie Sanders

## INDICATIONS/CONTRAINDICATIONS

Surgical management of ingrown toenails is generally reserved for cases in which optimal nonoperative management has failed (2,4,9). In some cases, the threshold for treatment should be lowered, as in diabetic patients or in patients with total joint replacements. In those instances, it is better to prevent recurrent infections and sepsis, and surgery should be performed sooner. Additional indications for surgical management include extremely deformed, fungal nails in which pressure from the surface of the shoe causes significant pain for the patient. Suppurative lesions with granulation tissue require initial decompression by removal of the marginal nail plate. This facilitates soft tissue healing so that definitive surgical treatment can be performed. If possible, all infection should be eradicated before proceeding with matricectomy to prevent seeding deeper tissues or the bone. The major contraindication for surgery is a dysvascular great toe.

## PREOPERATIVE PLANNING

Evaluation of the patient before the surgical procedure should include obtaining a history of the frequency of recurrent infections and determining how recalcitrant they have been to treatment. If there is concern about deep infection, anteroposterior and oblique radiographs of the great toe should be examined for evidence of periosteal elevation or bone erosion. Plain film radiographs usually are sufficient to reveal underlying unusual bony shapes, such as enchondromas, which may cause nail deformity or infection. In most cases, more involved and costly studies are unnecessary as a part of preoperative planning. Patients are encouraged to improve their general foot hygiene before surgery and specifically to clean the area at least daily with antiseptic for 3 days before surgery. Any medications that may prolong bleeding time, including vitamin E, should be stopped at an appropriate interval before the procedure.

M. Sanders, M.D.: Private Practice, OrthoIndy, Indianapolis, Indiana.

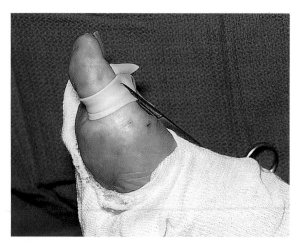

**Figure 1-1.** A large Penrose drain is used to exsanguinate the toe initially. It is then secured proximally with a hemostat to act as a tourniquet.

## SURGERY

The most common anesthetic for this procedure is a digital block, and the procedure is typically performed in the office. Some patients request general anesthesia or sedation because of anxiety. Regardless of the anesthetic used, it is desirable to perform a digital block with a long-lasting anesthetic agent at the end of the procedure to provide prolonged pain relief after surgery. With the patient supine, the foot should be prepped to the level of the ankle. If a temporizing partial nail avulsion is planned and gross infection is present, I do not exsanguinate the toe. If no acute infection is present, a large Penrose drain is used to exsanguinate the toe and used as a tourniquet at the base of the toe (Fig. 1-1). It is important to use a hemostat to secure the Penrose to avoid the possibility of leaving the Penrose drain in place at the end of the procedure when the dressing is applied. Another option is to use the proper size toe tourniquet.

### Technique

After a bloodless field is established, the toenail is approached from its distal end. A small, curved hemostat works well to separate the nail plate from the underlying nail bed. Removal of the entire nail can be accomplished with gentle and persistent blunt dissection to-

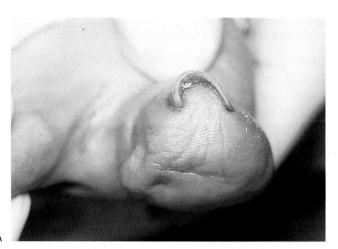
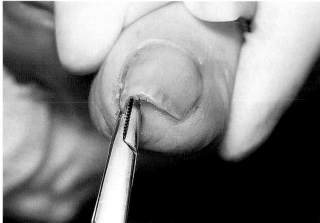

A                                                                                                              B

**Figure 1-2.   A:** Tubular nail. **B:** A small, curved hemostat is used to bluntly elevate the nail from the nail bed.

[Figure 1-3 image]

**Figure 1-3.** A nail splitter is introduced to cut the nail longitudinally.

ward the base of the nail (Fig. 1-2). This technique is carried out in a more limited fashion on the medial or lateral margins, or both, where only partial nail ablation is to be performed. In the case of partial nail ablation, a nail splitter is used to separate the margin of the nail from the central portion. This separation is carried up under the edge of the ungual fold (Fig. 1-3). The nail is then removed from the operative field (Fig. 1-4).

For the next stage of the operation, loupe magnification can be extremely helpful. Oblique incisions are made at the proximal corners of the ungual fold (Fig. 1-5). These incisions are carried only to the depth of the fatty tissue underlying the dermis, because their purpose is exposure of the underlying matrix. There is matrix tissue that can form nail plate under the edge of the ungual fold, curving around the base of the toenail and in the nail bed proximal to the lunula. It is necessary to excise this inferior surface of the ungual fold (Fig. 1-6). The scalpel blade is inserted parallel to the overlying ungual fold, sharply separating it from the underlying matrix. This technique is carried out along the lateral ungual fold as well. The nail bed is then cut horizontally at a level slightly distal to the lunula. In some patients, a change in coloration can be seen where the matrix darkens at its junction from a pale color to the normal pink or red of the nail bed. The transverse incision in the nail bed and matrix surface is carried down to the level of the bone. At this stage, the corner of the matrix is grasped gently with forceps, and a sharp instrument (i.e., no. 15 scalpel blade or a Beaver blade) is used to separate the matrix from the surrounding and underlying tissues (Fig. 1-7).

Partial matricectomy usually yields a piece of tissue that is approximately 0.75 × 0.75 cm (Fig. 1-8). It should be carefully examined to note whether there are any holes or rents

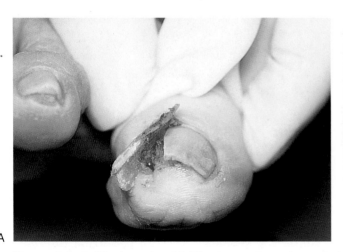

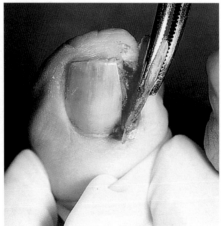

A                                                                                                                        B

**Figure 1-4.  A:** The lateral nail is lifted away from the underlying nail bed. **B:** Avulsion of the nail is completed.

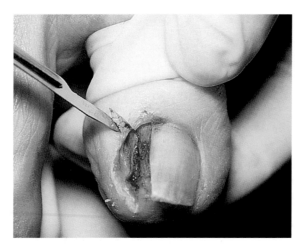

**Figure 1-5.** Oblique proximal incision.

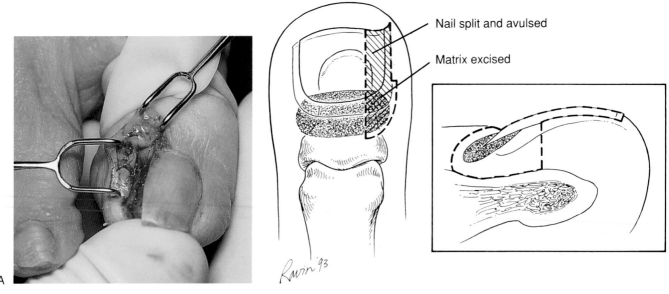

A

Nail split and avulsed

Matrix excised

B

**Figure 1-6. A:** Exposure of the matrix is complete. Notice the difference in color between the nail bed and the matrix. **B:** Extent of tissue resection needed for the marginal nail ablation procedure.

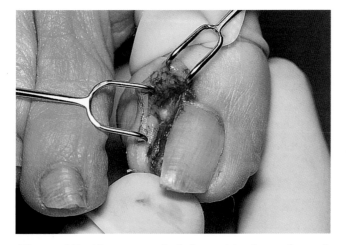

**Figure 1-7.** After removal of the matrix, the surface of the proximal phalanx is visible in the wound.

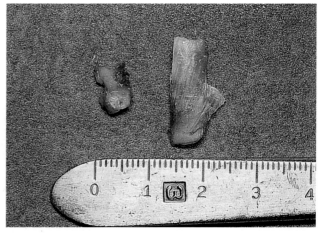

**Figure 1-8.** Specimens are from a partial matricectomy and the nail.

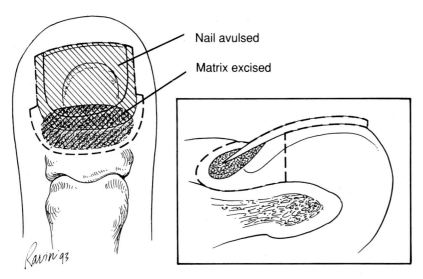

**Figure 1-9.** Extent of tissue resection needed for total nail-matrix ablation.

in the specimen. If such openings exist, a careful search for the missing tissue should be undertaken, although this is sometimes fruitless. If there is concern about whether the matrix was completely removed, I generally use a small curette to elevate the periosteum on the phalanx and to remove any fibrous tissue that may represent matrix. In some patients, the matrix extends deep in the corners medially and laterally, and it is helpful to use a small skin hook to elevate the matrix from the underlying tissue. It may also be helpful to extend the oblique incision slightly. The danger of extending the incision is that the matrix could be transected, leaving a corner of the matrix behind.

A complete matricectomy requires excision of the matrix across the entire base of the nail bed (Fig. 1-9). Typically, this is carried out at a level slightly distal to the distal edge of the lunula. Resection of this tissue creates a significant soft tissue defect, but it is necessary to remove all of the germinal tissue. The dorsal aspect of the nail bed in its central one third should be removed along with any germinal matrix that may be present. At this stage, irrigation with crystalloid solution usually is performed. Thermal or Bovie cautery may be used to minimize bleeding. A small piece of Gelfoam may be applied into the area of resected matrix (Fig. 1-10). The oblique incisions at the corners generally are closed with a mattress stitch using nonabsorbable nylon suture. The lateral edge of the ungual fold can also be sutured to the nail plate through a hole created by a large needle, if desired (Fig. 1-11).

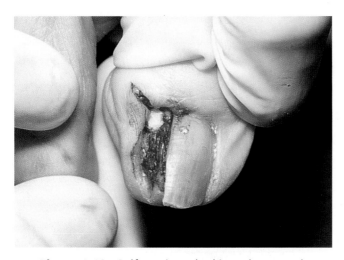

**Figure 1-10.** Gelfoam is packed into the wound.

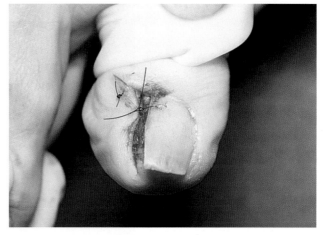

**Figure 1-11.** The wound is closed with nonabsorbable nylon suture.

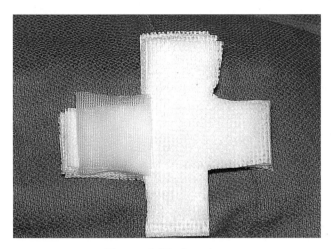

**Figure 1-12.** Dressing.

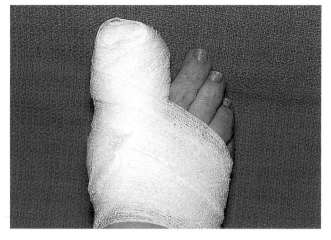

**Figure 1-13.** Completed dressing.

The dressing is first applied with a nonadherent material such as Xeroform. A bulky dressing, such as multiple 4 × 4 inch gauze pieces cut in the shape of a cross, is applied. When placed over the end of the toe, it results in a well-fitting dressing that is absorbent but not excessively bulky (Fig. 1-12). A 2-inch Kling is necessary to hold the gauze firmly and anchor the bandage (Fig. 1-13). The long-lasting digital block can be performed before or after the dressing is applied.

## POSTOPERATIVE MANAGEMENT

Patients are dismissed the day of the procedure in any shoe that can accommodate the dressing. A postoperative shoe is inexpensive and works well. Some patients are more comfortable in an old shoe or sandal as long as the surgical area is not compressed. This type of footwear is necessary for 2 to 4 days after surgery. Patients are sent home from the surgical procedure with instructions, including a warning to expect postoperative bleeding. Bleeding may sometimes saturate the dressing within 10 to 15 minutes of dressing application, requiring reinforcement. When the blood dries, the dressing can become rigid. Patients are instructed to change the dressing approximately 36 to 48 hours after surgery. Soaking the dressing in saline, hydrogen peroxide, or sterile water can assist in removing bandages that are adherent. Bleeding usually has subsided by the time of the dressing change, and the patient can put a smaller nonadherent dressing over the toe. Patients are cautioned against soaking or immersion of the foot, and they are asked to keep the surgical area clean and dry. Additional instructions include application of ice and elevation of the foot, particularly for the first 3 to 4 days.

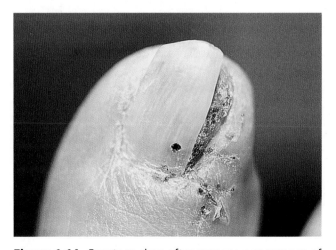

**Figure 1-14.** Fourteen days after surgery, appearance of the toe after suture removal.

Use of the digital block generally lessens the postoperative pain significantly, and patients are often able to discontinue pain medications after 1 or 2 days. If a surgical procedure is done in the presence of infection, oral antibiotics may be provided preoperatively and for several days postoperatively. The regimen is similar to that used for patients with total joint replacements, regardless of whether acute infection is present.

Patients return to the office about 10 days after surgery for suture removal (Fig. 1-14). Many patients come to the first postoperative follow-up visit wearing enclosed shoes and hose. Any deviation from steady recovery should raise concerns about problems such as a postoperative infection. The second follow-up visit, scheduled 2 to 3 months postoperatively, is used to assess the toe for signs of nail regrowth or nail spike.

## COMPLICATIONS

In a series with a mean follow-up of 10 years reported by Pettine et al. (6), results of marginal nail excision with surgical excision of the associated nail matrix had a recurrence rate of 6% (6 of 95 nail edges), and only 1 of the 6 patients required further surgical treatment. In the same report, after marginal nail excision with chemical matrix ablation, the recurrence rate was 20% (12 of 61 nail edges), and 8 of 12 required further surgical treatment.

The most common complication from the procedure is the persistence of nail horns or spikes after the ablation of the nail and matrix. They occur because remnants or islands of germinal matrix that form nail are left. In some instances, they are not particularly troublesome to the patient and are managed by periodic trimming or removal by the patient. In other cases, they are quite problematic and can result in the need for further surgery. Sometimes, adequate removal of the nail spike can be performed with an en bloc excision, but other cases require a more extensive procedure, such as a terminal Syme amputation (8). Some patients form a cornified layer of tissue overlying the nail bed that can appear to be nail plate but is not adherent to the nail bed and can be removed easily. In rare instances, a very thin remnant may regrow centrally after a total matricectomy.

When the nail and matrix are removed for fungal infection, the integumentary structures surrounding the nail may also be infected. The abnormalities of the skin usually respond to topical antifungal agents.

## ILLUSTRATIVE CASE

An ingrown toenail occurred in a 49-year-old male anesthesiologist. It was intermittently painful in the medial border of the nail for 27 years and was managed previously by placing cotton beneath the nail plate medially. About 1 week before presentation, he had an

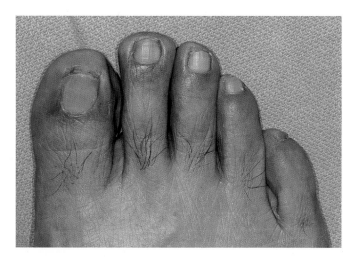

**Figure 1-15.** Appearance of the toe 11 years after surgery. (Copyright Mayo Clinic/Mayo Foundation.)

acute exacerbation of pain, accompanied by erythema, swelling, and tenderness. There was no purulent discharge.

Partial matricectomy was performed with digital block anesthesia. He returned to work the following day, and the wound healed uneventfully in 2 weeks. Figure 1-15 shows the appearance of the toe 11 years after surgical treatment, which produced a good clinical result and no recurrence of symptoms. He continues to be active in anesthesiology, teaching, and bodybuilding.

## RECOMMENDED READING

1. Ceilley RI, Collison DW: Matricectomy. *J Dermatol Surg Oncol* 18:728–734, 1992.
2. Dixon GL: Treatment of ingrown toenail. *Foot Ankle* 3:254–260, 1983.
3. Grieg JD, Anderson JH, Ireland AJ, et al.: The surgical treatment of ingrowing toenails. *J Bone Joint Surg Br* 73:131–133, 1991.
4. Heifetz CJ: Ingrown toenail: a clinical study. *Am J Surg* 38:298–315, 1937.
5. Leahy AL, Timon CI, Craig A, et al.: Ingrowing toenails: improving treatment. *Surgery* 107:566–567, 1990.
6. Pettine KA, Cofield RH, Bussey RM: Ingrown toenail: results of surgical treatment. *Foot Ankle* 9:130–134, 1988.
7. Siegle RJ, Stewart R: Recalcitrant ingrowing nails: surgical approaches. *J Dermatol Surg Oncol* 18:744–752, 1992.
8. Thompson TC, Terwillinger C: The terminal Syme operation for ingrown toenail. *Surg Clin North Am* 31:575–584, 1951.
9. Zadik FR: Obliteration of the nail bed of the great toe without shortening the terminal phalanx. *J Bone Joint Surg* 32:66–67, 1950.

# 2

# Phenol Matricectomy

Irwin L. Bliss and Steven J. Kavros

## INDICATIONS/CONTRAINDICATIONS

Onychocryptosis is one of the most common and disabling foot problems. Ingrown nails in children have been attributed to factors similar to those found in adults. Poorly fitting shoes, overzealous nail cutting, and onychophagia are often the cause (2). In adults, additional factors have been reported, such as abnormally long toes, hereditary conditions (excessive convexity of the nail plate), hyperhidrosis, imbalance of the width of the nail plate and nailbed, and the prominence of the nail folds (4). Most of the geriatric population has at least one toe with a symptomatic incurvating nail causing pressure in the offended nail groove (Fig. 2-1). Diabetic patients with deformed nails are at risk for infection (14). This concern can be obviated safely if ablation of the nail borders or total nail ablation is carried out before neuropathic or vascular compromise occurs. Specific indications for a partial or total phenol matricectomy are painful nails unresponsive to conservative therapy, severely deformed nails, failure with systemic oral antifungals (i.e., onychomycosis), and a desire for a reliable, permanent correction. Permanent phenol matricectomy should be accomplished in the absence of cellulitis or purulent drainage.

If an acute paronychia or cellulitis is present, a partial nail avulsion can be performed and the local infection treated. Tepid saline solution or Domeboro solution (i.e., aluminum sulfate and calcium acetate) can be used twice daily for 15 to 20 minutes. In the case of more extensive infection, a complete nail avulsion may be warranted. Oral antibiotics can be considered for patients that are medically compromised or carry comorbidities of concern.

Multiple approaches to the permanent partial or total nail ablation have been described (1,3,5). Some include soft tissue correction involving a variety of surgical procedures, but all include removal of the involved portion of matrix with the surrounding portion of the nail fold. Other techniques have included the use of electrocautery, thermal ablation with laser (11,13), and sodium hydroxide chemical matricectomy (18).

I. L. Bliss, M.D.: Department of Orthopaedic Surgery, University of California Los Angeles Medical Center, and Cedars Sinai Medical Center, Los Angeles, California.

S. J. Kavros, D.P.M.: Department of Orthopedic Surgery, Mayo Clinic, Rochester, Minnesota.

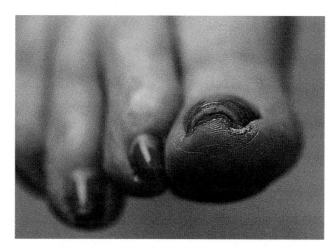

**Figure 2-1.** Painful callus in the nail groove.

Phenol ablation offers several advantages. The procedure does not require an incision, and sutures therefore are not needed. The procedure can easily be done in an office or outpatient facility. Postoperative pain is usually minimal. Small nerve fibers are desensitized by the phenol, reducing postoperative pain. It is a relatively quick procedure using routine instruments and materials commonly stocked in an office.

The normal nail plate and nail bed are flat or greatly curved. In a young patient with an ingrown nail, the edge of the nail turns in (incurvation), but the nail bed remains flat. In the older patient, the nail plate and nail bed deform almost symmetrically. Incurvation of the nail may be thought of as part of a continuum, with the end of the spectrum being a tubular nail, or *pincher nail* (Fig. 2-2). The hypertrophy of the nail plate and possible onychomycosis add to the deformity. The amount of nail removed should leave no residual incurvating corners. It is usually not necessary to remove as much nail border in the younger individual because hypertrophy and dystrophic changes are not as common. If the degree of incurvatum is so severe (i.e., pincher nail) that removing the borders leaves only a thin central portion, total nail ablation is recommended. A total matricectomy can be accomplished with this technique. In this instance, the entire nail plate is avulsed, and the undersurface of the eponychium is abraded along with the matrix that overlies the proximal aspect of the distal phalanx.

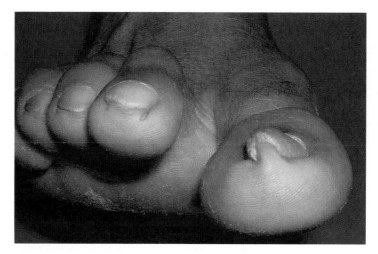

**Figure 2-2.** Severe incurvation deformity of the nail plate is also called a *pincher nail*.

As with any surgical procedure, some contraindications should be considered. Phenol is 89% carbolic acid. This procedure should be avoided in patients with a known allergy or sensitivity to phenol. A history of prolonged wound healing from a prior phenol procedure should be considered. Brittle diabetics and patients with vascular compromise need special attention before surgery. Patients with Raynaud's phenomenon, scleroderma, vasculitis, and immunodeficiencies are at higher risk because of poor wound healing from this elective chemical cauterization procedure. Traditional surgical wedge procedures may be preferable in patients with hypertrophic nail fold deformity. Plastic reduction of nail fold deformity is poorly resolved with the phenol procedure.

## PREOPERATIVE PLANNING

Pain, deformity, and swelling of the toe with nail plate deformity may suggest underlying pathology. Radiographs of the hallux or affected digits are helpful. A subungual exostosis is not uncommon with a history of trauma or a crush injury (Figs. 2-3 and 2-4). Osteomyelitis should be considered in patients with long-standing onychocryptosis and infection, diabetes, or arterial insufficiency (Fig. 2-5).

Fungal infection in conjunction with or as a cause of nail deformity is not a contraindication to phenol matricectomy (Fig. 2-6). Patients can be offered medical management with oral antifungals, such as terbinafine, itraconazole, or Diflucan, as an alternative or as concomitant therapy. A potassium hydroxide (KOH) wet mount or fungal culture can indicate the presence of a dermatophyte infection. Appropriate treatment protocols and outcomes are available for review with respect to oral antifungal agents (8,16,17). It is important to identify the presence of fungal infection before oral treatment. Psoriatic and dystrophic nails do not respond to these effective antifungal medications.

In the acutely infected ingrown nail (e.g., paronychia, cellulitis, abscess), partial or total nail plate avulsion is indicated before the definitive ablation procedure. After removal of the offending nail border, the infection usually subsides with appropriate local care. Postoperative care is important for a successful outcome after partial nail avulsion. The new advancing edge of the nail plate needs attention so it does not invade the nail fold. A cotton wisp can be placed under the nail edge to assist the process. Lloyd-Davis and Brill (12) reported a 47% recurrence rate of infection after partial nail plate avulsion. Keyes (9) reported a 77% incidence of recurrence. A permanent phenol matricectomy can be considered after the infection is cleared.

Diabetic and vascular patients who have absent palpable pulses are of concern in terms of wound healing. A handheld bidirectional Doppler device can allow the physician to as-

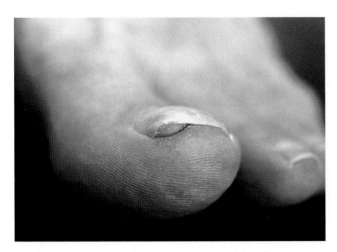

**Figure 2-3.** Subungual prominence resulting from an exostosis.

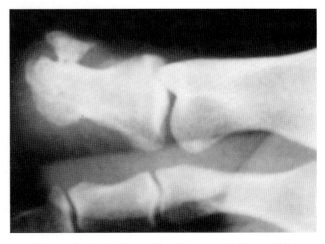

**Figure 2-4.** Radiograph of the toe in Figure 2-3.

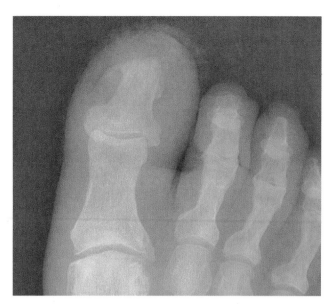

**Figure 2-5.** Osteomyelitis of a distal phalanx in a diabetic patient with long-standing onychocryptosis and infection.

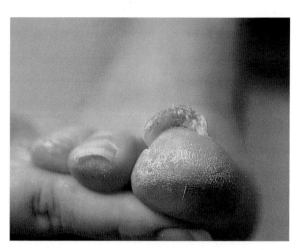

**Figure 2-6.** Subungual material can be debris or fungus.

sess the patency of the pedal vessels (dorsalis pedis and posterior tibial). Transcutaneous oximetry (TcPO$_2$) is of value in assessing blood flow to the skin. Values of 50 mm Hg and above usually indicate satisfactory blood flow for healing (15). TcPO$_2$ levels that are below 40 mm Hg may not be as favorable for predicted outcomes in wound healing. Semmes-Weinstein monofilament nylon can also be used to detect peripheral neuropathy. The circulatory and nerve evaluation can be of benefit in assessing preoperative risk.

## SURGERY

The patient is placed supine on the table and positioned comfortably. Some desire the hip and knee flexed so the foot is plantigrade or fully extended and the foot relaxed in plantarflexion. The foot and nails are scrubbed, nail is trimmed, and subungual debris is removed. Betadine or skin antiseptic of choice is used. The forefoot or toe is sterilely draped. A digital block with Lidocaine or bupivacaine is used. Block the toe at the base of the phalanx proximally. Usually, only two or three injections are needed. Avoid penetrating the ex-

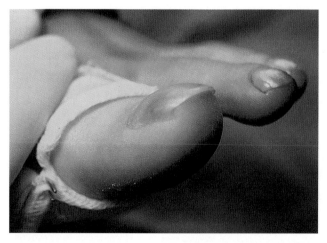

**Figure 2-7.** The toe is exsanguinated, and a Penrose drain is applied over the gauze sponge at the base of the toe.

tensor hallucis longus tendon. A 0.25-inch Penrose drain is wrapped around the base of the toe over a gauze sponge (Fig. 2-7). A commercially available Tourni-cot (Mar-Med, Grand Rapids, MI) in various sizes can be used as an alternative to a Penrose drain for hemostasis.

## Technique

The incurvated border of the nail (Fig. 2-8) is elevated with a spatula (Fig. 2-9) and is then cut with a nail clipper or splitter (Fig. 2-10). The cut portion of the nail is removed. The matrix, including the portion that is on the undersurface of the eponychium, is removed with a curette, as is the exposed portion of the nail bed under the removed segment of nail plate (Fig. 2-11). To facilitate access to the eponychial undersurface, apply digital pressure to the dorsum of the toe, proximal to the matrix and in a distal direction, because this often draws additional, inaccessible matrix into the field.

A petroleum-base ointment is applied to the surrounding skin for protection from the phenol. A cotton swab with approximately 50% of its bulk removed is dipped into 89% phenol (avoid excessive saturation of the swab) and then introduced under the eponychium into the area of the matrix. There it is rotated for approximately 30 seconds and removed (Fig. 2-12). This step is repeated three times. A copious amount of isopropyl alcohol is

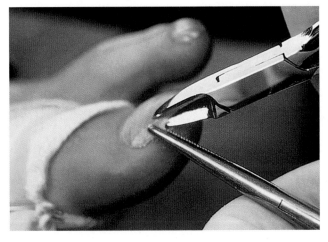

**Figure 2-8.** The medial border of the hallux nail plate has a 90° downward turn.

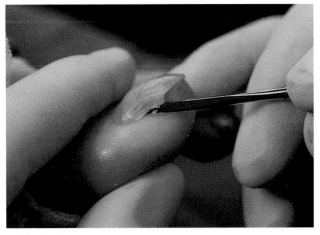

**Figure 2-9.** The incurvated border of the nail is elevated with a spatula.

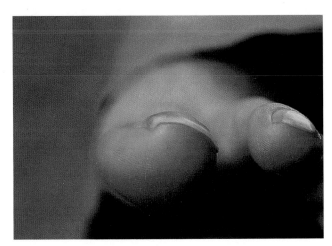

**Figure 2-10.** Nail cutter with clipper.

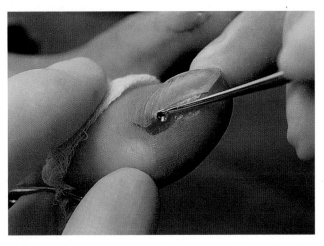

**Figure 2-11.** Matrix and nail bed are removed with a curette.

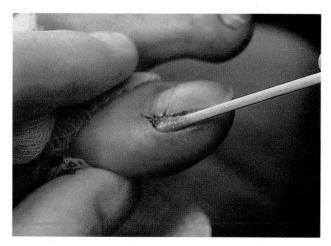

**Figure 2-12.** A debulked cotton swab is used to introduce phenol.

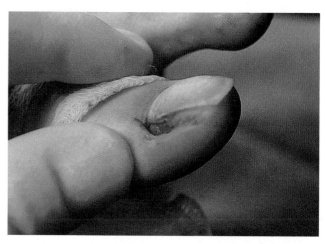

**Figure 2-13.** Appearance at the end of the procedure.

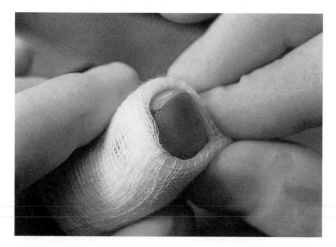

**Figure 2-14.** A bandage is applied and covered with a compressive dressing.

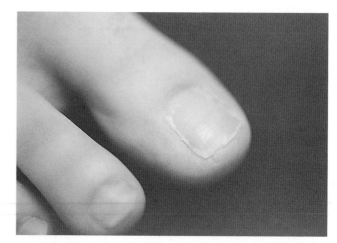

**Figure 2-15.** Appearance 1 year after lateral border ablation with phenol.

flushed in the surgical site. The isopropyl alcohol neutralizes the caustic effect of the phenol (Fig. 2-13). The surgeon can identify a gray color to the remaining matrix area. The phenol (an acid) denatures the matrix (a protein), leaving a grayish color. If the matrix is still pearl white after three applications of phenol, the surgical site is covered with antibiotic ointment and a compression dressing after the tourniquet is removed (Fig. 2-14). Figure 2-15 describes a patient with a partial phenol matricectomy who is 1 year postoperative without recurrence of symptoms.

## POSTOPERATIVE MANAGEMENT

Patients are advised to elevate the extremity immediately postoperatively. Acetaminophen or ibuprofen is usually satisfactory if analgesic control is necessary. Patients are advised to soak in tepid saline solution or Domeboro astringent solution for 15 to 20 minutes twice daily for 2 weeks. Drainage from the chemical burn can be expected. It is usually a clear, serous drainage. Approximately 1 week postoperatively, the patient has the surgical site gently debrided. The moist clot is removed, and this facilitates drainage and a more rapid healing. Antibiotic ointment and light gauze dressing is applied after soaks. Avoid occlusive dressings such as Band-Aids or tape, because they prolong healing. An open-toe shoe or sandal is preferable for the first few days and then a regular shoe as tolerated. If a total nail procedure is accomplished, encourage an open-toe shoe for a few weeks.

Multiple published reports validate outcomes with phenol cauterization procedures. Gem and Sykes (6) reported a 96% success rate over 20 years in the United Kingdom. Kuwada (10) reported a recurrence rate of 4.3% after partial matricectomy and 4.7% after complete matricectomy. His long-term analysis consisted of 733 cases.

## COMPLICATIONS

The most common entity postoperative is prolonged serous drainage. This is usually seen when patients are less vigilant with their instructed postoperative soaking. Recurrence after phenol matricectomy is less than 5% (6,10). Spicule formation is rare as is seen in surgical excision procedures. In cases of recurrence, the entire border is usually present. This can be reduced with careful examination of the nail bed after the serial applications of phenol. If the matrix remains glistening white after serial application, recurrence is likely. Ischemic necrosis with tourniquet application to the digits has been reported by Haas et al. (7).

Figure 2-16 describes a patient after a total phenol matricectomy. Postoperatively, the patient had a phenol reaction. Notice the hypertrophic granulation tissue of the nail bed. Additional debridement followed by aggressive soaking and silver sulfadiazine is recommended.

The matrix is formed embryonically from an epidermal invagination, and the underside of the eponychium therefore has growth cells, as does the dorsum of the phalanx (Fig. 2-17). Failure to remove the segment will result in regrowth of nail or spicule formation.

Phenol must be kept in a cool, dark area and changed on a regular basis because it deteriorates rather quickly after exposure to air. The surgical field must be dry because phenol mixed with blood alters the pH, compromising the effectiveness of the phenol and turning the area black. The phenol technique will fail if old phenol is used, if the phenol is not ap-

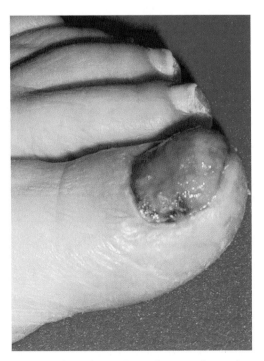

**Figure 2-16.** Phenol reaction after total matricectomy. Notice the hypertrophic granulation tissue of the nail bed.

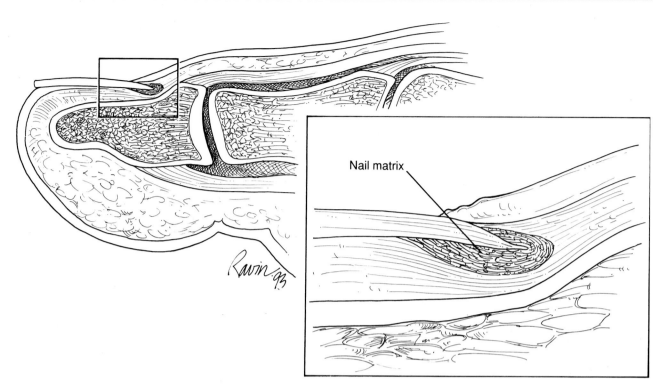

**Figure 2-17.** Drawing of the lateral view of the distal phalanx shows germinal cells under the eponychium and at the base of the nail bed.

plied to all the appropriate areas, or if an insufficient amount of nail is removed at the primary procedure.

## RECOMMENDED READING

1. Appelberg DB, et al.: Progress report on the use of carbon dioxide laser for nail disorders. *Curr Podiatry* 32: 29–31, 1983.
2. Bently PB, Cole I: Ingrown toenails in infancy. *Int J Dermatol* 22:113, 1983.
3. Burzotta JZ, Turri RM, Tsouris J: Phenol and alcohol chemical matrixectomy. *Clin Podiatr Med Surg* 6: 453–468, 1989.
4. Cohen PR, Scher RK: Nail changes in the elderly. *J Geriatr Dermatol* 1:45, 1993.
5. Dixon GL: Treatment of ingrown toenail. *Foot Ankle* 3:254–260, 1983.
6. Gem MA, Sykes PA: Ingrowing toenails: studies of segmental chemical ablation. *Br J Clin Pract* 44: 562–563, 1990.
7. Haas F, Moshammer H, Schwarzc F: Iatrogenic necrosis of the large toe after tourniquet placement. *Chirurgie* 70:608–610, 1999.
8. Hall M, Monka C, Krupp P, et al.: Safety of oral terbinafine. *Arch Dermatol* 133(10):1213–1219, 1997.
9. Keyes EL: The surgical treatment of ingrown toenails. *JAMA* 102:1458–1460, 1934.
10. Kuwada G: Long-term evaluation of partial and total surgical and phenol matrixectomies. *J Am Podiatr Med Assoc* 81:33–36, 1991.
11. Leshin B, Whitaker DC: Carbon dioxide laser matricectomy. *J Dermatol Surg Oncol* 14:608–611, 1988.
12. Lloyd-Davis RW, Brill GL: The etiology and outpatient management of ingrowing toenails. *Br J Surg* 50: 592–597, 1963.
13. Neev J, Nelson JS, Critelli M, et al.: Ablation of human nail by pulsed lasers. *Lasers Surg Med* 21:186–192, 1997.
14. Nicklas BJ: Prophylactic surgery in the diabetic foot. In: Frykberg R, ed. *The high risk foot in diabetes mellitus.* New York: Churchill Livingstone, 1990:513–516.
15. Rooke TW, Osmundson PJ: The influence of age, sex, smoking, and diabetes on lower limb transcutaneous oxygen tension in patients with arterial occlusive disease. *Arch Intern Med* 150:129–132, 1990.
16. Scher RK: Oncyhomycosis: therapeutic update. *J Am Acad Dermatol* 40(6 Pt 2):S21–S26, 1999.
17. Tausch I, Decroix J, Gwiezdzinski Z, et al.: Short-term itraconazole versus terbinafine in the treatment of tinea pedis and manus. *Int J Dermatol* 37:128–144, 1998.
18. Travers GR, Ammon RG: The sodium hydroxide chemical matricectomy procedure. *J Am Podiatr Assoc* 70: 476–478, 1980.

# 3

# Hallux Interphalangeal Arthrodesis

Ian J. Alexander

## INDICATIONS/CONTRAINDICATIONS

Arthrodesis of the hallux interphalangeal (IP) joint is primarily indicated for deformity and arthritis of this joint. In certain instances, it is used independently or as an adjunct to tendon transfers when the IP and metatarsophalangeal (MTP) joints are unstable or malaligned due to soft tissue deficiency or muscular imbalances. Examples include a claw hallux secondary to intrinsic muscle denervation (e.g., Charcot-Marie-Tooth disease), flexor hallucis brevis detachment after sesamoidectomy, and hallux varus deformity after bunionectomy. The IP arthrodesis stabilizes the joint when the extensor hallucis longus is transferred to the metatarsal neck in the Jones procedure or when it is transferred to the lateral aspect of the phalangeal base in the correction of hallux varus. When short flexor deficiency is the indication for IP fusion, arthrodesis of the IP joint addresses the flexion deformity at the joint, allowing the flexor hallucis longus to flex the hallux at the MTP joint, thereby restoring great toe function.

Contraindications include patients with a symptomatic clawing of the toes in which the cosmetic appearance is the main concern. Hallux varus associated with MTP arthritis is a contraindication for interphalangeal arthrodesis. This procedure should not be performed if there is an ulcer, infection, or questionable vascularity of the forefoot.

## PREOPERATIVE PLANNING

Preoperative examination of the foot should include a careful assessment of the circulatory status of the foot and the integrity of the skin in the area of the proposed surgery. Range of motion of IP and MTP joints must be assessed, particularly in patients with a claw toe deformity of the hallux. If the hallux MTP joint cannot be passively flexed to at least the neutral (plantigrade) position in the sagittal plane, surgery on the MTP joint at the time of the

I. J. Alexander, M.D.: Department of Orthopaedic Surgery, Northeastern Ohio Universities College of Medicine, Rootstown, Ohio.

IP fusion may be necessary to ensure good postoperative position of the hallux. In cases involving transfer of the extensor hallucis longus, care must be taken to assess function of the extensor hallucis brevis. Absence of the extensor hallucis brevis could result in a "drop hallux" if the longus is transferred.

Weight-bearing anteroposterior, lateral, and oblique radiographs of the foot are obtained, and the degree of deformity present at the IP joint of the great toe is assessed. Malalignment can result from fracture malunion or arthrosis. The alignment can be restored by adjusting the level of the resection of the joint surfaces. The degree of great toe shortening can also be estimated. The goal is to place the IP joint in neutral flexion-extension (sagittal plane), as well as neutral varus-valgus (transverse plane) and neutral eversion-inversion (coronal plane). The surgeon should plan to have several fixation techniques available. Internal fixation with a single compression screw is preferable.

The length of screw needed can be estimated by first measuring the combined length of the proximal and distal phalanges and then subtracting for bone resection of about 4 mm. The preoperative estimate of the desired screw length ensures that the longitudinally oriented screw will not penetrate the MTP joint.

## SURGERY

The IP joint surfaces are exposed and then resected with flat cuts using a sawblade or by denuding the articular surfaces.

### Technique

This procedure is best accomplished through a dorsal transverse incision across the joint with terminal curves or an L-shaped incision (Figs. 3-1 to 3-3). The dorsal capsule and medial and lateral collateral ligaments are divided to allow adequate visualization of the joint surfaces (Fig. 3-4). A saw can be used to resect joint surfaces to prepare the fusion site (Figs. 3-5 to 3-9), or the surfaces are prepared by removing only the articular cartilage and

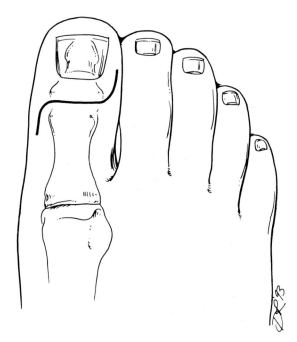

**Figure 3-1.** A sigmoid-shaped skin incision for hallux interphalangeal arthrodesis.

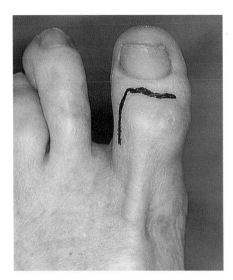

**Figure 3-2.** Skin marking for an L-shaped incision starting distal to the interphalangeal joint transversely and then running longitudinally in the dorsolateral aspect of the hallux.

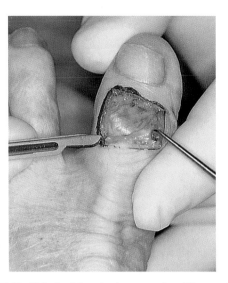

**Figure 3-3.** This incision is deepened, with special care taken to create and protect the full-thickness flap. Notice that the incision is just proximal to the growth matrix of the nail and that the extensor hallucis longus tendon is seen in the depths of the wound.

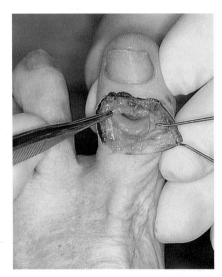

**Figure 3-4.** The joint is exposed by cutting the collateral ligaments of the joint and transection of about two thirds of the width of the extensor hallucis longus tendon. The medial one third of the tendon is kept intact on the medial side of the joint. Notice the thumb forceps pointing to the collateral ligament on the lateral side of the interphalangeal joint.

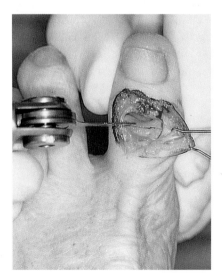

**Figure 3-5.** The joint surface of the proximal phalanx is removed with a saw, resecting about 2 mm.

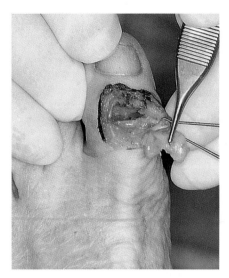

**Figure 3-6.** The resected bone from the distal end of the proximal phalanx is shown in the thumb forceps.

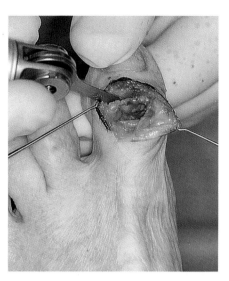

**Figure 3-7.** The joint surface of the distal phalanx is removed using a sagittal saw.

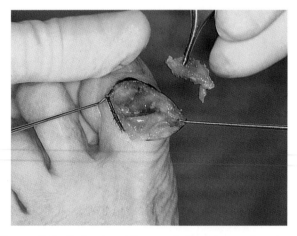

**Figure 3-8.** Only about 2 mm of the joint surface is removed, as seen in the thumb forceps.

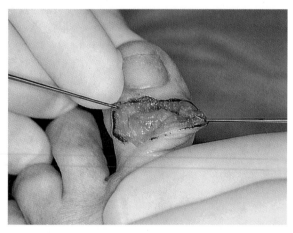

**Figure 3-9.** The two bony surfaces are apposed. The dorsal cortex of the proximal phalanx and the dorsal cortex of the distal phalanx should be well apposed.

dense subchondral bone following the contours of the joint surfaces. After removing the articular surfaces, a 3.5-mm drill hole is made in the distal phalanx in the antegrade direction, exiting the toe tip skin just below the nail (Figs. 3-10 and 3-11). The joint surfaces are apposed, and the position and bony contact are checked. A 2.0-mm drill bit is placed, entering the terminal phalanx distally through the previous hole, and the proximal phalanx is drilled (Figs. 3-12 and 3-13). Fixation is achieved with a 4.0-mm cancellous lag screw that compresses the fusion site, a technique described by Shives and Johnson (6) (Figs. 3-14 to 3-17). Limited rotational stability provided by the single screw has contributed to nonunion in a few of our patients despite excellent initial screw fixation. To improve rotational stability, an obliquely oriented 0.045-inch, threaded Kirchner wire may be used to transfix the joint (Fig. 3-18). Intraoperative radiographs in two planes are advisable to assess bone contact at the fusion site and to determine the screw and pin position. The stability of the fixation must be tested intraoperatively, and if questionable, alternative fixation is used. Another technique of fixing the IP joint when the screw is inadequate is to insert two parallel, threaded Steinmann pins, first antegrade through the distal phalanx and then retrograde almost to the MTP joint.

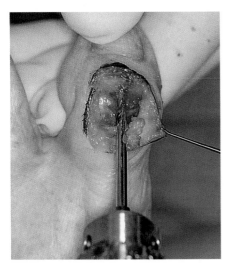

**Figure 3-10.** A 3.5-mm drill bit is used to drill the distal phalanx antegrade, starting from its proximal aspect through the wound.

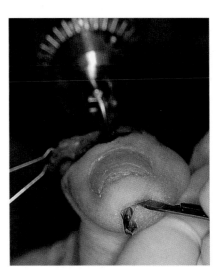

**Figure 3-11.** The skin on the tip of the toe is incised where the drill bit tents the skin.

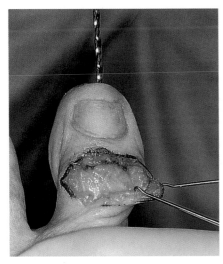

**Figure 3-12.** A 2.0-mm drill bit is placed in the drill hole retrograde in the distal phalanx while the arthrodesis site is held in the proper position.

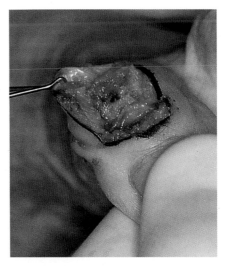

**Figure 3-13.** The drill bit should enter the resected end of the proximal phalanx in its midportion medial-lateral and dorsal-plantar.

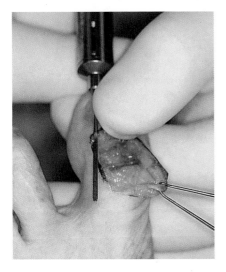

**Figure 3-14.** The length of screw to be used is measured with a depth gauge and compared with an estimate made from the preoperative radiograph.

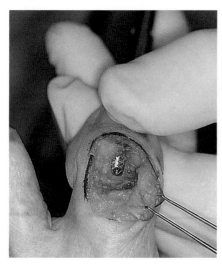

**Figure 3-15.** The appropriate 4.0-mm cancellous bone screw is advanced through the tip of the toe and out the proximal surface of the distal phalanx.

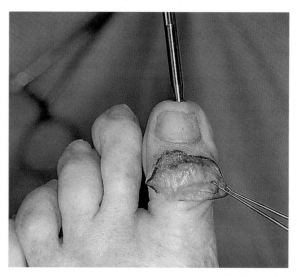

**Figure 3-16.** The screw is then tightened, closely apposing the two surfaces of the arthrodesis site.

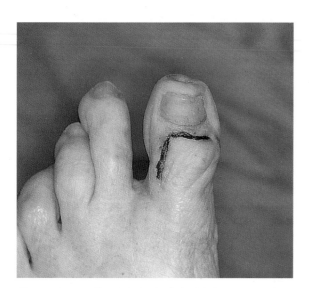

**Figure 3-17.** The skin is closed with interrupted sutures.

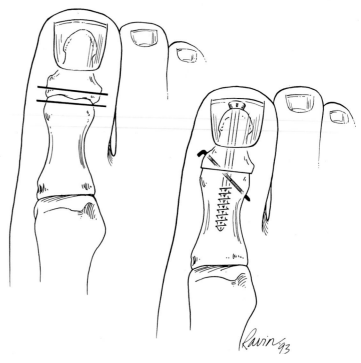

**Figure 3-18.** The drawing shows joint resection *(left)* and alternate fixation *(right)* using a screw with a threaded Kirschner wire that is oriented obliquely.

## POSTOPERATIVE MANAGEMENT

Postoperative shoe immobilization for 6 weeks is usually sufficient, but it is also advisable to limit activity and weight bearing on the hallux until union is apparent radiographically. The screw and wire can be removed under toe block anesthesia in the office at 3 months postoperatively if healing is complete. The 4.0-mm cancellous screw can be a challenge to remove if more than 3 months have elapsed since insertion, because it does not have back-cutting threads. In the original description of the technique by Shives et al. (6), a dramatic improvement in union rate was seen in 20 feet compared with Kirschner wire fixation in 166 feet. Asirvatham et al. (1) compared three methods of stabilizing the IP joint of the hallux and found the best results were obtained in 32 patients who had screw fixation, of which one required reoperation for nonunion. In the patients who had Kirschner wire fixation, nonunion occurred in 9 of the19. Tenodesis of the exterior hallucis longus to the exterior digitorum brevis tendon in 10 patients were unsatisfactory because of toe-drop.

Interphalangeal arthrodesis of the hallux is an important modification of the Jones operation with transfer of the extensor hallucis longus tendon to the first metatarsal neck and head. This procedure is applicable for claw toe deformity of the hallux due to problems such as Charcot-Marie-Tooth disease or poliomyelitis. M'Bamali (5) reported good results in 29 (80%) of 36 feet. Gould (4) recommended the Jones procedure for patients with advanced Charcot-Marie-Tooth disease. Faraj (2) reported very good results in 10 patients and fair results in 2 patients of the 12 patients total who underwent surgery for post-polio claw toe of the hallux. Success rates and patient satisfaction with the outcome of this procedure have been excellent.

## COMPLICATIONS

Less than optimal outcomes are usually the result of nonunion, which may be related to in-adequate fixation, failure to achieve adequate bony apposition, premature loading of the digit or severe osteopenia with fixation (i.e., "cutting out"). Subsequent treatment also in-volves revision arthrodesis. After revision arthrodesis, a non–weight-bearing cast is applied that extends over the hallux and is maintained until union is confirmed clinically and ra-diographically. An example of successful revision arthrodesis with alternate fixation is shown in Figure 3-19.

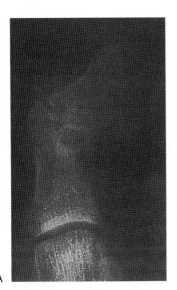 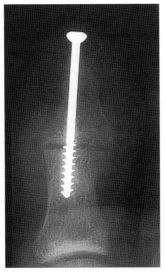

A                                                                                    B

**Figure 3-19. A:** Anteroposterior radiograph shows a painful deformity of the inter-phalangeal joint of the great toe in a 14-year-old boy after a stroke with concomitant valgus and flexion deformity. **B:** Postoperatively, the patient was extremely active, the screw loosened, and a painful nonunion ensued. *(continued)*

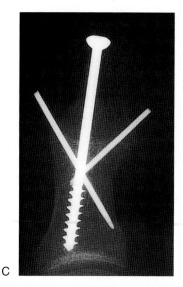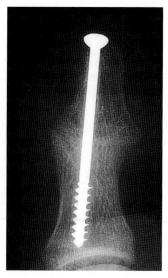

C                                                                                          D

**Figure 3-19.** *Continued.* **C:** Repeat arthrodesis involved further resection of the joint surfaces, insertion of a longer longitudinal screw, and supplemental fixation with crossed Kirschner wires. **D:** A solid arthrodesis occurred, and the percutaneous Kirschner wires were removed.

Malposition is occasionally a problem. Any degree of malrotation is easily detected. Screw removal sometimes is advisable, particularly if the screw head is prominent. This was reinforced by my own experience with an immunosuppressed woman with rheumatoid arthritis who stubbed her toe, dehisced the wound over the screw head, and subsequently developed osteomyelitis.

## RECOMMENDED READING

1. Asirvatham R, Rooney R, Watts HG: Stabilization of the interphalangeal joint of the big toe: comparison of three methods. *Foot Ankle* 13:181–187, 1992.
2. Faraj AA: Modified Jones procedure for post-polio claw hallux deformity. *J Foot Ankle Surg* 36:356–359, 1997.
3. Giannini S, Girolami M, Ceccarelli F, et al.: Modified Jones operation in the treatment of pes cavovarus. *Ital J Orthop Traumatol* 11(2):165–170, 1985.
4. Gould N: Surgery in advanced Charcot-Marie-Tooth disease. *Foot Ankle* 4:267–273, 1984.
5. M'Bamali EI: Results of modified Robert Jones operation for clawed hallux. *Br J Surg* 62:647–650, 1975.
6. Shives TC, Johnson KA: Arthrodesis of the interphalangeal joint of the great toe—an improved technique. *Foot Ankle,* 1:26–29, 1980.

# PART II

# Metatarsophalangeal Joints

# 4

# Chevron Osteotomy

Harold B. Kitaoka

## INDICATIONS/CONTRAINDICATIONS

The primary indication for a chevron osteotomy is pain over the medial eminence or bunion associated with a hallux valgus deformity. The pain is related to the use of enclosed shoes. The deformity may be flexible initially, and with the passage of time, become more rigid and more difficult to correct manually. There may be related forefoot disorders such as a hammer toe of the second, metatarsalgia of the second, soft corn in lateral hallux or medial second toe, and first metatarsophalangeal (MTP) degenerative arthritis. Most patients are improved with the use of appropriate footwear with a wider toe box, softer leather upper, low heel, and stretching the leather over the bunion with a ring and ball device. Convincing patients of the importance of footwear with these characteristics may be as challenging as the operative procedure.

Some surgeons advocate shoe inserts with an arch support because there may be an associated flatfoot deformity. Chevron osteotomy is indicated in patients with symptomatic mild to moderate hallux valgus deformity with no significant arthritis. Mild to moderate deformities are those with an intermetatarsal (IM) 1–2 angle of 16° or less in a weight-bearing anteroposterior radiograph of the foot (Fig. 4-1). More severe deformities may not be adequately corrected with this operation (Fig. 4-2). It is preferable if the patient has a painless, mobile MTP joint that may be passively corrected to anatomic alignment. The chevron osteotomy is occasionally indicated in patients who have failed hallux valgus operations, such as simple bunionectomy with medial capsulorrhaphy.

Chevron osteotomy is not indicated for patients who have general or local conditions that preclude operative treatment such as skin ulceration, local or remote infection, or dysvascular foot, or for patients who are unable to comply with required postoperative immobilization and protected weight bearing. Operating on patients with asymptomatic hallux valgus deformities is generally not advisable, nor is surgery because of anticipation of difficulty at some uncertain time in the future. Patients must understand that the conse-

H. B. Kitaoka, M.D.: Foot and Ankle Section, Department of Orthopaedics, Mayo Clinic and Mayo Foundation; and Mayo School of Medicine, Rochester, Minnesota.

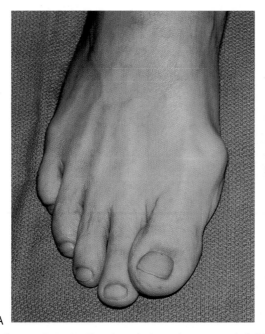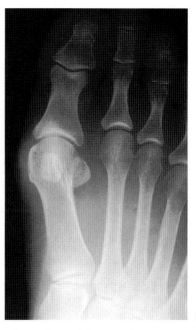

A                                                                      B

**Figure 4-1. A:** The dorsal view shows a painful hallux valgus deformity in a 36-year-old woman. The range of motion of the first metatarsophalangeal joint is 30° dorsiflexion and 34° plantarflexion relative to the plantar foot. The patient also has a painful bunionette. **B:** The anteroposterior radiograph of the right foot shows a moderate hallux valgus deformity with a hallux valgus angle of 25° and intermetatarsal 1–2 angle of 13°.

quence of returning to fashionable, constrictive footwear is a higher rate of recurrent deformity and symptoms. Significant MTP arthritis and severe hallux valgus with an IM 1–2 angle of more than 16° are also contraindications for the operation. Neuropathy is a relative contraindication. The patient's chronologic age is not as an important factor as physiologic age in considering this procedure. Although it was previously believed that the operation was not indicated in patients older than 50 years of age, this concept has been challenged

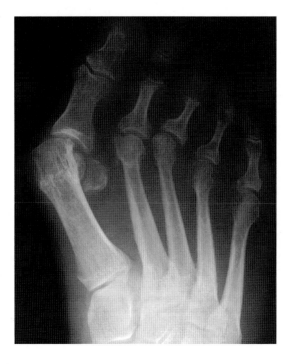

**Figure 4-2.** Radiograph of a patient with recurrent pain and hallux valgus deformity after a modified chevron procedure with an L-shaped osteotomy and screw fixation elsewhere. Seven weeks later, the screw was removed. The osteotomy was translated about 2 mm. The severity of the recurrent deformity was essentially unchanged from the preoperative status. Because of metatarsus adductus, the limited intermetatarsal 1–2 angle measurement of 13° is misleading and suggests a moderate deformity. The hallux valgus angle of 48° is consistent with a severe deformity. The recurrent hallux valgus resulted from multiple factors, including selection of the distal osteotomy technique.

by favorable clinical results in these patients. An MTP joint that is rigid, tender, has painful motion, or crepitus with motion and is not passively correctable to anatomic varus-valgus alignment has a worse prognosis.

## PREOPERATIVE PLANNING

Planning for a chevron osteotomy includes a history, examination of the foot, general health evaluation, radiologic interpretation, and consideration of expectations. An ideal patient for a chevron osteotomy describes the symptoms in realistic terms and has appropriate expectations. When the pain is excruciating, involves areas of the foot and ankle other than the bunion, or is present even without the use of shoes, a chevron osteotomy may not be the answer.

Besides noting the presence of the hallux valgus deformity, the foot examination should include measurement of MTP joint movement in dorsiflexion and plantarflexion relative to the plantar foot. Many patients with hallux valgus are unaware of their restricted MTP motion preoperatively, but they may recognize the limitation after the operation. It is also useful to determine flexibility of the hallux in the varus-valgus plane and notice whether the toe deformity is easily correctable. A deformity that is not passive correctable may be an indication of an arthritic joint or a laterally facing distal articular surface of the metatarsal (i.e., increased distal metatarsal articular angle) that is not effectively treated with a conventional chevron osteotomy. The neurovascular status of the foot should be documented. If posterior tibial and dorsalis pedis pulses are not palpable, additional investigation is warranted, such as a Doppler examination or noninvasive vascular studies.

The foot should be examined for any difficulties with lesser toe deformities or callus formation beneath the second metatarsal head, because they may be a source of symptoms after hallux valgus surgery. An adjunctive procedure for a lesser metatarsal is occasionally indicated with a chevron osteotomy of the first metatarsal. However, restoring the hallux alignment and first metatarsal head in an improved weight-bearing position with the chevron osteotomy may decrease the overloading of the second metatarsal and reduce in callus formation and pain.

A general health evaluation is important to anticipate difficulties that may occur. The presence of diabetes mellitus, peripheral vascular disease, peripheral neuropathy, and selected medications such as prednisone all have specific implications.

Radiologic evaluation should include weight-bearing anteroposterior and lateral views. The IM 1–2 angle is measured as the angle between lines drawn from the center of the head to the center of the base for the first and second metatarsals. This angular measurement may in some instances underestimate the magnitude of deformity, as occurs in feet with metatarsus adductus. The hallux valgus angle measured between the first metatarsal axis and the shaft of the proximal phalanx is also determined. Degenerative arthritis at the MTP joint can be evaluated on the anteroposterior and lateral radiographs.

A chevron osteotomy can be done under ankle block anesthesia as outpatient surgery. Patients who are particularly anxious can still tolerate an ankle block anesthetic with some degree of parenteral sedation. Occasionally, patients may prefer general anesthesia, and this is reasonable for bilateral surgery. Because of general health difficulties or for pain control, it may be necessary to admit a patient overnight.

Since the operation was described in early reports by Austin and Leventen (1) and by Johnson (6), it has been modified in more than a dozen ways in more than 50 publications in the orthopaedic and podiatric literature. These modifications include various shapes of medial capsular incisions, release of lateral capsular contractures, altering the position and angle of osteotomy in the sagittal plane, angling the axis of the osteotomy distally to maintain length, adding a closing wedge osteotomy component (biplanar osteotomy), combining it with a proximal phalangeal osteotomy, addition of fixation with a percutaneous pin or absorbable pin or with a staple or bone peg, fixation with a Herbert screw or compression screw or plate with screws or absorbable screws, and corrective soft dressing or slipper cast or short-leg cast. It is conceivable that the same successful result may be achieved by different modifications of the basic procedure.

This chapter describes a chevron osteotomy with percutaneous pin fixation to limit the potential for osteotomy displacement postoperatively. Although the chevron osteotomy has inherent stability, displacement can occur if the toe is traumatized, such as from a fall in the early postoperative period. Fixation ensures the metatarsal head will stay in the proper position and allows early weight bearing and range of motion exercises without osteotomy displacement.

## SURGERY

Ankle block anesthesia is usually administered. The patient is positioned supine on the surgical table. A 4-inch rubber Esmarch bandage is applied around the foot and ankle for exsanguination and is wrapped several times around the ankle for hemostasis. Applying a double-thickness stockinette over the skin before application of the Esmarch bandage provides padding to the skin and increases patient acceptance of the compression at the ankle.

### Technique

A longitudinal skin incision, about 7 cm long, is placed medially and centered over the medial eminence (Fig. 4-3). The subcutaneous tissue and bursal tissues are elevated from the capsule over the medial eminence, taking care to protect the dorsomedial sensory nerve and the plantar-medial nerve to the great toe. If the plantar-medial nerve is surgically injured, it is a significant problem because the subsequent end-bulb neuroma will be repetitively irritated with weight bearing. Iatrogenic trauma to the dorsomedial nerve may lead to hypesthesia in the dorsomedial hallux, irritation by footwear, and hypersensitivity.

When the medial capsule has been exposed, an L-shaped capsular incision is made with the horizontal limb plantar-medially and vertical limb several millimeters proximal to the MTP joint line. The capsular structures are dissected off the medial eminence (Fig. 4-4). Avoid injury to the dorsomedial and plantar-medial nerves to the great toe. This can be done by making the initial skin incision mid-medially. By dissecting the subcutaneous tissue and bursa dorsally and plantarward, the nerves can be protected from injury.

Excessive stripping of soft tissues from the lateral aspects of the metatarsal head may deprive the metatarsal head of part of its extraosseous blood supply and is not indicated. Releasing lateral joint contracture by perforating the lateral capsule under direct vision may aid in the realignment of the hallux. Multiple clinical and vascular anatomic studies (7,11) demonstrate that the distal chevron osteotomy with lateral capsulotomy may be accom-

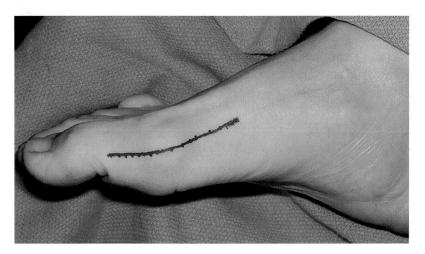

**Figure 4-3.** Placement of the midmedial, longitudinal skin incision.

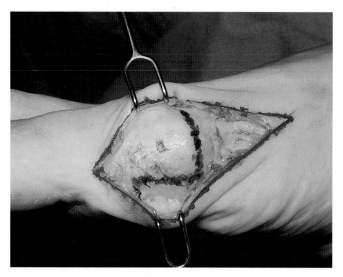

**Figure 4-4.** The bursa and subcutaneous tissues are dissected from the capsule. The L-shaped capsulotomy is marked with the horizontal limb placed plantar-medially, adjacent to the medial margin of the medial sesamoid.

plished without sacrificing the extraosseous blood supply to the metatarsal head and creating subsequent osteonecrosis.

The MTP joint is exposed with the L-shaped flap only enough to allow visualization of the sagittal groove of the medial eminence (Figs. 4-4 and 4-5). Starting at the sagittal groove, the medial eminence is removed parallel to the medial border of the foot (Fig. 4-6). A microsagittal saw with a thin blade is ideal for medial eminence removal, subsequent V-shaped osteotomy, and removing the uncovered portion of the metaphysis. Removal of the medial eminence along the medial border of the foot is performed to present a smooth, flat surface in an area typically in contact with footwear. If medial eminence resection is performed in a plane parallel to the shaft of the first metatarsal, there is a tendency to leave the

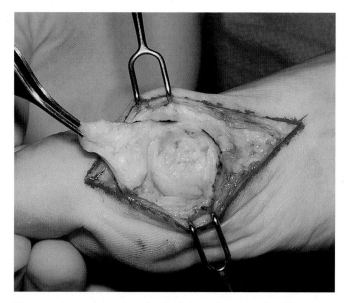

**Figure 4-5.** After capsular incision, the capsular flap is retracted distally. Capsular and ligamentous attachments to the medial eminence are carefully dissected proximally and retracted to expose the entire medial eminence.

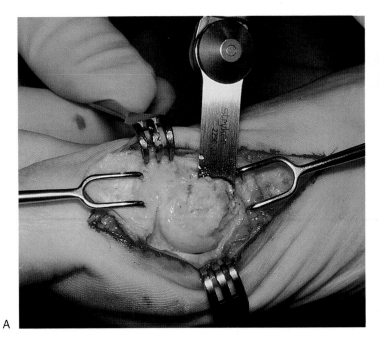

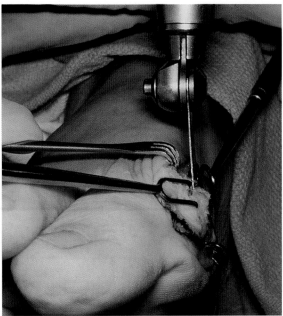

A     B

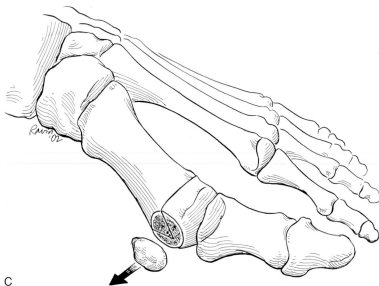

C

**Figure 4-6. A:** The prominent medial eminence is resected from dorsal to plantar with a microsagittal saw in the sagittal groove in a plane paralleling the medial border of the foot. The surface of the cut bone is carefully inspected for proper orientation. **B:** The anterior view shows the plane of resection. **C:** Schematic drawing of the procedure.

distal-medial aspect of the metatarsal head prominent, which could be a source of symptoms later. The plane of resection of the medial eminence must be correct, because the V-shaped osteotomy is oriented in relation to this bone cut.

Lateral capsulotomy may be performed by placing traction on the hallux distally using smooth retractors placed in the joint at the base of the proximal phalanx and manual traction on the hallux (Fig. 4-7). In this fashion, it is possible to consistently visualize the lateral capsule, which then is carefully incised at its attachment to the phalanx (Fig. 4-8). There is no attempt at adductor tenotomy and the capsulotomy is never performed unless it is easily visualized. As an alternative, the capsulotomy may be performed through a separate first web space incision. There is no need to deliver the entire metatarsal head out of the incision for exposure as this degree of soft tissue dissection increases the likelihood of joint stiffness and osteonecrosis.

The V-shaped osteotomy is performed at the head-neck level. The chevron osteotomy has been modified in several ways: the osteotomy is made with a more acute angle of 55°,

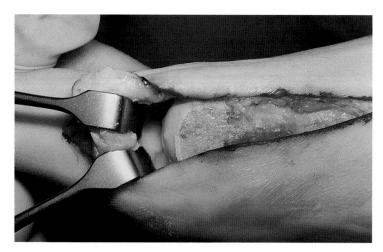

**Figure 4-7.** Traction is placed on the great toe by grasping the toe and by using two smooth retractors placed in the joint at the base of the proximal phalanx. This maneuver allows clear visualization of the lateral capsule of the metatarsophalangeal joint.

positioning the apex of the osteotomy 2 mm distal to the center of the head, lateral capsular perforation, and pin fixation of the osteotomy (Figs. 4-9 and 4-10).

The chevron osteotomy itself has some potential pitfalls. Placing the osteotomy too proximally in the neck region does not allow as much translation of the osteotomy, and less correction is therefore achieved. Placing the apex of the osteotomy 2 mm distal to the center of the head provides more surface area of cancellous bone, is more stable, readily unites, and the width of the head is greater, allowing more displacement. One of the more common pitfalls encountered is orienting the axis of the osteotomy obliquely instead of transversely. Slight dorsal angulation leads to dorsal displacement of the distal fragment and increases the likelihood of transfer metatarsalgia. If the apex is angled proximally, translating the distal fragment laterally is readily accomplished, but metatarsal shortening occurs. If one limb of the osteotomy is inadvertently angled dorsally or plantarward, optimal bony apposition does not occur. If there is a periosteal attachment that is not completely sectioned at the most proximal margin of the dorsal or plantar limbs of the osteotomy, the metatarsal head tends to rotate during translocation, causing the distal metatarsal articular surface to face more laterally. As a consequence, the hallux may gradually deform into a varus position.

The distal fragment of the osteotomy is translated laterally by grasping the shaft with a small towel clip with one hand, distracting the toe with the other hand, and applying a laterally directed force with the thumb to about one third of the width of the head (Fig. 4-11). Particular attention is given to translocating the capital fragment laterally without any tilt-

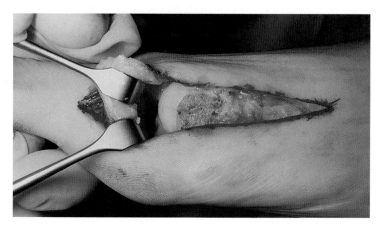

**Figure 4-8.** The lateral capsule is carefully perforated at its phalangeal attachment. The lateral capsular incision is shown.

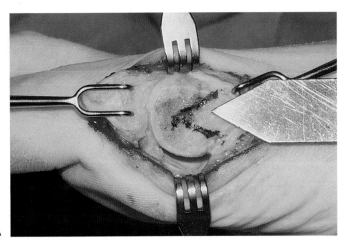
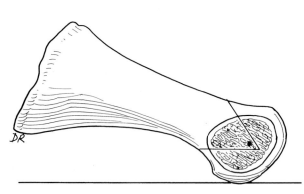

A                                                                                                                                                                     B

**Figure 4-9.  A:** The center of the metatarsal head is marked, as well as a second point positioned 2 mm distal to the first mark. The apex of the V-shaped osteotomy is centered at the more distal mark, and limbs of the proposed osteotomy are drawn using a simple jig or angle guide that has a 55°-tip. **B:** Schematic drawing shows the center of the metatarsal head, osteotomy placement, and osteotomy with dorsal and plantar limbs of equal length.

ing or angulation by noticing that the medial surface of the distal fragment is parallel to the medial surface of the proximal fragment after translocation. Gentle longitudinal compression on the great toe is performed; it should be inherently stable and not "spring back" to the original position.

Attention is directed to insertion of a smooth, 0.045-inch Kirschner wire from proximal and dorsal in the diaphysis, across the osteotomy, and through the head distally and plantarward (Fig.4-12A,B). The pin is advanced through the metatarsal head until the tip is visible and then withdrawn so the tip is just beneath the level of the articular cartilage. This orientation prevents the possibility of sesamoid impingement on the tip and allows weight bearing. The osteotomy is inherently stable, but the pin resists the medial-lateral shear force that can cause the distal fragment to move medially toward its original position. The pin provides adequate stabilization, although some surgeons prefer fixation with a screw, cortical bone peg, staple, absorbable pin, Herbert screw, or plate. Pin fixation does not require stripping of soft tissues

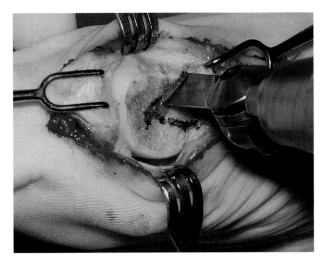

**Figure 4-10.** A chevron-shaped osteotomy is made in the head and neck with a microsagittal saw at an angle of 55°.

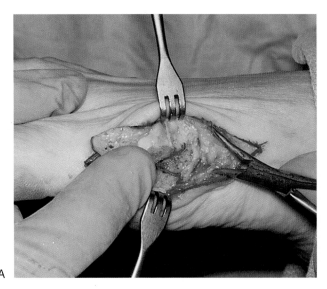
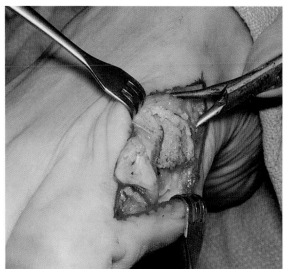

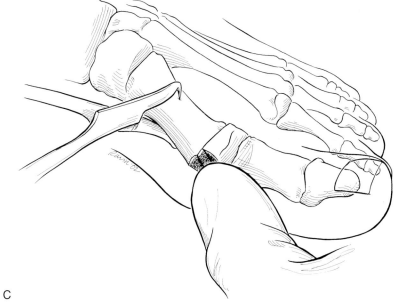

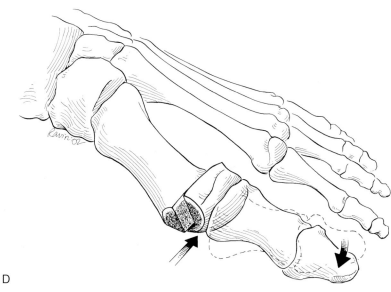

**Figure 4-11.  A:** A small towel clip stabilizes the metatarsal shaft, traction is placed on the hallux, and the distal fragment is displaced laterally by one third of the width of the metatarsal head. Care is taken to avoid excessive translation or angulation of the distal fragment. **B:** The anteromedial view shows the degree of displacement of the distal fragment. **C and D:** In the schematic drawings, an *arrow* indicates lateral displacement of the distal fragment.

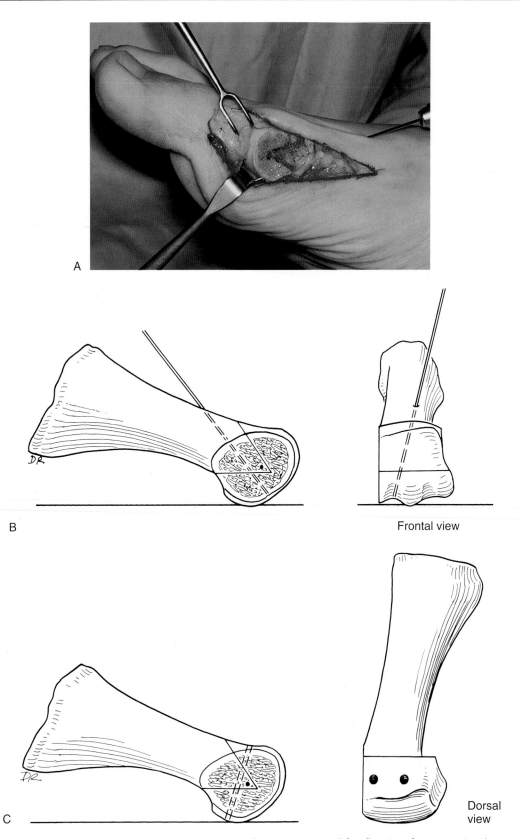

Frontal view

Dorsal
view

**Figure 4-12. A:** A percutaneous, 0.45-inch pin is inserted for fixation from proximal-dorsal to distal-plantar sites. The orientation of the pin is shown, and the tip of the pin is visible. The pin is then withdrawn until the tip is just beneath the articular surface. **B:** A schematic drawing shows pin placement. **C:** Alternate placement of fixation using two bioabsorbable pins from dorsal and medial views.

from the metatarsal neck and head dorsally, has a shorter operative time, and does not require an anesthetic to remove as other forms of internal fixation sometimes require. If it is observed during the soft tissue reconstruction and closure that the alignment is not optimal, minor adjustments in soft tissue tension may be attempted, but the osteotomy position may need to be revised. The pin can be removed and reinserted more readily than other forms of fixation. After removal of the percutaneous pin, there is no residual hardware that can become prominent after the swelling in the forefoot subsides and more normal footwear is used.

Fixation may also be accomplished with bioresorbable pins, such as a 1.3-mm Poly-P-Dioxanone (PDS) Pin (OrthoSorb, Johnson and Johnson Orthopaedics, Raynham, MA). Two pins may be placed from dorsal to plantar aspects (Fig. 4-12C). The bioresorbable pin eliminates the need for special cast padding when a cast is applied over the percutaneous pin with pin cap. Use of the bioresorbable pin does require additional dissection of soft tissues from the dorsal head and neck and somewhat longer operative time, and the pin is significantly more expensive than a stainless steel pin with cap.

Resection of the uncovered portion of metaphysis is now performed in a plane parallel to the medial border of the foot (Fig. 4-13). Directing the saw blade from the dorsal aspect

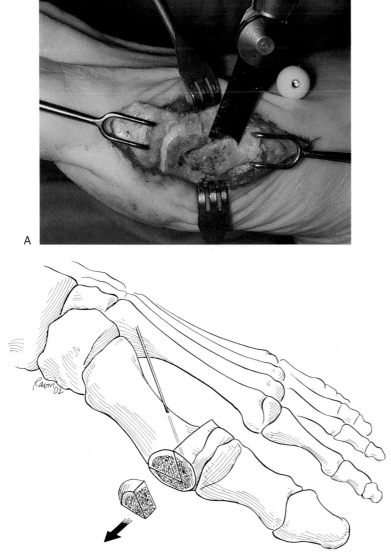

A

B

**Figure 4-13. A:** The remaining head and neck prominence is removed with a microsagittal saw in a plane parallel to the medial border of the foot. **B:** Schematic drawing of the procedure.

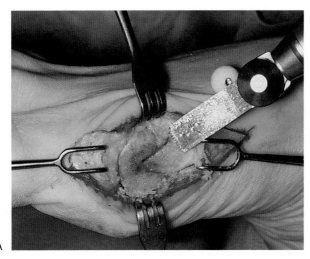
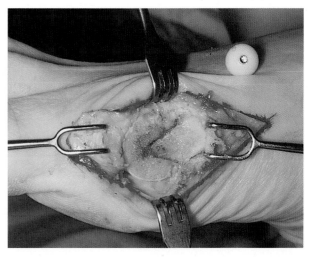

A                                                                                                                                                    B

**Figure 4-14. A:** Prominent dorsomedial margin of the distal metatarsal head and neck is removed with a microsagittal saw. **B:** The osteotomy is seen before closure, with the medial sesamoid correctly positioned under metatarsal head.

of the metatarsal facilitates a smooth, straight resection along the medial border of the foot (Fig. 4-13B). Directing the saw blade from distal to proximal aspects in continuity with the medial margin of the distal fragment leads to scalloping of the distal metatarsal. A small, needle-nosed bone rongeur or saw is used to smooth off the dorsomedial aspect of the metatarsal head so it will not be prominent with footwear (Fig. 4-14A). The medial and dorsal forefoot is palpated to detect any bony prominence. Before capsular closure, the medial sesamoid can be seen in its correct position beneath the metatarsal head (Fig. 4-14B).

Soft tissue reconstruction after completion of the osteotomy is important. With the L-shaped incision in the medial capsule followed by removal of the medial eminence and osteotomy displacement, excess capsular tissue will be recognized. A small portion of redundant capsule tissue is removed from the horizontal and vertical limbs of the capsulotomy before closure. The amount of capsule to be removed is determined by placing a 4 × 4 inch

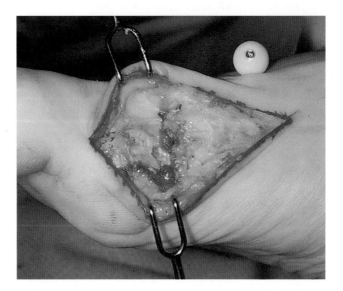

**Figure 4-15.** A portion of the redundant capsule is excised from the horizontal and vertical limbs, and the capsule is closed tightly. A 4 × 4 inch gauze is placed between the first and second toes, with the hallux in slight varus and neutral dorsiflexion-plantarflexion during capsular repair. The skin is closed in layers, followed by application of a compressive dressing with a plaster splint.

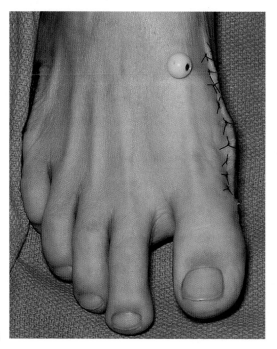
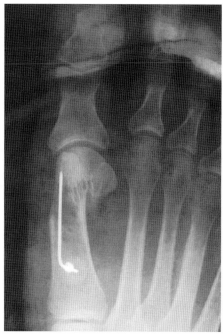

A                                                                    B

**Figure 4-16. A:** Position of the toe intraoperatively in neutral to slight varus. **B:** Immediately postoperatively, the anteroposterior radiograph shows pin placement and desired alignment.

gauze in the first web space to slightly overcorrect the hallux position in 5° of varus while the MTP joint is in a neutral dorsiflexion-plantarflexion position. Using a thumb forceps on each capsular flap, the capsule is overlapped and an estimate made of the width of capsule to be resected, which is usually about 2 mm wide. With the great toe again held in the overcorrected position of about 5° of varus, the medial capsular closure is made with 2-0 Vicryl sutures. After the first two or three sutures have been placed, the tension on the medial capsule is checked by removing the gauze from the web space and observing the toe in a resting position (Fig. 4-15). The toe should rest unsupported at about neutral to slight varus while it is in neutral flexion-extension alignment. At this point, if the great toe position is clearly in valgus or excessive varus, a judgment is made regarding whether the position can be improved with the medial capsular reconstruction or whether the osteotomy displacement is optimal. If necessary, the capsular sutures are removed, the pin removed, and the osteotomy position corrected. The final unsupported position of the great toe when the medial capsule is tightly closed should be about neutral with the phalanx in line with the first metatarsal (Fig. 4-16A). Appropriate soft tissue balancing of the vertical limb of the L-shaped capsulotomy helps maintain the position of the great toe in valgus-varus plane. Soft tissue balancing of the horizontal limb of the capsulotomy will aid in restoring sesamoid alignment beneath the metatarsal head and correcting hallux pronation. Closing the capsule tightly in this manner helps to maintain the sesamoid position beneath the metatarsal head. Skin closure is usually accomplished with absorbable sutures in the subcutaneous tissues and nylon in the skin.

The wound is dressed with a Xeroform strip and multiple 4 × 4 inch gauze sponges unfolded to 4 × 8 inches. A Robert Jones compressive dressing is applied with plaster splints. There is an effort to apply the compressive dressing without inadvertently forcing the hallux into a valgus position. Anteroposterior and lateral radiographs of the foot are taken in the recovery room (Fig. 4-16B).

## POSTOPERATIVE MANAGEMENT

The Robert Jones dressing provides immobilization, compression without constriction, and comfort. The patient can bear partial weight on the dressing. Crutches are used for balance as well as for limiting pressure on the painful foot.

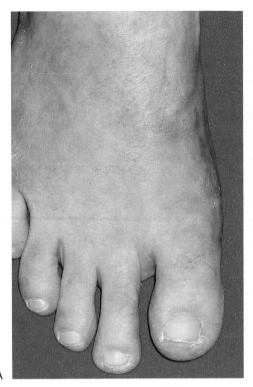
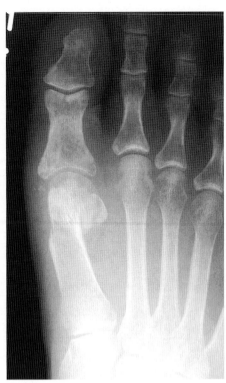

A

B

**Figure 4-17. A:** Clinical photograph obtained postoperatively. **B:** Postoperatively, the anteroposterior radiograph shows good alignment and correct sesamoid position beneath the lateral head.

The day after surgery, the compression dressing is removed, and a short-leg cast is applied. The forward edge of the cast should protrude beyond the great toe and support it inferiorly. The patient is allowed to bear partial weight on the cast. A "doughnut" constructed of 0.25-inch felt is used to pad around the pin cap before application of the cast padding.

The cast is removed about 3 weeks after surgery, sutures are removed, and the percutaneous pin is easily removed with a needle holder. A soft hallux valgus splint and a postoperative shoe are used for an additional 3 weeks. The patient is instructed in flexion-extension exercises for the great toe. At 5 to 6 weeks postoperatively, anteroposterior and lateral radiographs of the foot are obtained, and if they demonstrate union of the osteotomy, use of a closed toe shoe is resumed. The patient will continue to have some swelling during the rehabilitation period, and comfortable, loose-fitting footwear is advised (Fig. 4-17).

The results of chevron osteotomy depend to a large degree on proper patient selection. If the procedure is done for the patient group already described, the clinical results should be about 90% successful. There is consistent relief of pain over the medial eminence, improved comfort with footwear, and improved alignment. Unfortunately, is not unusual for patients to use increasingly more constrictive footwear with increasing heel height and then complain of aching in the foot. If cosmetic appearance seems to be an important aspect during preoperative discussions, caution should be exercised in suggesting surgical care. Providing nonoperative treatment recommendations as described earlier will provide symptomatic relief in some patients to the extent that surgery may not be necessary and provides insight about the likelihood of compliance with management after the operation.

The perceived length of recuperation from any foot surgical procedure varies among patients. When the question arises regarding how long it will take to recover, an answer of several months to complete recovery seems reasonable.

## COMPLICATIONS

As with any operative procedure, failures and complications can occur after chevron osteotomy. These include recurrent deformity, hallux varus, infection, osteonecrosis, stiffness, transfer metatarsalgia, degenerative arthritis, and unfulfilled patient expectations.

*Recurrent hallux valgus* may be caused by several factors. The original deformity may have been too severe and not adequately corrected by the distal osteotomy. The osteotomy may have displaced toward its original position or not displaced enough. There may be a laterally facing distal metatarsal articular surface angle. The patient may have chosen to resume the use of constrictive fashionable footwear. Systemic ligamentous laxity may be a factor. The medial capsular reconstruction may have been insufficient from attenuation of the capsule, medial capsular tissue fragmentation during the operation, or dehiscence of the capsular sutures. Careful patient selection and operative technique are important in minimizing the potential for recurrence. Rarely, a revision procedure, such as a proximal metatarsal osteotomy with distal soft tissue reconstruction, may be performed for recurrent symptoms.

*Hallux varus* is a complication that may occur from overzealous displacement of the osteotomy, from tightening the medial capsule excessively, or from removing too much of the medial eminence. If the capital fragment inadvertently tips laterally, the toe may begin to deviate into varus. Hallux varus may or may not be symptomatic and can be avoided. If the deformity is caused by malposition of the osteotomy and the patient is significantly symptomatic, the osteotomy may be revised in selected cases.

*Osteonecrosis* rarely occurs with this operation. Multiple clinical and laboratory-based studies demonstrate that lateral capsulotomy may be performed with the distal chevron osteotomy without the complication of avascular necrosis. Jones and Cracchiolo (7) found that an extensive network of extraosseous vasculature to the metatarsal head is present and is preserved when the osteotomy is done properly. Technical problems appear to be a greater threat to the viability of the metatarsal head, such as cutting of the first dorsal metatarsal artery by overpenetration of a saw blade or incorrect placement of the osteotomy (7). Patients who had simple bunionectomy with medial capsulorrhaphy along with lateral capsulotomy had better alignment at an average of 5 years after surgery compared with others who had the same operation without lateral capsulotomy (8).

*MTP joint stiffness* commonly occurs after surgery. However, critical analysis of the patient preoperatively will indicate that most of these patients have asymptomatic restriction of MTP dorsiflexion-plantarflexion motion preoperatively, and this should be documented. Some patients may exhibit signs of overloading of the second ray, such as metatarsalgia, intractable plantar keratosis, MTP synovitis, metatarsal stress fracture, or hypertrophy of the second metatarsal. It is important to document these findings preoperatively because they may persist even after successful chevron osteotomy surgery. Degenerative arthritis rarely occurs as a consequence of the operation.

The preoperative discussion should include the expectations of the patient. When cosmetic concerns or the desire to wear fashionable shoes is the main motivation to have surgical care, a cautious approach by the surgeon is suggested. Trying to explain in detail appropriate expectations can avoid or make conflict later.

## ILLUSTRATIVE CASE

This 36-year-old woman complained of pain at the medial eminence region of her right foot (Fig. 4-18A). She had no lesser toe symptoms or plantar forefoot pain. A hallux valgus deformity was observed. The range of motion of the first MTP joint was painless but restricted. There was no tenderness of the MTP joint. There was mild erythema over the prominent medial eminence. The valgus malposition was passively correctable.

The radiographs on the anteroposterior weight-bearing view (Fig. 4-18B) demonstrated a hallux valgus deformity and satisfactory cartilage space. The IM 1–2 angle measured 13°, and the MTP angle was 28°. The medial sesamoid was subluxated beneath the metatarsal head and lateral sesamoid uncovered.

A chevron osteotomy was performed under ankle block anesthesia as an outpatient. The patient went home the same day with the foot in a compressive dressing and had a short-leg cast applied the next day. The cast was removed in 3 weeks along with sutures and the

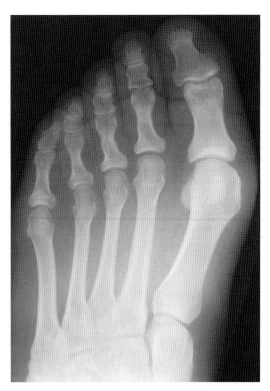

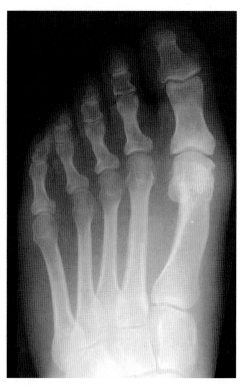

**Figure 4-18.** The anteroposterior radiograph demonstrates a hallux valgus deformity.

**Figure 4-19.** Follow-up radiograph at 5 years shows good alignment and no significant arthritis.

percutaneous pin. She used a postoperative shoe and soft hallux valgus splint for an additional 3 weeks, and performed range of motion exercises of the MTP joint.

At follow-up 5 years later, she had no pain, no restriction of activities, and no difficulty with footwear. She was graded a good result and was satisfied. Radiographs showed good alignment and no significant arthritis (Fig. 4-19). The IM 1–2 angle was 7°, and the hallux valgus angle was 16°.

## RECOMMENDED READING

1. Austin D, Leventen E: A new osteotomy for hallux valgus. *Clin Orthop* 157:25–30, 1981.
2. Chou LB, Mann RA, Casillas MM: Biplanar chevron osteotomy. *Foot Ankle Int* 19:579–584, 1998.
3. Donnelly RE, Saltzman CL, Kile TA, et al.: Modified chevron osteotomy for hallux valgus. *Foot Ankle Int* 15:642–645, 1994.
4. Gill LH, Martin DF, Coumas JM, et al.: Fixation with bioabsorbable pins in chevron bunionectomy. *J Bone Joint Surg Am* 79:1510–1518, 1997.
5. Hattrup S, Johnson K: Chevron osteotomy: analysis of factors in patients' dissatisfaction. *Foot Ankle* 5: 327–332, 1985.
6. Johnson K, Cofield R, Morrey B: Chevron osteotomy for hallux valgus. *Clin Orthop* 142:44–47, 1979.
7. Jones KJ, Feiwell LA, Freedman EL, et al.: The effect of chevron osteotomy with lateral capsular release on the blood supply to the first metatarsal head. *J Bone Joint Surg Am* 77:197–204, 1995.
8. Kitaoka HB, Franco MG, Weaver AL, et al.: Simple bunionectomy with medial capsulorrhaphy. *Foot Ankle* 12:86–91, 1991.
9. Leventen E: The chevron procedure. *Orthopedics* 13:973–978, 1990.
10. Zilberfarb JL, Greene MA, Peterson DA, et al.: Avascular necrosis of the first metatarsal head: incidence in distal osteotomy combined with lateral soft tissue release. *Foot Ankle Int* 15:59–63, 1994.

# 5

# Hallux Metatarsophalangeal Arthrodesis

Ian J. Alexander

## INDICATIONS/CONTRAINDICATIONS

Although surgeons and patients may shy away from the thought of first metatarsophalangeal (MTP) arthrodesis as an option in treatment of disorders of the MTP joint, their concerns in many cases are unjustified. Unquestionably, arthrodesis of the first MTP joint has an effect on foot mechanics, but in situations in which first MTP mechanics are already abnormal, fusion of the joint to eliminate pain or severe deformity may improve foot function.

Indications for first MTP arthrodesis include painful degenerative, inflammatory, or posttraumatic arthritis; marked deformity; and occasionally, chronic instability. Arthrodesis in many cases is the optimal means of salvaging failed first MTP joint surgery. When systemic disease such as rheumatoid arthritis or previous surgery has created a bony defect at the first MTP joint, a solid arthrodesis with a well-positioned hallux of reasonable length may be achieved with special techniques such as an interposition bone graft method.

Contraindications to first MTP arthrodesis include impaired vascularity and significant neuropathy. Arthrodesis of the first MTP joint should also be cautiously considered if there is coexistent arthritis of the interphalangeal (IP) joint of the hallux. Performing an MTP arthrodesis while ignoring an arthritic IP joint can lead to accentuation of IP joint symptoms. Fusing both joints simultaneously creates a stiff first ray that is prone to overloading the toe tip and metatarsocuneiform joint. Under these circumstances, in selected patients, combining an MTP joint resection arthroplasty with an IP fusion may be a reasonable option.

Alternatives to first MTP arthrodesis include resection or implant arthroplasty. Resection arthroplasty is a reasonable choice for patients with combined advanced hallux valgus and arthritis who are reluctant to have an arthrodesis because of limitations placed on their footwear selection postoperatively and in patients who are not able to comply with weight-bearing restrictions or immobilization requirements after arthrodesis. First MTP joint im-

I. J. Alexander, M.D.: Department of Orthopaedic Surgery, Northeastern Ohio Universities College of Medicine, Rootstown, Ohio.

plants should be approached with caution. I think there are no indications for unipolar Silastic implants. The use of bipolar Silastic implants for the first MTP joint in rheumatoid arthritis patients may be considered, but the popularity of these devices is declining, perhaps related to problems of silicone synovitis or to litigation related to other types of silicone implants. Implants with metal and polyethylene components should be viewed as experimental; the poor track record of designs similar to those currently being promoted should dampen any enthusiasm. If they fail, the bone deficiency associated with their insertion presents a difficult reconstructive problem.

Achieving a successful outcome with first MTP arthrodesis depends on careful preoperative planning to avoid predictable problems and intraoperative attention to detail to ensure rigid fixation, good cancellous bone contact, and optimal position.

## PREOPERATIVE PLANNING

Preoperative examination of the patient should ensure adequate circulation, sensation, and integrity of the skin over the sight of the proposed surgical incision. Patients with MTP arthritis have painful and restricted MTP motion, crepitus, and tenderness of the joint, and there may be deformity in valgus, varus, or extensus that should be documented. Pain, tenderness, motion, and stability of the IP joint should be recorded. Presence of other pathology such as transfer metatarsalgia or lesser toe problems should be noted.

Preoperative weight-bearing anteroposterior and lateral radiographs of the feet are mandatory. Several angles should be measured: hallux valgus angle, intermetatarsal (IM) 1–2 angle, and angle of inclination of the first metatarsal relative to the floor. If narrowing of the IM 1–2 angle is part of the objective of the first MTP fusion, as in severe hallux valgus, attention should be paid to the appearance of the base of the first metatarsal and metatarsocuneiform joint. The presence of a facet on the lateral aspect of the first metatarsal base abutting against the second metatarsal should make the surgeon aware that normal reduction of the IM 1–2 angle (usually 8° to 9°) will not occur (6).

It is important that the most desirable position of the hallux in the three primary planes is determined before surgery. Failure to position the hallux well in the sagittal (flexion-extension) plane is the positioning error. Excessive hallux extension results in dorsal toe irritation by the shoe at the IP joint. Reduced hallux function predisposes the patient to secondary metatarsalgia. Excessive plantarflexion may result in overloading of the hallux and painful plantar callosities at the plantar aspect of the IP joint region. This is particularly apt to occur when an IP sesamoid is present by the flexor hallucis longus tendon just proximal to its insertion. The sagittal position is optimal in most cases when the sagittal axis to the proximal phalanx is parallel to the floor when the foot is plantigrade. If the hallux is fused in a position parallel to the floor, elevation of the first metatarsal head by the sesamoids and the normal shape of the plantar surface of the proximal phalanx will result in proximal phalanx clearing the floor by about 4 to 8 mm (Fig. 5-1). This clearance allows for relatively normal roll-off during walking without hallux overload, and dorsal toe irritation is rarely a problem. This position also gives women some leeway in terms of shoe heel height. Another way to assess proper sagittal position after fixation is to palpate the contour starting proximal to the ankle, over the surface of the foot, and over the dorsal surface of the great toe. If there is a "ski jump" effect of the toe or a prominence as the hand palpates the dorsal surface of the hallux, the toe is probably placed in too much extension, and dorsal toe irritation is likely to occur.

The optimal sagittal arthrodesis angle (AA) is widely quoted as 25° to 30°. This is usually correct, because most individuals have a metatarsal inclination angle (MIA) relative to the floor of 25° to 30° (Fig. 5-2). In the case of pes planus and pes cavus, however, routinely fusing the hallux at 25° to 30° results in malposition. For example, if the MIA is 15° (pes planus) and the AA is 30°, the hallux fuses at 15° of dorsiflexion, and dorsal toe irritation will almost certainly result. If the MIA is 45° (pes cavus) and the AA is 30°, the hallux will be plantarflexed 15°, and overload may result. To achieve a hallux that is parallel to the floor the AA should be about equal to the MIA. The MIA can be easily determined from the preoperative standing lateral radiograph by measuring the angle between the floor and

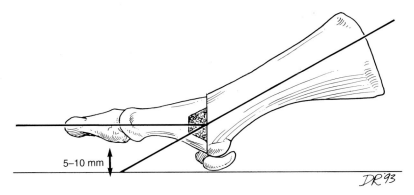

**Figure 5-1.** Proper position in the sagittal plane.

a line intersecting the top of the head and the base of the first metatarsal (Fig. 5-2). To intraoperatively assess sagittal plane position, pressure is applied to the plantar aspect of the foot with a flat rigid surface (Fig. 5-3). With this load-bearing simulation, the tip of the proximal phalanx should clear the flat surface by 4 to 8 mm. If the toe tip rests against the flat surface, the position is too plantarflexed. If the surgeon's index fingertip passes easily under the tip of the toe, the position is too dorsiflexed. Observation of the toe position from the medial side of the foot should demonstrate the hallux in a parallel position relative to the flat surface or in very slight plantarflexion.

Two clinical problems result from transverse (valgus-varus) plane malposition. Excessive valgus results in painful great toe–to–second toe impingement, and excessive varus may lead to IP joint degeneration. Recommending a specific hallux valgus angle of 15° to 20° as optimal for all cases is inappropriate. In many hallux rigidus patients, the hallux valgus angle is only 0° to 5°, with the second toe parallel to and resting against the hallux (Fig. 5-4). If the hallux is fused at 15° to 20° of valgus, painful great toe–to–second toe impingement and crossover toe deformity predictably occur (Fig. 5-5). In this instance, the optimal transverse plane fusion angle is the same as the preoperative hallux valgus angle. A good rule is to fuse the great toe in a transverse plane position that avoids second toe impingement if the preoperative hallux valgus angle is less than 15°. If the preoperative hallux valgus angle exceeds 15°, the hallux is best fused at approximately 10° to 15° of valgus. Correction of a malaligned second toe may also be necessary to prevent impingement problems if preoperatively it is deviated in a varus position.

To confirm that impingement between first and second toes will not be a problem postoperatively, a small gap should be present between the great and second toe during the load-bearing simulation intraoperatively.

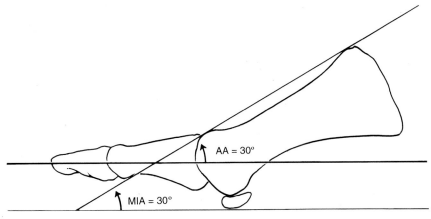

**Figure 5-2.** Measurement of the metatarsal inclination angle (*MIA*) and arthrodesis angle (*AA*).

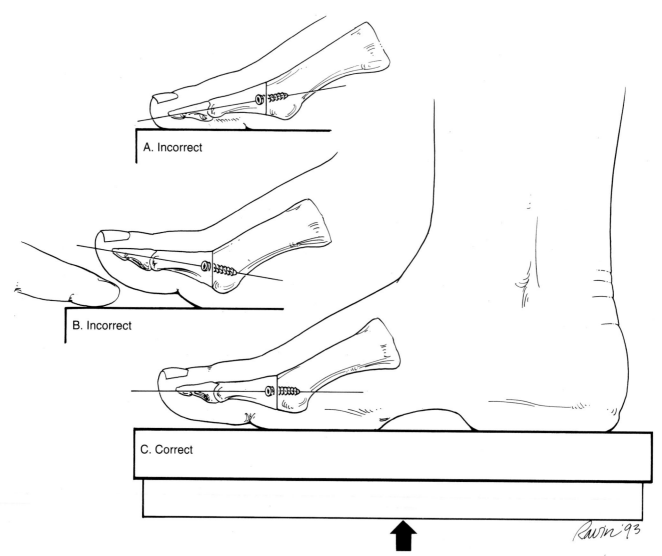

A. Incorrect

B. Incorrect

C. Correct

**Figure 5-3.** Intraoperatively, the surgeon checks for positioning in the sagittal plane: excessive plantarflexion **(A)**, excessive dorsiflexion **(B)**, and the correct position **(C)**.

Coronal plane rotation, often referred to as pronation or supination of the hallux, also influences outcome but may not be as critical as alignment in the other two planes. The most frequent problem in this plane is excessive pronation, which is usually encountered when severe hallux valgus is being corrected with an arthrodesis. The lateral capsular tightness resists hallux derotation. The consequence of fusing the hallux in pronation is that terminal push-off occurs on the plantar-medial aspect of the hallux at the IP joint rather than on the fleshy pulp of the great toe, potentially causing a painful callus at the IP joint. With hallux malrotation, IP flexion-extension occurs at an angle oblique to the normal sagittal plane. Proper hallux rotation is checked intraoperatively by carefully observing nail plate alignment of all the toes from a dorsal view and an end-on view. It is helpful also to be certain that IP flexion-extension occurs in the sagittal plane to avoid malpositioning the toe in the coronal plane.

Obtaining a solid arthrodesis is important to achieve a successful result. Factors that contribute to reliable healing of first MTP fusions include extensive cancellous bone contact, inherent stability of the fusion configuration, and rigid fixation.

Cancellous bone contact and inherent stability are related to the technique used to prepare the surfaces of the phalangeal base and the metatarsal head. Surface preparation that results in good inherent stability such as interlocking conical or truncated cone shapes re-

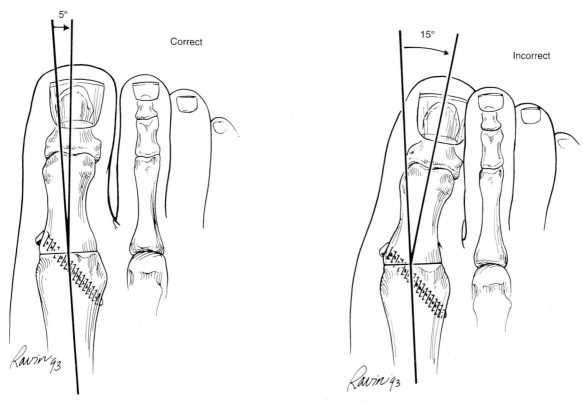

**Figure 5-4.** Position in the transverse plane, showing correct fusion alignment.

**Figure 5-5.** Position in the transverse plane, showing excessive valgus alignment.

quires less fixation compared with flat bone surfaces. With these techniques, fixation with a single, small fragment screw usually provides excellent positional control (Fig. 5-6). Crossed screws are advisable if there is less inherent stability, as with flat cuts on even dome surface preparation, or if the bone is osteoporotic (Fig. 5-7). Other methods of fixation have been advocated. These include use of two longitudinal, heavy threaded pins that

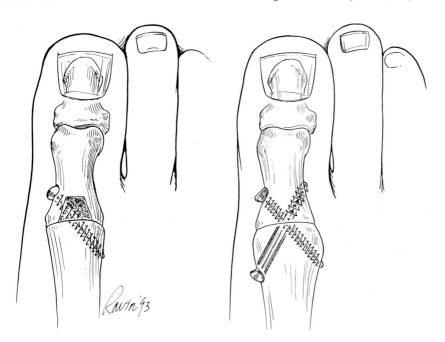

**Figure 5-6.** Fixation of fusion with a single bone screw (**left**) and with two screws (**right**).

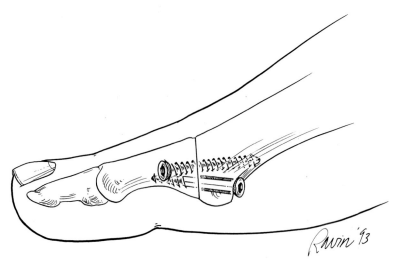

**Figure 5-7.** Two-screw fixation technique.

traverse the IP and MTP joints, dorsal plate and screws, and multiple small Kirschner wires. Although the use of heavy threaded longitudinal pins is indicated when the bone is extremely osteoporotic or in salvage situations when screw fixation is not possible, they can contribute to the later development of IP joint arthritis. If longitudinal pin fixation is required, a single, longitudinal, threaded Steinmann pin works well when supplemented with a smaller, obliquely smooth, 0.062- or 0.045-inch Kirschner wire crossing the MTP fusion site (not IP joint) to control rotation. In my hands, the dorsal plate and screw fixation is useful mainly when the fusion technique includes an interposition bone graft. For routine fusion operations, a plate on the dorsal (compression) side of the fusion is prone to failure and often requires removal because of the prominence. Multiple small pins may be used in salvage situations but removing them may not be an enjoyable experience.

Methods of preparing inherently stable surfaces that provide extensive cancellous contact include dome-shaped surfaces prepared with a rongeur, curettes, and a burr or the Coughlin small joint fixation system (Stryker Howmedica Osteonics Corp., Allendale, NJ). A second method uses conical shaped reamers such as those described by Marin (7) to create conical surfaces. A third method uses a truncated cone reamer system (Biomet, Inc., Warsaw, IN).

Although surface preparation with a rongeur and curettes may be tedious, it requires no special instrumentation and it has a distinct advantage of allowing the toe to be easily positioned and repositioned as desired. It is more stable than flat bone cuts. The disadvantage of this technique is that it is time consuming.

The Marin reamers are manual instruments that provide a more stable arthrodesis than that provided by a dome created by a rongeur, curettes, and a burr. The conical reamers prepare the bony surfaces in the shape of a pointed cone after initial surface joint debridement. Problems encountered with this method include significant shortening of the hallux and difficult surface preparation if the bone is dense. The acute angle of the conical reamers results in a removal of a significant portion of the cancellous bone in the phalanx.

The truncated cone reamer system was designed to use power instrumentation to prepare the articular surface in a reproducible manner based on measurements taken from preoperative foot radiographs. Cancellous apposition and inherent stability is maximized by the accurately machined Morse taper configuration of the prepared surfaces. There is less bone loss and shortening using a truncated cone compared with a full cone-shaped surface preparation. The system consists of guides, templates, and a series of Kirschner wire–guided reamers that facilitate accurate positioning and surface preparation (Fig. 5-8). This system provides a reliable, reproducible means of achieving a well-positioned solid arthrodesis. Potential problems with the technique include phalangeal fracture of osteopenic bone during reaming and some difficulty changing the fusion position after initial reaming.

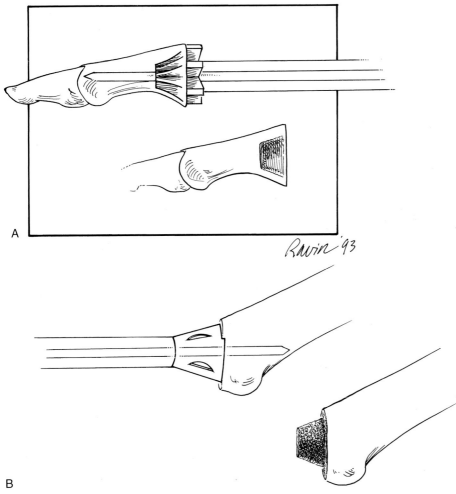

**Figure 5-8.** Overall plan for phalanx base **(A)** and metatarsal head **(B)** preparation using specialized reamers.

## SURGERY

The patient is positioned supine on the operating table. Ankle block anesthesia or general or spinal anesthesia may be used. If an ankle tourniquet is to be used, a few wraps of sterile cast padding are placed in the supramalleolar area, and the foot is exsanguinated with a 4-inch Esmarch bandage starting from the toes. The bandage is wrapped with even tension in three to four layers on top of the cast padding at the supramalleolar level. A thigh tourniquet can be employed in patients under general or spinal anesthesia.

### Standard Dome Technique

A straight medial incision is centered over the MTP joint of the great toe. Flaps of tissue are not developed, but instead the incision is brought directly through the skin and subcutaneous tissue, through the medial joint capsule, and down to the medial cortical surface of the first metatarsal and the base of the proximal phalanx. The base of the proximal phalanx is mobilized enough to provide easy access to the proximal phalanx base with an end-on view. Any articular cartilage is removed with a curette, and the hard subchondral bone is removed with a pineapple-shaped burr until a porous cancellous bone surface is exposed. Rongeurs are then employed to remove the articular cartilage and subchondral bone of the metatarsal head. The two surfaces are then shaped until they are congruent when apposed.

Fixation is achieved with two screws such as 4.0-mm cancellous screws, 3.5-mm cortical screws, or cannulated small-fragment screws of a similar size (4.0 mm). The first drill bit is inserted from the medial aspect of the proximal phalanx at the midpoint (dorsal-plantar) at the distal margin of the flare of the phalangeal base and is angled slightly dorsally into the MT head. The second drill bit is inserted from the plantar-medial aspect of the first MT neck just proximal to the articular surface and directed distally and laterally to engage the cortex of the plantar-lateral aspect of the phalangeal base. With the drill bits in place, a hard flat surface (e.g., the metal top of the small fragment set) is held against the plantar aspect of the foot to assess the position of the hallux in all three planes as previously outlined. It is also advisable to check bony surface congruity visually or even with fluoroscopy because bony contact dorsally as a continuous cortical rim does not ensure central cancellous bone apposition. If position and bony apposition are good, both holes are tapped, and 3.5-mm cortical screws are inserted. If cannulated screws are used, hallux alignment and bony apposition are checked after placing the guide wires. Simulated weight bearing with the instrument box top should be repeated after screw placement because the position may shift as the screws are tightened, particularly if the bone is soft as in rheumatoid arthritis patients.

### Truncated Cone Reamer System Technique

The surgical approach and exposure is an outline in the preceding paragraph. Initially, a guide wire is placed down the center of the proximal phalanx joint surface. Over this guide wire, the base of the proximal phalanx is prepared with the specialized reamers (Fig. 5-9A–C) to create a truncated cone-shaped bone surface.

The metatarsal head is then exposed, and a guide pin is inserted into the metatarsal head at the appropriate angle using the dorsal aspect of the first metatarsal as a reference (Fig. 5-9D). The guide pin should be placed in line with the desired final position of the toe. When the guide pin is properly placed, the reamer system is used to produce a truncated cone configuration in the distal metatarsal (Fig. 5-9E,F).

The two bony surfaces are apposed, and an obliquely oriented screw is placed from distal to proximal, starting from the medial base of the proximal phalanx, extending across the arthrodesis site, and extending into the plantar-lateral cortex of the metatarsal neck (Fig. 5-9G–I). A fully threaded, 4.0-mm cancellous screw or a 3.5-mm cortical screw is used for fixation, depending on the density of the cortical bone, which can be estimated by the resistance of the bone of the far cortex during drilling. This screw should be countersunk to avoid a medial prominence of the screw head and cracking of the cortical shelf or bridge on the medial base of the proximal phalanx. The final position of the toe is checked in flexion-extension, varus-valgus, and rotation by simulating weight bearing on a flat, rigid surface.

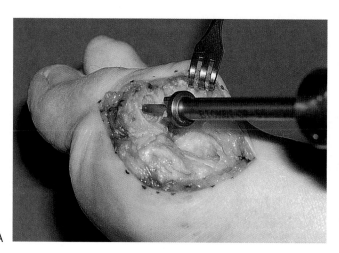

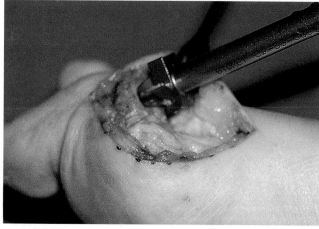

A

B

**Figure 5-9. A:** Preparing the phalangeal base with the end-cutting reamer. **B:** Cutting the truncated cone with the side-cutting reamer. *(continued)*

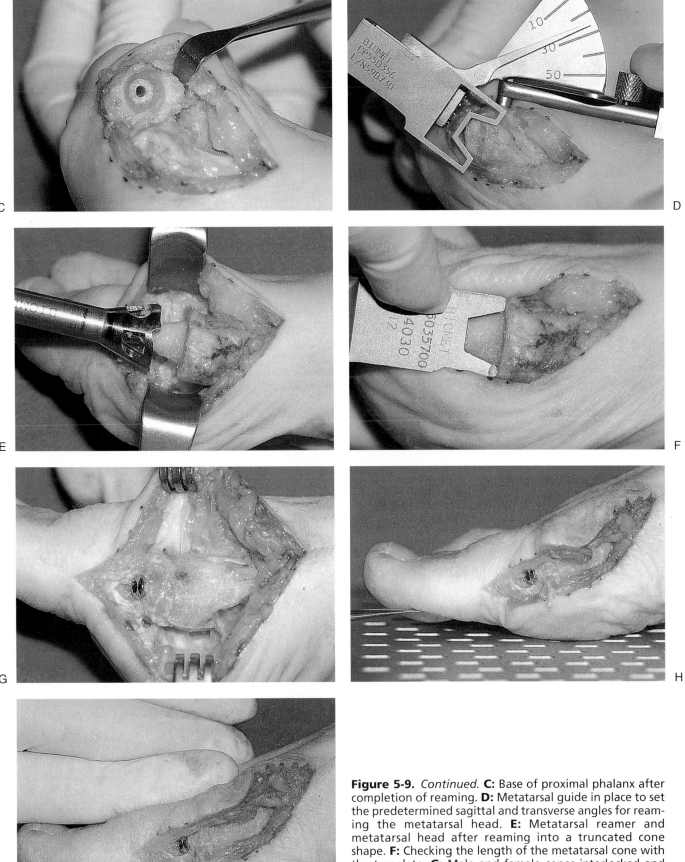

**Figure 5-9.** *Continued.* **C:** Base of proximal phalanx after completion of reaming. **D:** Metatarsal guide in place to set the predetermined sagittal and transverse angles for reaming the metatarsal head. **E:** Metatarsal reamer and metatarsal head after reaming into a truncated cone shape. **F:** Checking the length of the metatarsal cone with the template. **G:** Male and female cones interlocked and fixed with a single oblique screw. **H:** Ensuring adequate hallux clearance under the phalangeal head. **I:** Checking the dorsal line of the first ray to ensure the prominence of the phalangeal head is not excessive.

The wound is closed with absorbable sutures in the capsule and subcutaneous tissue and nonabsorbable sutures for the skin.

### First Ray Reconstruction with Interposition Bone Graft

When pain, deformity, or instability at the first MTP joint is associated with bone deficiency because of erosive arthritis or previous surgical resection of bone, the usual technique of apposition of existing bone surface to obtain a stable, well-aligned and pain-free hallux may result in an unacceptable degree of first ray shortening. Under these circumstances, filling the defect with autogenous iliac crest bone graft often allows the surgeon to meet the objectives of an arthrodesis while restoring first ray length and more normal foot geometry.

The basic structural component of the interposition bone graft is a tricortical block of iliac crest. This block is fashioned to fit the size, shape, and cortical deficiency of the defect to be filled (Fig. 5-10). The surgical approach to the joint in these individuals is usually dictated by previous surgical incisions. Often, there have been multiple previous surgical approaches to the first MTP joint. Patients must be carefully assessed preoperatively to determine if there are other sources of medial forefoot pain such as incisional neuromas of the dorsal proper digital nerve or medial plantar nerve. It may be necessary to address incisional neuromas operatively to avoid these potential sources of persistent postoperative pain.

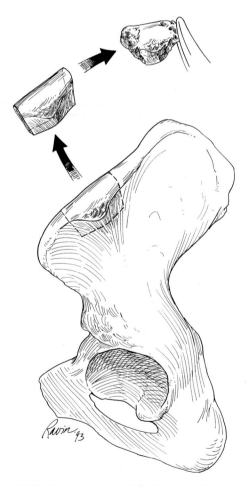

**Figure 5-10.** Harvesting and fashioning the tricortical graft.

The bone surfaces should be debrided of soft tissues such as fibrous tissue, which is commonly observed in the bone defects. Initially, all bone attached solidly to the metatarsal or phalanx should be left intact, even if it is a relatively thin cortical shell. Efforts should be made to preserve periosteal blood supply whenever possible. If the defect is asymmetric (e.g., dorsal cortical erosion associated with a double-stem Silastic implant), it may be possible to appose the residual cortices (in this case on the plantar aspect) to maintain length. Adjusting the contour of these surfaces and apposing them provides a bony bridge in direct contact that may enhance stability and healing.

The tricortical iliac crest bone graft is fashioned to fill the defect. Cortex should be removed from the graft to provide cancellous contact with existing bone, but whenever possible, cortex should be left on the graft surface, where it can bridge cortical defects or windows. This cortical strut provides structural support and a surface for fixation. A large piece of intercalated bone graft in which the cortical bone has been removed may be predisposed to collapse or late stress fracture.

Fixation of these fusions depends on the size and shape of the interposition graft. Crossed-threaded Kirschner wires, Steinmann pins, and/or screws may provide excellent stabilization if the interposition graft is short, but fixation with a plate and screws is frequently necessary for longer segmental grafts. These plates are usually placed on the dorsal surface and are mechanically under compression and therefore prone to failure when subjected to repetitive dorsiflexion bending forces.

## POSTOPERATIVE MANAGEMENT

Patients undergoing primary arthrodesis are routinely asked to wear a wooden postoperative shoe, to walk flat-footed, and are specifically cautioned not to load the hallux. Every 2 weeks, until 6 weeks postoperatively, the integrity of the fusion is checked, and the bandage is changed. If any movement is present at these intervals, the patient should be immobilized in a cast. A cast is also advisable if the patient is unreliable, osteoporotic, has difficulty using ambulatory aids, or the stability of fixation is thought to be tenuous.

In patients who undergo arthrodesis with interposition graft, complete healing is a much longer process, and weight bearing is usually avoided for 3 months. After that, weight bearing is allowed in a cast with a posterior locking heel until solid healing is demonstrated on radiographs.

In our follow-up of patients who underwent arthrodesis with interposition graft we found excellent subjective results in terms of patient satisfaction with position, stability, and pain relief, but dynamic foot pressure analysis in almost all cases showed little or no significant hallux function.

## COMPLICATIONS

The most frequent complications of first MTP arthrodesis are malposition and nonunion. Salvage of these complications may consist of revision arthrodesis, if necessary, taking all the precautions discussed previously to ensure good position and to maximize the potential for solid healing. Prominent hardware may be a problem with any technique and may require removal. Damage to the dorsal proper digital nerve can cause pain and a sensitive incisional neuroma. If nerve desensitization fails to resolve the problem, the nerve may need to be transected and its terminal end buried into a dorsomedial drill hole in the first metatarsal.

## ILLUSTRATIVE CASES

A 67-year-old, retired dentist presented with severe hallux valgus and painful prominence of the medial eminence. The hallux was markedly pronated, and the valgus deformity was

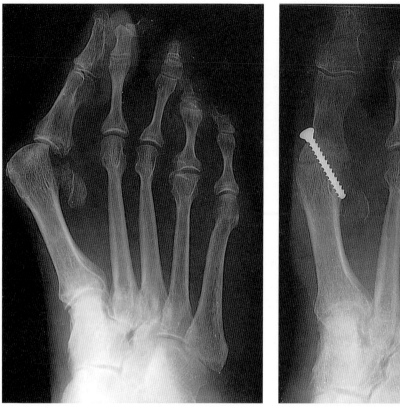
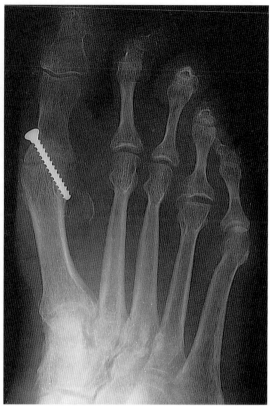

A          B

**Figure 5-11.** Case presentation. Preoperative **(A)** and postoperative **(B)** metatarsophalangeal arthrodesis.

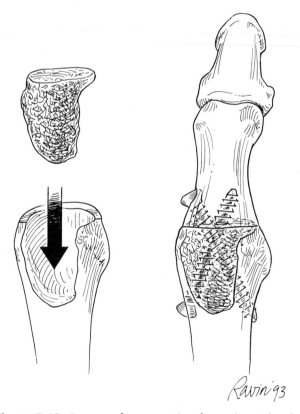

**Figure 5-12.** Bone graft preparation for an irregular defect.

not passively correctable. After discussing possible options, the patient chose a first MTP arthrodesis to obtain reliable correction without risk of recurrence. The significant decrease in the IM 1–2 angle is easily appreciated (Fig. 5-11).

A woman with rheumatoid arthritis presented with pain in the first MTP joint. Radiographs showed a large lytic defect in the first metatarsal head with a thin cortical shell (Fig. 5-12). At surgery, the cyst was curetted, and the articular surface and subchondral bone of the base of the phalanx and the remaining metatarsal articular surface were removed. An entirely cancellous graft was fashioned to fill the defect, and stable fixation was provided by cross screws.

Another patient had a painful MTP joint after a double-stem Silastic implant (Fig. 5-13). At surgery, almost the entire cortical rim was intact circumferentially, but no cancellous bone remained in the phalangeal base or the distal metatarsal. The bone ends were planed with a saw to provide flat apposing surfaces, and a football-shaped totally cancellous graft was fashioned to fill the defect. Chips of cancellous bone were placed proximal and distal to the interposition graft to fill the defect, and cross screws provided excellent fixation.

A woman with a painful nonfunctional great toe presented after previous bunion surgery (Fig. 5-14). Although the shape of the phalangeal base was unusual, this patient had apparently undergone a previous Keller resection arthroplasty. To maintain hallux length, a full tricortical graft with cancellous surfaces facing proximally, distally, and medially was interposed and fixed with longitudinally threaded Kirschner wires using a technique described by Coughlin and Mann (3).

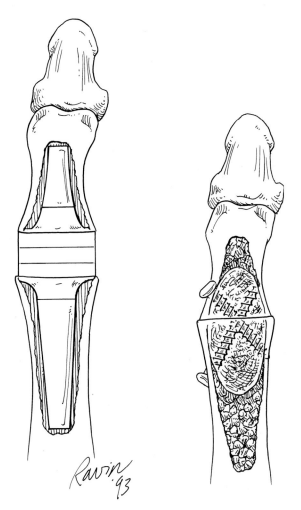

**Figure 5-13.** Combination of cortical and cancellous bone to fill an extensive defect.

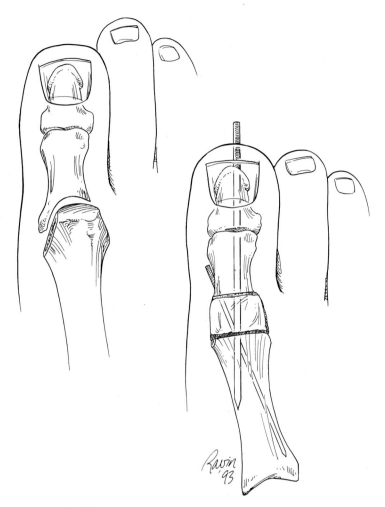

**Figure 5-14.** This block type of graft was used with Kirschner wire fixation.

In another case, a woman presented with a flail, malpositioned, and painful great toe after removal of a double-stem Silastic implant that had caused extensive dorsal bone destruction and perforation of the IP joint (Fig. 5-15). At surgery, the residual phalangeal condyles surprisingly had intact articular cartilage. An extensive tricortical graft was fashioned to fill a defect, and at its distal end, cortical bone was removed, and a dome of cancellous bone was fashioned to fit the proximal surface of the remaining phalanx. Proximal fixation was obtained with a dorsal plate, and two crossed Kirschner wires were placed distally to hold the phalanx to the interposition graft (Fig. 5-16).

Coughlin and Mann (3) concluded that MTP arthrodesis was a useful salvage procedure for failed Keller resection arthroplasty in 16 feet. Smith et al. (10) reported results of 7 MTP arthrodeses in 34 feet with threaded, 0.062-inch Kirschner wires. Union was achieved in 97%. Coughlin and Abdo (2) described a high rate of success of MTP arthrodesis with cone-shaped or cup-shaped reamers and plate-screw fixation in 58 feet. Solid union was achieved in 98%. Hecht et al. (4) reported success in arthrodesis of the first MTP joint to salvage failed silicone implant arthroplasty with interposition bone graft in 5 patients. Brodsky et al. (1) achieved union in 11 of 12 patients who had MTP arthrodesis with structural iliac crest bone graft and plate fixation. Myerson et al. (8) performed arthrodesis with bone graft to restore length, and union was achieved in 19 (79%) of 24 patients. Postoperative infection occurred in three.

In our follow-up of these and other interposition graft patients, we found an excellent subjective outcome in terms of patient satisfaction with position, stability, and pain relief, but dynamic foot pressure analysis in almost all cases showed little or no significant hallux function.

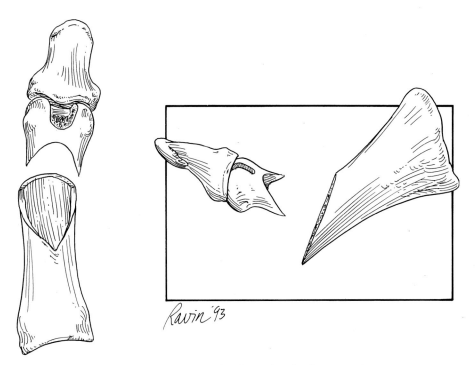

**Figure 5-15.** Extensive bone loss had occurred.

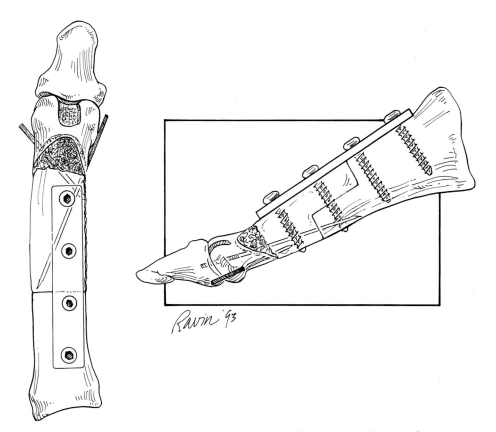

**Figure 5-16.** Repair required cortical and cancellous bone with plate fixation.

## RECOMMENDED READING

1. Brodsky JW, Ptasek AJ, Morris SG: Salvage fist MTP arthrodesis utilizing ICBG: clinical evaluation and outcome. *Foot Ankle Int* 21:290–296, 2000.
2. Coughlin MJ, Abdo RV: Arthrodesis of the first metatarsophalangeal joint with Vitallium plate fixation. *Foot Ankle Int* 15:18–28, 1994.
3. Coughlin MJ, Mann RA: Arthrodesis of the first metatarsophalangeal joint as salvage for the failed Keller procedure. *J Bone Joint Surg Am* 69:68–75, 1987.
4. Hecht PJ, Gibbons MJ, Wapner KL, et al.: Arthrodesis of the first metatarsophalangeal joint to salvage failed silicone implant arthroplasty. *Foot Ankle Int* 18:383–390, 1997.
5. Johnson KA: *Surgery of the foot and ankle*. New York: Raven Press, 1989:202–208.
6. Mann RA, Katcherian DA: Relationship of metatarsophalangeal joint fusion on the intermetatarsal angle. *Foot Ankle* 10:8–11, 1989.
7. Marin GA: Arthrodesis of the first metatarsophalangeal joint for hallux valgus and hallux rigidus. *Int Surg* 50:174–178, 1968.
8. Myerson MS, Schon LC, McGuigan FX, et al.: Result of arthrodesis of the hallux metatarsophalngeal joint using bone graft for restoration of length. *Foot Ankle Int* 21:297–306, 2000.
9. Shereff MJ, Baumhauer JF: Hallux rigidus and osteoarthrosis of the first metatarsophalangeal joint. *J Bone Joint Surg Am* 80:898–908, 1998.
10. Smith RW, Joanis TL, Maxwell PD: Great toe metatarsophalangeal joint arthrodesis: a user-friendly technique. *Foot Ankle* 13:367–377, 1992.

# 6

# Hallux Proximal Phalanx Osteotomy—The Akin Procedure

Carol Frey

## INDICATIONS/CONTRAINDICATIONS

In 1925, Akin (1) described a procedure for correction of hallux valgus that involved resection of the medial prominence of the first metatarsal head and a medial wedge osteotomy of the proximal phalanx of the great toe. Akin also described removal of the hypertrophic bone on the medial aspect of the base of the proximal phalanx of the great toe and lateral capsular release if necessary. In the following years, various modifications were added to the basic procedure described by Akin. The operation was popularized by Melvin H. Jahss, who also provided insight with respect to its application and limitations.

Indications for the Akin procedure include painful hallux valgus interphalangeus deformity and selected cases of hallux valgus. The hallux valgus interphalangeus deformity may be painful over the prominent medial condyle of the proximal phalanx. The deformity may cause a painful corn in the lateral hallux, where it contacts the second toe or even pain in the hallux toenails from impingement with the second toe. The Akin procedure can be used with success in those patients who present with second toe problems related to the deformed hallux, such as pain, soft corn, hammer toe, valgus second toe, or painful toenail (Fig. 6-1). The procedure may also be used in cases of residual valgus deformity after previous hallux valgus surgery. The osteotomy is applicable in patients who have a combined valgus deviation at the metatarsophalangeal (MTP) and interphalangeal (IP) joints in whom the MTP deformity is mild and a simple procedure is desirable. In patients with more complex valgus deformities, such as a congruent MTP joint with laterally facing distal metatarsal articular angle (DMAA) or juvenile bunion, it may be combined with other procedures. Surgeons have combined the Akin procedure with a distal chevron osteotomy (8), proximal closing wedge osteotomy (7), and proximal metatarsal osteotomy with cuneiform osteotomy (2).

C. Frey, M.D.: Department of Orthopaedic Surgery, University of California Los Angeles, Los Angeles, California; Foot and Ankle Surgery, West Coast Sports Performance, Manhattan Beach, California.

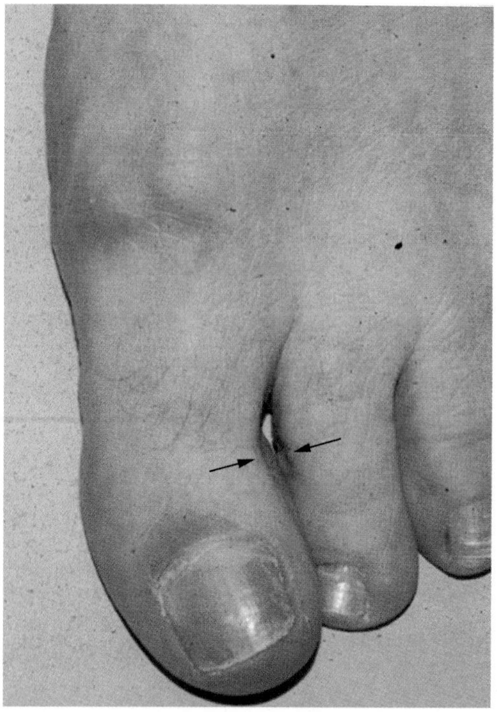

**Figure 6-1.** The patient has a hallux valgus interphalangeus deformity. Notice the distal phalanx of hallux overlapping the second toe and the soft corns on the lateral hallux and medial second toe *(arrows).* (Courtesy of the Mayo Clinic and Mayo Foundation, Rochester, Minnesota.)

Contraindications include patients with infection, skin ulceration, neuropathy, dysvascular extremity, MTP degenerative arthritis, hallux valgus with an incongruent MTP joint, or hallux valgus with metatarsus primus varus. An incongruent MTP joint with a rounder shape than the metatarsal articular surface is more likely to continue to subluxate after surgery.

## PREOPERATIVE PLANNING

It is important to obtain the specific patient concerns to determine how to direct treatment. The patient criterion for an Akin procedure is similar to that of other bunion procedures. Patients become candidates for surgery only after they have failed an adequate course of nonoperative treatment, which includes a shoe with a high, wide toe box; a soft leather upper; and adequate room for all the toes to fully extend. Stretching the leather upper in the region of the forefoot prominence is useful. If the main concern is painful, soft corns in the lateral hallux and medial second toe, various foam pads, tubular sleeves, and instructions on debriding the corns are effective.

During physical examination, it is important to notice the degree and level of the toe deformity. It should be determined to what extent the valgus deformity is present at the IP versus the MTP joint. Hallux pronation should be noted because only a limited degree of rotatory deformity can be corrected at the time of surgery. Range of motion of the hallux MTP and IP joints should be measured. It is not unusual for patients with hallux deformities to have asymptomatic joint stiffness, and this condition should be documented before the surgery. Tenderness, swelling, and painful joint motion should be documented.

Preoperatively, all patients should have weight-bearing anteroposterior, lateral, and

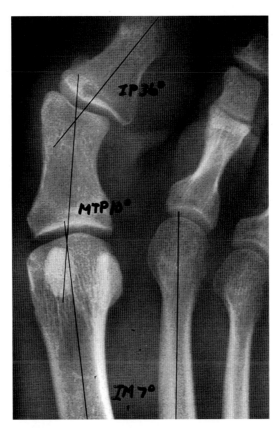

**Figure 6-2.** Radiologic measurements in a patient with an abnormal hallux IP angle but a normal metatarsophalangeal angle and normal intermetatarsal 1–2 angle. (Courtesy of the Mayo Clinic and Mayo Foundation, Rochester, Minnesota.)

oblique radiographic views of the foot taken. Radiographic measurements include intermetatarsal angle to determine the degree of metatarsal primus varus, the first MTP angle to determine the amount of hallux valgus, and the great toe IP angle to determine the amount of hallux valgus interphalangeus (Fig. 6-2). The hallux valgus interphalangeus angle may appear nearly normal if there is significant toe pronation; clinical examination is required to determine this pronation. The degree of MTP and IP arthritis should be assessed.

The position of the sesamoids should be measured on the anteroposterior view of the foot. Displacement of the sesamoids, such as an uncovered lateral sesamoid is concerning as this observation is consistent with a moderate or severe hallux valgus deformity and may not be adequately corrected by the Akin procedure.

The degree of congruity of the MT joint is noted. Radiographs should be examined to determine the DMAA of the metatarsal. The DMAA is defined as the angle formed between a line that subtends the medial and lateral edges of the articular surface of the metatarsal to a line that is perpendicular to the longitudinal axis of the first metatarsal. The DMAA is normally less than 10°. In patients with a DMAA of greater than 10°, the Akin procedure may be indicated to prevent resultant incongruity of the articular surfaces of the first MTP joint during the correction of a valgus deformity.

It is generally not advisable to use the isolated Akin procedure on the hallux deformity associated with an abnormal intermetatarsal 1–2 angle of more than 10°, degenerative changes in the MTP or IP joints, or incongruity of the MTP joint. The decision to incorporate the Akin proximal phalangeal osteotomy with another primary bunion procedure is often best made at the time of surgery.

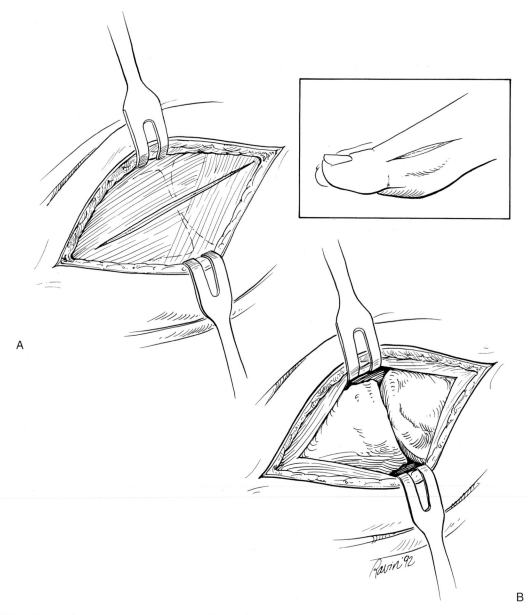

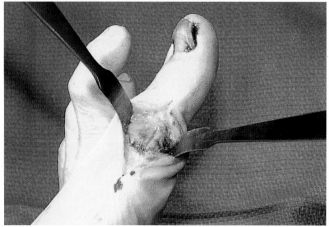

**Figure 6-3. A:** A straight medial skin and capsular incision is centered over the proximal phalanx base. **B:** After the capsular incision is complete, the metatarsal head and phalanx base are uncovered. **C:** An intraoperative view shows the exposed metatarsophalangeal joint.

## SURGERY

The Akin procedure may be performed in an outpatient setting with ankle block anesthesia. Sterile surgical preparation to just below the knee is recommended. The patient is placed in the supine position, and an ankle tourniquet may be used.

### Technique

The operative technique is initiated with a longitudinal medial incision made over the first MTP joint and carried down through the bursa and the capsule onto the metatarsal head (Fig. 6-3). Longitudinal capsular flaps are elevated with a scalpel and Freer elevator. Small retractors can be used to protect the flexor hallucis longus and extensor hallucis longus tendons. Care should be taken to avoid stripping the soft tissue attachment to the phalangeal base fragment as much as possible.

If prominent or symptomatic, the medial eminence of the metatarsal head is resected in line parallel with the medial border of the foot. The same incision is extended distally to expose the basilar portion of the proximal phalanx. A 3-mm, medially based closing wedge osteotomy is performed in the metaphyseal region of the proximal phalanx within 5 to 7 mm of the metatarsal joint line using a sharp sawblade and a microsagittal saw (Fig. 6-4). Approximately 8° of correction can be expected with this size of wedge resection. Care is

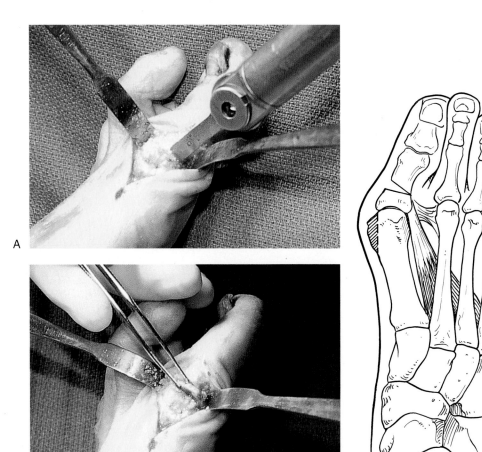

A

C

Ravin '92    B

**Figure 6-4.  A:** A small sagittal saw is used to make the phalanx osteotomy. **B:** Position of the osteotomy. **C:** The medially based bone wedge is removed from the proximal phalanx.

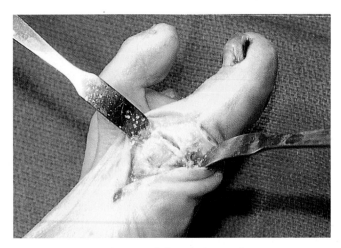

**Figure 6-5.** Closure of the phalangeal osteotomy.

taken to keep the lateral cortex and periosteum intact. The wedge is closed (Fig. 6-5), hinged on the medial cortex and periosteum. The osteotomy position is maintained by two crossed, 0.062-inch Kirschner wires placed from distal to proximal. The Kirschner wires are then bent to 90° and left protruding through the skin (Fig. 6-6). Pin caps are applied. The capsule is repaired and the skin incision is closed and a bunion dressing applied to maintain the corrected position.

An example of a patient with progressive, painful hallux valgus interphalangeus deformity and hammer toe is shown in Figure 6-7. The intermetatarsal 1–2 angle is 9°, hallux valgus angle is 17°, IP angle is 15°, and DMAA is 13°. The patient had a successful

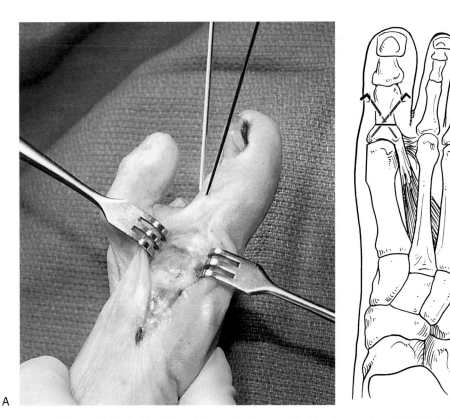

A     B

**Figure 6-6.  A:** Fixation of the osteotomy with Kirschner wires. **B:** Detail view shows the positions of the Kirschner wires. *(continued)*

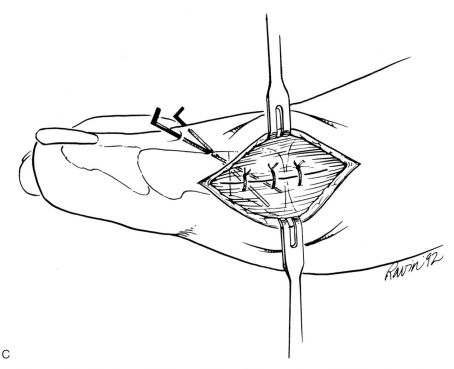

C

**Figure 6-6.** *Continued.* **C:** Lateral view of the positions of the Kirschner wires.

result after Akin osteotomy and hammer toe correction. The technique has been modified in various ways, such as the fixation with one or more sutures, wire suture, staples, or compression screw. The osteotomy has been modified as well, such as an obliquely oriented closing wedge, crescentic closing wedge performed in the midshaft or distal portion of the proximal phalanx, and derotational osteotomy. It has been combined with distal chevron metatarsal osteotomy, proximal closing wedge metatarsal osteotomy, and proximal closing wedge osteotomy with opening wedge cuneiform osteotomy (i.e., triple osteotomy).

Technical pitfalls include fixation failure, poor bone apposition, and plantar angulation (apex plantar) at the osteotomy site (Fig. 6-8). Poor bone apposition can lead to the un-

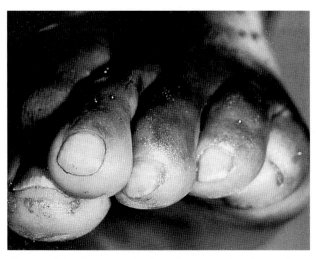
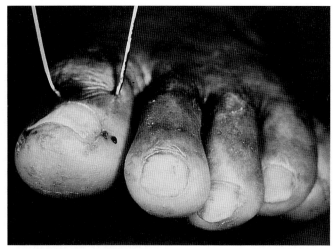

A                                                                                                 B

**Figure 6-7. A:** Preoperative photograph of a patient with hallux valgus interphalangeus deformity and metatarsophalangeal joint synovitis in the subluxated second toe. **B:** Postoperative photograph of the same patient after a successful Akin procedure and hammer toe correction.

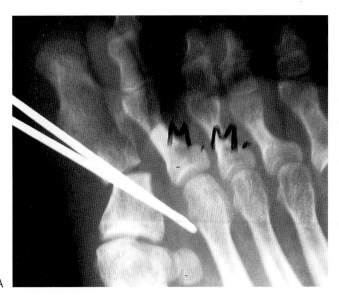

A

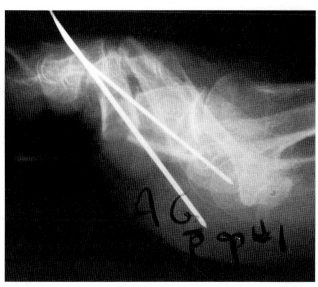

B

**Figure 6-8. A:** Poor bone apposition resulted in this malpositioned osteotomy. **B:** Lateral view shows plantar angulation of the apex.

common complication of nonunion. To avoid this complication, it is recommended that the surgeon obtain intraoperative radiographs to check the position and apposition of bone, use some form of secure fixation, use care in performing the osteotomy accurately, and limit the soft tissue dissection about the osteotomy.

A common technical problem is plantar angulation at the osteotomy site. This occurs because of the action of the extensor hallucis longus with resultant apex plantar angulation across the osteotomy site or, more likely, malposition of the distal fragment at the time of surgery. Intraoperative radiographs are of value to check the position of the osteotomy and fixation. This problem, however, may not lead to any long-term complications.

## POSTOPERATIVE MANAGEMENT

The patient is instructed to remain non–weight bearing, with elevation of the involved extremity for the first 3 to 5 days until the initial inflammatory phase has passed. The patient is then allowed to heel walk as tolerated in a postoperative shoe with a bunion dressing. The bunion dressing maintains the great toe in a neutral position and is changed at regular intervals for 6 weeks, allowing the osteotomy and the soft tissues to heal. The sutures are removed at 2 weeks, and the pins are removed at 3 weeks in the office.

Healing is usually adequate enough to allow gentle active range of motion exercises to begin at 3 weeks. Some gentle passive range of motion exercises may be started at 4 to 6 weeks as tolerated. Radiographs are taken in the office at the first postoperative visit and at 6 weeks postoperatively. The osteotomy site is usually clinically healed at 4 to 6 weeks, but radiographic healing may not occur for 3 or more months.

If patients are carefully selected, approximately 85% should have good or excellent results. Most patients wear a large, soft shoe at 6 weeks postoperatively. Patients should be advised not to expect to fit into a more fashionable shoe for 3 months after surgery. As with other bunion procedures, patients should expect some postoperative swelling for up to 6 months after surgery.

## COMPLICATIONS

Complications include nonunion, shortening of the toe, and recurrence of deformity. Nonunion is rare (reported in less than 5% of cases) but can occur particularly if there is

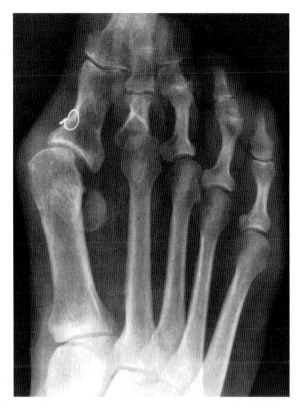

**Figure 6-9.** Typical appearance of recurrent hallux valgus in a patient who underwent an Akin osteotomy for moderate hallux valgus deformity with an incongruous joint. Notice the lateral subluxation of the base of the phalanx. The patient also had a recurrent hammer toe of the second toe. (Courtesy of the Mayo Clinic and Mayo Foundation, Rochester, Minnesota.)

poor bone apposition. Shortening of the hallux occurs in all cases and is unavoidable when performing a closing wedge osteotomy. However, shortening can be limited if a small amount of bone is removed from the proximal phalanx. Because the microsagittal saw blade results in approximately 1 mm of bone loss with each cut, to make a 3-mm wedge, only 1 to 2 mm of bone needs to be removed. The need to remove a larger wedge to achieve correction causes concern because it suggests that the procedure was used to correct a larger magnitude of deformity.

Recurrence of deformity is the most common complication and usually occurs when the indications for the procedure are being stretched (Fig. 6-9). Plattner et al. (9) reported the results of 26 Akin proximal phalangeal osteotomies and recommended that it not be performed in a hallux valgus deformity with an incongruent joint because of recurrent hallux valgus.

Degenerative arthritis may occur from intraarticular extensions of the Akin osteotomy. Avascular necrosis of the base of the phalanx may occur from excessive stripping of soft tissues from the proximal fragment. Rarely is an Akin procedure alone indicated for the correction of a hallux valgus deformity. In most patients with hallux valgus, the proximal phalangeal osteotomy needs to be performed in combination with some other procedure, such as a distal or proximal metatarsal osteotomy, to correct all components of the hallux valgus deformity.

## RECOMMENDED READING

1. Akin OF: The treatment of hallux valgus: a new operative procedure and its results. *Med Sentinel* 33: 678–679, 1925.

2. Colloff B: Proximal phalangeal osteotomy in hallux valgus. *J Bone Joint Surg Am* 48:1442–1443, 1966.

3. Coughlin M, Carlson R: Treatment of hallux valgus deformity with an increased distal metatarsal angle: evaluation of double and triple first ray osteotomies. *Foot Ankle Int* 20:762–770, 1999.

4. Frey C, Jahss M, Kummer FJ: The Akin procedure: an analysis of results. *Foot Ankle* 12:1–6, 1991.

5. Goldberg I, Bahar A, Yosipovitch Z: Late results after correction of hallux valgus deformity by basilar phalangeal osteotomy. *J Bone Joint Surg Am* 69:64–67, 1987.

6. Goldberg I, Bahar A, Yosipovitch Z: Correspondence [letter]. *J Bone Joint Surg Am* 69:950, 1987.

7. Granberry WM, Hickey CH: Hallux valgus correction with metatarsal osteotomy: effect of lateral distal soft tissue procedure. *Foot Ankle Int* 16:132–138, 1995.

8. Mitchell LA, Baxter DE: A Chevron double osteotomy for correction of hallux valgus. *Foot Ankle* 12:7–14, 1991.

9. Plattner PF, Van Manen JW: Results of Akin-type osteotomy for correction of hallux valgus deformity. *Orthopaedics* 13:989–996, 1990.

10. Seelenfruend M: Correction of hallux valgus deformity by basal phalanx osteotomy of the big toe. *J Bone Joint Surg Am* 55:1411–1415, 1973.

11. Silberman FS: Proximal phalangeal osteotomy for the correction of hallux valgus. *Clin Orthop Rel Res* 85:98–100, 1972.

# 7

# Proximal First Metatarsal Osteotomy

## Michael J. Coughlin

## INDICATIONS/CONTRAINDICATIONS

The primary indication for a distal soft tissue realignment (DSTR) with a proximal first metatarsal osteotomy (PMO) is a symptomatic hallux valgus deformity of a moderate or severe nature (i.e., a hallux valgus angle ≥35° and an intermetatarsal [IM] angle ≥13°).

Initially, McBride described a technique involving a lateral metatarsophalangeal (MTP) joint capsular release, an adductor tendon transfer into the lateral metatarsal head, a lateral sesamoid excision, medial eminence resection, and a medial capsulorrhaphy. DuVries and, later, Mann modified this technique significantly, and the term *distal soft tissue realignment* is therefore preferred. Likewise, the limitations of this procedure were defined by further experience. A DSTR procedure alone achieves an average correction of the hallux-valgus angle of 17° and an average correction of the 1–2 IM angle of 5.2° (8). The addition of a proximal metatarsal osteotomy allows a greater diminution of the 1–2 IM angle (average of 8°) and hallux valgus angle (average of 30° for severe deformity) as well. This correction is achieved without a lateral sesamoid excision, which decreases the incidence of a postoperative hallux varus deformity. For a mild and low-moderate deformity (IM 1–2 angle <15°, hallux valgus angle <25°), a DSTR alone may be sufficient to attain a complete correction; for more severe deformities (IM 1–2 angle >16°, hallux valgus angle >35°), a DSTR with a PMO may be used to achieve a correction of the hallux valgus angle. For intermediate deformities, the use of the osteotomy with DSTR depends on the surgeon's preference and the ease with which an alignment is achieved.

Age does not seem to be a contraindication for this procedure, although in a younger patient with an open epiphysis, a proximal metatarsal osteotomy should avoid the proximal first metatarsal epiphysis. In the older patient or the patient with a more severe deformity, decreased MTP joint range of motion may develop postoperatively; however, this does not appear to influence patient satisfaction. Metatarsocuneiform hypermobility is a contraindi-

M. J. Coughlin, M.D.: Department of Orthopaedic Surgery, Oregon Health Sciences University, Portland, Oregon; and Private Practice, Boise, Idaho.

cation to this procedure, and fusion of the metatarsocuneiform joint may be necessary in this situation. This condition is relatively uncommon.

A subluxated or noncongruent MTP joint is a necessary precondition for performing a DSTR with a PMO. Radiographic evaluation can assist the surgeon in determining the congruency of the joint. A varus-valgus stress test can be used to clinically evaluate congruency as well. Manually dorsiflexing and plantarflexing the hallux MTP joint in varus and valgus will help to determine if the toe can be realigned with an intraarticular repair. Diminution of motion may indicate a congruent joint, which is a contraindication to this specific surgical repair.

Close inspection of the MTP joint articulation on the preoperative anteroposterior radiograph is necessary to determine the orientation of the metatarsal and phalangeal articular surfaces and to distinguish a subluxated from a congruent articulation.

Pain over the medial eminence is the major preoperative complaint of patients in over three fourths of cases. Another frequent complaint is a second toe hammer toe deformity or metatarsalgia beneath the second metatarsal head.

Occasionally, a patient has no pain but is concerned with the cosmetic appearance of his or her foot. Surgery is ideally deferred in these patients until pain becomes a major complaint. The examiner should be aware of the patient's occupation, footwear requirements, and athletic activity because certain stressful physical activities may not be compatible with a successful surgical result. An athlete may find minor postoperative restricted range of motion much more annoying than the preoperative discomfort that led her or him to surgery. Degenerative arthritis or hallux rigidus is a relative contraindication to surgery, depending on the magnitude of the arthritic changes. Prior hallux valgus surgery is not necessarily a contraindication and this procedure may be used to salvage a previous surgical failure.

Specific contraindications for this procedure include MTP joint arthritis, significant metatarsus adductus, active infection, and a congruent MTP joint with significant distal metatarsal articular angle (DMAA $>15°$).

## PREOPERATIVE PLANNING

Decision making in bunion surgery starts with an in-depth history and careful physical examination. A patient's symptoms help to define the area of pain.

During the physical examination, an assessment of the neurovascular status is important to help predict healing capacity and the absence of diabetes or peripheral vascular disease. The foot is examined with the patient in a sitting and standing position and inspected for pes planus, intractable plantar keratosis, other areas of callous formation, lesser toe deformities, and the presence or absence of an interdigital neuroma. The skin overlying the medial eminence is assessed for blistering or potential skin breakdown. Range of motion of the hallux is evaluated, and the magnitude of pronation of the great toe is assessed.

Weight-bearing anteroposterior radiographs, lateral radiographs, and sesamoid views are obtained. The 1–2 IM angle is quantified (normal $<9°$). The hallux valgus angle is also measured (normal $<15°$) (Fig. 7-1).

The first MTP joint is inspected for evidence of degenerative arthritis. Because an intraarticular realignment with a distal soft tissue realignment may lead to postoperative stiffness and therefore with hallux rigidus, this procedure is contraindicated. The forefoot is inspected for the presence of significant metatarsus adductus. A significant hallux valgus deformity may occur even if the 1–2 IM angle is measured as normal because of significant metatarsus adductus. In this situation, a first metatarsal osteotomy cannot realign the first ray because there is insufficient room for a lateral displacement of the first metatarsal with the osteotomy.

The congruency of the first MTP joint is assessed. This is the relationship between the corresponding articular surfaces of the first metatarsal head and the base of the proximal phalanx. The DMAA quantitates the angle of slope between the longitudinal axis of the first metatarsal and the distal metatarsal articular surface. The angle is formed by a perpendicular line connecting points defining the medial and lateral edges of the articular surface of the metatarsal head and the longitudinal axis of the first metatarsal (Fig. 7-2). The DMAA relates the inclination of the metatarsal head articular surface to the longitudinal axis of the

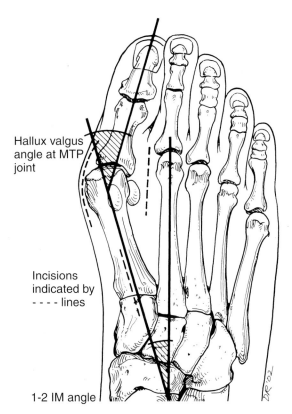

**Figure 7-1.** The hallux valgus angle is the magnitude of the angular deformity at the first metatarsophalangeal joint. The 1–2 intermetatarsal angle is the magnitude of divergence between the first and second metatarsals.

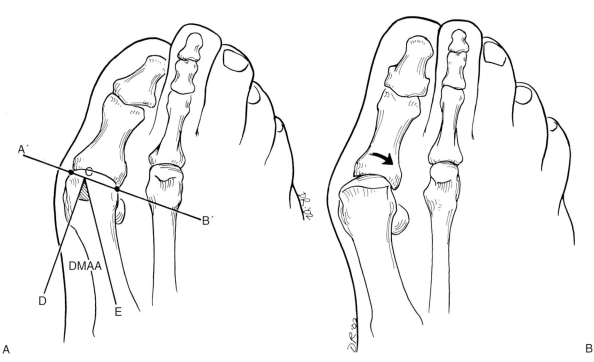

**Figure 7-2. A:** The distal metatarsal articular angle (*DMAA*) defines the slope of the distal metatarsal articular surface. A line is drawn connecting the medial (*A'*) and lateral extent (*B'*) of the metatarsal articular surface. A perpendicular line is then drawn in reference to this line (*C,D*). The angle formed between this line (*C,D*) and the longitudinal axis (*C,E*) of the first metatarsal constitutes the DMAA. **B:** Subluxated first metatarsophalangeal joint.

first metatarsal. Normally, this angle varies from 0° to 8° (10). An examiner must assess the magnitude of the DMAA as a hallux valgus deformity may result entirely from this inclination. When a significant DMAA is present, a surgical attempt to reduce or realign the proximal phalanx on the laterally inclined metatarsal articular surface will create an abnormal articulation that may eventually result in recurrence of deformity, MTP joint stiffness, or degenerative arthritis of the first MTP joint.

The magnitude of the hallux valgus angle must be correlated with whether the first MTP joint is congruent or incongruent (subluxated) and with the magnitude of the DMAA (1). With a congruent joint, the proximal phalangeal articular surface is centered on the articular surface of the first metatarsal head (Fig. 7-3A). With an incongruent joint, the proximal phalanx is subluxated or displaced in relation to the first metatarsal articular surface (5) (Fig. 7-3B). If the first MTP joint articulation is incongruent (or subluxated), the proximal phalanx can be realigned on the metatarsal head articular surface with an intraarticular realignment such as a distal soft tissue realignment.

The size of the medial eminence is determined on the radiograph by drawing a line along the medial border of the first metatarsal shaft. The medial eminence varies considerably in size. The position of the sagittal sulcus (Fig. 7-4) is a less reliable reference for the medial eminence resection because it appears to be positioned more laterally in feet with more severe valgus deformity. With severe deformities, a sagittal sulcus may be located close to the midportion of the metatarsal head and could lead to an excessive resection if used as a landmark for the medial eminence resection.

In a normal foot without deformity, the sesamoids are located beneath the metatarsal head. With increasing deformity, the fibular sesamoid lies exposed or uncovered on an anteroposterior radiograph and is seen along the lateral border of the first metatarsal head. The magnitude of this exposure depends on the severity of the hallux valgus deformity and the amount of pronation of the great toe.

To achieve a successful and stable correction of a hallux valgus deformity, an attempt must be made to correct all elements of the deformity present, including an increased 1–2

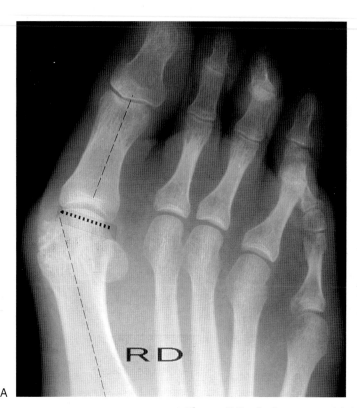
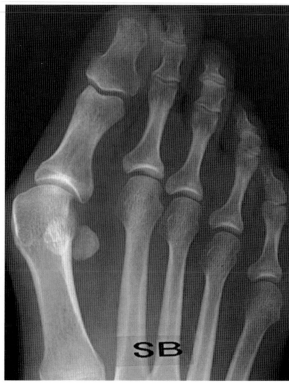

A                                                                                                    B

**Figure 7-3. A:** A congruent joint with a lateral sloping distal metatarsal articular angle. **B:** The radiograph demonstrates a subluxated metatarsophalangeal joint.

**Figure 7-4. A:** Sagittal sulcus as seen at surgery. The sagittal sulcus is an unreliable reference point for the medial eminence resection. **B:** With a small eminence, the sulcus may be the site of the osteotomy. With a more severe deformity, the sulcus is positioned more laterally and, if used as a landmark, may lead to excessive resection.

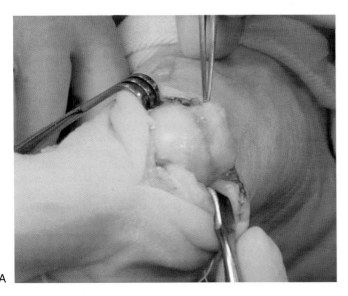

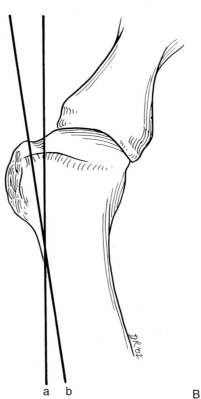

A

a  b                                B

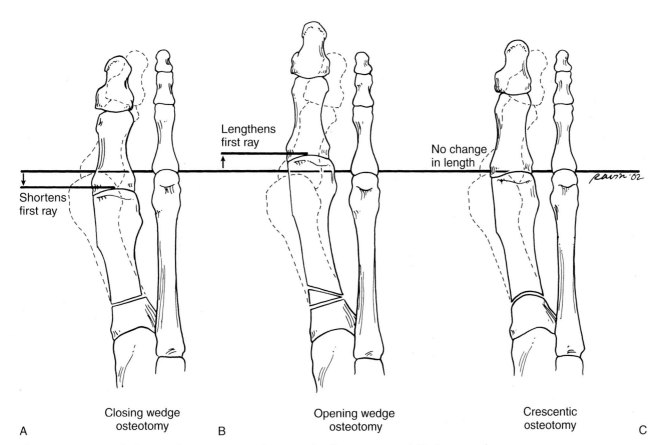

Shortens first ray

Lengthens first ray

No change in length

Closing wedge osteotomy

Opening wedge osteotomy

Crescentic osteotomy

A                                B                                                    C

**Figure 7-5. A:** A closing wedge osteotomy shortens the first metatarsal. **B:** An opening wedge osteotomy tends to lengthen the first metatarsal. **C:** A crescentic osteotomy tends to maintain the first metatarsal length.

luxation, and pronation of the great toe. Incomplete correction of these elements may lead to recurrence of the deformity.

A DSTR with PMO may be performed on an outpatient or inpatient basis, depending on the patient's condition and on the patient's and surgeon's preference. The procedure may be performed under general or regional anesthetic; however, a foot block or popliteal block achieves adequate anesthesia and provides long-lasting pain relief and is my preference.

Techniques of proximal first metatarsal osteotomy include a crescentic osteotomy, opening wedge and closing wedge osteotomy, as well as a proximal chevron osteotomy. A closing or opening wedge osteotomy alters the metatarsal length, and it is typical that the first and second metatarsals are about the same length. A crescentic osteotomy is my preference because it can correct an increased 1–2 IM angle without significantly altering the length of the first metatarsal (Fig. 7-5). Locating the osteotomy at the proximal first metatarsal level provides a broad contact area that is characterized by rapid healing because of its large surface area.

## SURGERY

The patient is placed in a supine position on the surgical table. The foot and lower leg are cleansed in a routine fashion. The foot is exsanguinated with an Esmarch bandage. Padding is placed around the ankle, and the Esmarch bandage is used as a tourniquet. With peripheral anesthesia, the patient is usually comfortable with an ankle tourniquet; however, intravenous sedation occasionally may be used to augment patient relaxation. The surgeon sits on a stool next to the contralateral leg, across the table from the operative foot. This position is used for the intermetatarsal approach. For the medial approach and the metatarsal osteotomy, the surgeon sits on the ipsilateral side looking down on the operative foot.

### Intermetatarsal Technique

A 3-cm, dorsal, longitudinal incision is centered on the first intermetatarsal web space, beginning at the distal extent of the web space and extending proximally (Fig. 7-6). The sub-

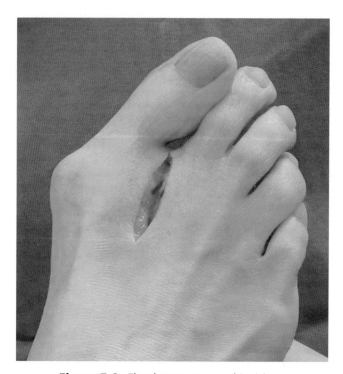

**Figure 7-6.** First intermetatarsal incision.

cutaneous tissue is sharply incised, and the first and second metatarsals are distracted with a Weitlaner retractor, exposing the conjoined adductor tendon. The tendon is dissected free from the lateral border of the sesamoid. The lateral sesamoid is completely freed up *but is not excised*. The sesamoid is freed up on its lateral and plantar border and is released from its dorsal attachments. The metatarsal-sesamoid ligament is detached on the superior aspect of the lateral sesamoid (Fig. 7-7). The distal adductor tendon insertion is left attached to the base of the proximal phalanx with a stump of approximately 2 cm of tendon remaining. The tendon is released at the level of the musculotendinous junction and the adductor hallucis muscle is allowed to retract (Fig. 7-8). A suture is placed in the tendon stump, and this is later repaired to the lateral metatarsal capsule (Fig. 7-9). The transverse intermetatarsal ligament is incised with care taken to avoid injury to the common digital nerve that lies directly beneath the transverse intermetatarsal ligament or the flexor hallucis longus tendon. The lateral MTP joint capsule is then perforated several times with a scalpel blade, and the toe is angulated medially, causing a disruption of the lateral capsule. It is important to avoid an abrupt incision in the lateral capsule, because this may leave a paucity of scar tissue. This tissue is needed to help provide postoperative stability on the lateral aspect of the first MTP joint. The stump of conjoined tendon that is preserved and later sutured into the lateral MTP capsule helps to minimize the possibility of a postoperative hallux varus deformity. Three interrupted 2-0 absorbable sutures are placed to reef the first and second MTP joint capsules and are later tied at the conclusion of the surgery.

## Medial Technique

A longitudinal medial incision is centered over the medial eminence, beginning at the midportion of the proximal phalanx and extending 1 cm above the medial eminence. The dissection is carried directly down to the medial capsule. Care is taken to protect the medial dorsal and medial plantar digital nerves, which are swept in a dorsal and plantar direction and protected with retractors. With a midline incision, deepened directly to the capsule, the dorsomedial sensory nerve is protected and retracted (Fig. 7-10). It lies right on the capsule and may be inadvertently injured if it is not located and protected. An L-shaped distally based

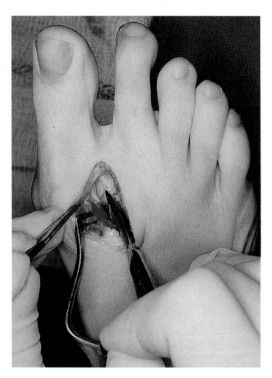

**Figure 7-7.** The sesamoid is completely freed on the superior aspect.

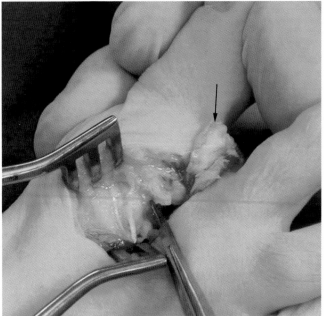

A

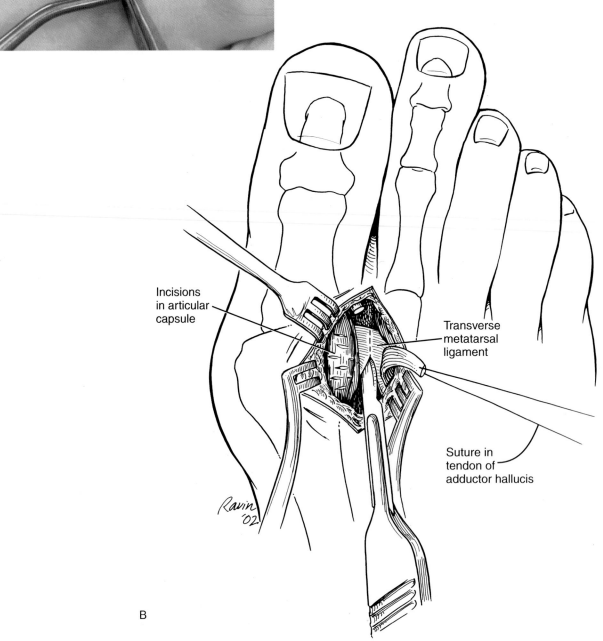

B

**Figure 7-8. A:** A lateral capsular release has been performed, and a 2-cm stump of adductor tendon *(arrow)* is retained for a later repair, creating a cuff of capsule on the lateral aspect of the metatarsophalangeal joint. **B:** Perforation of the lateral capsule, adductor tendon release, and release of the transverse metatarsal ligament.

Incisions in articular capsule

Transverse metatarsal ligament

Suture in tendon of adductor hallucis

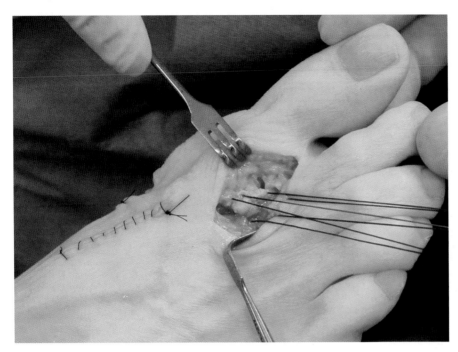

**Figure 7-9.** Three interrupted sutures are placed between the first and second metatarsophalangeal capsule. A fourth suture is placed in the stump of adductor tendon.

capsular flap is developed, releasing the capsule on the dorsal and proximal aspect (Fig. 7-11). The weakest attachments of the capsule are on the proximal and dorsal aspects. The strongest attachments, on the plantar and distal aspects, are preserved. This allowed excellent visualization of the first metatarsal shaft for the osteotomy of the medial eminence.

The capsule is retracted, and the medial eminence is resected with an oscillating saw in a line parallel with the diaphyseal cortex of the first metatarsal (Fig. 7-12). Excessive resection is the most common cause of a postoperative varus deformity. The medial capsular exposure described gives a good distal view of the metatarsal shaft. A retractor can be

*(Text continues on page 83.)*

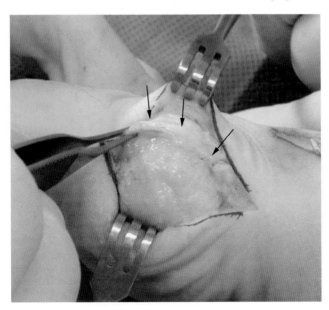

**Figure 7-10.** The dorsal sensory nerve located on the superior aspect of the capsule is identified and protected.

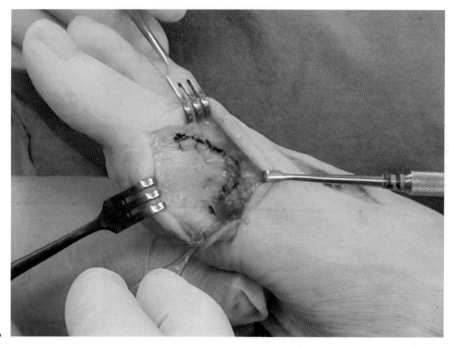

A

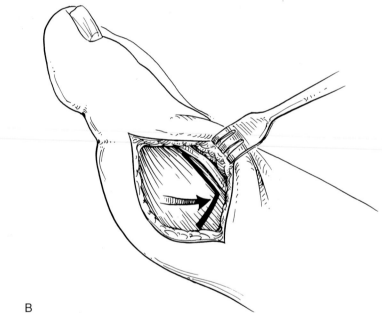

B

**Figure 7-11. A and B:** An L-shaped capsular release is carried out on the dorsal and proximal aspects of the medial capsule. *(continued)*

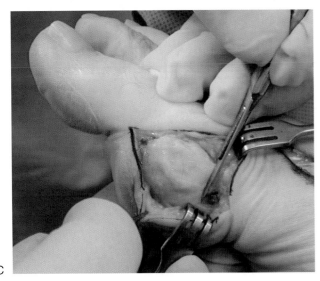

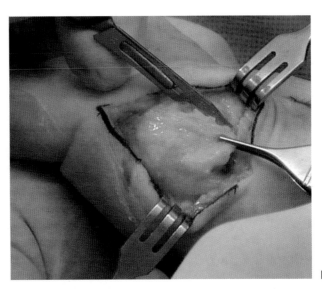

C

D

**Figure 7-11.** *Continued.* **C:** The proximal aspect of the capsule is incised vertically. **D:** The dorsal aspect of the capsule is incised longitudinally.

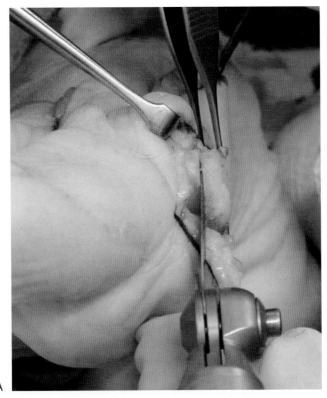

A

**Figure 7-12. A:** The capsular flap is turned downward, and a sagittal saw is used to remove the medial eminence in line with the medial cortex of the first metatarsal. *(continued)*

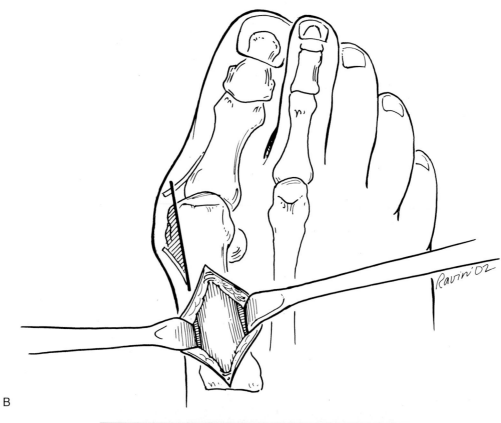

B

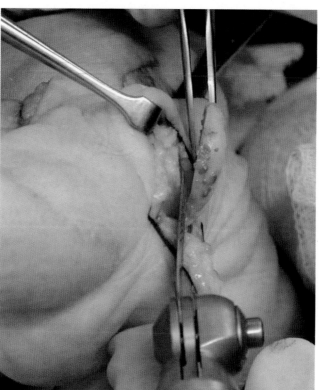

C

**Figure 7-12.** *Continued.* **B:** The proximal shaft is exposed through the proximal incision as a reference point for this osteotomy. **C:** The medial eminence resection osteotomy is in line with the medial aspect of the first metatarsal cortex.

placed in the proximal metatarsal incision, and the proximal first metatarsal shaft can be delineated. By visualizing the first metatarsal shaft when resecting the medial eminence, an osteotomy in line with the medial border of the first metatarsal shaft is performed. If the sagittal sulcus is located lateral to the medial eminence osteotomy, the prominent edge of the sulcus can be beveled with a rongeur. Use of the sagittal sulcus as a landmark for the medial eminence resection is unreliable, and in severe deformities, it may lead to an excessive resection.

### Proximal Metatarsal Technique

Probably the most difficult aspect of the procedure is the first metatarsal osteotomy. A 3-cm, dorsal, longitudinal incision is centered over the dorsal proximal first metatarsal along the medial border of the extensor hallucis longus tendon. The dissection is carried down to the first metatarsal shaft, and the periosteum is stripped medially and laterally. The metatarsocuneiform joint is identified. A mark is placed on the first metatarsal 1 cm distal to the metatarsocuneiform joint, and this is the location of the most proximal extent of the crescentic osteotomy. A Stryker microsaw provides an easily adaptable power source that can be used for the sagittal saw, a curved saw, power drill, and Kirschner wire driver. A curved saw blade (no. 5053-176, Zimmer Co., Warsaw, IN; no. 2296-31-416S7 or 277-31-416S1, Stryker Corp., Kalamazoo, MI) is used for the crescentic osteotomy. The osteotomy is oriented in a dorsal-plantar direction at a 120°-angle to the metatarsal shaft.

There has been considerable debate regarding the orientation of the saw blade. It may be placed concave distal or in a concave proximal direction. The concavity facing distally allows the osteotomy to displace easily; however, it is easier also to overcorrect the osteotomy (Fig. 7-13) with this orientation. Although at one time the concave surface was oriented distally, I now prefer an orientation in a proximal direction. The use of intraoperative radiography enables the surgeon to ensure that he or she is not overcorrecting the osteotomy site

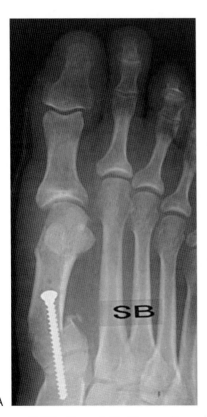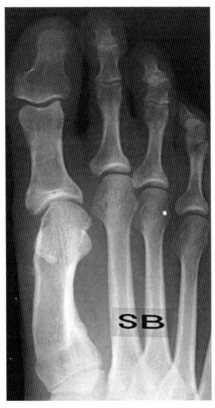

A                                                                                              B

**Figure 7-13. A and B:** The radiographs show overcorrection after a proximal metatarsal osteotomy with the concave saw surface oriented distal (i.e., old technique).

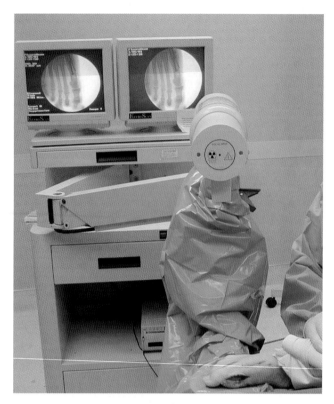

**Figure 7-14.** Intraoperative fluoroscopy helps to ensure that the alignment of the osteotomy site is appropriate.

(Fig. 7-14). With the concavity facing proximally, osteotomy is more difficult to displace but does appear to decrease the chance of overcorrection. Internal fixation with this osteotomy (concavity facing proximally) is placed approximately 8 mm distal to the osteotomy site on the metatarsal shaft, which may necessitate closer approximation of the surgical incisions. One tip to aid the osteotomy displacement is to distract the osteotomy using a small osteotome. With a small rongeur, the lateral proximal edge of the distal metatarsal fragment is removed to avoid impingement as the osteotomy is "dialed medially."

The direction of the saw can be varied in the distal-proximal (sagittal) and medial-lateral (coronal) planes. Medial orientation of the saw blade may cause pronation of the toe and elevation of the distal metatarsal fragment (Fig. 7-15A). Lateral orientation of the saw blade may cause supination of the toe and depression of the metatarsal head (Fig. 7-15B). It is desirable to maintain the saw in a neutral medial-lateral plane (Fig. 7-15C).

Distal-proximal inclination of the saw blade may occur as well. A distal inclination creates an osteotomy at close to a 90°-angle with the metatarsal shaft and decreases the surface contact area. This may cause an increased incidence of dorsiflexion malunion at the osteotomy site. A proximal inclination creates a more oblique osteotomy (approximating 135°) and is more difficult to cut, requiring a longer osteotomy. It may also be more difficult to displace (Fig. 7-16).

Ideally, an osteotomy at an angle of approximately 110° to 120° is desired in relation to the metatarsal shaft. The osteotomy is displaced by dialing or rotating the distal fragment. Most of the correction of the hallux valgus deformity occurs here. If the first metatarsal metaphysis is unusually thick, an osteotome may be needed to complete the plantar cut or continue the cut medially or laterally. Any prominent bone is removed with a rongeur. The proximal fragment is displaced medially with a small elevator and the distal fragment is then rotated in a lateral direction 2 to 3 mm to reduce the 1–2 IM angle (Fig. 7-17). Care must be taken not to overcorrect the osteotomy site and create a negative 1–2 IM angle.

The osteotomy is initially fixed with a 0.062-inch Kirschner wire. A lag compression screw is then used to fix the osteotomy. The screw is typically not countersunk, so that it
*(Text continues on page 89.)*

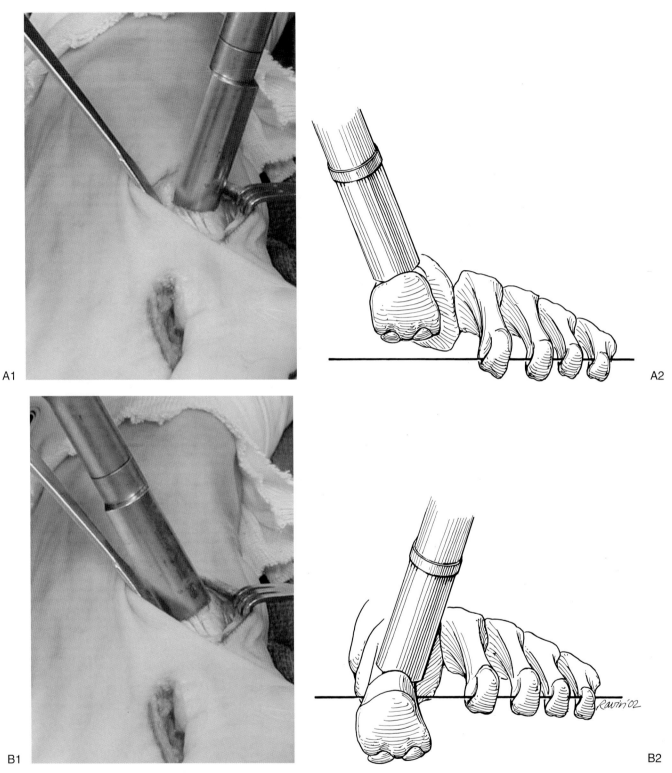

A1

A2

B1

B2

**Figure 7-15. A1:** Medial orientation of the saw blade may cause pronation of the toe and elevation of the distal metatarsal fragment. **A2:** Schematic diagram of the malpositioned saw shows elevation of the first metatarsal. **B1:** Lateral orientation of the saw blade may cause supination of the toe and depression of the metatarsal head. **B2:** Schematic diagram demonstrates depression of the first metatarsal head. (*continued*)

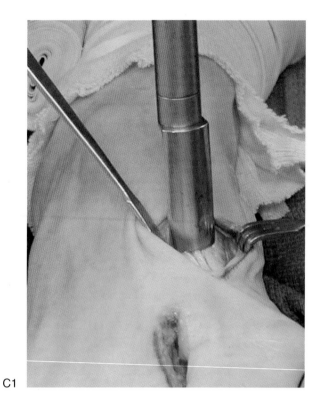

C1

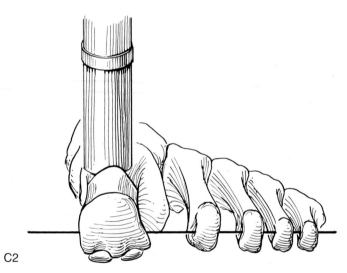

C2

**Figure 7-15.** *Continued.* **C1:** Neutral orientation of the saw blade in a neutral plane tends to neither elevate it nor depress it. **C2:** Schematic diagram shows the first metatarsal head in a neutral position.

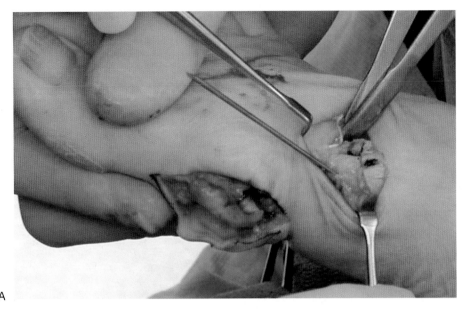

A

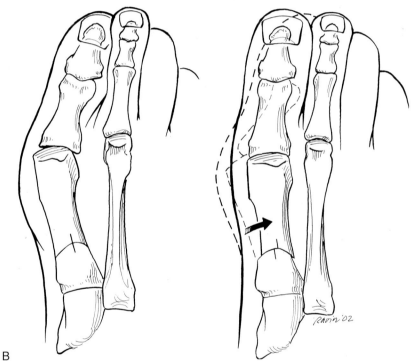

B

**Figure 7-17. A:** Marks on the proximal and distal first metatarsal fragment demonstrate the 2- to 3-mm displacement of the distal fragment in a lateral direction. A Kirschner wire has been used to stabilize the osteotomy site. **B:** The diagram demonstrates rotation of the osteotomy site.

may be easily removed. The Kirschner wire and screw fixation give rotational stability and help to reduce the tendency for dorsiflexion at the osteotomy site. A 3.5-mm drill hole is placed in the distal fragment, and a 2.5-mm drill hole is placed in the proximal fragment. The fixation hole is tapped, and a compression screw fixes and compresses the osteotomy site (Fig. 7-18). Buried internal fixation minimizes the occurrence of pin tract infections. Typically, internal fixation pins are removed 6 weeks after surgery.

After stabilization of the osteotomy, the transverse metatarsal arch is compressed, and the intermetatarsal sutures are tied (Fig. 7-9), after which the adductor hallux tendon is su-

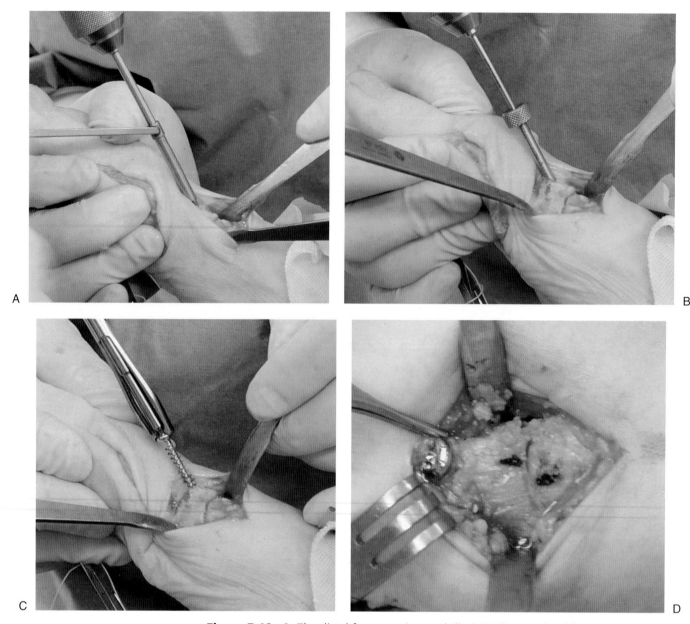

**Figure 7-18. A:** The distal fragment is overdrilled. **B:** The proximal fragment is under-drilled and tapped. **C:** The osteotomy site is stabilized with a fully threaded compression screw. **D:** The screw and pin stabilize the displaced osteotomy site.

tured to the lateral metatarsal capsule (Fig. 7-19A). A further reinforcing suture may be added, reefing the lateral capsule (Fig. 7-19B).

Intraoperative fluoroscopy or radiographs help in evaluating the correction of the 1–2 IM angle, the position of the internal fixation, and the correction of the hallux valgus angle. On visual inspection during surgery, the first ray may appear to be well aligned, but the MTP articulation may be undercorrected or overcorrected. Intraoperative radiographic evaluation of the alignment is helpful to decrease the incidence of recurrence and overcorrection.

With the toe held in a (de-rotated) corrected position, the medial capsule is repaired with interrupted 2-0 Vicryl suture. A fixation hole may be placed in the dorsal proximal metaphysis to give an anchor hole for the capsular repair (Fig. 7-20A). The L-shaped medial

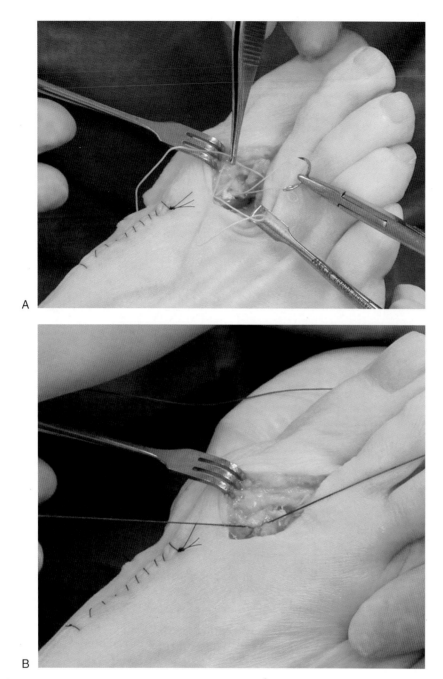

**Figure 7-19. A:** The adductor tendon is sutured into the lateral metatarsal capsule.
**B:** Further reinforcement of the lateral capsule may be achieved with an absorbable
2-0 suture.

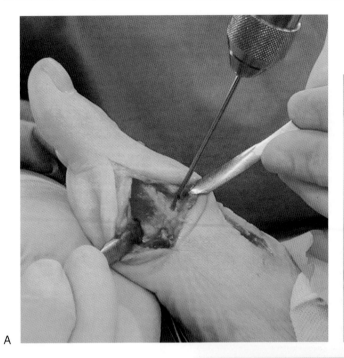
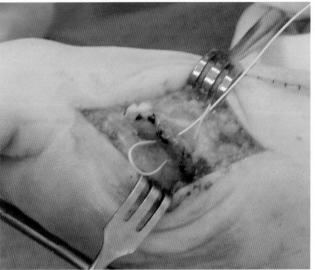
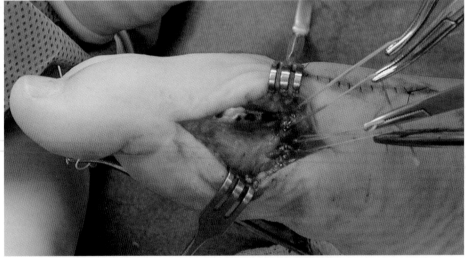

**Figure 7-20. A:** A fixation drill hole is placed in the proximal medial metaphysis. **B:** The medial capsule is reefed with several interrupted sutures. **C:** Completion of the capsular reefing allows realignment of the hallux.

capsular cuff is a very strong anchor that can de-rotate as well as correct valgus malalignment of the great toe (Fig. 7-20B). The medial capsular repair is critical to the MTP joint realignment. A subtotal repair risks recurrence while an overcorrection may lead to a hallux varus deformity. At the completion of the procedure, the great toe rests in a corrected position without any dressing support (Fig. 7-20C).

## POSTOPERATIVE MANAGEMENT

After completion of the surgical procedure, the foot is enclosed in fluffed gauze and wrapped in a 2-inch Kling compression dressing (Figs. 7-21 and 7-22). The patient is instructed to elevate the foot on two pillows and use ice as tolerated. Crutches or a walker is used, depending on a patient's preference. The patient bears weight initially on the heel and

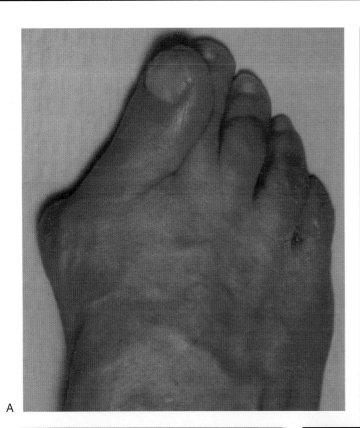

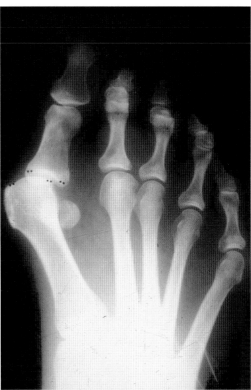

A

B

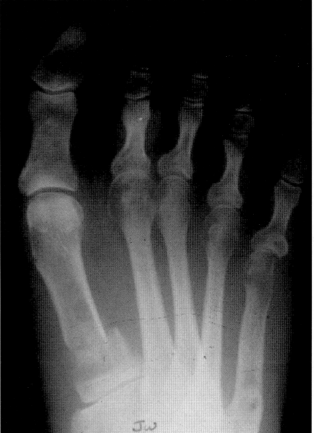

C

D

**Figure 7-21.  A:** Preoperative clinical appearance. **B:** Preoperative radiograph. **C:** Post-operative clinical appearance. **D:** Postoperative radiograph.

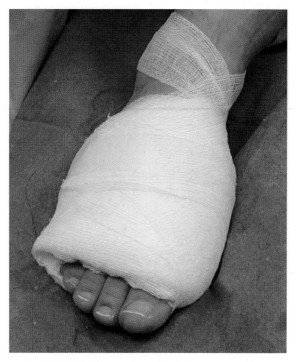

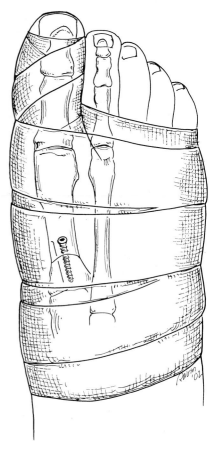

A                                                                                                    B

**Figure 7-22. A and B:** A bulky gauze and tape compression dressing is applied post-operatively.

later on the outside of the foot. Six weeks after surgery, a flat-footed gait is permitted.

One to two days after surgery, the dressing is changed. A gauze-and-tape toe spica dressing is applied and changed on a weekly basis for 7 more weeks. The patient is allowed to ambulate in a postoperative shoe. At about 6 weeks, a roomy sandal is permitted. At 3 weeks after surgery, the patient is instructed to start dorsiflexion-plantarflexion stretching exercises of the toe within the confines of the tape dressing. After the discontinuance of dressings at 8 weeks, a more aggressive range of motion and stretching is initiated.

A frank preoperative discussion with the patient is important to cover the patient's expectations and the surgeon's goals. Reported patient satisfaction with this procedure ranges from 78% to 93% (1,8,9). The average hallux valgus correction has been consistently reported to be 23° to 24°. The degree of improvement is directly proportional to the severity of the preoperative deformity, but for more severe deformities, the average correction is 30°. The average correction of the 1–2 IM angle varies from 8° to 11°.

Two thirds of patients are able to wear the shoes that they desire (9); however, one third of patients may still have footwear restrictions. Pain relief is uniformly good and relief of associated metatarsalgia is common.

## COMPLICATIONS

Complications unique to the DSTR and PMO can occur. Some of the major complications include recurrence of deformity, hallux varus or overcorrection, malalignment of the osteotomy, and delayed union. Each is described, and prevention is considered along with suggested management of the complication.

*Recurrent hallux valgus deformity* may occur for a variety of reasons. A distal soft tissue reconstruction should be avoided in the presence of a congruent MTP joint because there is a high possibility of recurrence (2,5). Recurrence may result from an insufficient lateral release, lack of reduction of the sesamoids, inadequate osteotomy correction, insufficient correction of the soft tissue, inadequate medial capsular plication, or inadequate correction of pronation. Complete correction at the time of surgery is the best insurance against recurrence of deformity. A revision operation may be necessary if a significant recurrence occurs.

Overcorrection, or *hallux varus*, may occur for a number of reasons (Fig. 7-23): overplication of the medial capsule, excessive medial eminence resection, lack of sufficient lateral capsular tissue reformation to stabilize the lateral joint, and overcorrection of the osteotomy. Intraoperative radiography helps to ensure proper alignment of the first metatarsal osteotomy and the MTP joint realignment. Depending on the cause, correction of a hallux varus deformity may be achieved with a soft tissue realignment, revision of the osteotomy, tendon transfer (2), or MTP joint arthrodesis.

*Osteotomy delayed union* is infrequently encountered with a first metatarsal osteotomy. The major symptoms are continued swelling and vague aching at the osteotomy site. Adequate internal fixation is probably the most important factor to avoid dorsiflexion malunion or delayed union and the lateral metatarsalgia associated with malunion. If a delayed union occurs, the application of a below-knee walking cast usually enables an expeditious healing of the osteotomy site. Excessive soft tissue stripping should also be avoided at the osteotomy site (Fig. 7-24).

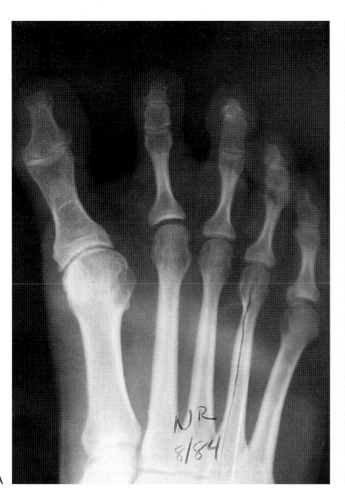

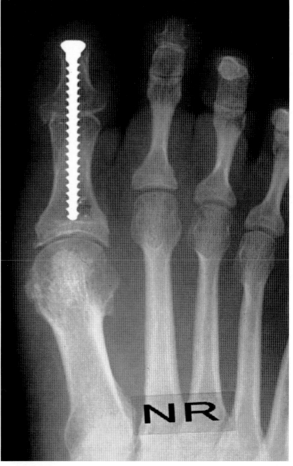

A                                                                                          B

**Figure 7-23. A:** Postoperative hallux varus deformity. **B:** Postoperative correction after extensor hallucis longus tendon transfer with interphalangeal arthrodesis. *(continued)*

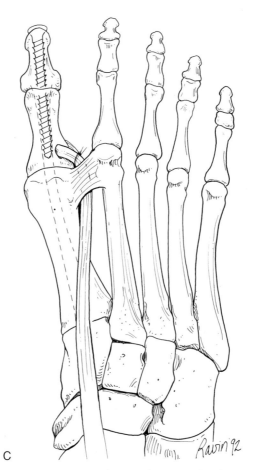

**Figure 7-23.** *Continued.* **C:** Technique of soft tissue correction with interphalangeal joint fusion (6).

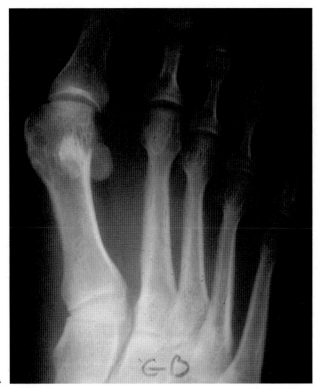

**Figure 7-24. A:** Preoperative radiograph demonstrates hallux valgus deformity. *(continued)*

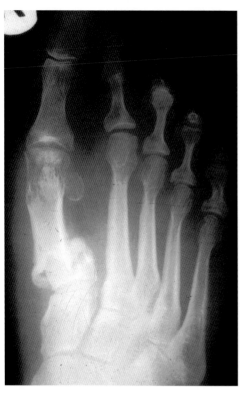
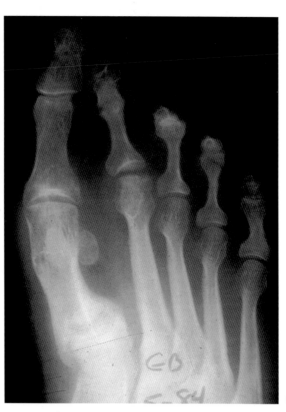

B

C

**Figure 7-24.** *Continued.* **B:** Postoperative radiograph demonstrates delayed union of proximal metatarsal osteotomy. **C:** Postoperative radiograph shows successful healing of the osteotomy site.

*Malunion of the osteotomy site* can be a difficult problem to treat. Overcorrection, if severe, may lead to a hallux varus deformity. The surgical salvage requires a complex and extensive revision procedure with a bone cut through the previous osteotomy site, realignment, and medial capsule release. Lateral capsular reefing may be necessary. The best treatment of this difficult problem is prevention. Intraoperative radiography may help to diminish the incidence of overcorrection of the osteotomy site. Dorsiflexion malunion also may occur. Rigid internal fixation with a lag screw and Kirschner wire prevents rotation, gives increased stability, and decreases the incidence of a dorsiflexion malunion.

Proximal metatarsal osteotomy combined with a distal soft tissue reconstruction is a technically demanding surgical procedure. In the treatment of moderate and severe hallux valgus deformities characterized by subluxation of the MTP joint, meticulous attention to the operative technique coupled with careful preoperative planning can minimize postoperative complications.

## RECOMMENDED READING

1. Coughlin M: Hallux valgus: an instructional course lecture. *J Bone Joint Surg Am* 78:931–966, 1996.
2. Coughlin M: Hallux valgus in men: effect of the distal metatarsal articular angle on hallux valgus correction. *Foot Ankle Int* 18:463–470, 1997.
3. Coughlin M: Juvenile bunions. In: Mann R, Coughlin M, eds. *Surgery of the foot and ankle*, 6th ed. St. Louis: Mosby–Year Book, 1992:297–340.
4. Coughlin M: Juvenile hallux valgus: etiology and treatment. *Foot Ankle Int* 16:682–697, 1995.
5. Coughlin M, Carlson R: Treatment of hallux valgus with an increased distal metatarsal articular angle: evaluation of double and triple first ray osteotomies. *Foot Ankle Int* 20:762–770, 1999.
6. Johnson K, Spiegl P: Extensor hallucis longus transfer for hallux varus deformity. *J Bone Joint Surg Am* 66:681–686, 1984.
7. Mann R: Decision making in bunion surgery. *Instr Course Lect* 40:3–13, 1992.

8. Mann R, Coughlin M: Adult hallux valgus. In: Mann R, Coughlin M, eds. *Surgery of the foot and ankle*, 7th ed. St. Louis: Mosby–Year Book, 2000:150–269.
9. Mann R, Rudicel S, Graves S: Repair of hallux valgus with a distal soft tissue procedure and proximal metatarsal osteotomy. *J Bone Joint Surg Am* 74:124–129, 1992.
10. Richardson E, Graves S, McClure J, et al.: First metatarsal head shaft angle: a method of determination. *Foot Ankle* 14:181–185, 1993.
11. Thordarson D, Leventen E: Hallux valgus correction with proximal metatarsal osteotomy: two year follow-up. *Foot Ankle* 13:321–326, 1992.

# 8

# Cuneiform-Metatarsal Arthrodesis for Hallux Valgus

Lew C. Schon and Mark S. Myerson

## INDICATIONS/CONTRAINDICATIONS

Fusion of the first metatarsal-cuneiform joint in conjunction with realignment of the great toe for correction of a hallux valgus deformity was promoted by Lapidus during the 1930s to the 1960s. In the past four decades since Lapidus last reported his work, the indications for performing this procedure and the operative technique have significantly changed. The goals of this operation have nevertheless remained the same: to correct and stabilize the first metatarsal at the apex of the deformity.

The primary indication for this procedure remains metatarsus primus varus that is associated with a hypermobile first ray. The hypermobility may occur in the horizontal (Fig. 8-1) or sagittal (Fig. 8-2) plane or in both. Other indications for this operation are hallux valgus and severe metatarsus primus varus associated with generalized ligamentous laxity or metatarsocuneiform (MTC) arthritis. The adolescent bunion with moderate to severe deformity is at a high risk for recurrence and has been successfully treated with the first MTC fusion when the epiphysis has closed (Fig. 8-3). Patients who have failed previous bunionectomy are often good candidates for the procedure. Severe deformities that occur in osteopenic feet may fare better with fixation at the MTC level than the proximal aspect of the first metatarsal. Although this is a good choice of operation for correction of severe hallux valgus, it should be used only if the metatarsophalangeal (MTP) joint is mobile.

The procedure is generally used in the younger age group, and less frequently used in the elderly population. The older patients often fare better with other procedures with less potential morbidity, with which they may be ambulatory immediately postoperatively. Noncompliant patients should not undergo the operation given the potential for nonunion and

L. C. Schon, M.D. and M. S. Myerson, M.D.: Department of Orthopaedics, Union Memorial Hospital, Baltimore, Maryland.

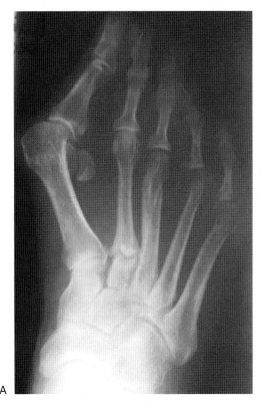
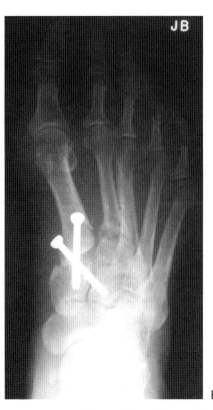

A                                                    B

**Figure 8-1. A:** Horizontal instability of the first metatarsocuneiform joint with a wide intermetatarsal angle is demonstrated on this anteroposterior radiograph. Notice the second and third metatarsal stress fractures. There is also narrowing of the second metatarsophalangeal joint. **B:** Notice the improvement of the intermetarsal angle and the correction of the hallux valgus after performing the Lapidus procedure.

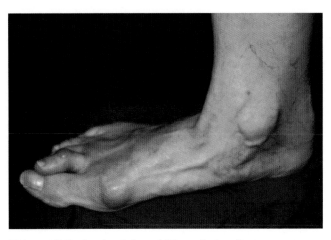

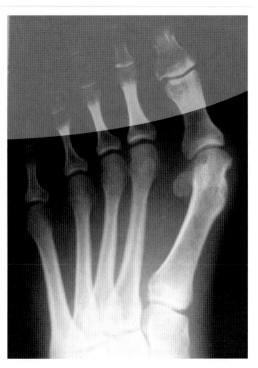

**Figure 8-2.** Sagittal instability of the first metatarso-cuneiform joint is seen in this patient with pes planus and hallux valgus.

**Figure 8-3.** Recurrent valgus after a bunionectomy that was done when the patient was an adolescent. The patient subsequently underwent a first metatarsocuneiform fusion and hallus valgus correction.

malunion. The procedure should not be performed in dancers or athletes, who typically require maximum joint flexibility during their desired activities.

Other relative contraindications include patients who have symptomatic arthritis of the first MTP joint as realignment may exacerbate the pain. In these cases, fusion of the first MTC, which may ultimately be necessary, may result in a transfer of stress to the adjacent joints causing the first MTP to become more symptomatic. Patients that have short first metatarsals may suffer from additional inherent shortening from the Lapidus procedure that may precipitate symptoms from second MTP overload. Preexisting sesamoiditis may be a relative contraindication to this surgery because the absence of mobility and stress dissipation from the first MTC joint will result in increased pain underneath the first metatarsal head.

The MTC arthrodesis is generally performed when the intermetatarsal (IM) angle is 14° or more (Fig. 8-4). If metatarsus adductus is present, however, the IM 1–2 angle may measure less than 14°, even though the position of the first metatarsal with respect to the longitudinal axis of the foot is in marked varus (Fig. 8-5). Rarely, on the anteroposterior radiograph, medial translation of the MTC may be appreciated (Fig. 8-6). On the weight-bearing lateral radiographs, several findings are indicative of first MTC instability, including loss of alignment between the first metatarsal and the medial cuneiform resulting in dorsal translation of the first metatarsal (Fig. 8-7) and a break in the axis of the medial column that occurs at the first metatarsal–medial cuneiform joint resulting in a plantar gap or widening between the joint surfaces (Fig. 8-8). Hypermobility is suggested radiographically as increased cortical hypertrophy along the medial border of the second metatarsal shaft (Fig. 8-9).

Further radiographic indication for a Lapidus procedure would be arthritis of the first MTC when it occurs in the presence of symptomatic hallux valgus. The optimal procedure would

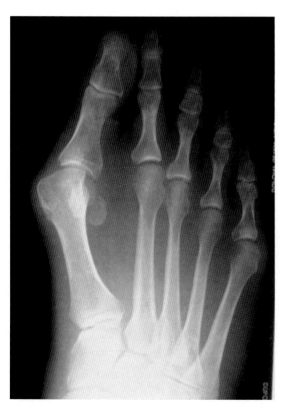

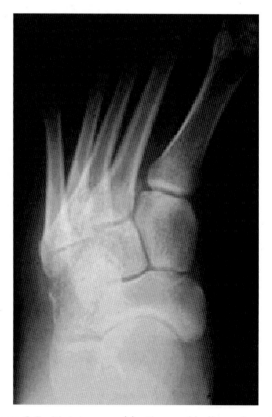

**Figure 8-4.** Anteroposterior radiograph demonstrates a wide intermetatarsal angle.

**Figure 8-5.** Metatarsus adduction and hallux valgus. Notice the medial deviation of the metatarsals relative to the longitudinal axis of the foot. Correction required Lapidus and proximal metatarsal osteotomies.

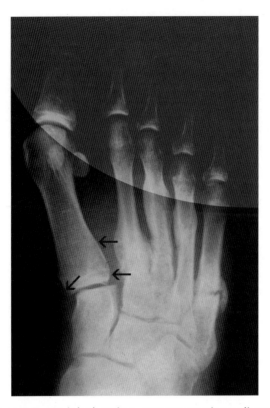

**Figure 8-6.** Weight-bearing, anteroposterior radiograph demonstrates medial translation *(arrows)* of the metatarsal relative to the cuneiform. Notice the stress fractures of the second through fifth metatarsals. These fractures occurred from medial to lateral sides after development of the instability.

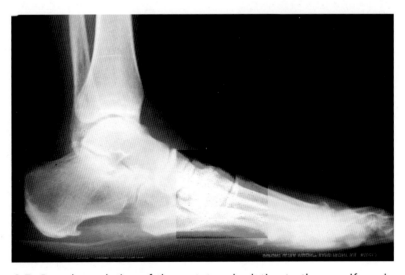

**Figure 8-7.** Dorsal translation of the metatarsal relative to the cuneiform is seen in this lateral, weight-bearing radiograph. The midfoot is highlighted to enhance the image.

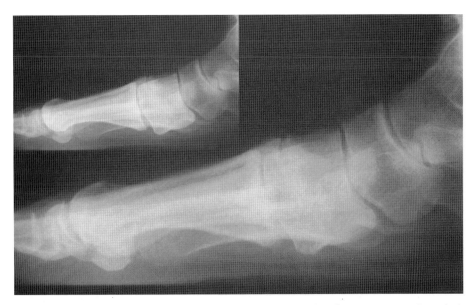

**Figure 8-8.** Widening of the plantar gap between the first metatarsal and the cuneiform. **Inset:** The first metatarsal and medial cuneiform are highlighted to demonstrate instability.

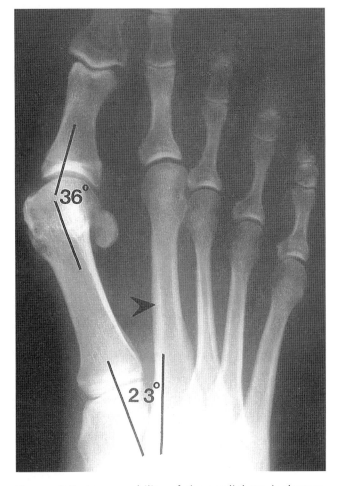

**Figure 8-9.** Hypermobility of the medial ray is demonstrated radiographically with hypertrophy of the medial border of the second metatarsal shaft. Appreciate the width and thickness of this metatarsal relative to the third, fourth, and fifth metatarsals.

address both these problems simultaneously. The radiographs should be reviewed to help determine the presence of a short first ray and to provide some insight into the bone density.

## PREOPERATIVE PLANNING

A general assessment of a patient's alertness and mental status will help determine his or her compliance for the surgical reconstruction. A patient who is less likely to be compliant should undergo a more patient-proof technique, or the technique used must be adjusted (i.e., add additional hardware) to accommodate the situation. Ligamentous laxity observed throughout the musculoskeletal system lends support to choosing a MTC fusion over a proximal first metatarsal osteotomy. Overall alignment of the lower extremity should be observed statically and dynamically to identify etiologic factors that may influence the outcome. Patients with acquired flatfoot deformity may need to have a reconstruction of their dysfunctional posterior tibial tendon with operations such as calcaneal osteotomy and flexor digitorum longus tendon (FDL) transfer. Those with malalignment due to malunion or arthritis at any location in their lower limb may need these elements addressed before or after their Lapidus procedure. Check the height of the medial arch while weight bearing. If there is a pes planus deformity from medial cuneiform–navicular or medial cuneiform–first metatarsal instability, the arch is flattened, but there is less valgus of the hindfoot than what would be observed with other causes of flatfoot, such as posterior tibialis dysfunction or talonavicular instability. Palpation of the pulses is critical to determine whether there is adequate vascularity and to assess the position of the dorsalis pedis relative to the MTC joint. It is often possible to palpate the medial dorsal cutaneous nerve, which is vulnerable to iatrogenic injury.

In addition to observing parameters such as the size and shape of the foot, the range of motion of the entire foot and ankle is assessed. Crepitus and restricted mobility in adjacent joints should be determined, because these joints may become more symptomatic after MTC fusion. The second and third MTC joints should be evaluated, because it is occasionally necessary to extend the fusion to incorporate these joints. Hypermobility of the first ray is evaluated by grasping the first metatarsal with the examiner's hand while stabilizing the rest of the foot with the other hand. While the midfoot is held stable, the thumb and forefinger of the opposite hand manipulate the first metatarsal in a dorsal-plantar plane. (Fig. 8-10A–E) The joint then is placed through a rotational arc (supination-pronation). Particular attention is paid to the increased arc of motion in the dorsal direction, which is associated with dorsal elevation or prominence of the first metatarsal and weight transfer to the second metatarsal. By abducting and adducting the metatarsal, medial-lateral stability is checked. When the metatarsal is held reduced to proper alignment, the first MTP should also be positioned. With both joints in more normal alignment, the range of motion of the MTP joint in the sagittal plane should be noted and compared with the motion of these joints in their deformed positions (Fig. 8-11).

Incongruity of the MTP and/or tightness of the lateral capsule may contribute to restricted motion. This incongruity, sometimes caused by a distal metatarsal articular surface angle of more than 15°, will cause a decrease in the range of motion postoperatively. If incongruity is present, correction may require a medial closing wedge distal metatarsal osteotomy or a proximal phalangeal medial closing wedge osteotomy. One additional sign of first MTC instability is a callosity under the second metatarsal head (Fig. 8-12).

Because this operation is often performed for recurrent hallux valgus following previous surgery, careful thought should be given to assessing the reasons for previous surgical failure. Was the correct procedure performed for the right indications? Did the bone, soft tissues, or joints fail and result in the deformity? Was the fixation adequate? Did the initial correction address the pathology? Were there adjacent joint malalignments that were unrecognized? Was the patient compliant? Was the immobilization and weight bearing postoperatively appropriate? Were there systemic factors such as neuropathy, metabolic disease, arthritis, or congenital abnormalities that led to recurrence? If factors are identified that contributed to failed surgery, attempts should be made to avoid or address these factors at the time of the revision operation.

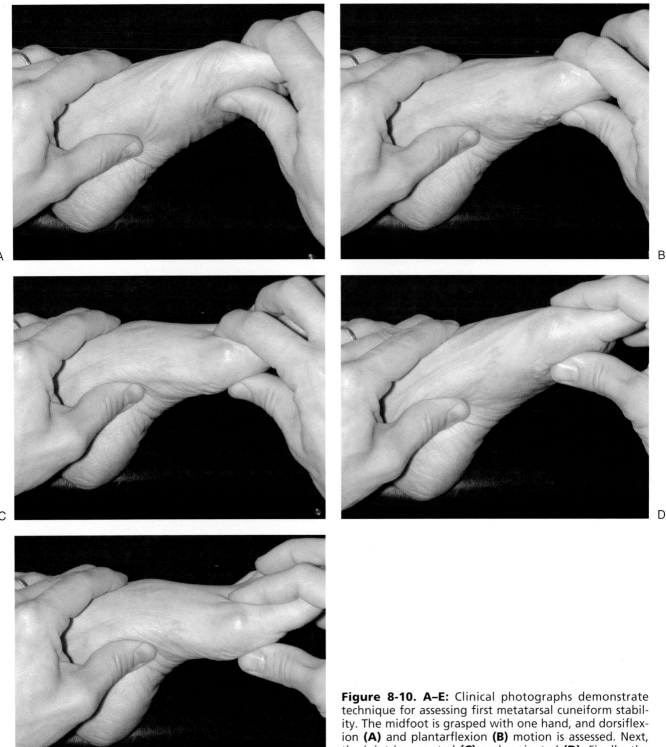

**Figure 8-10. A–E:** Clinical photographs demonstrate technique for assessing first metatarsal cuneiform stability. The midfoot is grasped with one hand, and dorsiflexion **(A)** and plantarflexion **(B)** motion is assessed. Next, the joint is pronated **(C)** and supinated **(D)**. Finally, the metatarsal is abducted **(E)** and adducted.

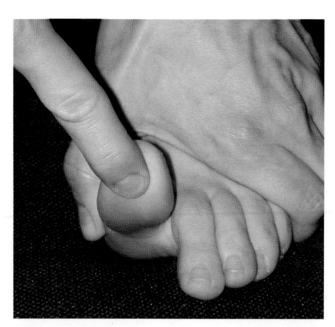

**Figure 8-11.** With the metatarsocuneiform and the metatarsophalangeal (MTP) joints held in proper alignment, the MTP joint is put through a range of motion to determine the anticipated postoperative stiffness and assess the congruency of the MTP joint.

Weight-bearing radiographs should be obtained. Measurements of the 1–2 IM angle, first MTC angle, and hallux valgus angle are made. The presence of metatarsus adductus, the lengths of the first and second metatarsals, and the congruity of the hallux MTP joint are noted. A laterally facing metatarsal joint surface with increased distal metatarsal articular angle should be determined preoperatively and addressed as described previously.

Preoperatively, it is important to educate the patient. The nature of this operation as well as the various alternative treatments should be explained. This operation involves potential problems that are unique to the arthrodesis. Patients need to be aware of the potential for complications including prolonged recovery time, nonunion, and malunion. After arthrode-

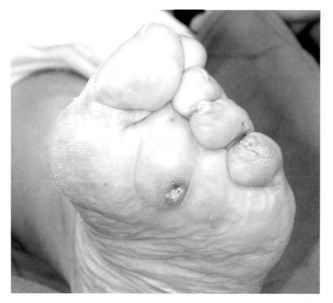

**Figure 8-12.** Callus under the second metatarsal head is associated with metatarsocuneiform instability.

sis, patients experience more discomfort and swelling than with other procedures for severe hallux valgus. I tell patients that, by 3 months postoperatively, the bone is 75% healed, and by 6 months, it is 90% healed. Swelling is the last symptom to improve, and various aches and pains may take more than a year for resolution. Joint stiffness and pain beneath the sesamoids, problems with wound healing, infection, incisional neuromas, and the need for hardware removal should be discussed and are otherwise similar to other bunion operations that require internal fixation.

## SURGERY

The patient is positioned supine on the operating table. Bilateral procedures are not performed simultaneously. Surgery is performed with intravenous sedation under ankle block anesthesia using 20 mL of 0.5% bupivacaine without epinephrine. A popliteal block may also be used. We do not use a tourniquet, and hemostasis is controlled and bleeding minimized with the use of small hemostat clamps.

### Technique

A mid-medial longitudinal incision is made over the hallux MTP joint (Fig. 8-13). An L-shaped capsular incision is made, with the apex dorsal and proximal (Fig. 8-14A). The capsule is dissected subperiosteally off of the metatarsal neck, exposing the entire medial eminence (Fig. 8-14B). The advantage of this flap is the broad exposure of the medial eminence, subsequent ease of capsular closure under the appropriate amount of tension, and its ability to reduce pronation of the hallux. If there is little soft tissue along the dorsomedial aspect of the metatarsal neck to reattach the capsule, then a small hole is made with a 0.062-inch Kirschner wire to attach the capsule with sutures through bone.

A soft tissue release, including an adductor tenotomy with partial lateral capsulotomy is performed through a separate dorsal incision over the distal 1–2 IM space (Fig. 8-15). In some patients with marked hypermobility of the first ray, the adductor release may not be necessary. By squeezing the forefoot (medial-lateral compression), the change in position of the hallux may indicate whether the adductor tenotomy is needed. If the hallux assumes a corrected position without pushing it into varus, a soft tissue release is probably unnecessary. The adductor tendon is dissected off the lateral border of the sesamoids and the flexor brevis tendon. A longitudinal capsulotomy is made dorsal to the fibular sesamoid,

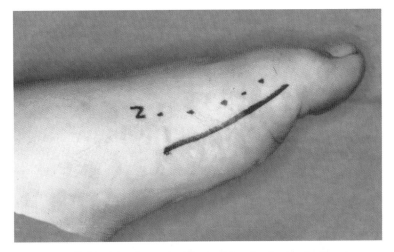

**Figure 8-13.** A medial incision is made. The incision is plantar to the dorsomedial hallucal nerve (drawn on the foot and labeled with *n*) and dorsal to the plantar medial cutaneous nerve, which courses over the junction of the medial sesamoid and the first metatarsal head.

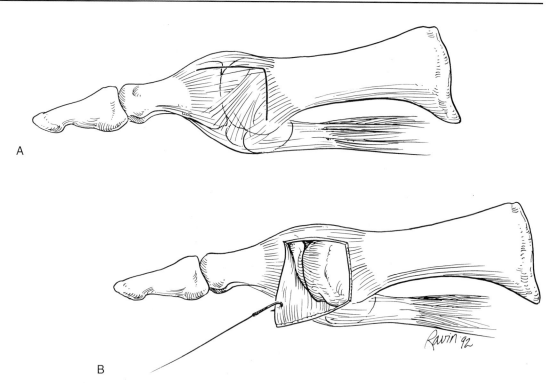

**Figure 8-14. A:** The capsular incision is demonstrated. **B:** The capsule is reflected to expose the medial eminence.

between it and the metatarsal head and neck. This lateral release should permit the sesamoid mechanism–metatarsal head relationship to be restored as the metatarsal is repositioned. With severe hallux valgus, the sesamoid mechanism is severely displaced, and unless it is freed from its scarred attachments, accurate repositioning of the sesamoid mechanism is not possible. If the deformity is very severe, the lateral portion of the flexor brevis tendon is sometimes sectioned to address the contracture. The lateral capsule is then perforated with a no. 15 scalpel blade. The hallux is passively manipulated into varus to complete the capsulotomy. Reduction of the MTP joint is critical during this maneuver to avoid levering the base of the phalanx into the metatarsal head and crushing a portion of the cartilage. The range of motion at the hallux MTP joint is again assessed in the neutral position to evaluate for any incongruity. If the joint is truly incongruent, a medial closing wedge distal metatarsal osteotomy is performed.

A third incision is made proximally, medial to the extensor hallucis longus tendon, to expose the MTC joint (Fig. 8-16). Care should be taken to avoid injury to the distal branch of the medial dorsal cutaneous nerve, which originates proximally from the superficial peroneal nerve. In the original description of this procedure, a biplanar wedge resection of the joint was recommended. The wedges were based laterally and plantarward, thereby adducting and plantarflexing the metatarsal (Fig. 8-17). Our current recommendation is to try to avoid resection of any bone if possible, minimizing shortening of the first metatarsal and preserving higher density periarticular bone for optimal fixation. Only the lateral and plantar articular cartilage is removed, and the medial aspect of the joint is left intact (Fig. 8-18), which can result in more natural movement of the foot (Fig. 8-19). Because of the unusual shape of the joint, optimal correction of deformity is not always easy to achieve. The correction depends on the presence of the usual slight concave-convex configuration, which can also be saddle shaped or bean shaped but not flat. Numerous configurations of the joint surfaces are encountered, some of which enhance and some block the repositioning of the metatarsal. Occasionally, there are two separate facets on the base of the metatarsal. The plane of this concavity is toward the second cuneiform, and the convexity faces medially. The depth of the articular surface is deep and sometimes difficult to reach even with a long

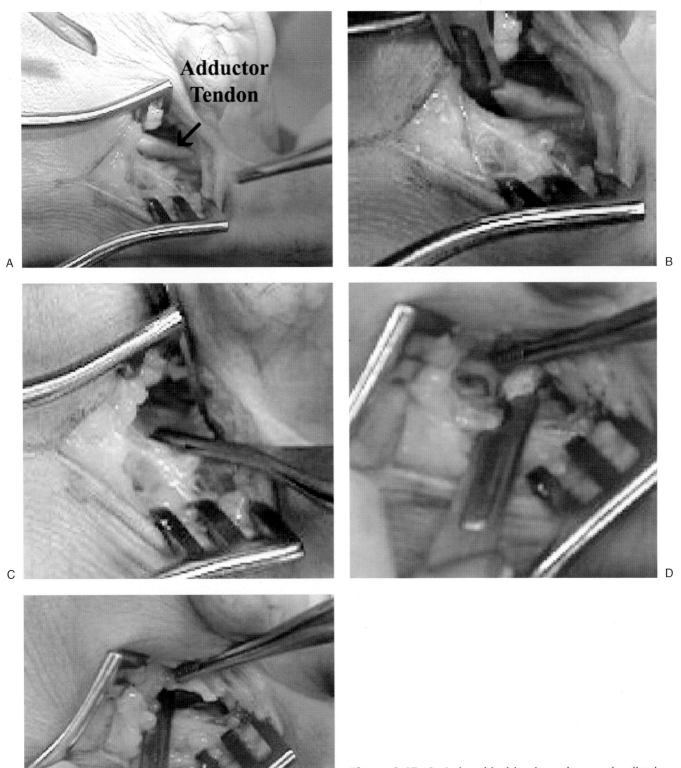

**Figure 8-15. A:** A dorsal incision is made over the distal intermetatarsal space of the left foot. **B:** A longitudinal capsulotomy is made dorsal to the fibular sesamoid, between it and the metatarsal head and neck. **C:** The distal end of the adductor tendon is transected near the base of the proximal phalanx. **D and E:** The adductor is freed up off the lateral border of the sesamoids and the flexor brevis tendon.

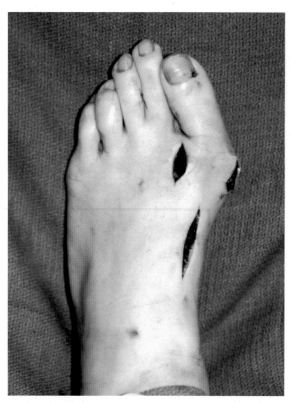

**Figure 8-16.** The third incision is made dorsally over the metatarsocuneiform joint, medial to the extensor hallucis longus tendon.

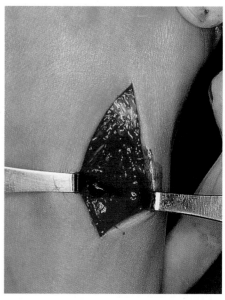

**Figure 8-17.** Resection of a biplanar wedge at the metatarsocuneiform joint is not recommended unless the smaller resection of the plantar lateral surfaces fails to permit reduction of the deformity.

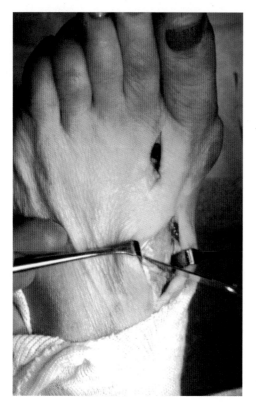

**Figure 8-18.** The chisel is placed within the joint to begin the minimal resection of the plantar-lateral aspects of the metatarsocuneiform joint.

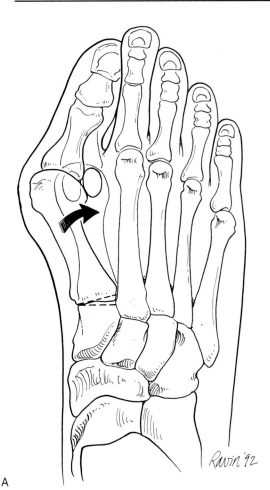

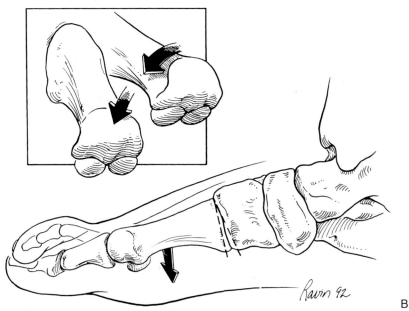

**Figure 8-19. A and B:** The first metatarsal is adducted and plantarflexed.

A

B

curette. There is a tendency to remove insufficient bone from the deeper (plantar) metatarsal and cuneiform joint surfaces, and careful inspection is needed when removing the deeper parts of the metatarsal with a long rongeur, curette, or thin chisel (Fig. 8-20). To complete the preparation of the joint surfaces, a sharp osteotome is used to fish-scale and cross-hatch the subchondral bone. If the correction cannot be achieved by simply sliding

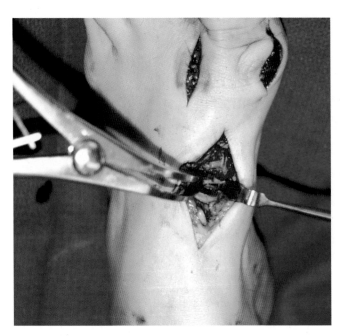

**Figure 8-20.** A laminar spreader improves visualization when removing the plantar-most portion of the metatarsocuneiform surfaces. Be careful not to crush the bone in osteopenic cases.

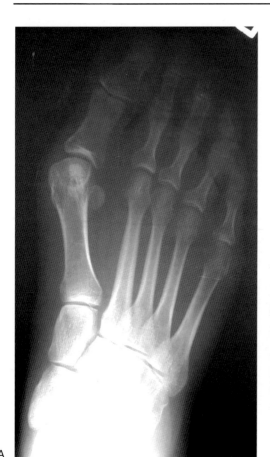

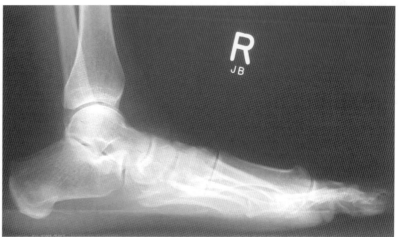

A

B

C

**Figure 8-21.** Preoperative anteroposterior (AP) radiograph of a patient with a collapsed arch and hallux valgus deformity from metatarsocuneiform instability **(A)**. The preoperative lateral radiograph shows the dorsal elevation of the first ray **(B)**. Postoperative oblique **(C, left)**, AP **(C, right)**, and lateral **(D)** radiographs display the positioning of the screws. *(continued)*

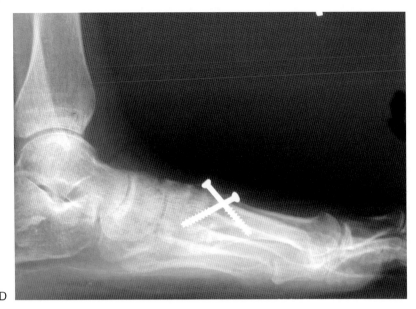

**Figure 8-21.** *Continued.*

the metatarsal on the cuneiform, then a small wedge may be resected from the joint. To avoid removing an excessively large wedge of bone at the tarsometatarsal joint, first resect a small wedge, hold the metatarsal in adduction and plantarflexion, and then secure it with a guide wire for a cannulated screw set or a Kirschner wire for temporary fixation.

Intraoperative anteroposterior and lateral radiographs should be obtained to confirm correction. Evaluate for the presence of overcorrection, undercorrection, and dorsal-plantar translation of the first metatarsal. Care is taken not to overcorrect the first metatarsal; if a negative IM angle is created, a hallux varus deformity may result. If the correction is unacceptable, remove the temporary fixation and attempt further reduction with or without resection of more bone.

Once the alignment is judged to be acceptable, screw fixation is performed using 4.0- or 4.5-mm, cannulated screws. There are several good options and combinations for screw placement. The first screw is inserted from proximal-dorsal across the arthrodesis site and angulated distally and plantarward into the first metatarsal. The second screw is placed starting from the base of the first metatarsal dorsally, across the arthrodesis site, and into the plantar aspect of the medial cuneiform (Fig. 8-21). A third screw may be warranted to increase stability. This is typically placed from the medial aspect of the base of the first metatarsal into the middle cuneiform or into the base of the second metatarsal (Fig. 8-22). While the first two screws are placed with a lag effect, the medial-to-lateral screw is placed as a neutralization screw. When this screw is inserted, it is important to ensure that the tip of the screw does not push against and displace the second metatarsal. This will tend to separate the first and second metatarsals and may affect stability of fixation at the MTC joint. Although this problem can be obviated by inserting the screw in a lag fashion, unnecessary compression of the first and second metatarsals may compromise the arthrodesis.

Two options exist for filling any voids at the arthrodesis site and decreasing the nonunion rate: the stress-relieving bone graft, as introduced by Hansen, or a sliding wedge bone graft. The stress-relieving bone graft is performed by using a burr to create small dorsal and medial troughs across the joint. Local bone graft harvested from the bunionectomy or from removal of a prominent cuneiform or metatarsal bone is used to fill the trough. If there is no available source of local bone or if the void is too great, a calcaneal bone graft may be harvested from the lateral heel through a 12-mm incision plantar and posterior to the sural nerve using a trephine. The other alternative (LCS's choice) is to perform a sliding bone graft. In this technique, two parallel osteotomies are created perpendicular to the MTC joint

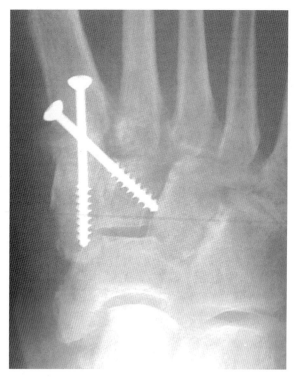

**Figure 8-22.** An anteroposterior radiograph shows a medial to lateral neutralization screw used in conjunction with a distal dorsal to proximal plantar lag screw.

away from the purchase point of the screw heads (Fig. 8-23A,B). They are begun as shallow cuts, and as they approach the opposite joint surface, they become progressively deeper (Fig. 8-23C). Next, an osteotome with a width that matches the distance between the parallel cuts is used to create a wedge, beginning shallow and becoming progressively deeper as the opposite joint surface is encountered (Fig. 8-23D). This wedge is then tamped across the void and recessed (Fig. 8-23E).

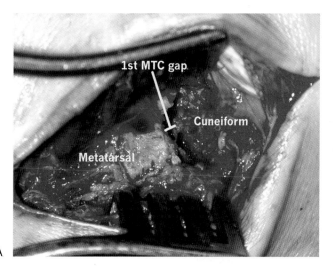
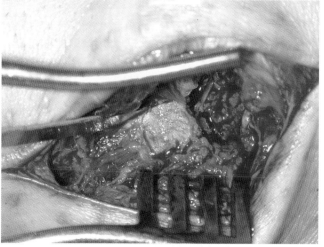

A

B

**Figure 8-23. A:** A sliding bone graft at the metatarsocuneiform joint. First, an osteotomy is created perpendicular to the metatarsocuneiform joint and away from the purchase point of the screw heads. **B:** The second osteotomy is made parallel to the first. *(continued)*

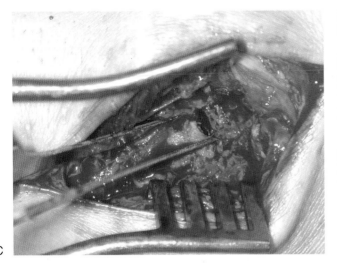

C

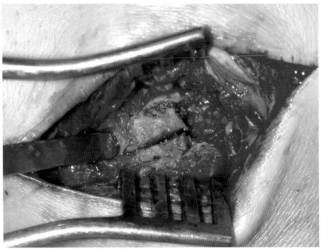

D

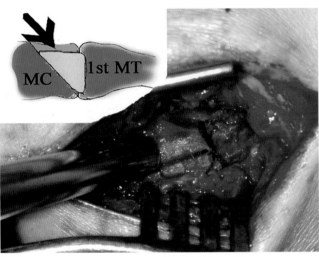

E

**Figure 8-23.** *Continued.* **C:** These osteotomies are begun as shallow cuts, and as they approach the opposite joint surface, they become progressively deeper. **D:** A chisel whose width matches the distance between the parallel cuts is used to create a wedge that begins shallowly and becomes progressively deeper as the opposite joint surface is encountered. **E:** The wedge is tamped across the void and recessed. **Inset:** Diagram of the sagittal plane of the metatarsocuneiform joint demonstrates how the triangular block of bone slides across the gap.

Once the metatarsal has been stabilized, attention is again directed toward the distal alignment. The congruity of the MTP joint is again evaluated. If the range of motion of the MTP joint is diminished in the corrected position, this indicates that here is a potential for medial impingement and incongruity. It is then preferable to leave the metatarsal in this position and perform a closing wedge osteotomy at the base of the proximal phalanx or neck of the metatarsal. The hallux should rest in a neutral position, and closure made without relying on the capsulorraphy to realign the toe. The capsulorraphy is performed as described earlier by using the L-shaped flap, and if necessary, it is attached by suture passed through a hole in the metatarsal neck made with a Kirschner wire. Nonabsorbable 2-0 suture is used in the capsular repair, and nylon mattress or nonabsorbable subcuticular sutures are used in the skin.

## POSTOPERATIVE MANAGEMENT

Patients use crutches until comfortable, followed by weight bearing as tolerated in a short-leg cast or a stiff postoperative shoe. Unless the patient is very active and noncompliant, a postoperative shoe is used. If a cast is warranted, it is removed by the sixth week, and the foot is placed into a postoperative shoe until 3 months after the operation. A soft bunion splint or a narrow elastic bandage is used until 3 months from the surgery to maintain the hallux in neutral alignment. Some patients are able to advance into a comfortable sneaker by 8 to 10 weeks, typically bearing weight on the lateral side of the foot. As healing progresses, they apply more weight medially. In the last few weeks of the 3-month postoperative period, they often wear a shoe with a spacer placed between the first and second toes to help maintain the position of the hallux. By 4 months postoperatively, they are allowed to use any footwear, but most patients find that the foot is too swollen to return to their usual shoes until approximately 4 to 8 months. During the postoperative period between the second and sixth months, patients are encouraged to manipulate their MTP joint or to undergo a course of physical therapy to improve the motion.

Our combined experience with the procedure involves well over 275 cases treated with this procedure. We estimate that 80% are completely satisfied, 15% are satisfied with some reservations, and 5% are dissatisfied. Pain, function, appearance of the foot, and footwear restrictions after surgery dramatically improve in more than 90% of the cases. The alignment also improves radiologically with an average decrease in IM 1–2 angle of 14° and an average decrease of 30° in the hallux valgus angle.

## COMPLICATIONS

In our experience, loss of some correction ($>10°$) from the initial postoperative radiographs occurred in 20% of the cases at the MTP joint during medium and longer-term follow-up. Most of these cases remained asymptomatic, and revision operations for recurrence were therefore rare. Loss of correction at the MTC joint ($>5°$) occurred in 5% of the cases and was rarely symptomatic. Dorsal elevation occurred in 8%, and this typically was apparent within the first 4 months. Revision operations for this complication were unusual, although symptoms of second metatarsal stress transfer were common but tolerable. Hallux varus was seen in 10% of the radiographs but clinically was not consistently symptomatic. Nonunions were seen in less than 5%, and only 20% of these required additional fixation and/or bone grafting. Delayed unions were observed in 15% and typically resolved with immobilization in a walking boot (i.e., prefabricated AFO).

Shortening of the first metatarsal averaged 3 to 4 mm. Because care was taken to plantarflex or translate the first metatarsal plantarward, shortening was often not symptomatic. Sesamoid pain occurred in 15% of cases but was often well managed with appropriate footwear and orthotic devices. Surgery to address this problem was performed in 15% of these symptomatic cases and included sesamoid shaving, sesamoid resection, or rarely, a first metatarsal osteotomy. A dorsal bunion develops in about 8% of feet in association with nonunion or malunion of the first metatarsal. Although most are asymptomatic, decreased range of motion of the hallux MTP joint is present in nearly all patients. Stiffness, however, was only reported in 10% and was treated nonoperatively or occasionally with cheilectomy.

A revision arthrodesis was rarely warranted in our series. Although it may seem that revision of the arthrodesis is a major undertaking, it is easily accomplished by a simple opening wedge osteotomy of the arthrodesis site and interposition of a tricortical bone graft. This osteotomy/arthrodesis is quite stable, and patients tend to recover quickly. The most common reason for additional surgery was hardware removal, which occurred in 25% of the patients. Although hardware breakage occurred in 10%, the reason screws were removed usually related to the prominence of the head of the screw.

## ACKNOWLEDGMENTS

We would like to thank Ted Hansen for inspiring us both during the 1980s to perform this surgery with appropriate rigid internal fixation. We offer special appreciation to Jennifer Shores and Lyn Camire for helping with the preparation of this chapter.

This chapter is dedicated in honor of our dear mentor at the Hospital for Joint Diseases Orthopaedic Institute, Melvin Jahss, who taught us what he had learned from his mentor, Paul Lapidus. Dr. Jahss' loving devotion to advancing the knowledge of the foot and ankle has inspired many of today's leaders in our field. We reflect on his unique wit and encyclopedic wisdom daily.

## RECOMMENDED READING

1. Catanzariti AR, Mendicino RW, Lee MS, et al.: The modified Lapidus arthrodesis: a retrospective analysis. *J Foot Ankle Surg* 38:22–332, 1999.
2. Clarke HR, Veith RG, Hansen ST: Adolescent bunions treated by the modified Lapidus procedure. *Bull Hosp Joint Dis* 47:109–122, 1987.
3. Faber FW, Kleinrensink GJ, Verhoog MW, et al.: Mobility of the first tarsometatarsal joint in relation to hallux valgus deformity: anatomical and biomechanical aspects. *Foot Ankle Int* 20:651–656, 1999.
4. Klaue K, Hansen ST, Masquelet AC: Clinical, quantitative assessment of first tarsometatarsal mobility in the sagittal plane and its relation to hallux valgus deformity. *Foot Ankle Int* 15:9–13, 1994.
5. Lapidus PW: The operative correction of the metatarsus varus primus in hallux valgus. *Surg Gyneol Obstet* 58:183–191, 1934.
6. Lapidus PW: A quarter of a century of experience with the operative correction of the metatarsus varus in hallux valgus. *Bull Hosp Joint Dis* 17:404–421, 1956.
7. Lapidus PW: The author's bunion operation from 1931 to 1959. *Clin Orthop* 16:119–135, 1960.
8. Myerson MS: Metatarsocuneiform arthrodesis for treatment of hallux valgus and metatarsus primus varus. *Orthopedics* 13:1025–1031, 1990.
9. Myerson MS, Allon S, McGarvey W: Metatarsocuneiform arthrodesis for management of hallux valgus and metatarsus primus varus. *Foot Ankle* 13:107–115, 1992.
10. Schon LC, Acevedo JI, Mann MR: Technique tip: the sliding wedge local bone graft for midfoot arthrodesis. *Foot Ankle Int* 20:340–341, 1999.

# 9

# Cheilectomy

Glenn B. Pfeffer

## INDICATIONS/CONTRAINDICATIONS

Hallux rigidus is a degenerative condition of the great toe metatarsophalangeal (MTP) joint characterized by decreased dorsiflexion, osteophyte proliferation, and painful motion. First described by Davies-Colley in 1887, J. M. Cotterill later coined the term *hallux rigidus* (1). After hallux valgus, it is the most common painful affliction of the great toe, occurring in approximately 2% of the population between the ages of 30 and 60 years. As the degenerative process progresses, proliferation of bone on the dorsal aspect of the metatarsal head increases the size of the joint and blocks dorsiflexion of the proximal phalanx. These changes are possibly initiated by previous occult trauma (5). Patients usually present with unilateral symptoms, but it is common for stiffness and the degenerative process to affect the opposite foot.

Initial treatment should be nonoperative in an effort to decrease joint inflammation and to protect the toe from painful motion. A nonsteroidal antiinflammatory agent, contrast baths, and a stiff-soled, low-heeled shoe are helpful. An intraarticular injection of a steroid preparation may decrease acute synovitis, but repeated injections are not recommended. Shoe modification includes a selection of shoes with a wide toe box or stretching the shoe upper in the area of the painful dorsal prominence. A rocker-bottom sole, a stiff fiberglass or steel shank in the sole, or an orthotic device can also be used to limit dorsiflexion of the MTP joint. These modifications can have variable patient compliance when prescribed.

When nonoperative treatment fails, surgical intervention with cheilectomy should be considered. The specific indication for cheilectomy is pain due to abutment of the proximal phalanx of the great toe against degenerative osteophytes on the dorsal aspect of the first metatarsal (Fig. 9-1). Another indication is pain from skin ulceration or abrasion overlying large dorsal osteophytes. The term *cheilectomy* is derived from the Greek *cheilos*, meaning lip. The goal of surgery is to excise the proliferative bone on the "lip" of the joint, thereby allowing dorsiflexion motion. Other surgical options include MTP resection arthroplasty

G. B. Pfeffer, M.D.: Department of Orthopaedics, University of California, San Francisco; and California Pacific Medical Center, San Francisco, California.

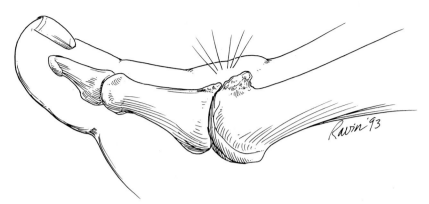

**Figure 9-1.** Medial view of a foot with hallux rigidus. Dorsal osteophytes on the first metatarsal head block normal extension of the proximal phalanx.

such as a Keller procedure, implant arthroplasty, osteotomy about the joint of either the proximal phalanx or first metatarsal, and MTP arthrodesis. Cheilectomy offers the advantage of preserving the length, stability, and flexion-extension strength of the great toe that are often sacrificed with these other procedures. An arthroplasty or arthrodesis can always follow a failed cheilectomy, but not vice versa. Contraindications to cheilectomy include very advanced degeneration of the joint, local infection, skin ulceration, and a foot with impaired vascularity. A relative contraindication is a previous failed operation for hallux rigidus.

## PREOPERATIVE PLANNING

It is essential to differentiate hallux rigidus from other causes of great toe pain. The hallmark of the physical examination of hallux rigidus is restricted active and passive dorsiflexion of the toe with reproduction of the patient's pain (3). The MTP joint is rarely rigid, and a firm end point to dorsiflexion can be appreciated. Passive range of MTP motion is measured with a goniometer in dorsiflexion and plantarflexion in relation to the shaft of the first metatarsal or in relation to the plantar foot. Compensatory hyperextension at the interphalangeal (IP) joint may occur and should be documented, including whether the IP joint is tender or has painful motion or crepitus. Plantarflexion of the MTP joint is usually not as restricted, although passive motion may cause dorsal pain by stretching the inflamed capsule or extensor tendon over a prominent osteophyte (4) (Fig. 9-2). A large osteophyte along the dorsal aspect of the metatarsal head may irritate a sensory nerve to the hallux and cause dysesthesias or paresthesias with palpation.

Radiographic evaluation should include standing anteroposterior and lateral views of the foot. The standing lateral view is most helpful because it demonstrates the dorsal osteophytes and reveals the extent of joint space narrowing. The upper portion of the joint may be destroyed while the lower one half may have preserved articular cartilage space. If the inferior portion of the joint space is not preserved in more severe disease, cheilectomy will not be successful. The anteroposterior radiograph may demonstrate lateral osteophytes, subchondral sclerosis, or cyst formation. Occasionally, an oblique view of the great toe helps to visualize early joint space narrowing dorsally. The sesamoids are rarely involved in the degenerative process of hallux rigidus, and an axial view to visualize them is not usually obtained. Specialized diagnostic studies usually are unnecessary.

Based on the plain film radiographic findings, the grade of hallux rigidus should be determined. Grade I is defined as mild to moderate osteophyte formation with joint space preservation (Fig. 9-3). Grade II is moderate osteophyte proliferation with joint space narrowing and subchondral sclerosis (Fig. 9-4). Grade III is severe osteophyte formation and

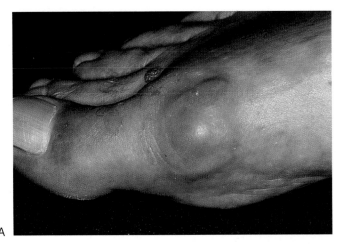
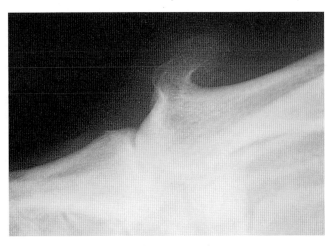

A                                                                                B

**Figure 9-2. A:** Photograph of a patient with hallux rigidus shows enlargement about the metatarsophalangeal joint from soft tissue inflammation and osteophytes. **B:** A large, prominent dorsal osteophyte is observed on the lateral radiograph.

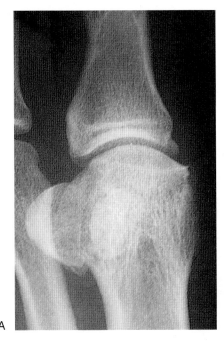

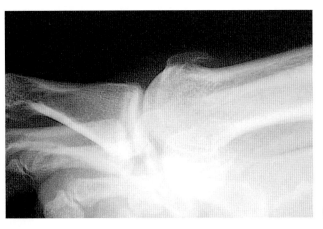

**Figure 9-3. A and B:** Grade I or mild hallux rigidus with small osteophyte and no joint space narrowing.

A                                                                                B

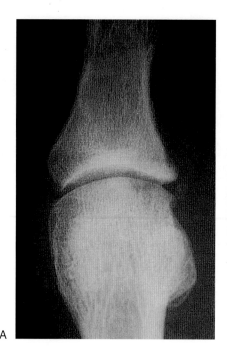

A

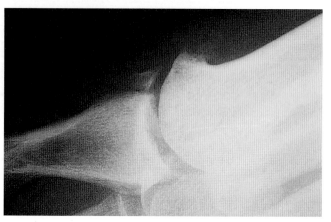

B

**Figure 9-4. A and B:** Grade II or moderate hallux rigidus with osteophytes dorsally and laterally and with joint space narrowing.

loss of joint space, including the inferior portion of the joint. Marked sclerosis and cyst formation are also present (Fig. 9-5). Patients with grade I or II changes are excellent candidates for cheilectomy (2). Patients with grade III changes are candidates for alternative procedures such as an arthrodesis or a Keller resection arthroplasty. Occasionally, the final decision of the specific operation is made at the time of surgery, such as the patient who has a higher grade II disease. The patient should be counseled preoperatively that the appropriate procedure will be chosen after the joint cartilage is examined.

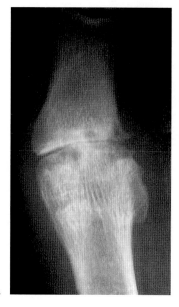

A

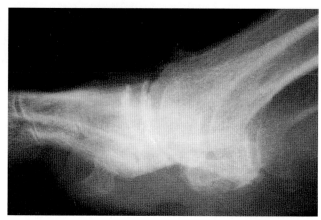

B

**Figure 9-5. A and B:** Grade III or advanced hallux rigidus with osteophytes dorsally and laterally and with severe joint destruction with loss of joint space.

## SURGERY

A cheilectomy is usually performed under regional anesthesia with intravenous sedation. An ankle block using 20 to 25 mL of 0.25% or 0.5% bupivacaine hydrochloride (Marcaine) mixed with 1% lidocaine, both without epinephrine, is appropriate. The patient is placed supine on the operating table. A pneumatic ankle tourniquet is applied over two or three layers of cast padding. After the foot in exsanguinated with a 3-inch Esmarch bandage, the tourniquet is inflated to 250 mm Hg.

### Technique

Using a no. 15 blade scalpel, a 5- to 6-cm longitudinal incision centered over the first MTP joint is made dorsally along the medial border of the extensor hallucis longus tendon (Fig. 9-6). Care is taken to protect the dorsocutaneous sensory nerve, although they are not routinely visualized in this approach (Fig. 9-7). The extensor hood is divided 2 mm medial to the border of the extensor hallucis longus tendon, thereby keeping the tendon within its sheath (Fig. 9-8). This lessens the occurrence of postoperative adhesions. The tendon is retracted laterally, and the joint capsule is divided longitudinally. A proliferative synovitis may be encountered, and a plane between the capsule and the synovium is developed. A complete synovectomy is performed. Cartilaginous loose bodies may be present and should be removed. A no. 15 blade or a no. 64 Beaver blade is then used to carefully dissect the joint capsule to expose the medial, dorsal, and lateral aspects of the metatarsal head and the base of the proximal phalanx (Fig. 9-9).

The toe is plantarflexed at the MTP joint approximately 45° to allow complete inspection of the joint surface (Fig. 9-10). Further dissection of the capsule may be required to

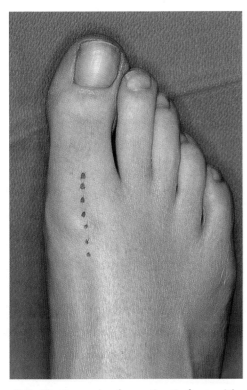

**Figure 9-6.** Photograph of a patient's foot with painful hallux rigidus. A 5- to 6-cm longitudinal incision is made along the medial border of the extensor hallucis longus tendon.

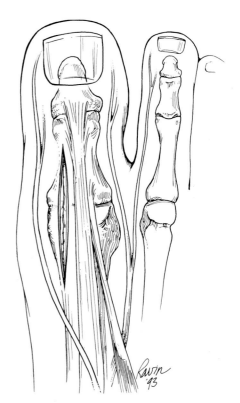

**Figure 9-7.** Drawing shows incision placement dorsally and the dorsal sensory nerves to the hallux, although they are not routinely visualized in this approach.

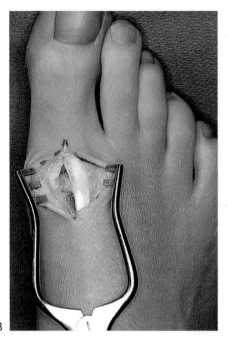
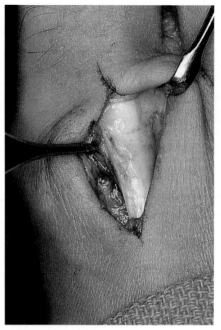
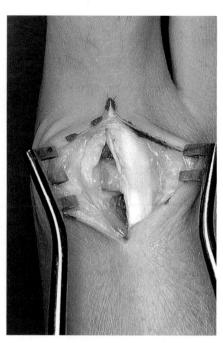

A, B

C

**Figure 9-8. A:** The extensor hallucis longus sheath is divided 2 to 3 mm medial to the border of the tendon, thereby keeping the tendon within its sheath. **B:** The medial border of the extensor hallucis longus sheath is held in the forceps. **C:** The capsule is divided longitudinally.

gain adequate exposure. The large dorsal osteophyte and the predominant lateral osteophytes are readily apparent (Fig. 9-11). The pathologic changes of the cartilage on the metatarsal head can now be appreciated fully. The changes are often worse than expected based on preoperative radiographs. The cartilage on the proximal phalanx is usually better preserved, although changes centrally and dorsally can occur. A prominent dorsal ridge of

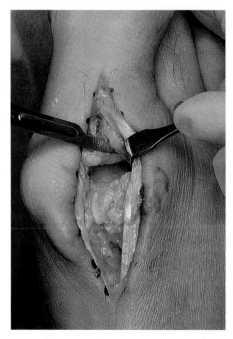

**Figure 9-9.** The capsule is dissected away from the metatarsal head and the base of the proximal phalanx to expose dorsal and lateral osteophytes.

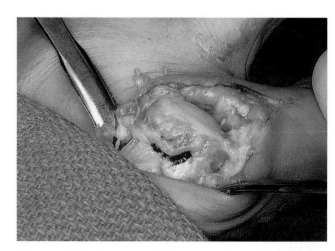

**Figure 9-10.** Dorsal-medial view of the metatarsophalangeal joint. The toe is plantarflexed 45° to expose the metatarsal head.

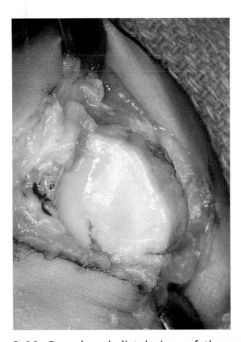

**Figure 9-11.** Dorsal and distal view of the metatarsophalangeal joint with the toe flexed to expose dorsal osteophyte. In this case, approximately 35% of the metatarsal head is damaged with fissuring and softening of the dorsal cartilage.

bone at the base of the proximal phalanx is frequently present. This is removed with a needle-nosed rongeur.

The dorsal bony prominence of the metatarsal is excised obliquely along with up to one third of the metatarsal head (Fig. 9-12). The amount of metatarsal head that is excised largely depends on the amount of bone removal that is required to allow passive dorsiflexion of the toe. Even in the mildest of cases, at least 20% of the dorsal metatarsal head should be removed for adequate dorsiflexion. From distal to proximal, the line of resection slopes upward, usually extending from a level just dorsal to the edge of viable cartilage to just proximal to the dorsal prominence (Fig. 9-13). Exposed bone surface that remains on the metatarsal head could be drilled multiple times with a small Kirschner wire to induce formation of fibrocartilage. Any small irregularities along the cartilage edges should be carefully trimmed using a no. 15 blade or small rongeur.

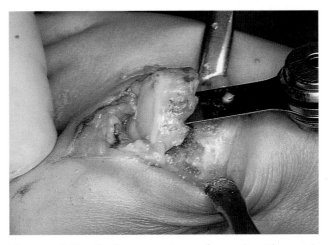

**Figure 9-12.** Cheilectomy is performed with a microsagittal saw from proximal to distal.

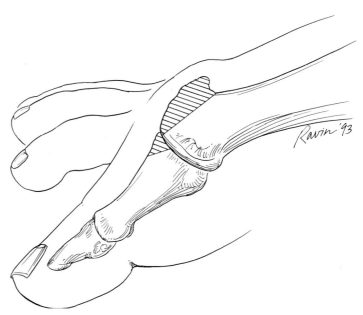

**Figure 9-13.** The line of resection extends from just dorsal to the edge of the viable cartilage to just proximal to the dorsal prominence of the metatarsal head. Use of resection of the dorsal osteophyte at the base of the proximal phalanx is shown.

A microsagittal saw is used, such as the Zimmer Micro-Aire saw (Zimmer Co., Warsaw, IN) with a fine-toothed sagittal blade (no. ZS-038), which is approximately 1.25 inches long, 0.37 inches wide, and 0.015 inches thick. A small amount of crystalloid solution is used for irrigation so as not to cause thermal necrosis of the bone and cartilage. A 6-mm osteotome can also be effective, although fragmentation of the bone may occur. The bone cut is most easily performed from proximal to distal, especially if 25% or more of the head is to be removed. When less than 25% of the head is excised, it is more difficult to place the sawblade parallel to the metatarsal shaft, and the cut is better made from distal to proximal (Fig. 9-14).

After the metatarsal prominence is excised, the marginal osteophytes are addressed. Two small Hohmann retractors placed medially and laterally provide exposure of the metatarsal head while protecting the adjacent tendons and neurovascular structures. A microsagittal saw is used to resect the osteophytes flush with the medial and lateral margins of the metatarsal shaft unless there is loss of medial or lateral cartilage (Fig. 9-15). In such a case,

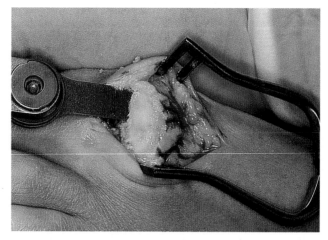

**Figure 9-14.** If a more limited portion of the metatarsal head is resected, the cut can be readily made from distal to proximal.

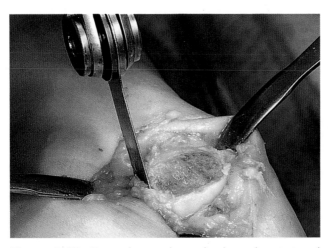

**Figure 9-15.** Osteophytes along the lateral metatarsal head should be excised with a saw or rongeurs. Hohmann retractors are used to protect the neurovascular structures and tendons. If there is loss of articular cartilage on the lateral aspect of the joint, that portion of the metatarsal head should be excised as well.

2 to 3 mm of the metatarsal head should be removed in the sagittal plane. If such articular cartilage loss occurs, it is usually on the lateral aspect of the joint where the most prominent osteophytes occur (Fig. 9-16). Osteophytes medially are unusual and can easily be excised with a small needle-nose rongeur. The sharp borders left by the saw cuts should be rounded using a rongeur or a microreciprocating rasp or can be feathered with a sawblade. A prominent dorsal lip on the proximal phalanx should be trimmed down in a similar fashion, using a rongeur or microreciprocating rasp.

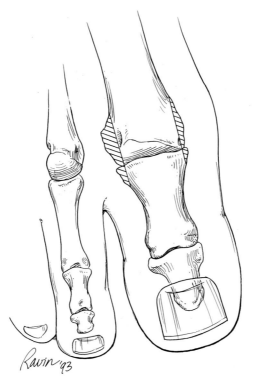

**Figure 9-16.** The drawing shows excision of lateral osteophytes and a small portion of metatarsal head and phalangeal base with cartilage loss. Bony prominences may be resected medially as well.

After the bony cuts have been made, the sesamoid complex should be examined. There are rarely degenerative changes present. A small Freer elevator can be used to release adhesions between the sesamoid mechanism and the plantar aspect of the metatarsal head. At this point, the surgeon should be able to passively dorsiflex the phalanx about 70° relative to the plantar foot (Fig. 9-17). If this degree of dorsiflexion is not obtainable, the joint should be reassessed for probable further bony resection (Fig. 9-18). The joint is then copiously irrigated with crystalloid solution, and the capsule is closed using absorbable suture. Selection of a nonabsorbable suture would cause less of an inflammatory reaction postoperatively, but the suture knots can be noticeable after swelling subsides and footwear is used. One or two 4-0 absorbable sutures are used to repair and realign the extensor mechanism. The tourniquet is deflated and hemostasis obtained with compression and cautery. No subcutaneous sutures are required. The skin is closed with interrupted 4-0 nylon horizontal mattress sutures. An antibiotic ointment and nonadherent 4 × 4 inch gauze are placed over the wound, and a sterile, bulky compressive dressing is applied.

Cheilectomy is not a complicated operation. Results depend on careful patient selection and surgical technique, as well as judgments made intraoperatively such as extent of bony resection. Variations on the surgical approach have been recommended by different authors. The procedure can be successfully accomplished through a medial longitudinal incision and longitudinal capsulotomy. An approach based on the medial side of the extensor hallucis longus tendon provides excellent visualization of the joint and avoids dissection of

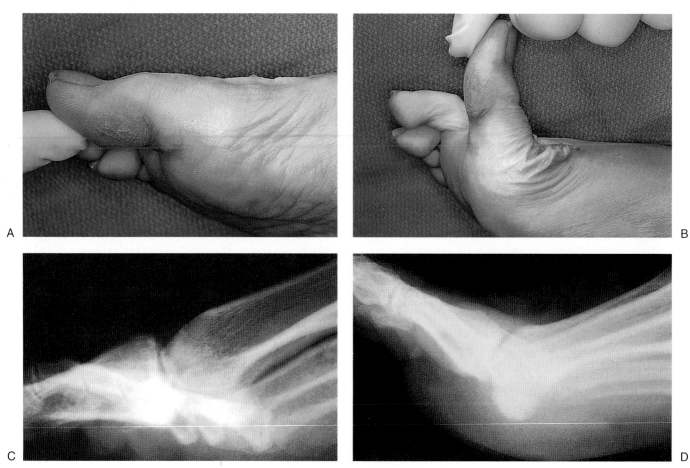

**Figure 9-17.  A:** Photograph shows a medial view of the foot before cheilectomy, with dorsiflexion limited to 20° relative to the plantar foot. **B:** Intraoperative photograph after cheilectomy demonstrates about 80° of dorsiflexion. **C:** Lateral radiograph after approximately 30% of the metatarsal head was excised. **D:** Postoperative lateral radiograph of the foot in dorsiflexion. The proximal phalanx can now move more freely on the metatarsal head, because it is no longer blocked by a prominent dorsal osteophyte.

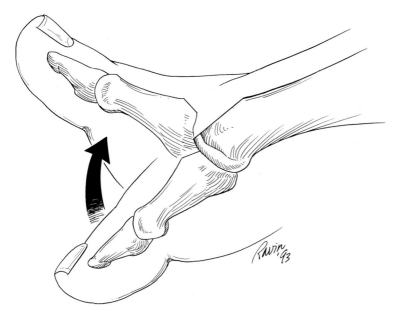

**Figure 9-18.** Adequate resection of the metatarsal head and phalangeal base is necessary to gain adequate motion.

the extensor hallucis brevis tendon. By leaving the extensor hallucis longus in its sheath, the potential for postoperative adhesions is lessened. Aggressive bony resection of the dorsal osteophyte and diseased portion of the metatarsal head is essential. Excision of the prominent lateral osteophytes with "squaring off" of the metatarsal is required to adequately decompress the joint.

## POSTOPERATIVE MANAGEMENT

After surgery, the patient is immobilized in a stiff postoperative shoe for 10 days until the wound is healed and the sutures are removed. Gentle range of motion exercises are started by the patient as early as the second postoperative day as pain allows. At the first visit, 3 to 5 days postoperatively, the dressing is changed, and a new compressive dressing is applied. Three or four sterile 4 × 4 inch gauzes and a 3-inch Kling are used, beginning the circumferential compressive dressing just distal to the tibialis anterior insertion. By the 14th postoperative day, the patient should be back into a flexible closed-toe athletic shoe.

Active and passive MTP range of motion exercises are encouraged. A home therapy program of passive motion should include 10 minutes of dorsiflexion exercises every 1 to 2 hours while awake. A nonsteroidal antiinflammatory medication, ice, massage, and contrast baths can help decrease inflammation. The patient may use a mild analgesic rather than forego range of motion exercises.

If no significant progress is obtained with the home program, formal occupational or physical therapy is initiated at 3 weeks postoperatively up to three times each week, as needed. I have found that a dynamic extension splint, similar to that used in selected hand surgery procedures, can be helpful in regaining motion (Fig. 9-19). The dynamic splint is worn at night and is used for approximately 1 month, as tolerated. Manipulation of the joint in the office could be considered 8 to 10 weeks after surgery in carefully selected patients if significant disparity exists between intraoperative and postoperative motion.

It is expected that a substantial degree of dorsiflexion motion obtained intraoperatively will be lost in the early postoperative period. Without aggressive therapy, the patient can expect to gain one half or even less of the motion obtained during surgery. The degree of intraoperative motion achieved may or may not be directly related to the final outcome. There is certainly no reason to lose what has been gained by a careful surgical technique. Most patients will plateau in terms of progress with their therapy program approximately 4

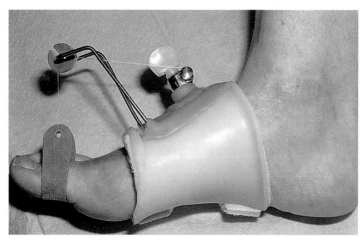

**Figure 9-19.** A dynamic extension splint for the great toe's metatarsophalangeal joint.

months postoperatively, with little increase in range of motion seen after that time. The symptoms often continue to abate for up to 6 months or even a year after surgery. Most patients have pain relief postoperatively, even if range of motion is not increased significantly (6). There is no clear correlation in fact between the degree of pain relief and the percentage increased of motion obtained.

## COMPLICATIONS

Some patients may be dissatisfied with persistent pain and MTP stiffness after cheilectomy. Usually, it is advisable to defer a reoperation until 1 year after cheilectomy. Rather than undergoing another operation, the patient should be encouraged to pursue shoe modifications, antiinflammatory medications, and exercises.

Keller resection arthroplasty or an arthrodesis of the MTP joint can be performed for failed cheilectomy. Before the original cheilectomy, patients should be advised about the possibility of a second procedure in the future. The cheilectomy relieves the dorsal impingement of the joint but does not alter the underlying degenerative process that may ultimately progress and later require further operative intervention.

There are complications reported that are specific to this procedure. Excessive metatarsal head resection can produce an unstable painful MTP joint with progressive arthrosis. Iatrogenic injury to the extensor hallucis longus tendon during the operative procedure is a difficult complication to manage. If the tendon is inadvertently cut, it should be repaired with a 3-0 or 4-0 nonabsorbable suture. Initiating rigorous range of motion exercises in the early postoperative period may compromise the integrity of a repaired tendon laceration.

## ILLUSTRATIVE CASE

This 42-year-old, heavy laborer with bilateral grade II hallux rigidus (Fig. 9-20) had an implant arthroplasty of the right MTP joint performed elsewhere (Fig. 9-21). Before implant arthroplasty, his MTP range of motion was 20° of dorsiflexion, and 6 months postoperatively it was 30° of dorsiflexion with relief of pain. He had continued pain of the left first MTP joint due to hallux rigidus and underwent surgery. Preoperatively, his range of motion was 20° of dorsiflexion. Six months postoperatively, he had 30° of dorsiflexion on the operative side with complete relief of pain. He had continued pain on the left and chose to have a cheilectomy performed. Large dorsal and lateral osteophytes were excised along with approximately 30% of the dorsal metatarsal head (Fig. 9-22). A small osteophyte on

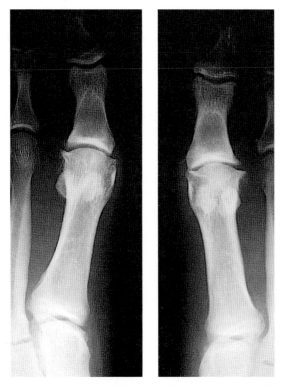

**Figure 9-20.** Preoperative standing, anteroposterior radiographs of a patient with moderate hallux rigidus.

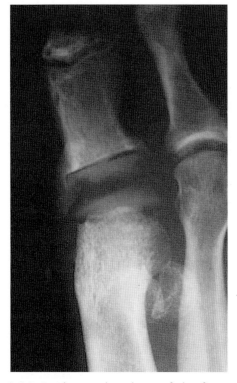

**Figure 9-21.** Implant arthroplasty of the first metatarsophalangeal joint was performed elsewhere in the right foot.

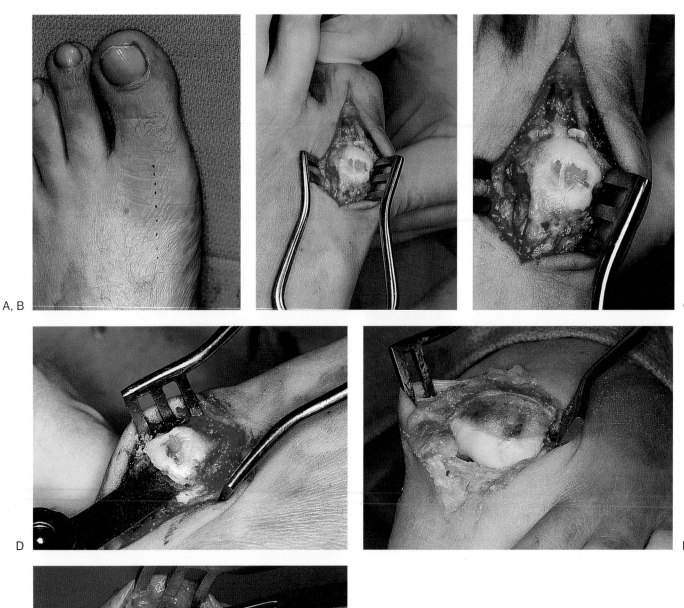

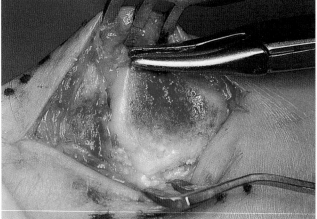

**Figure 9-22. A:** The dorsal longitudinal incision is based on the medial aspect of the extensor hallux longus. **B and C:** Plantarflexion of the great toe exposes significant cartilage loss and osteophyte proliferation on the dorsal aspect of the metatarsal head. **D:** Diseased portion of metatarsal head is excised with a microsagittal saw. **E:** The metatarsal head is carefully assessed. Medial and lateral osteophytes are excised, and if necessary, drilling of small cartilage defects is performed. **F:** A small, dorsal-medial osteophyte is excised with a rongeur. *(continued)*

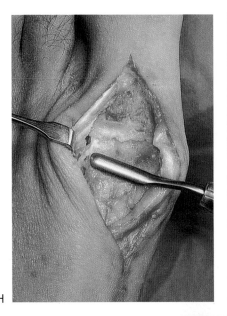
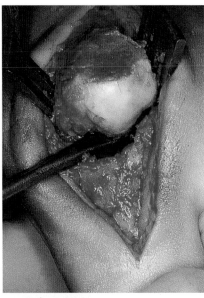
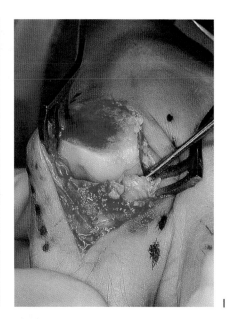

G, H

I

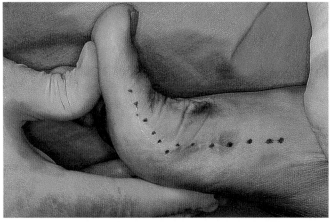

J

**Figure 9-22.** *Continued.* **G:** A microreciprocating rasp is used to smooth out prominent bone edges. **H:** A Freer elevator is used on the plantar aspect of the metatarsal head to release any adhesions that may restrict dorsiflexion of the great toe. **I:** Prominent osteophytes on the lateral aspect of metatarsal head are removed. **J:** After cheilectomy, dorsiflexion is increased to approximately 70° on the operative table.

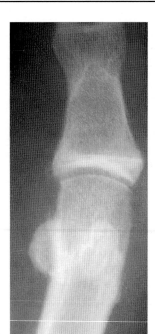

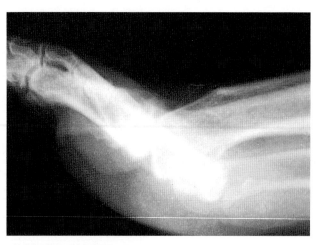

A                                                                                                                B

**Figure 9-23.** Postoperative anteroposterior radiograph **(A)** and lateral dorsiflexion radiograph **(B)** of the left first metatarsophalangeal joint after cheilectomy. Radiographs demonstrate resection of the osteophytes was performed laterally and medially, and about one third of the metatarsal head has been resected dorsally.

the dorsal aspect of the base of the proximal phalanx was also excised. He obtained 65° of passive dorsiflexion on the operating table, and 5 months postoperatively he had 40° of active dorsiflexion on the left and was pain free (Fig. 9-23).

## RECOMMENDED READING

1. Davies-Colley N: Contraction of the metatarsophalangeal joint of the great toe (hallux flexus). *Br Med J* 1: 728, 1887.
2. Easley ME, Davis WH, Anderson RB: Intermediate to long-term follow-up of medial approach dorsal cheilectomy for hallux rigidus. *Foot Ankle Int* 20:147–152, 1999.
3. Hattrup SJ, Johnson KA: Subjective results of hallux rigidus following treatment with cheilectomy. *Clin Orthop Rel Res* 226:182–191, 1988.
4. Hawkins BJ, Haddad RJ: Hallux rigidus. *Clin Sports Med* 7:37–49, 1988.
5. Karasick D, Wapner KN: Hallux rigidus deformity: radiologic assessment. *AJR Am J Radiol* 157:1029–1033, 1991.
6. Mann RA: Hallux rigidus. *Instr Course Lect* 39:15–21, 1990.
7. Mann RA, Clanton TO: Hallux rigidus: treatment by cheilectomy. *J Bone Joint Surg Am* 70:400–405, 1988.
8. Mulier T, Steenwerckx A, Thienpent E, et al.: Results of cheilectomy in athletes with hallux rigidus. *Foot Ankle Int* 20:232–237, 1999.

# 10

# Proximal Phalangeal (Moberg) Osteotomy

Javad Parvizi and Harold B. Kitaoka

## INDICATIONS/CONTRAINDICATIONS

Hallux rigidus is a painful degenerative joint disease affecting the first metatarsophalangeal (MTP) joint and is associated with osteophyte formation and limitation of motion, especially in dorsiflexion.

Nonoperative treatment of the hallux rigidus includes activity modification, administration of nonsteroidal antiinflammatory medications, footwear alteration, and intraarticular injection of corticosteroids. Shoe modification includes wide and deep toe box to reduce skin abrasion from dorsal osteophytes and irritation of the dorsomedial cutaneous nerve. A stiff-soled shoe with rocker-bottom, steel or fiberglass shank built in the sole can also help by minimizing the first MTP motion at toe-off (10).

When conservative measures fail to control the symptoms, operative intervention is warranted. A variety of surgical treatment options have been reported. Cheilectomy, resection arthroplasty, implant arthroplasty, and MTP arthrodesis constitute the main surgical treatment options. There have also been reports of osteotomies about the first MTP joint, attempting to address the pain and stiffness of the affected first MTP. These osteotomies included closing wedge proximal phalangeal osteotomy, proximal metatarsal osteotomy, and distal metatarsal osteotomy (5).

Closing wedge osteotomy of the proximal phalanx for hallux rigidus was first proposed by Bonney and Macnab (2) in 1952, and short-term results were reported by Kessel and Bonney (8) in 1958. Closing wedge proximal phalanx osteotomy is, however, best known as the Moberg osteotomy since he popularized this technique (9). The aim of the operation is to move the limited arc of motion at the affected joint to a more dorsiflexed position so that the function is improved. It is applicable in patients with mild to moderate degenerative disease of the first MTP joint due to hallux rigidus. We advocate this procedure for pa-

J. Parvizi, M.D.: Department of Orthopaedic Surgery, Mayo Clinic, Rochester, Minnesota.

H. B. Kitaoka, M.D.: Foot and Ankle Section, Department of Orthopaedics, Mayo Clinic and Mayo Foundation; and Mayo School of Medicine, Rochester, Minnesota.

tients with grade II hallux rigidus and reserve the isolated cheilectomy for grade I disease with prominent symptomatic dorsal osteophytes.

The indications for this procedure are hallux rigidus, which is painful, disabling, and refractory to nonoperative treatment. Additional indications include stiff, painful range of motion of the MTP joint, difficulty with footwear, and recurrent bursitis or skin callosity over prominent osteophytes. It may be indicated for recurrent abrasion or skin ulceration over the prominent osteophytes once the ulcer is healed.

The contraindications are a foot with vascular insufficiency, infection or ulceration, and sensory neuropathy. A relative contraindication is a patient who is noncompliant.

## PREOPERATIVE PLANNING

The clinical features of hallux rigidus includes pain in the first MTP joint region, with restricted active and passive range of motion. Osteophytes, particularly on the dorsal aspect, cause mechanical block to dorsiflexion and are easily palpable. The patient may complain of difficulty with footwear because of the enlargement of the joint and osteophyte formation. Occasionally, the osteophytes may reach a large size and cause irritation of adjacent sensory nerves such as the dorsomedial cutaneous nerve to the hallux. In this circumstance, the patient may complain of dysesthetic pain. Painful motion and crepitus may occur with sagittal motion. The range of motion of the first MTP should be measured with goniometer and recorded. We use the plantar surface of the foot and the axis of the proximal phalanx for range of motion measurements (Fig. 1). Other physicians measure the position of the toe relative to the metatarsal axis, recognizing that the angular measurement obtained is influenced by the height of the arch. Dorsiflexion of 25° in a cavus foot is of more concern than in a flat foot. During clinical evaluation, care should be taken to note the posture and the range of motion of the interphalangeal (IP) joint. This joint often develops compensatory hypermobility in dorsiflexion. Failure to recognize hyperextension of the IP joint can result in poor outcome and patient dissatisfaction if this joint becomes painful and arthritic postoperatively. The IP joint should be held in a neutral position when measuring MTP motion (Fig. 10-1), or the degree of the dorsiflexion will be overestimated.

Radiographs should be obtained to evaluate the severity of the joint degenerative disease and to determine the presence of concurrent pathology. Radiograph evaluation should include standing anteroposterior and lateral views (Fig. 10-1 and 10-2). The anteroposterior view can be useful in evaluating medial and lateral osteophytes, toe alignment, joint space

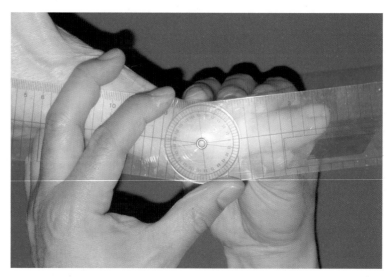

**Figure 10-1.** Clinical photo of a patient with painful hallux rigidus, showing restriction of dorsiflexion as measured with a goniometer.

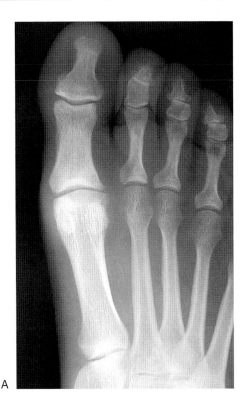

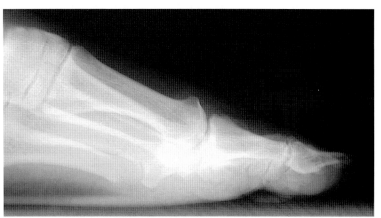

**Figure 10-2.** Radiographs of a 62-year-old man with painful grade II hallux rigidus and with prominent dorsal osteophytes. Anteroposterior **(A)** and lateral **(B)** standing radiographs of the foot.

A

B

narrowing, and condition of the adjacent joints. The standing lateral view is helpful because it demonstrates the dorsal osteophytes and reveals the extent of joint space narrowing. Hyperextension of the IP joint can be appreciated in this view, but this usually is determined clinically. The oblique view of the foot can help visualize early joint space narrowing (Fig. 10-2C). Based on the radiographic findings, the grade of the hallux rigidus can be determined (Table 10-1). Advanced diagnostic studies could be performed but are rarely indicated.

## SURGERY

The closing wedge osteotomy with cheilectomy can be performed using ankle block, spinal, or general anesthesia. It is usually performed as outpatient procedure. Patient is placed supine, and the extremity is prepared and draped up to the knee. The extremity is exsanguinated over a sterile, double stockinet using a 4-inch, rubber Esmarch bandage. In most cases, when ankle block anesthesia is administered, the rubber bandage is then wrapped at the ankle level several times for hemostasis. As an alternative, a sterile tourni-

**Table 10-1.** *Grading system for hallux rigidus*

| Grade | Finding |
|-------|---------|
| I | Mild to moderate osteophyte formation |
|   | Minimal joint space narrowing |
| II | Moderate osteophyte proliferation |
|   | Subchondral sclerosis |
|   | Mild joint space narrowing |
| III | Marked osteophyte formation |
|   | Marked joint space narrowing |

Data from Regnauld, B.: The foot: pathology, aetiology, semiology, clinical investigation, and treatment. Berlin: Springer-Venlag, 1986:335–350. R. Elson, translator.

quet may be used at the ankle. In patients who have general or spinal anesthesia, a thigh tourniquet may be used.

## Technique

The preoperative range of motion in the first MTP joint is again tested. The 5- to 6-cm skin incision is made over the medial aspect of the toe and centered over the first MTP joint (Fig. 10-3). The capsule is then longitudinally incised to expose the underlying first MTP joint and the base of the proximal phalanx (Figs. 10-4 and 10-5). Cheilectomy is performed with a microsagittal saw, resecting the dorsal one fourth of the metatarsal head approximately in line with the dorsal cortex of the metatarsal shaft (Fig. 10-6). The range of motion is improved in dorsiflexion after cheilectomy. The prominent medial eminence, medial and lateral osteophytes may then be resected. The base of the proximal phalanx is exposed sharply with a no. 15 blade scalpel, avoiding circumferential resection of the base. Right-angle retractors, such as Senn retractors, may be used for retraction. A closing wedge osteotomy is marked with a skin scribe, designed to remove about a 6-mm wedge of bone. Using a microsagittal saw with a thin, sharp blade, the osteotomy is performed. The proximal cut is aligned parallel with the phalangeal joint surface, and the distal cut is fashioned obliquely (Fig. 10-7A–D). Although the proximal cut should be placed close to the joint, the concave joint surface of the proximal phalanx and its preoperative radiographic morphology should be taken into account to avoid penetrating the joint surface with the first cut. The osteotomy cuts should extend to but not through the plantar cortex, and the tendon of flexor hallucis longus should be protected during the osteotomy cuts with a retractor. The plantar cortex should be left intact at the completion of these cuts and excision of the wedge (Fig. 10-7E). Occasionally, we use a 0.045-inch Kirschner wire to create multiple perforations in the plantar cortex that facilitate completion of the osteotomy (Fig. 10-7F). The osteotomy is then gently closed, hinging on the plantar cortex and the plantar periosteum (Fig. 10-7G).

A 1.5-mm drill or a 0.062-inch Kirschner wire is used to make two small drill holes in the dorsal aspect of the proximal phalanx on either side of the osteotomy (Fig. 10-8A). The drill holes should be placed 2 mm from the edge of the osteotomy so that an adequate bone bridge is left to allow tightening of the flexible wire fixation. We typically use a flexible, 22-gauge, stainless steel wire (Ethicon Inc., Johnson and Johnson, Westbury, MA). The wire is passed through distal hole first, and then the wire is fed into the tip of an 18-gauge needle to facilitate passage. Alternatively, steel wire on a cutting needle (Ethicon Inc., Johnson and Johnson, Westbury, MA) may be used. After placement of the dorsal wire, a second wire is placed dorsomedially in a similar fashion (Fig. 10-8B). Both wires are then tightened gently using a needle holder (Fig. 10-8C,D). Care must be exercised to avoid overtightening, which may cause the wire to break or cut through the bone bridge.

*(Text continues on page 142.)*

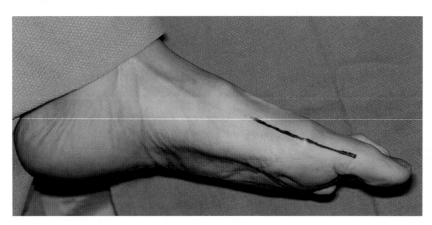

**Figure 10-3.** The medial longitudinal incision is marked.

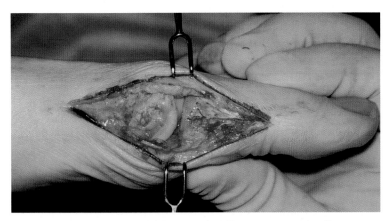

**Figure 10-4.** The capsule is incised longitudinally to expose the first metatarsopha-langeal joint, the proximal phalanx, and metatarsal head.

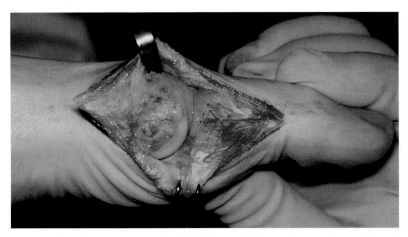

**Figure 10-5.** The soft tissues are carefully dissected from the metatarsal head and the base of proximal phalanx. The osteophytes then become visible.

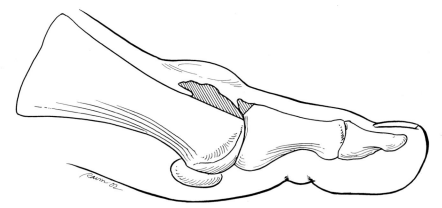

**Figure 10-6.** Schematic drawing of cheilectomy, removing the dorsal one fourth of the metatarsal head. When present, osteophytes on the dorsal base of the proximal phalanx and loose osteochondral fragments are removed.

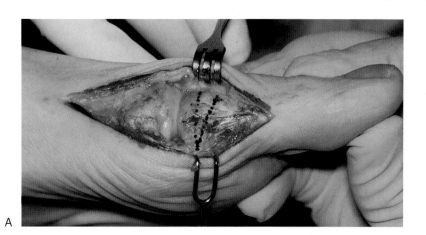

A

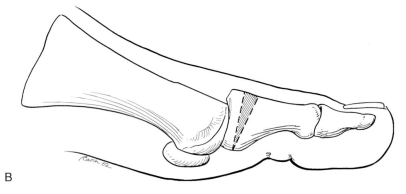

B

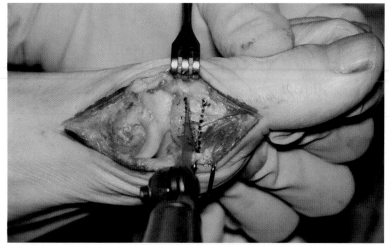

C

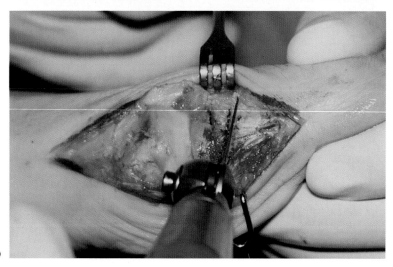

D

**Figure 10-7. A:** Osteotomy cuts are marked. The base of the wedge should measure approximately 6 mm. **B:** The drawing shows the planned osteotomy. The proximal cut is parallel to the joint surface **(C)**, and the distal cut is oblique **(D)**. *(continued)*

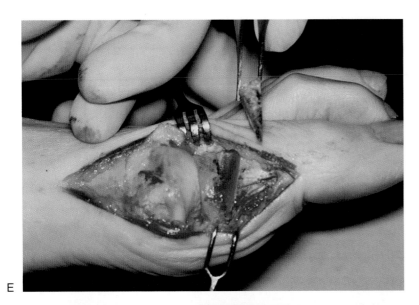

E

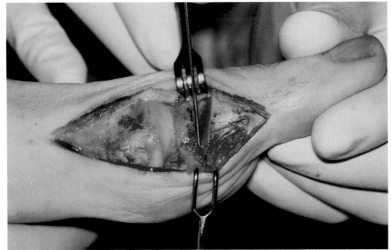

F

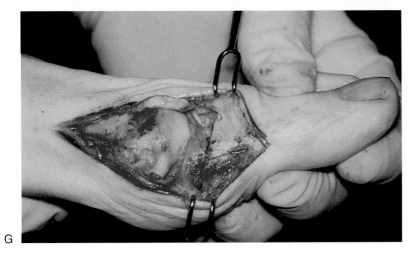

G

**Figure 10-7.** *Continued.* **E:** The dorsal wedge is excised, ensuring that the plantar cortex and the periosteum remain intact. The plantar cortex is perforated with a Kirschner wire **(F)** and then gently closed **(G)**.

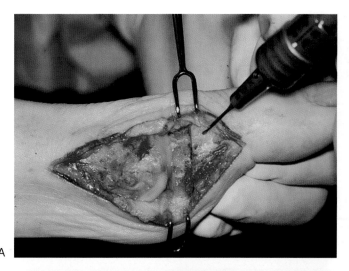

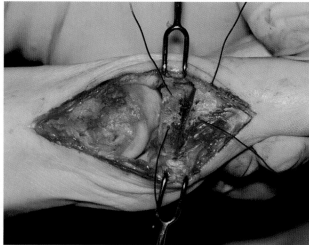

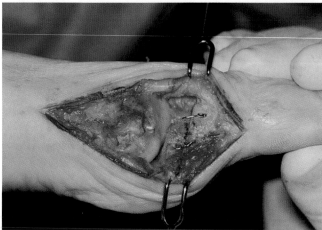

**Figure 10-8. A:** Two drill holes are made on the dorsal surface of the phalanx on either side of the osteotomy cuts, and two drill holes are made dorsomedially. The holes are placed approximately 2 mm from the bone cuts to leave an adequate bone bridge. **B:** Two 22-gauge, stainless steel wires are passed through the drill holes dorsally and dorsomedially. **C:** The osteotomy is closed, the toe is supported, and the wires are tightened. The ends of the wires are buried in bone. **D:** Closing wedge osteotomy of the proximal phalanx with cheilectomy.

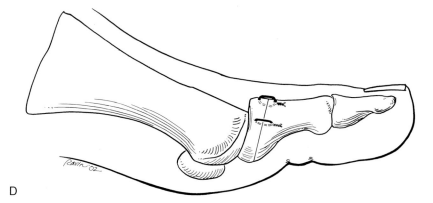

Once the wires are tightened, the stability of fixation is tested. In cases of questionable stability, one or two supplementary Kirschner wires may be used. The toe is then tested for adequacy of motion, which should be approximately 70° to 75° of dorsiflexion relative to the plantar foot (Fig. 10-9). The tourniquet is released, the joint irrigated, and hemostasis obtained. We use 2-0 Vicryl suture to close the capsule and the subcutaneous tissues. The skin is closed using 4-0 nylon sutures in interrupted horizontal mattress fashion. A sterile dressing and Robert Jones compressive splint are applied. Radiographs are obtained intraoperatively and postoperatively to assess bony apposition and fixation placement (Fig. 10-10).

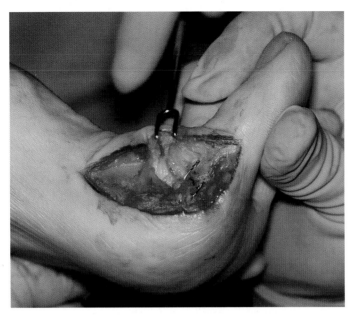

**Figure 10-9.** The toe is tested for range of motion and stability of the fixation. Approximately 70° to 75° of dorsiflexion is obtained at the end of the procedure.

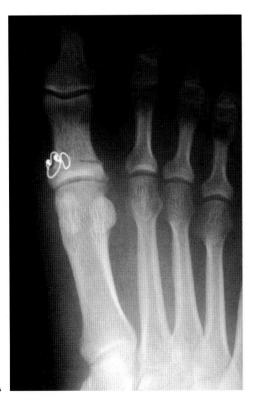

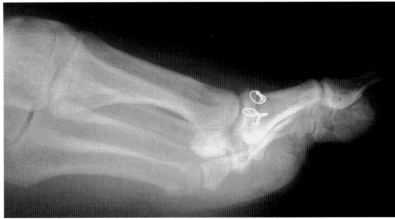

**Figure 10-10.** Postoperative anteroposterior **(A)** and lateral **(B)** radiographs.

A

B

## POSTOPERATIVE MANAGEMENT

The surgery is performed on an outpatient basis. The patient is instructed to continue elevating the operated extremity, and the wound is inspected 24 to 48 hours after the surgery. At this time, the dressing is changed, and the foot is immobilized in a rigid postoperative shoe or walking boot. At 3 weeks postoperatively, the sutures are removed, and the patient is allowed to weight bear as tolerated. Gentle passive range of motion exercises are initiated 3 weeks postoperatively. At 6 weeks postoperatively, radiographs are obtained, and if the osteotomy is united, the patient is allowed to wear loose-fitting, closed-toe shoes.

Results of combined cheilectomy and closing wedge osteotomy have been reported to be superior compared with cheilectomy alone (14). Based on the review of 24 toes undergoing combined cheilectomy and closing wedge osteotomy, Thomas and Smith (14) concluded that addition of the dorsal-closing wedge osteotomy of the proximal phalanx increases patient satisfaction and functional outcome in patients with moderate hallux rigidus.

Other studies have confirmed satisfactory results after closing wedge osteotomy. Citron and Neil (3) reported the long-term results of dorsal wedge osteotomy in eight women (ten toes) with a mean age of 23 years. All the patients had relief from pain soon after the surgery. At 22 years of follow-up, five toes were completely symptom free, four others had slight discomfort but were able to engage in all activities of daily living, and only one had required MTP fusion. Blyth et al. (1) reported excellent or good results, at an average follow-up of 4 years, in 14 of 18 toes that underwent dorsal wedge osteotomy. Others have reported good functional outcome after 10 closing wedge osteotomies (13).

The osteotomy is technically more challenging than isolated cheilectomy. It includes a period of protected weight bearing and does carry potential of additional complications compared with cheilectomy. However, there is growing concern regarding persistent pain and MTP joint stiffness in patients with hallux rigidus after cheilectomy. There are also reports confirming progression of the underlying degenerative disease process (4,6,11), and abnormal MTP motion patterns have been noted following cheilectomy (7). In a cadaveric model, the increase in dorsiflexion after cheilectomy was found to be caused by pivoting of the proximal phalanx on the metatarsal head at the level of the cheilectomy (7). The abnormal MTP kinematics may account for the progression of the disease after cheilectomy. Mulier et al. (11) observed that 7 of 13 of their young patients exhibited radiologic progression of the disease within 4 years of their cheilectomies. Similarly, clinical and radiologic progression of the disease of at least one grade was seen in 32 of 68 feet in patients who underwent cheilectomy (4). Fifteen (88%) of the 17 feet with grade I disease before surgery progressed one or two grades, and 24 (62%) of 39 feet with grade II hallux rigidus progressed to grade III (4). The outcome of cheilectomy for hallux rigidus is thought to be more favorable in patients with milder disease (6).

## COMPLICATIONS

The complications of proximal phalangeal osteotomy with cheilectomy include nonunion, delayed union, or malunion. Avascular necrosis of the base of the phalanx and flexor hallucis longus tendon injury have been observed after other proximal phalangeal osteotomies, such as the Akin osteotomy procedure, and are potential problems associated with the Moberg osteotomy. Persistent stiffness and limited increase in motion could result from an inadequate wedge resection. Inadvertent penetration of the phalangeal joint surface by the saw blade can also occur. This complication can be avoided by careful examination of the morphology of the phalanx and by placing a Kirschner wire parallel to the joint surface to orient the first bone cut.

## RECOMMENDED READING

1. Blyth MJ, MacKay DC, Kinninmonth AW: Dorsal wedge osteotomy in the treatment of hallux rigidus. *J Foot Ankle Surg* 37:8–10, 1998.

2. Bonney G, Macnab I: Hallux valgus and hallux rigidus: a critical survey of operative results. *J Bone Joint Surg Br* 34:366, 1952.

3. Citron N, Neil M: Dorsal wedge osteotomy of the proximal phalanx for hallux rigidus: long-term results. *Bone Joint Surg Br* 69:835–837, 1987.

4. Easley ME, Davis WH, Anderson RB: Intermediate to long-term follow-up of medial approach dorsal cheilectomy for hallux rigidus. *Foot Ankle Int* 20:147–152, 1999.

5. Haddad SL: The use of osteotomies in the treatment of hallux limitus and hallux rigidus. *Foot Ankle Clin* 5:629–661, 2000.

6. Hattrup SJ, Johnson KA: Subjective results of hallux rigidus following treatment with cheilectomy. *Clin Orthop* 226:182–191, 1988.

7. Heller WA, Brage ME: The effects of cheilectomy on dorsiflexion of the first metatarsophalangeal joint. *Foot Ankle Int* 18:803–808, 1997.

8. Kessel L, Bonney G: Hallux rigidus in the adolescent. *J Bone Joint Surg Br* 40:668, 1958.

9. Mann RA, Coughlin MJ, DuVries HL: Hallux rigidus: a review of the literature and a method of treatment. *Clin Orthop* 142:57–63, 1979.

10. Moberg E: A simple operation for hallux rigidus. *Clin Orthop* 142:55–56, 1979.

11. Mulier T, Steenwerckx A, Thienpont E, et al.: Results after cheilectomy in athletes with hallux rigidus. *Foot Ankle Int* 20:232–237, 1999.

12. Regnauld B: *The foot: pathology, aetiology, semiology, clinical investigation and treatment.* Berlin: Springer-Verlag, 1986:335–350. Elson R, translator.

13. Southgate JJ, Urry SR: Hallux rigidus: the long-term results of dorsal wedge osteotomy and arthrodesis in adults. *J Foot Ankle Surg* 36:136–140, 1997.

14. Thomas PJ, Smith RW: Proximal phalanx osteotomy for the surgical treatment of hallux rigidus. *Foot Ankle Int* 20(1):3–12, 1999.

# 11

# Realignment of Lesser Toe Deformities

## Harold B. Kitaoka and E. Greer Richardson

## INDICATIONS/CONTRAINDICATIONS

A variety of lesser toe (i.e., toes two through five) deformities, such as the hammer toe, claw toe, crossover toe, and mallet toe, may be associated with pain and footwear restrictions. Although much attention has been focused on the treatment of problems of the great toe (e.g., hallux valgus, hallux varus), deformities of the lesser toes often cause severe, debilitating symptoms even when there is no association with a hallux valgus deformity. Deformities of the lesser toes may involve the metatarsophalangeal (MTP) or interphalangeal (IP) joint or both and may involve single or multiple digits. The incidence of pain and impairment due to second MTP synovitis, MTP joint instability and dislocation has become more evident in recent years.

The many causes of lesser toe deformities include neuromuscular diseases and peripheral neuropathies such as Charcot-Marie-Tooth disease; connective tissue diseases; inflammatory arthritides (e.g., rheumatoid arthritis, Reiter's disease, psoriatic arthritis); traumatic injuries; compartment syndrome, congenital anomalies, and iatrogenic causes. Anatomic factors and constricting footwear also play roles in the development of lesser toe deformities. A long second toe is at risk for becoming a mallet toe or hammer toe. Irregularity in the shape of the middle phalanx can cause deviation of the distal phalanx. Extrinsic pressure of the hallux against the second toe may result in hammer toe deformity, subluxation, or dislocation of the MTP joint.

Choosing the appropriate surgical procedure for individual deformities can be difficult, and recommendations in the literature often are conflicting. Elements from several soft tissue and bony procedures are usually combined to completely correct the deformity. According to Kelikian (12), "the main function of the toes is to contact the proffered surface and exert strong enough pressure on it to obtain purchase, a fixed point from which the

H. B. Kitaoka, M.D.: Foot and Ankle Section, Department of Orthopaedics, Mayo Clinic and Mayo Foundation; and Mayo School of Medicine, Rochester, Minnesota.

E. G. Richardson, M.D.: Orthopaedic Surgery, Campbell Clinic-University of Tennessee, Germantown; and Foot and Ankle Service and Fellowship, Department of Orthopaedic Surgery, University of Tennessee Teaching Hospital, Memphis, Tennessee.

body can be propelled." Treatment should aim to restore this function to the lesser toes, to alleviate pain, and to allow a reasonable variety of footwear. Thorough evaluation and careful treatment choices can obtain these goals in most patients with lesser toe deformities, remembering that these deformities often are multiplanar and complete correction of the deformity while maintaining full motion of the joints of the involved digit may not be possible. Before surgery, patients must be made aware of the complexity of these seemingly straightforward deformities.

The term *hammer toe* is used most often to describe an abnormal flexion posture of the proximal interphalangeal (PIP) joint of one of the lesser four toes. The flexion deformity may be fixed (i.e., not passively correctable to the neutral position) or flexible (i.e., passively correctable). If the flexion contracture at this middle joint of the digit is severe and of long enough duration, the MTP joint becomes deformed in the opposite direction (i.e., extension). The distal interphalangeal joint (DIP) may stay supple, but it too may develop an extension or a flexion deformity.

*Claw toe* and *hammer toe* are sometimes used interchangeably, but most physicians generally differentiate the deformities by the following:

1. Claw toes frequently are caused by neuromuscular diseases, and often a similar deformity is present in all toes, whereas a hammer toe deformity usually affects only one or two toes.
2. Claw toes always have extension deformity at the MTP joint, but in hammer toe deformity, abnormal extension of the MTP joint may or may not be present.
3. Claw toes often have a flexion deformity at the DIP joint, but this usually does not occur in hammer toes.

Three areas may be painful in lesser toe deformity. The most common area is the dorsum of the PIP joint in the hammer toe and crossover toe or at the DIP joint in the mallet toe. A corn caused by pressure from the toe box or vamp of the shoe develops. When a flexion posture of DIP joint is present, a painful callus will develop just plantar to the nail end. This is called an *end corn*. A painful callus may develop beneath the metatarsal head if the proximal phalanx subluxates dorsally. In patients who have conditions that result in decreased sensibility, such as diabetes mellitus or myelomeningocele, ulceration and deep infection can develop at one or more of these areas of pressure, complicating the treatment plan and endangering the toe or foot.

Nonoperative treatment of lesser toe deformities can be disappointing. Various pads and straps are commercially available to reduce the deformity and relieve pressure over painful points. If the deformity is of short duration and an extension deformity at the MTP joint is not present, daily manipulation and taping the toe have been attempted to improve MTP extension and PIP flexion. However, recurrence is likely after the passive stretching and taping ceases, and many patients with symptomatic hammer toes eventually require surgery. Only the symptomatic toe should undergo surgery. An unattractive deformity that is painless is not an indication for surgical correction.

## PREOPERATIVE PLANNING

The use of soft tissue reconstruction procedures alone may or may not result in permanent correction of lesser toe deformities (Table 11-1). However, in a skeletally immature foot with symptomatic flexible hammer toes or a young adult foot with dynamic flexible deformities of one or more toes (e.g., prominent hammering only with weight bearing) that interfere with footwear, flexor-to-extensor tendon transfer may be appropriate.

The most commonly used procedure for the correction of hammer toe is hemiphalangectomy, which involves resection of the condyles of the proximal phalanx. Hammer toe encompasses a spectrum of deformities, and the indicated procedure varies, depending on the stage of the deformity when first seen and the diagnosis.

Treatment of hammer toe deformity should focus on the PIP joint and sometimes the MTP joint. Any fixed deformity of the PIP joint exerts a linkage effect at the MTP joint, and maximal active and passive flexion of the MTP joint will be slowly but relentlessly de-

**Table 11-1.** *Classification of lesser toe deformities*

| Deformity | Characteristics | Treatment |
|---|---|---|
| Flexible hammer toe | No fixed contracture at MTP or PIP joint | Usually nonoperative. Rarely, flexor to extensor transfer using FDL |
| Rigid hammer toe with MTP subluxation | Fixed flexion contracture at PIP; MTP subluxation in extension | Resection of condyles of proximal phalanx, dermodesis. Lengthening of EDL, tenotomy of EDB; MTP capsulotomy, collateral ligament sectioning |
| Claw toe | | |
| Rigid hammer toe with MTP dislocation | Fixed flexion contracture at PIP; complete MTP dislocation | Resection of condyles of proximal phalanx, dermodesis. Lengthening of EDL, tenotomy of EDB; MTP capsulotomy, collateral ligament sectioning. MTP arthroplasty or Weil osteotomy |
| Crossover toe | Fixed flexion contracture at PIP; MTP subluxation in varus or valgus | Resection of condyles of proximal phalanx, dermodesis. Collateral ligament/capsular repair. EDB transfer |
| Mallet toe | Fixed flexion contracture at DIP | Resection of condyles of middle phalanx, dermodesis. FDL tenotomy |

DIP, distal interphalangeal joint; EDB, extensor digitorum brevis; EDL, extensor digitorum longus; FDL, flexor digitorum longus; MTP, metatarsophalangeal joint; PIP, proximal interphalangeal joint.

creased. Over a lengthy period, the plantar plate (probably at the metatarsal neck origin) also becomes attenuated (i.e., cystic-mucoid degeneration of collagen). This attenuation decreases the ability of the plantar plate to prevent minor degrees of dorsal subluxation of the base of the proximal phalanx. The stage is set for an instability pattern in the sagittal plane to develop at the MTP joint.

After the base of the proximal phalanx with the first and second dorsal interossei insertions (in the second toe) subluxates dorsally, the flexion moment of the interossei at the MTP joint is decreased markedly because of their normal proximity to the instant center of rotation of the MTP joint on the metatarsal head. The interosseous tendons pass only a few millimeters plantar to this instant center of rotation. A weakened flexion moment at the MTP joint begins to surrender to intrinsic and extrinsic extensor forces at the MTP joint, and the MTP joint gradually deforms in extension and eventually become fixed. As the MTP joint postures into extension, the flexion forces at the PIP and to some degree DIP joints increase. Visualizing these pathologic mechanisms of deformity is helpful in surgical planning.

The mild, flexible hammer toe is often associated with limited symptoms and may be addressed with loose-fitting footwear with an adequate toe box, patient education, and observation. Occasionally, flexor-to-extensor transfer may be indicated. Operative treatment usually is performed in patients with lesser toe deformities for pain relief; these symptomatic patients are more likely to have rigid hammer toe without MTP subluxation, rigid hammer toe with MTP subluxation, rigid hammer toe with MTP dislocation, rigid crossover toe, or mallet toe. The operative approach to each is unique and is addressed separately.

## SURGERY

### Technique: Correction of Rigid Hammer Toe without Metatarsophalangeal Subluxation

Make an elliptical incision over the PIP joint. Remove the skin only initially, and cauterize the vessels. Remove a similar elliptically shaped segment of extensor tendon and dorsal capsule of the PIP joint. The proximal end of the extensor tendon usually retracts beneath the proximal skin flap, but it can be easily pulled distally during closure. Flex the PIP joint about 20° while putting traction on the distal and middle phalanges. Then, using a small-blade knife, section the collateral ligaments from outside in on both sides of the joint by placing the blade between the skin and the ligament and then turning the cutting edge toward the joint and lifting the capsule and tendon. The medial collateral ligament may also be sectioned by placing the blade in the joint transversely and carefully following the margin of the condyle medially and proximally. Similarly, the lateral collateral ligament may be sectioned by placing the blade in the joint transversely and carefully following the margin of the condyle laterally and proximally. Now the PIP joint can be flexed to 90°, and the head and neck (condyles) of the proximal phalanx are clearly exposed. With a rongeur or small-blade power saw, remove the head and neck of the proximal phalanx and smooth any sharp points of bone with a rasp or rongeur. Extend the ankle to neutral position (i.e., the push-up test), and feel for tightness with abutment of the articular surface of the middle phalanx on the distal end of proximal phalangeal remnant. If it feels tight, remove 2 or 3 mm more of bone. The push-up test should indicate that the PIP deformity is corrected and that there is no significant MTP subluxation. Use a 3-0 or 4-0 nonabsorbable suture for a vertical mattress suture, entering the proximal skin edge and then the proximal extensor tendon. Next, enter the distal extensor tendon on its joint surface and distal skin. Enter the distal skin near the edge and the proximal skin near the edge to complete the vertical mattress suture. Two of these stitches may be placed centrally, and a simple stitch in each corner. When the ankle is held in neutral position, if the MTP joint rests in a neutral position with no significant extension deformity, a supportive dressing to the tip of the toe may be applied.

This technique usually holds the PIP joint in acceptable alignment with only a few degrees of flexion. It is usually unnecessary to insert a Kirschner wire for fixation because of the dermodesis.

### Technique: Correction of Rigid Hammer Toe with Metatarsophalangeal Subluxation or Claw Toe

A more severe hammer toe deformity has a fixed flexion contracture at the PIP joint as well as a fixed extension contracture at the MTP joint; both joints require correction (Fig. 11-1). The toe deformity may be corrected starting at the PIP joint or at the MTP joint. The same operative treatment for the rigid hammer toe with MTP subluxation is applicable to the symptomatic claw toe.

Begin at the MTP joint with an angled or, alternatively, a straight longitudinal incision centered over the MTP joint (Fig. 11-1B,C). Cauterize or retract the dorsal veins to expose the extensor tendons. The extensor digitorum brevis (EDB) is located more lateral and deep to the extensor digitorum longus (EDL). The EDB will join the EDL and extensor expansion at the neck of the metatarsal (Fig. 11-1D). Before this confluence, dissect the EDB from the EDL, and remove a 2- to 3-mm segment of EDB (Fig. 11-1F). Then perform a Z-plasty lengthening of the EDL (Fig. 11-1G). The use of a small blade (no. 67 Beaver or similar) is helpful. Lift the tendon away from other soft tissue attachments. This maneuver lengthens the EDL and improves the MTP subluxation.

With the ankle held at 90°, if the toe then rests in neutral position at the MTP joint, this is all that is required to correct this joint, except for suturing the EDL in its lengthened position with 3-0 absorbable suture after the PIP joint deformity has been addressed. However, if after this procedure, the toe still rests in extension, a dorsal MTP capsulotomy is done transversely (Fig. 11-1I). After the capsule is divided, position the ankle to 90°, observing the resting posture of the toe. If the MTP posture is acceptable with no MTP subluxation, all that is needed is to suture the EDL in its lengthened position. If the toe still has an unacceptable extension posture, acutely flex the toe and incise the collateral ligaments on both sides of the MTP joint down to but not through the plantar plate of the joint. This should allow the toe to assume a neutral position (i.e., no MTP subluxation with the push-up test) at the MTP joint even if the toe was severely subluxated dorsally.

The operation to remove the condyles of the proximal phalanx is performed as described previously, and it can address the PIP flexion deformity. It is usually advisable to fix the

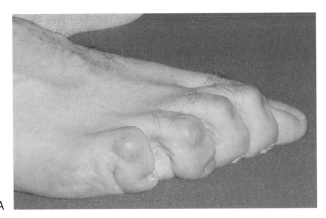

A

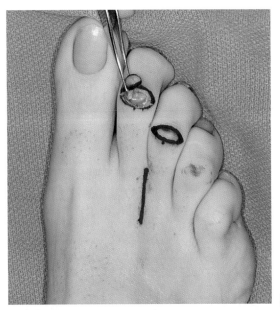

B

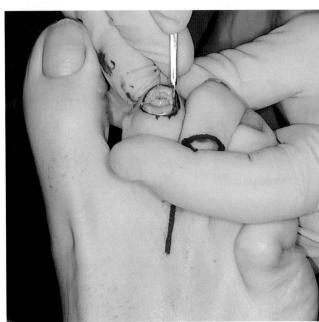

C

D

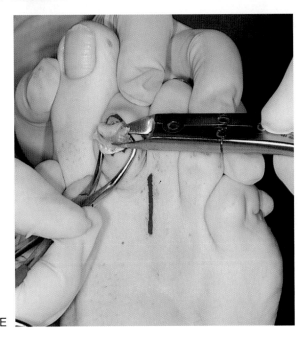

E

**Figure 11-1.** Correction of rigid hammer toe with metatarsophalangeal (MTP) subluxation or claw toe. **A:** Preoperative photograph shows multiple claw toes with end corns. **B:** Placement of incisions over the proximal interphalangeal (PIP) joint of second and third toes. For second and third MTP joint exposure, a single longitudinal incision may be made between the distal second and third metatarsals. An elliptical incision is made through the skin and extensor mechanism of the second PIP joint. **C:** The dorsal PIP capsulotomy is made transversely. **D:** Collateral ligaments are sectioned to expose the head and neck of the proximal phalanx. **E:** A towel clip placed over the phalanx provides excellent exposure for resection of the head and neck (condyles) with a bone cutter and rongeur. *(continued)*

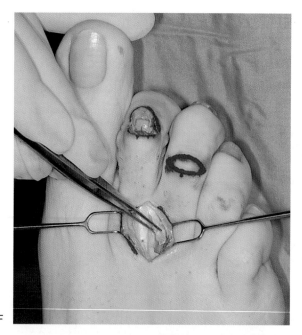

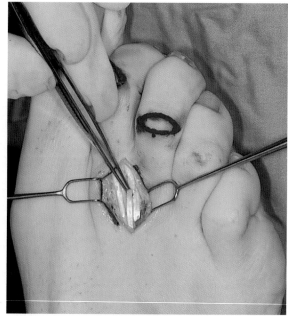

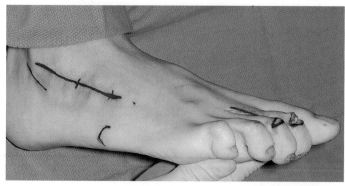

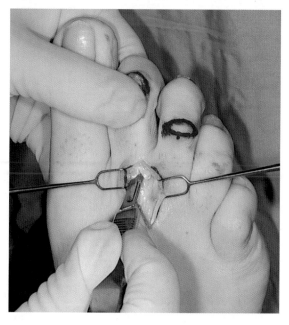

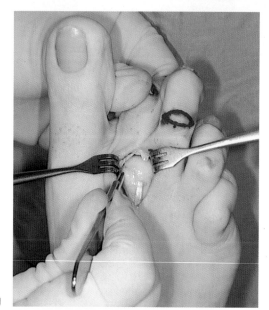

**Figure 11-1.** *Continued.* **F:** A longitudinal incision is made to expose the second MTP joint. The extensor digitorum brevis (EDB) tendon is seen lateral to the extensor digitorum longus (EDL) tendon and is sectioned. **G:** The EDL tendon is lengthened in Z-plasty fashion. **H:** Push-up test. Dorsiflexion of the ankle to neutral demonstrates persistent dorsal subluxation of the MTP joint even after tendon lengthening, indicating a need for further MTP reconstruction. **I:** The dorsal MTP capsulotomy is performed transversely, and the push-up test is repeated. **J:** Collateral ligaments of the MTP are joint sectioned. *(continued)*

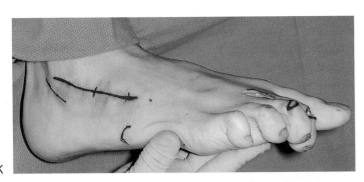

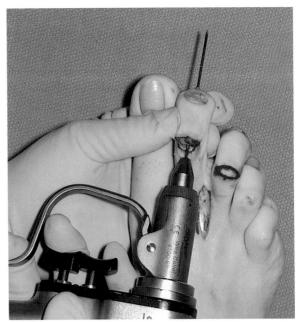

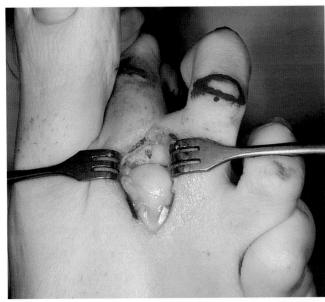

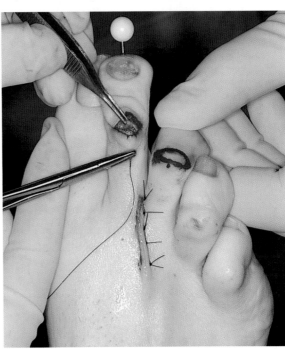

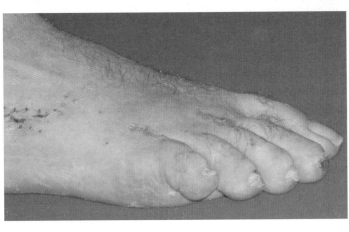

**Figure 11-1.** *Continued.* **K:** The push-up test now shows no subluxation of the MTP joint. **L:** A 0.062-inch K wire is inserted antegrade through middle and distal phalanges to exit 2 to 3 mm below nail plate distally. **M:** With the PIP joint fully extended, the Kirschner wire is advanced retrograde through proximal phalanx to exit in the center of the joint surface. **N:** The Kirschner wire is advanced retrograde across the MTP joint and into metatarsal while holding the MTP joint in a reduced position. The extensor mechanism and skin over the PIP joint are closed with a horizontal mattress stitch. **O:** Appearance of the toe after wound closure. *(continued)*

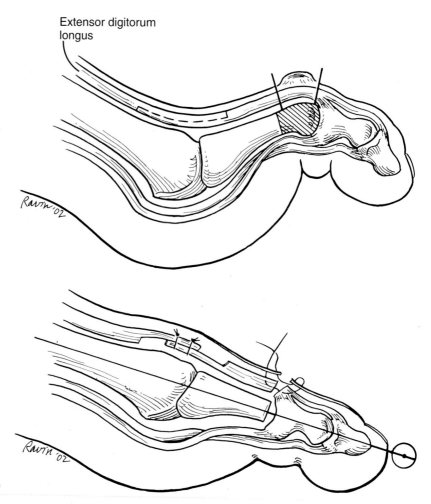

Extensor digitorum longus

**Figure 11-1.** *Continued.* **P:** Drawing of selected components of the hammer toe or claw toe correction. Upper part shows a deformity at the PIP and MTP joints and the level of resection of the head and neck of the proximal phalanx. Lower part shows the vertical mattress stitch at the PIP level, Z-lengthening of the EDL tendon, and Kirschner wire placement with the PIP and MTP joints in the corrected position. (**A–O,** Copyright the Mayo Clinic and Mayo Foundation, Rochester, Minnesota.)

toe with a 0.062-inch Kirschner wire. The technique of pinning can vary, but one suggestion is to place the pin from distal to proximal through the middle and distal phalanges, exiting in the midline 2 to 3 mm plantar to the nail plate (Fig. 11-1L). The pin then is passed from distal to proximal through the shaft of the proximal phalanx to the base of the phalanx with the PIP joint reduced. The pin exits the articular surface of the proximal phalanx near the center of the joint surface, and while holding the MTP joint reduced, advance the pin into the metatarsal. Sometimes, aligning the pin through the medullary canal of the proximal phalanx and exiting the center of the joint surface are difficult. Predrilling the proximal phalanx with a 0.062-inch Kirschner wire allows the wire to find its way without exiting the cortex before reaching the proximal articular surface. After pin placement, suture the EDL, and close the PIP extensor mechanism and skin as described previously.

### Technique: Correction of Rigid Hammer Toe with Metatarsophalangeal Dislocation Using Metatarsophalangeal Arthroplasty

This deformity can be difficult to correct, to the extent that some surgeons have performed toe amputation. All the earlier recommendations are applicable, including resection of the condyles of the proximal phalanx, EDL lengthening, EDB tenotomy, dorsal MTP capsulotomy, and bilateral MTP collateral ligament release. Decompression of the MTP joint usually is required. This can be done on the phalangeal or metatarsal side of the joint. Resecting the base of the proximal phalanx is simple, but it is currently not recommended, because the MTP joint often becomes unstable, and the toe subluxates or dislocates dorsally with recurrent symptoms. There is no acceptable salvage procedure for failure. This recurrent deformity occurs even after the toe is pinned for several weeks.

The MTP joint can be decompressed at the metatarsal side of the dislocated joint. Resecting and contouring the distal margin of the metatarsal head, including its plantar projection, can help to reduce the MTP joint; this is the so-called DuVries procedure. This does not return the joint to a normal condition, but it usually restores acceptable MTP alignment, allows limited motion, and results in sufficient stability for the joint to remain reduced. Contouring the metatarsal head enough to allow reduction of the MTP joint and passively total joint motion of 30° to 40° provides an acceptable result. Usually, the MTP and PIP joints are stiff even before surgery, but the patient may not be aware of it.

The operation is performed through the same angled or, alternatively, longitudinal incision to the MTP joint that was used for the MTP capsulotomy. The MTP joint is flexed to expose the metatarsal head (Fig. 11-2). The most distal margin of the condyles of the metatarsal head are resected with a sharp, 8- or 10-mm-wide osteotome, preserving the plantar condyles. The margins of the bone cut are rounded or contoured. If the MTP joint reduction is not stable with the push-up test, more bone is removed. A long-standing toe dislocation results in erosion of the dorsal margin of the metatarsal head by the base of the proximal phalanx, which may require slightly more bone to be resected than the usual 3 to 6 mm to create a stable reduction.

The toe alignment is maintained for 3 to 4 weeks with a longitudinal, 0.062-inch Kirschner wire pinned in neutral to slight extension and neutral varus-valgus position while holding the ankle at 90°. After contouring the metatarsal head, if the MTP joint still feels tight with the proximal phalanx grating on the contoured metatarsal head, more bone should be removed until the grating stops.

Remove the tourniquet and obtain hemostasis. Suture the EDL in a lengthened position. Close the skin with 4-0 nonabsorbable suture, and place a forefoot dressing, being careful not to constrict the toes.

In the chronically dislocated toe, reducing deformities and contractures at both the MTP and PIP joints may place tension on the neurovascular bundles. The reoperated toe is particularly vulnerable, with attendant scarring and compromised dorsal venous return. If the appearance of the toe is a concern after realignment, loosen the dressing and "piston" the toe proximally on the pin in case the toe and vessels are inadvertently distracted along the pin. Observe the toe closely for 10 minutes. If necessary, remove the Kirschner wire, and the toe will "pink up." Removing the pin early is a concern, and the surgeon needs to maintain the toe in an acceptable position. Some prefer to use only the dressing to hold the joint in the desired position for 3 weeks without the routine use of a pin. A patient who requires extensive dissection on adjacent joints (e.g., PIP, MTP) of the same toe, particularly a reoperated toe, must be advised preoperatively that loss of the toe from vascular compromise could occur.

## Technique: Correction of Rigid Hammer Toe with Metatarsophalangeal Dislocation Using a Weil Osteotomy

Nearly all of the previous recommendations for the rigid hammer toe with complete MTP dislocation are applicable: resection of condyles of proximal phalanx, EDL lengthening, EDB tenotomy, dorsal MTP capsulotomy, and MTP collateral ligament release (Figs. 11-3 and 11-4). Some form of decompression of the MTP joint is required. Some concerns have been raised that the MTP arthroplasty described earlier may cause excessive MTP stiffness. Although restoring MTP joint stability is essential, if motion is too restricted, patients may become aware of the MTP stiffness postoperatively. An oblique osteotomy of the metatarsal neck (i.e., Weil) is designed to shorten the metatarsal and decompress the

*(Text continues on page 159.)*

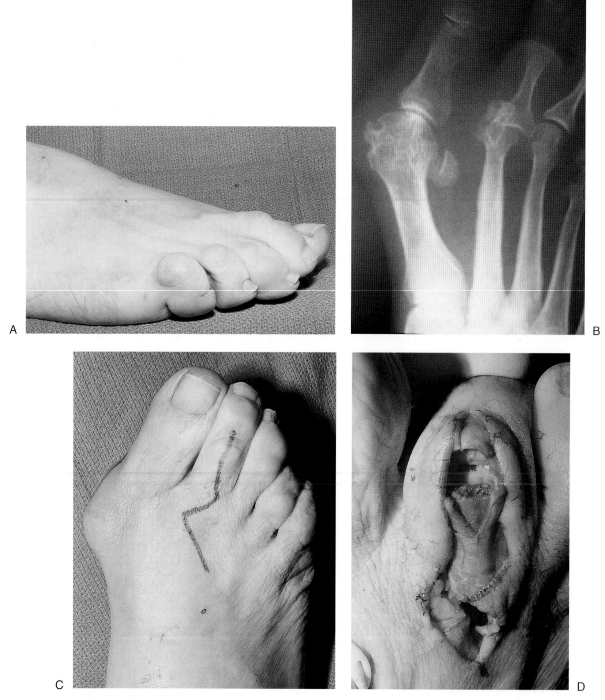

**Figure 11-2.** Correction for rigid hammer toe with metatarsophalangeal (MTP) dislocation using MTP arthroplasty. **A:** Clinical appearance, lateral view. Notice the hammer toe of the second and the dorsal prominence at the base of the toe, representing the dislocated base of the proximal phalanx tenting the skin. **B:** An anteroposterior radiograph shows hammer toe of the second with complete dislocation of the MTP joint. **C:** Dorsal view of foot shows a planned V-shaped incision over the MTP joint, extending proximally over the proximal phalanx and proximal interphalangeal (PIP) joint. **D:** After resection of the head and neck of the proximal phalanx, the extensor digitorum longus (EDL) tendon is lengthened, and the extensor digitorum brevis (EDB) tendon is sectioned. Dorsal MTP capsulotomy and sectioning of MTP collateral ligaments are performed. The base of the proximal phalanx remains dislocated even after extensive soft tissue release about the MTP joint, indicating a need for MTP arthroplasty. *(continued)*

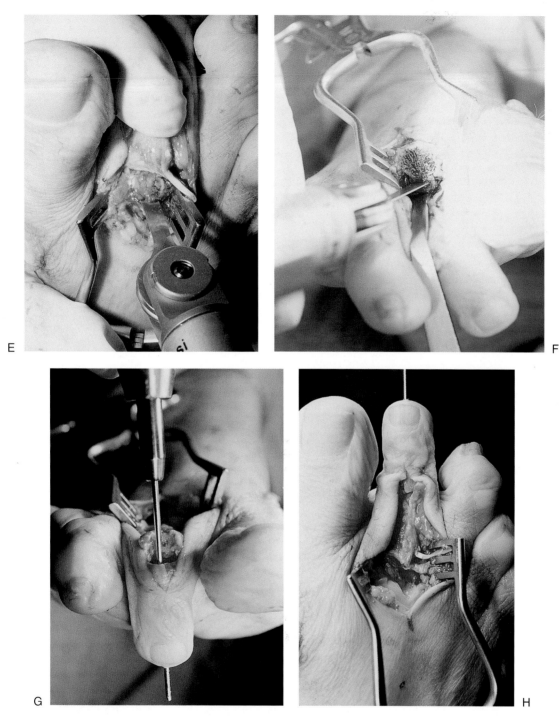

**Figure 11-2.** *Continued.* **E:** Resection of the distal portion of the metatarsal head with a microsagittal saw or sharp osteotomy. **F:** The toe is flexed to expose plantar condyles of the metatarsal. Plantar condylectomy of the metatarsal head is performed with a microsagittal saw or sharp osteotome. The head is then contoured with a rongeur to a rounded shape. **G:** Antegrade pinning through middle and distal phalanges with 0.062-inch Kirschner wires. **H:** Retrograde pinning through the proximal phalanx across the PIP and MTP joints with the toe held in a corrected position. *(continued)*

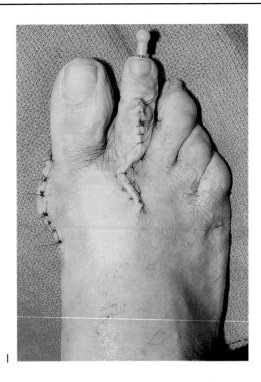

**Figure 11-2.** *Continued.* **I:** Postoperative appearance. (From Murphy GA, Richardson EG: Lesser toe abnormalities. In: Canale ST, ed. *Campbell's operative orthopaedics*, 9th ed. St. Louis: Mosby–Year Book, 1998:1746–1783, with permission.)

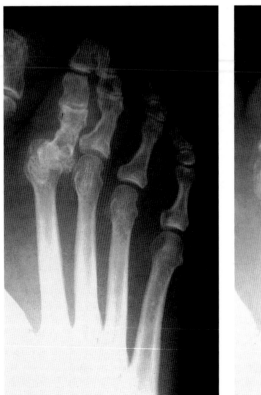
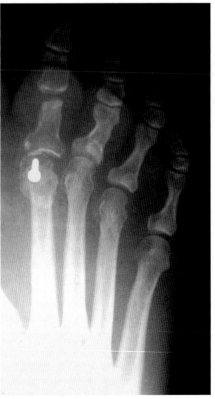

A                                                                                          B

**Figure 11-3.  A:** Correction for rigid hammer toe with metatarsophalangeal (MTP) dislocation using the Weil osteotomy. Anteroposterior radiographs show the hammer toe with long-standing MTP dislocation. **B:** Anteroposterior radiograph after a Weil osteotomy shows the MTP joint reduced, a shortened second metatarsal, and screw fixation.

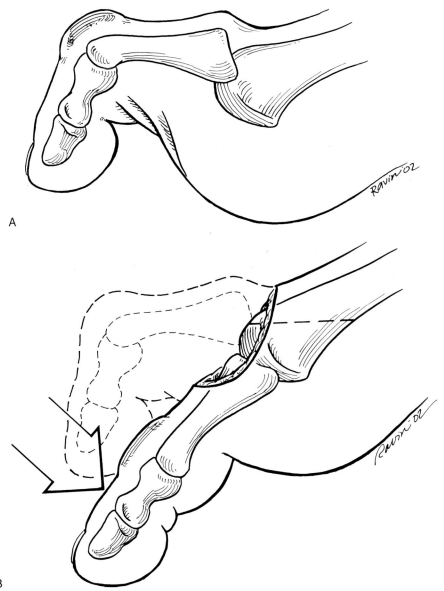

**Figure 11-4.** Weil osteotomy. **A:** Dislocated metatarsophalangeal joint. **B:** Toe flexed, with an oblique osteotomy marked from the dorsal margin of the metatarsal head proximally in a plane parallel to the plantar surface of the foot. *(continued)*

MTP joint, resulting in a more stable reduction while preserving the metatarsal articular surface.

The operation may be accomplished by extending the longitudinal MTP incision proximally, exposing the metatarsal head and neck. An oblique osteotomy is performed with a microsagittal saw from distal to proximal, starting at the dorsal margin of the metatarsal articular surface (Fig. 11-3). The saw blade is angled in a plane parallel to the plantar surface of the foot. The osteotomy is displaced proximally about 6 to 8 mm. For the second metatarsal, it is usually desirable to shorten the metatarsal length to match the third metatarsal. This amount of shortening is usually adequate to restore MTP stability and to relieve the metatarsalgia with limited risk of transfer metatarsalgia.

Fixation is accomplished with a single, 2.0-mm cortical screw oriented obliquely from proximal to distal. A twist-off screw also provides good fixation. Before placing the screw, temporary fixation may be achieved with a 0.035-inch Kirschner wire, which is removed after screw fixation. A longitudinal, 0.062-inch Kirschner wire may be used to supplement

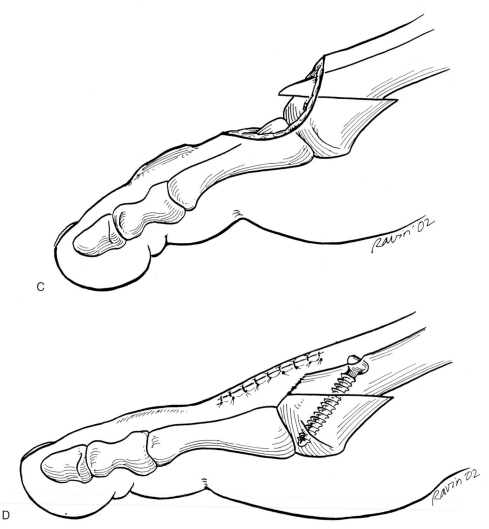

**Figure 11-4.** *Continued.* **C:** Osteotomy is shortened about 6 mm proximally. **D:** Fixation with a 2.0-mm cortical screw from proximal to distal. Dorsally, the uncovered metatarsal head and neck fragment is removed. A twist-off screw may also be used for fixation.

fixation, if desired. The MTP joint capsule and skin are closed. Patients are immobilized in a stiff postoperative shoe for 3 weeks, at which time the sutures and pin are removed. The postoperative shoe is continued for an additional 2 to 3 weeks until osteotomy union occurs. There has not been a study comparing the Weil osteotomy with the DuVries MTP arthroplasty for the dislocated MTP joint, but results of the osteotomy appear to be favorable for a difficult problem. The concern about transfer metatarsalgia is viable, although many of the patients with long-standing MTP dislocation and hammer toe have painful intractable plantar keratosis under the metatarsal head, which will be relieved by this operation. Some surgeons perform osteotomy on multiple metatarsals simultaneously for other primary diagnoses such as metatarsalgia without dislocation, but we usually apply it to a single osteotomy for the completely dislocated MTP joint associated with a hammer toe.

### Technique: Correction of Crossover Toe

A hammer toe may be associated with deviation in the varus-valgus plane. This deformity is called a crossover toe, because it crosses the adjacent toe or toes. The indications for surgery vary with the severity of the deformity. There are two common complaints that may require surgery. The first is pain in the second MTP joint from chronic synovitis (5). This usually occurs with mild or moderate deformities. The second complaint is mechanical impingement of the toe on the adjacent hallux in the toe box of the shoe. With time, the MTP synovitis symptoms subside, while the impingement symptoms deformities over the dorsal PIP joint increase (Fig. 11-5).

The inciting event is thought to be synovitis of the second MTP joint in which the fibular collateral ligament, lateral capsule, and even the second dorsal interosseous tendons are weakened through incremental attrition. The deformity progresses in direct proportion to the laxity of the lateral supporting capsular structures and finally results in plantar plate insufficiency.

The physical examination should not only focus on the obvious deformity, but also on the rest of the foot. A fixed varus deformity of the third toe may require correction to allow space for realignment of the corrected second toe. Similarly, if the hallux is in so much valgus that there is no space for the repositioned second toe, it is likely that the second toe deformity will recur. In some instances, addressing the hallux valgus deformity operatively is reasonable even if it is not a primary complaint. Any fixed toe contractures such as MTP joint extension or PIP joint flexion should be noted and corrected.

The test popularized by Thompson and Hamilton (8) for evaluation of the competence of the plantar plate and MTP joint involves stabilizing the second metatarsal with one hand and attempting to translate the base of the proximal phalanx dorsally, similar to a Lachman test of the knee. The test should be performed on an uninvolved toe for comparison. The second MTP joint should be inspected for loss of the skin extension creases suggestive of a joint effusion or slight subluxation or rotation of the second toe (i.e., splaying of the toes). The examiner should sense the ease with which the MTP joint can be reduced and how readily it returns to its dislocated position. Likewise, the stability and mobility of all of the MTP joints should be tested in multiple planes.

The plantar surface of the foot should be inspected for painful callosities beneath the metatarsal head. A callosity is one sign of an altered loading caused by an MTP extension posture, with or without a fixed contracture. Flexion contractures may be observed at the PIP and DIP joints in the overlapping toe.

In mild deformities, serial taping or splinting of the second toe in a reduced position, antiinflammatory medications, and selective use of an intraarticular corticosteroid injection may avoid the need for surgery. The indication for surgery is a painful, rigid crossover toe. A contraindication for surgical repair of this deformity is insufficient vascular supply to the toe. Relative contraindications are severe, rigid deformities of the hallux (in valgus) and third toe (in varus) to the extent that the second toe cannot be adequately realigned.

The second MTP joint is approached through a chevron incision with its apex at the MTP joint or by a longitudinal incision. The distal limb of the incision crosses obliquely over the proximal half of the proximal phalanx, and the proximal limb crosses the second metatarsal obliquely at the neck–distal metaphysis level (Fig. 11-6A). The subcutaneous tissues are dissected from the extensor apparatus and the interval between the EDL and the EDB tendons is identified in the proximal portion of the wound. The EDB approaches the MTP joint from lateral to medial and becomes confluent with the EDL at the level of the metatarsal neck (Fig. 11-6B). By detaching the EDB tendon from its confluence with the EDL more distally over the base of the proximal phalanx, a longer tendon is available for later transfer. The EDL is lengthened in a Z-plasty fashion (Fig. 11-6C).

The MTP capsule is inspected carefully with an angled probe, and any weakness in the capsule is identified. An abnormality is usually found in the integrity of the dorsolateral and lateral aspects of the capsule to the extent that the lateral base of the proximal phalanx and adjacent lateral surface of the metatarsal head may be completely exposed. If the entire lateral capsule is disrupted, the second dorsal interosseous tendon usually is disrupted as well because of its intimate course towards the base of the proximal phalanx.

With small right-angle (Ragnell) retractors placed laterally, the proximal phalanx is displaced medially and dorsally, and the joint is further inspected and palpated with the probe to evaluate the integrity of the plantar plate. If the plantar plate is disrupted from the neck of the metatarsal, soft tissue realignment procedures will often fail to maintain reduction in the long term. An intact plantar plate allows extreme MTP extension without disruption.

The phalanx is reduced congruously on the metatarsal head, and its stability is evaluated.

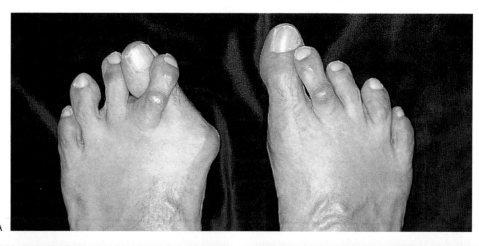

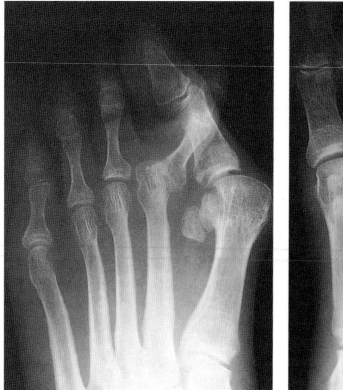

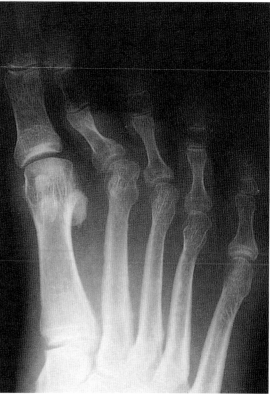

**Figure 11-5. A:** The photograph shows a severe crossover toe deformity in the left foot with hallux valgus. The hallux is contacting the third toe on the left. **B:** Anteroposterior radiograph of the left foot shows severe crossover deformity with the metatarsophalangeal joint almost dislocated. This is severe hallux valgus. **C:** An anteroposterior radiograph of the right foot shows varus malalignment of all the toes, particularly the second.

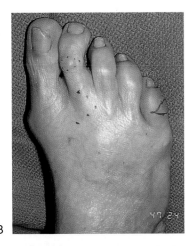
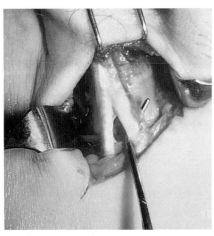
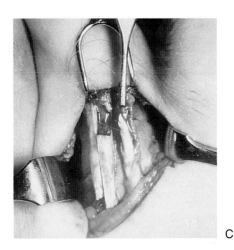

A, B                                                                          C

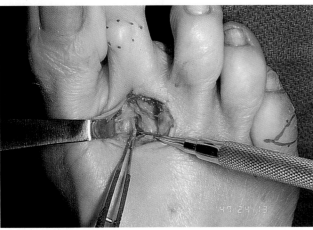
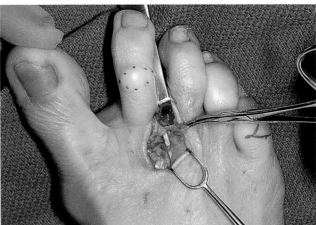

D                                                                            E

**Figure 11-6.** Crossover toe realignment operation. **A:** Dorsal view of the foot with crossover toe of the second (i.e., varus metatarsophalangeal [MTP] malalignment), hammer toe of the second, and synovitis of the second MTP joint. Skin incisions are marked. Notice the angled incision for MTP joint exposure, which has its apex at the fibular border of the MTP joint. **B:** Probe beneath the extensor digitorum brevis (EDB) tendon, and notice the junction with the extensor digitorum longus (EDL) at the MTP joint. **C:** The EDL has been lengthened in a Z fashion, and the EDB has been dissected and released about 1 cm distal to the MTP joint. **D:** Probe beneath thickened tibial collateral ligament and intrinsic muscle tendon. **E:** EDB tendon is passed through a tunnel in the extensor expansion and sutured to itself after remaining fibular capsular structures have been sutured.

If it springs back into its original position, the medial capsule is examined. In a severe, long-standing overlapping toe, the medial capsule may be very thick and contracted, and it should be released, usually along with the tibial collateral ligament. The dorsal capsule is incised transversely if the second MTP joint cannot be easily flexed to a neutral position. Even with extensive soft tissue release about the MTP joint (except for the plantar plate), the toe may still tend to deviate medially. Even the skin may be contracted in long-standing deformities.

Any fixed contractures of the PIP joint must be addressed as described previously for the hammer toe correction, removing the head and neck of the proximal phalanx. After the PIP and MTP contractures have been addressed, the EDB tendon is transferred through a tunnel in the lateral extensor hood as far plantarward as possible. Having an assistant translate the toe dorsally while the tunnel is made and the tendon is transferred makes this step easier. After the tendon is passed through the tunnel of tissue on the lateral base of the proximal phalanx, the MTP joint is overreduced in valgus of about 10°, and the tendon end is brought proximally and sutured back to itself. A sharp retractor is used to pull the third metatarsal head laterally, and a suture is placed as far plantar as possible toward the plantar plate of the second MTP joint, beginning proximally and passing the needle distally to tissue near the lateral side of the base of the proximal phalanx. If possible, another suture is placed in the same area dorsal to the EDB transfer, which is approximately in the midline.

After the EDB transfer and repair of the lateral capsule, the reduction is examined. The toe should rest congruously on the metatarsal head, the toe is held in 10° to 20° of flexion, and the EDL is sutured in a lengthened position. The dorsomedial capsule is not repaired. The skin is closed with interrupted absorbable sutures.

### Technique: Correction of Mallet Toe

Mallet toe refers to a flexion posture of the DIP joint (Fig. 11-7); it can occur as an isolated entity or in conjunction with hammer toe deformity, in which the deformity occurs at the PIP joint. The cause of mallet toe is uncertain; however, it occurs most often in the second toe, which is frequently the longest toe. This projection of the second toe distal to the other toes can cause pressure at the tip of the toe and buckling at the DIP joint in a shoe with a narrow or short toe box. With time, this flexion posture can attenuate the EDL tendon until it can no longer effectively extend the distal joint. Moreover, the flexor digitorum longus (FDL), in the absence of a strong antagonist, holds the DIP joint in flexion as the deformity eventually becomes fixed. In feet with normal sensibility, the most frequent complaint is a painful end corn just beneath the nail. In patients with peripheral neuropathy such as diabetics, the tip of the toe can ulcerate before the patient is aware of the problem. The conservative treatment of mallet toe with pads and splints is generally unrewarding.

Surgery usually involves resection of the condyles of the middle phalanx with dorsal dermodesis. A tenotomy of the FDL can be added if the bony resection and dermodesis do not hold the toe in the corrected position. Occasionally, other procedures may also be indicated, such as amputation of the distal half of the distal phalanx, which includes the nail and the matrix. Transfer of the deforming FDL to the extensor mechanism to correct a flexion deformity this far distal is technically difficult and not recommended. In elderly patients, a flexor tenotomy at the DIP flexion crease may be adequate to relieve the symptoms. Flexor tenotomy usually is combined with manual correction of any fixed flexion contracture at this joint. The wound is closed with one or two sutures, and a wooden-soled shoe is recommended until the sutures are removed at 2 weeks. The patient is encouraged to wear adequately long shoes with wide toe boxes after the sutures are removed.

If the mallet toe deformity is painful, of long duration, and fixed in severe flexion, resection of a portion or all of the middle phalanx, dorsal dermodesis, with or without tenotomy of the flexor digitorum longus effectively corrects the malalignment. Center a dorsal, transverse, elliptical incision over the DIP joint through skin and extensor mechanism (Fig. 11-7B). The dorsal capsule is incised transversely and collateral ligaments are divided (Fig. 11-7C). Acutely flex the distal phalanx to expose the middle phalanx and remove the head and neck of the middle phalanx. If the toe is still flexed, an FDL tenotomy is performed through the same dorsal incision or a separate plantar incision. (Fig. 11-7D) A 5-mm transverse incision in the flexion crease of the DIP joint can be made, being careful to avoid the neurovascular bundles at the ends of the incision. Using a small, single-pronged hook, bring the FDL into the wound and sharply divide it. Alternatively, the FDL tenotomy can be performed through the dorsal incision after bony resection by incising the plantar plate of the DIP joint sharply and spreading it longitudinally with a small hemostat, bringing the tendon into the wound with a hemostat and then sectioning the tendon. If a tourniquet has been used, secure hemostasis before wound closure.

Close the dorsal incision with horizontal mattress stitches in the center and simple sutures on each side. This will provide enough stability that a pin may not be required. Close the plantar wound with simple interrupted sutures, and apply a dressing that maintains the toe in the desired position.

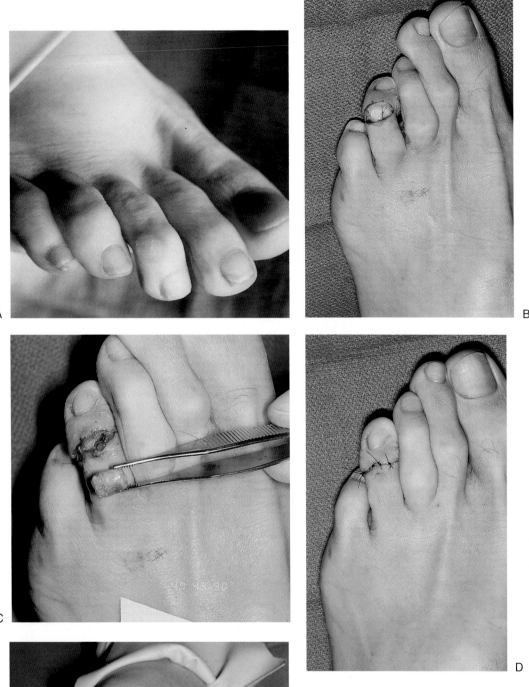

**Figure 11-7.** Procedure for correction of rigid mallet toe. **A:** Typical appearance of a painful mallet toe deformity of the third toe of the right foot. Notice the flexion deformity at the distal interphalangeal (DIP) joint and dorsolateral corn. **B:** Mallet toe correction of the fourth toe of the left foot. An elliptical skin incision is made over the distal interphalangeal (DIP) joint, through skin and extensor mechanism. **C:** Middle phalanx is exposed by dorsal capsulotomy, flexing the DIP joint and sectioning the collateral ligaments. The head and neck of the middle phalanx are resected. **D:** If necessary, a flexor digitorum longus tenotomy is performed. Kirschner wire fixation is used if desired. The extensor mechanism and skin are closed. A dorsal view of the postoperative alignment is shown. **E:** Appearance of the toe postoperatively. *(continued)*

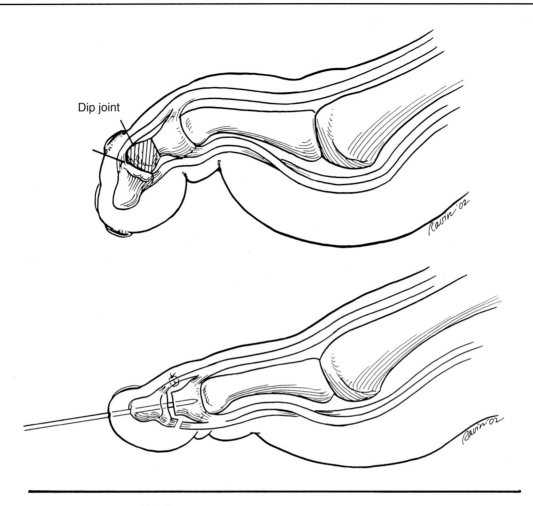

Dip joint

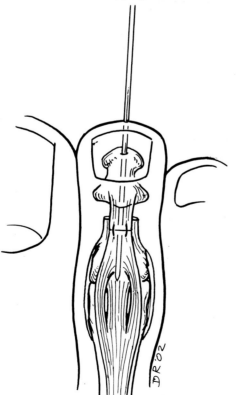

F

**Figure 11-7.** *Continued.* **F:** Drawing of selected components of mallet toe correction. Upper part shows mallet toe deformity at the DIP joint and the typical level of resection of the head and neck of the middle phalanx. Lower part shows the realigned DIP joint, repair of the extensor mechanism, a flexor tenotomy, and Kirschner wire placement.

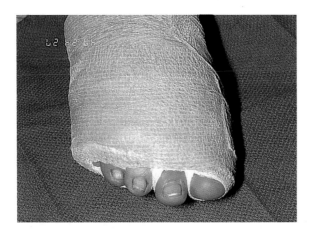

**Figure 11-8.** Form-fitting dressing for maintaining the position after lesser toe procedures.

## POSTOPERATIVE MANAGEMENT

Postoperative management principles are similar for the lesser toe realignment procedures. Weight bearing to tolerance is allowed in the early postoperative period, mostly on the heel. A stiff postoperative shoe is worn for 4 weeks. The sutures are removed at 2 to 3 weeks. Kirschner wires are usually removed at about 3 weeks postoperatively. As an alternative, a carefully applied corrective dressing or taping is used to maintains the toes in the corrected position for 4 weeks (Fig. 11-8). After hammer toe operations, the PIP joint retains a small amount of movement and is aligned in a gently flexed position, which seems to be more pleasing than a fused, straight toe at the PIP joint.

A closed-toe shoe with an adequate toe box is used after lesser toe procedures. It is common to have residual swelling for months after lesser toe procedures, and patients should be reminded of this. For the Weil osteotomy patients, a stiff postoperative shoe is used, and then at 3 weeks postoperatively, the pin is removed (when used). The postoperative shoe is continued for another 2 to 3 weeks until radiographs show osteotomy union.

## COMPLICATIONS

Recurrence of the toe deformity and reduced voluntary control of the digit may occur. Delayed wound healing and vascular compromise of the digit are less common but are more troublesome complications.

*Recurrence of the deformity* can be caused by several factors. If extrinsic, deforming forces are not addressed there is a higher likelihood of recurrence, such as severe hallux valgus or severe varus deviation of the of the third toe. Recurrent deformity may also result from the resumption of constrictive, fashionable footwear postoperatively. It may be caused by inadequate initial correction. The toe deformity should be fully corrected before placement of a longitudinal Kirschner wire. If it is less than optimal correction, removing the wire will result in rapid recurrence of malposition. There may also be recurrence if the wrong procedure is selected.

*Reduced voluntary control* of the digit is almost inevitable and should probably not be thought of as an operative complication. Nonetheless, the patient will notice this and must be advised before surgery that it will occur. If the patient is shown how little voluntary control actually is present at each joint of the toe *before surgery* compared with the other toes, this "complication" is more acceptable. Use of Kirschner wires for more than several weeks after surgery can contribute to stiffness. If excessive bone is removed, the toe may become flail. Certain operations that are known to create instability of the toe, such as removing the base of the proximal phalanx, should rarely be used.

*Delayed wound healing* at the MTP incision is most common in severe deformities such as MTP dislocation if the joint is not decompressed by an arthroplasty or osteotomy. After the MTP joint is reduced, marked tension remains at the skin edges. Limited debridement in the office and the continued use of the stiff postoperative shoe or even a walking boot reduce skin tension from movement of the foot and ankle and allow eventual healing.

*Vascular compromise of the digit* can be seen in revision lesser toe procedures or after reduction of the completely dislocated MTP joint with the use of Kirschner wire fixation. Should the toe not "perk-up" 10 minutes or so after the tourniquet is released, any constrictive dressing such as gauze placed between the toes is removed. If necessary, the pin is removed and a dressing applied to maintain position.

*Kirschner wear breakage* occurs infrequently, usually in a noncompliant patient who ambulates excessively. Zingas et al. (22) reported breakage of 33 Kirschner wires in 1002 wires used in 565 consecutive patients (failure rate of 3.2%). All wires that broke were 0.045-inch wires placed across lesser MTP joints, and most broke between 4 and 6 weeks after surgery. Zingas et al. (22) suggested that breakage might be prevented by using larger wires when possible and removing the wires earlier. If a broken Kirschner wire interferes with MTP joint function, it should be removed; however, most wires break just proximal to the joint surface and removal of the proximal portion is unnecessary.

## RECOMMENDED READING

1. Coughlin MJ: Crossover second toe deformity. *Foot Ankle* 8:29–39, 1987.
2. Coughlin MJ: Operative repair of the mallet toe deformity. *Foot Ankle Int* 16:109–116, 1995.
3. Coughlin MJ: Second metatarsophalangeal joint instability in the athlete. *Foot Ankle Int* 14:309–319, 1993.
4. Davies MS, Saxby TS: Metatarsal neck osteotomy with rigid internal fixation for the treatment of lesser toe metatarsophalangeal joint pathology. *Foot Ankle Int* 20:630–635, 1999.
5. Davis WH, Anderson RB, Thompson FM, et al.: Technique tip: proximal phalanx basilar osteotomy for resistant angulation of the lesser toes. *Foot Ankle Int* 18:103–104, 1997.
6. Fortin PT, Myerson MS: Second metatarsophalangeal instability. *Foot Ankle Int* 16:306–313, 1995.
7. Gazdag A, Cracchiolo A III: Surgical treatment of patients with painful instability of the second metatarsophalangeal joint. *Foot Ankle Int* 19:137–143, 1998.
8. Helal B: Metatarsal osteotomy for metatarsalgia. *J Bone Joint Surg Br* 57:187–192, 1975.
9. Idusuyi OB, Kitaoka HB, Patzer GL: Oblique metatarsal osteotomy for intractable plantar keratosis: 10-year follow-up. *Foot Ankle Int* 19:351–355, 1998.
10. Jahss MH: *Disorders of the Foot and Ankle,* 2nd ed, vol 2. Philadelphia: WB Saunders, 1991:1217–1221.
11. Johnson JB, Price TW: Crossover second toe deformity: etiology and treatment. *J Foot Surg* 28:417–420, 1989.
12. Kelikian H: Deformities of the lesser toes. In: *Hallux valgus and allied deformities of the forefoot and metatarsalgia.* Philadelphia: WB Saunders, 1965:382–387.
13. Mann RA, Coughlin MJ: Lesser toe deformities. *Instr Course Lect* 36:137–159, 1987.
14. Mann RA, Mizel MS: Monarticular nontraumatic synovitis of the metatarsophalangeal joint: a new diagnosis? *Foot Ankle* 6:18–21, 1985.
15. Mizel MS, Michelson JD: Nonsurgical treatment of monarticular nontraumatic synovitis of the second metatarsophalangeal joint. *Foot Ankle Int* 18:424–426, 1997.
16. Mizel MS, Yodlowski ML: Disorders of the lesser metatarsophalangeal joints. *J Am Acad Orthop Surg* 3:166–173, 1995.
17. Richardson EG: Lesser toe abnormalities. In: Crenshaw AH, ed. *Campbell's operative orthopaedics,* 8th ed. St. Louis: Mosby–Year Book, 1992.
18. Thompson FM, Hamilton WG: Problems of the second metatarsophalangeal joint. *Orthopedics* 10:83–89, 1987.
19. Trnka H-J, Mülbauer M, Zetti R, et al.: Comparison of the results of the Weil and Helal osteotomies for the treatment of metatarsalgia secondary to dislocation of the lesser metatarsophalangeal joints. *Foot Ankle Int* 20:72–79, 1999.
20. Vandeputte G, Dereymaeker G, Steenwerckx A, et al.: The Weil osteotomy of the lesser metatarsals: a clinical and pedobarographic follow-up study. *Foot Ankle Int* 21:370–374, 2000.
21. Weil LS: Weil head-neck oblique osteotomy: technique and fixation. Presented at Techniques of Osteotomies on the Forefoot, Bordeaux, France, October 20–22, 1994.
22. Zingas C, Katcherian DA, Wu KK: Kirschner wire breakage after surgery of the lesser toes. *Foot Ankle Int* 16:504–509, 1995.

# PART III

# Metatarsals, Midtarsal

# 12

# Primary Interdigital Neuroma Resection

Norman S. Turner and Harold B. Kitaoka

## INDICATIONS/CONTRAINDICATIONS

Pain in the forefoot is a common reason for presentation to health care providers. Numerous disorders can cause central forefoot symptoms that need consideration. One of these conditions is plantar interdigital neuroma, a condition in which a plantar interdigital nerve becomes compressed or entrapped as it courses in the plantar forefoot toward the toes.

Patients complain of burning pain or aching in the region of the second, third, and fourth metatarsophalangeal (MTP) joints plantarward. Patients can sometimes point to a specific web space where the pain is most intense, and at other times, it is a more ill-defined, diffuse aching. The pain can extend into the toes. It is more bothersome with footwear. According to Melvin H. Jahss, a pioneer in the orthopedic foot and ankle specialty, patients typically experience pain relief by sitting down, removing the shoe, and massaging the foot. He further states that pain from a neuroma does not extend proximally past the ankle.

Other sources of forefoot pain can be misdiagnosed as an interdigital neuroma, including MTP synovitis, rheumatoid arthritis, synovial cyst, or local infection. Metatarsalgia and plantar keratosis can give similar clinical presentations, although they generally are less painful with footwear and are more painful with barefoot ambulation. Lesser metatarsal stress fracture and Freiberg's disease should be considered. The surgeon should consider the possibility of a more proximal neurologic problem such as lumbar radiculopathy or tarsal tunnel syndrome. Nerve tumors such as neurilemoma and neurofibroma may occasionally occur in the forefoot.

Nonoperative measures for a Morton's neuroma include footwear modification (i.e., wide, soft shoes), metatarsal pads, orthotics or inlays, and cortisone injection in the web space. Despite these measures, it has been estimated that about one half of patients ultimately require excision of the interdigital neuroma as the definitive treatment.

The indication for resection of an interdigital neuroma is forefoot pain and impairment

N. S. Turner, M.D.: Department of Orthopedic Surgery, Mayo Clinic, Rochester, Minnesota.

H. B. Kitaoka, M.D.: Foot and Ankle Section, Department of Orthopaedics, Mayo Clinic and Mayo Foundation; and Mayo School of Medicine, Rochester, Minnesota.

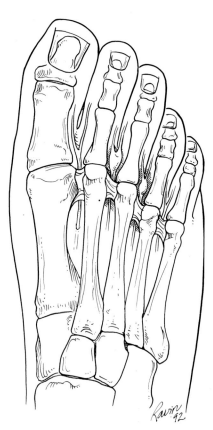

**Figure 12-1.** Central forefoot anatomy. Anteroposterior view of the foot shows a neuroma in the second web space and its location relative to the intermetatarsal ligaments.

recalcitrant to nonoperative measures. The pain is usually localized to the third web space, representing about 80% to 90% of interdigital neuromas (Fig. 12-1). The second web space accounts for the other 10% to 20%.

Contraindications are patients with diffuse forefoot pain or symptoms in a web space other than the third or second. This condition does not occur in the first or fourth web space. When considering a diagnosis of second web space neuroma, other causes must also be evaluated.

## PREOPERATIVE PLANNING

It is essential that the diagnosis is accurate before a resection of an interdigital neuroma. The usual complaint of a patient with an interdigital neuroma is central forefoot pain that is worse with footwear, especially tight-fitting shoes. It is usually described as a burning pain that is slowly relieved by resting the foot and exacerbated by activity. Patients often experience relief by removing the shoe and rubbing the foot. However, absence of this historical description does not exclude interdigital neuroma as the diagnosis.

These patients may describe a vague, slowly progressive forefoot pain that has persisted for a few months to many years. They may have difficulty in localizing the pain and may describe it by pointing to the entire forefoot. Less commonly, the pain may be localized to a specific web space. Sometimes, the only area where the patient perceives pain is in a toe adjacent to the involved web space. Other complaints are the sensation of a mass under the forefoot, described as a pebble in the shoe.

The physical examination is performed with the patient sitting, standing, and walking.

The neuroma may cause splaying between two of the lesser toes. However, this is a non-specific sign, because there are other causes of splayed toes, such as MTP synovitis. The patient may have a forefoot avoidance gait. Careful examination of the forefoot is mandatory because various disorders can cause forefoot pain, and they are often differentiated by the examination. It is sometimes difficult to determine a specific diagnosis when the patient is not having severe symptoms at the time of the examination. There should be an effort to recreate the pain during the examination.

The examination should include range of motion of the MTP joints, stability testing of the MTP joints with a Lachman-type test, and palpation of the metatarsal head, tenderness of the metatarsal dorsally, tenderness of the MTP joint dorsally, and tenderness of the web space. Swelling, erythema, toe deformities, and plantar keratoses should be noted.

A Mulder's click should be tested but is not always found. A Mulder's click is elicited by palpating from the distal and plantar forefoot between the toes, thereby trapping the mass between the metatarsal heads. The metatarsal heads are next compressed with the other hand from medial to lateral. This can result in a palpable and even audible click as the mass is forced plantarward (Fig. 12-2) with reproduction of pain. The presence of the click in association with recreation of the patient's symptoms is of clinical significance and strongly supports the diagnosis. There may also be paresthesias extending into the two adjacent toes with this maneuver. A nonpainful click can be observed in asymptomatic feet. The Mulder's click is helpful when it is present, but when it is not present, a diagnosis of interdigital neuroma is not excluded. Repeat examination on more than one occasion can help ensure accurate localization of the pain.

Sensory and motor function testing should be performed. Occasionally, patients have hypesthesia in the distribution of the affected common digital nerve. Percussion in the region of the common digital nerve usually does not cause paresthesias, but it is useful in other areas such as the posterior tibial nerve when other diagnoses are being considered, such as tarsal tunnel syndrome.

Standing anteroposterior, lateral, and oblique radiographs of the foot are essential to exclude any bony pathology that may be present. In more difficult cases, a bone scan may help to exclude occult bony processes that may be suspected, such as an early Freiberg's infraction. There are differing reports of the accuracy of diagnosis with magnetic resonance

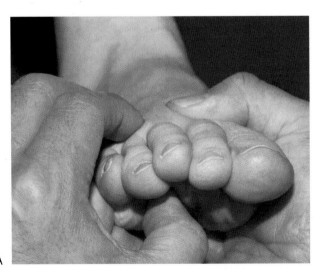
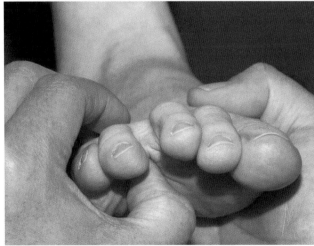

A                                                                                      B

**Figure 12-2.** Mulder's test. **A:** Deep palpation of the plantar forefoot in the third web space with the thumb of the left hand and no compression of the forefoot applied by the right hand. **B:** Deep palpation of the plantar forefoot in the third web space with the thumb of the left hand continues. On compression of the forefoot with the right hand, there is a detectable click, recreating the characteristic pain. This provocative test can sometimes cause paresthesias to extend into third and fourth toes as well. (Copyright the Mayo Clinic and Mayo Foundation, Rochester, Minnesota.)

imaging. Ultrasound is a more economical alternative, but the results are operator dependent and have not been reproduced. Electromyographic nerve conduction studies may be helpful in ruling out other neurologic causes of the presenting pain, but they are rarely indicated for neuromas.

Injection of corticosteroid and local anesthetic can be useful for treatment and for providing support for the diagnosis of interdigital neuroma. The injection is done by angling the needle from dorsal-distal to plantar-proximal directions, starting in the web space between the toes. Usually, a longer-acting anesthetic such as bupivacaine is used. Cortisone may be used at the same time if a longer-term conservative result is being sought in addition to the diagnostic information from the injection. The total amount of the injection should be approximately 1 mL of 0.5% bupivacaine and celestone Soluspan (4 mg/ml), or alternative corticosteroid suspension. The needle is palpated subcutaneously as it is advanced toward the plantar aspect. If cortisone is injected, the physician must ensure that the needle placement is accurate. Crossover toe deformities have resulted from injection of cortisone directly into a collateral ligament of the MTP joint and subsequent ligament rupture.

Before an injection, the patient should be instructed about its purpose. Results of an injection of a local anesthetic agent can help support the diagnosis. If the symptoms are not alleviated by an accurately performed injection, alleviating the problem by excising the affected nerve is less predicable. Diagnostic injections may also help differentiate pathology if two web spaces within the same foot seem to be affected. The patient should have consistent pain present at the time of injection to verify that the injection at least temporarily relieved the symptoms. Otherwise, there is a question about how to interpret the findings. There is also a concern regarding how to interpret the results if the central forefoot is flooded with a local anesthetic agent in multiple web spaces and the pain is relieved. If the injection does not alleviate the pain or other symptoms, it is possible that the injection was not accurately placed or an interdigital neuroma in that web space is not the proper diagnosis. Side effects from a single injection are rare but can include atrophy of the fat pad.

Rasmussen and Kitaoka (9) described results of a single corticosteroid injection for interdigital neuroma in the third web space in 51 feet of 43 patients. Most of the patients experienced initial pain relief from the injection. However, the symptoms recurred to the extent that 24 feet (47%) eventually underwent third web space neuroma resection. Symptoms were still present in the remaining patients who did not have surgery; they were irritating but not severe. The investigators concluded that the injection cannot be recommended as a cure for plantar interdigital neuroma, but it can be offered as temporizing measure or as nonoperative treatment. It is useful in patients who are not candidates for surgery because of local or general medical conditions.

The concept that an interdigital neuroma is caused by compression of the proper digital nerves and some surgeons recommend neurolysis one-centimeter distal to the transverse metatarsal ligament and three centimeters proximal. Okafor (8) reported his results in 35 patients and found that 72% of the patients with isolated interdigital neuroma had complete relief with neurolysis alone. Diebold et al. (4) report an excellent result in 37 of 40 patients after neurolysis, with 35 having normal toe sensation. An advantage to this procedure is the elimination of the stump neuroma. However, the standard operative treatment is resection of the neuroma and common digital nerve.

It is not unusual for patients to have forefoot pain from more than one source. Symptoms related to other problems such as MTP synovitis or metatarsalgia should be treated before considering operative treatment. In some instances, it is possible to avoid surgery if appropriate treatment of the other disorder is initiated and the patient experiences enough relief.

## SURGERY

This type of surgery can be done in an ambulatory surgery center or in a formal operative suite. The patient is placed in the supine position, facilitating the dorsal approach. A 4-inch Esmarch rubber bandage is wrapped around the ankle. A sterile supramalleolar tourniquet may also be used. Ankle block or local anesthesia is usually performed. Ankle block anesthesia performed by an anesthesiologist can be supplemented with light sedation. This is usually preferable to general anesthesia.

## Technique

A dorsal longitudinal incision is started in the appropriate web space between the toes and extended proximally 2 to 3 cm to about the level of the metatarsal heads (Fig. 12-3). It is important not to follow the extensor tendons, but to keep the incision between the metatarsals.

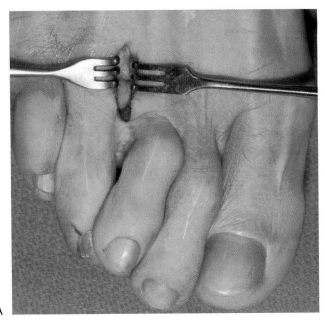

A

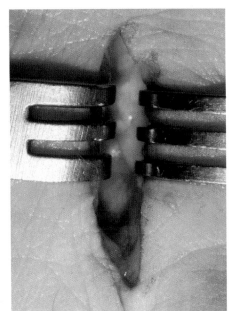

B

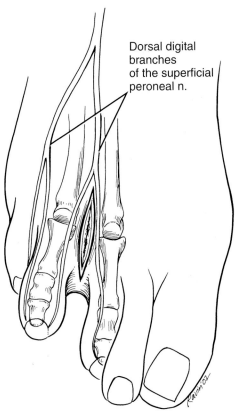

Dorsal digital
branches
of the superficial
peroneal n.

C

**Figure 12-3. A:** Placement of the incision in the third web space. **B:** Close-up view shows fascia between metatarsal heads. **C:** Illustration of the incision. (Figures 12-3A and 12-3B copyright the Mayo Clinic and Mayo Foundation, Rochester, Minnesota.)

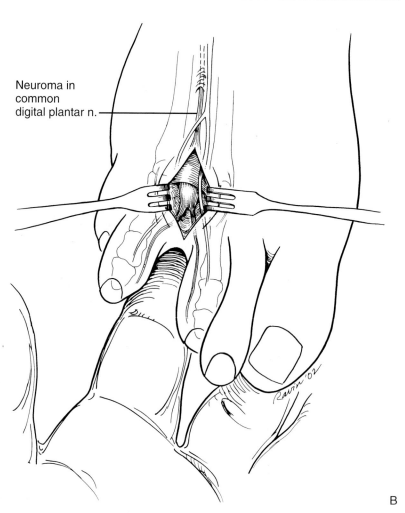

Neuroma in
common
digital plantar n.

**Figure 12-4. A:** Close-up view of third web-space with Freer elevator beneath transverse metatarsal ligament. **B:** Diagram showing deeper dissection of the third web space. The transverse metatarsal ligament is seen. (Figure 12-4A copyright the Mayo Clinic and Mayo Foundation, Rochester, Minnesota.)

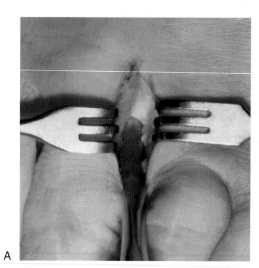

A

B

The dissection is deepened to the level of the metatarsal. A layer of fascia is located superficial to the intermetatarsal ligament and is transected (Fig. 12-3). Two sharp Senn retractors are used to separate the metatarsal heads. As an alternative, a self-retaining retractor such as a Weitlaner or neuroma retractor may be used between the metatarsal heads, which improves visualization and increases tension on the intermetatarsal ligament (Fig. 12-4). A Freer elevator is placed under the ligament to protect the underlying structures (Fig. 12-6). The ligament is then transected (Fig. 12-5). A bursa may be present.

Dorsally directed pressure can be applied to the plantar skin between the toes, distal to the metatarsal head level, and the neuroma should become obvious (Fig. 12-6). Bursa-like soft tissue may be present about the nerve and can be removed to allow better visualization. A fine, right-angle clamp or hemostat is carefully placed beneath the nerve to further improve visualization (Fig. 12-7). This method also has the advantage of minimizing trauma to the underlying fat pad. The common digital blood vessels are dissected away from the nerve. The nerve is then dissected distally to expose the bifurcation. Gentle tension is placed on the common digital nerve with the hemostat and the proper digital nerves are then sectioned distally (Figs. 12-8 and 12-9). Gentle traction is placed on the neuroma distally, and the common digital nerve is then sectioned at a level just proximal to the metatarsal heads (Figs. 12-10 and 12-11). More vigorous traction on the neuroma either during the division of the digital nerves or the common digital nerve will cause fragmentation of the mass. The specimen is sent for histologic examination. Structures that have been reportedly mistaken for the nerve include the lumbrical tendon, which passes to the medial portion of

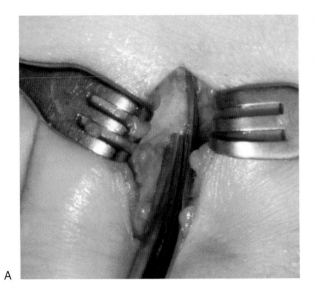

A

**Figure 12-5. A:** Transecting the transverse metatarsal ligament with scissors. **B:** Sectioning of the ligament. (Figure 12-5A copyright the Mayo Clinic and Mayo Foundation, Rochester, Minnesota.)

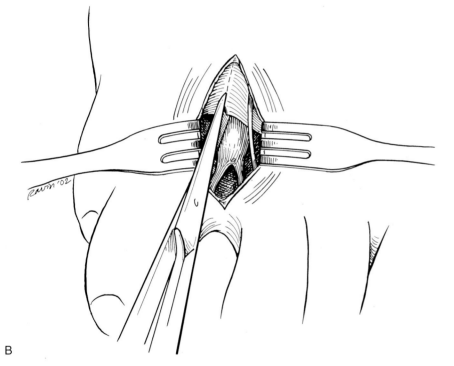

B

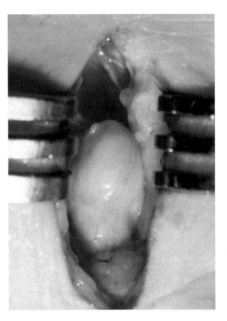

**Figure 12-6.** Close-up view of the third web space after the transverse metatarsal ligament is sectioned. The neuroma is clearly seen. (Copyright the Mayo Clinic and Mayo Foundation, Rochester, Minnesota.)

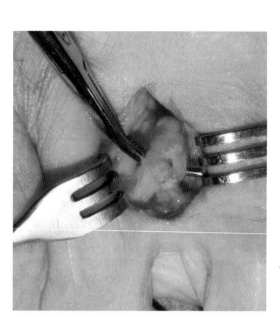

**Figure 12-7.** With gentle traction placed on the neuroma with the right-angle hemostat, each digital nerve is seen. (Copyright the Mayo Clinic and Mayo Foundation, Rochester, Minnesota.)

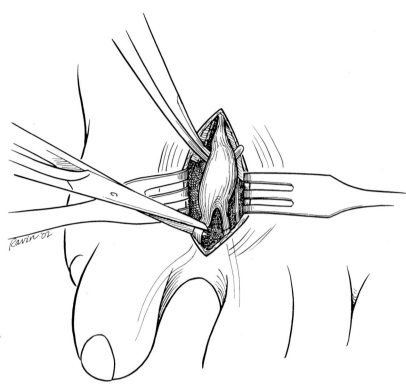

**Figure 12-8.** A hemostat placed deep to the neuroma and common digital nerve brings the neuroma and digital nerve branches into view.

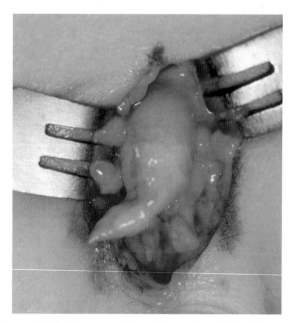

**Figure 12-9.** Close-up view of neuroma following transection of digital branches. (Copyright the Mayo Clinic and Mayo Foundation, Rochester, Minnesota.)

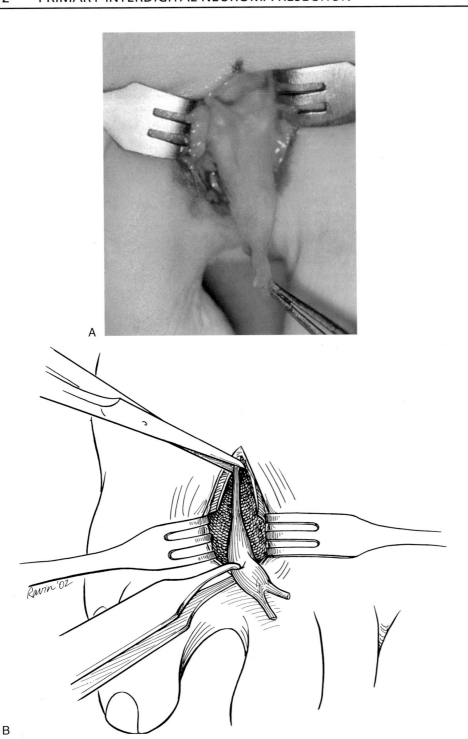

**Figure 12-10.** **A:** Gentle traction is placed on the neuroma and the common digital nerve distally with the hemostat. The common digital nerve is carefully dissected proximally. **B:** Transection of the common digital nerve proximally is performed under tension so the cut end of the nerve retracts proximally. (Figure 12-10A copyright of the Mayo Clinic and Mayo Foundation, Rochester, Minnesota.)

the adjacent proximal phalanx, and the common digital artery, which is adjacent to the nerve. If the artery is identified, it should be dissected away from the nerve and preserved.

The tourniquet is released and hemostasis is obtained. The wound is closed with interrupted 2-0 Vicryl suture subcutaneously and 4-0 nylon suture in the skin (Fig. 12-11). A compressive dressing is applied. Weight bearing as tolerated is permitted in a postoperative shoe.

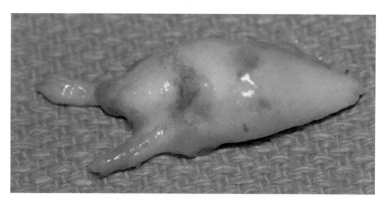

**Figure 12-11.** The neuroma is sent for histologic evaluation. (Copyright the Mayo Clinic and Mayo Foundation, Rochester, Minnesota.)

## POSTOPERATIVE MANAGEMENT

Patients are instructed to elevate the affected extremity and limit activities to lessen the pain, swelling, and wound drainage. Patients are allowed to bear weight as tolerated, initially on the heel in a stiff postoperative shoe. The dressing is changed during the first 2 to 3 days. The sutures are removed about 2 to 3 weeks after surgery.

By 2 to 3 weeks postoperatively, the patient resumes the use of loose-fitting, closed-toe shoes such as an athletic shoe or walking shoe. Patients should be advised that it may take months for swelling to completely resolve and for them to resume the use of their usual footwear. Patients are allowed to resume activities as tolerated starting at about 3 weeks postoperatively.

Results of surgery have been favorable. In a study of 305 feet in 259 patients, Friscia et al. (5) reported that 79% were satisfied or satisfied with minor reservations. Ninety-one percent of the neuromas were in the third web space. Results were better when it was localized to a third web space neuroma (90% successful) but worse in those with second web space neuromas (60% successful), worse in those with multiple web space operations in the same foot (59% successful), and worse in those with bilateral operations. Rasmussen and Kitaoka (9) reported a high rate of success for patients with only third web space neuromas who had recurrent symptoms after a single corticosteroid injection and subsequently underwent third web space neuroma resection. Of the 23 feet, patients were satisfied or satisfied with minor reservations in 22 feet (96%). Patients rated the improvement after surgery of more than 50% in 20 feet (87%). This study also demonstrated that previous corticosteroid injection did not preclude successful surgical treatment.

Several investigators reported lower success rates in feet that had surgery for recurrent interdigital neuroma. Johnson et al. (6) studied 33 patients who had reoperation for persistent pain after excision of interdigital neuroma, and 22 patients (67%) had complete relief or marked improvement in pain. This underscores the importance of accurate diagnosis prior to the primary neuroma resection.

## COMPLICATIONS

Neuroma resection is not a complex operation, but complications occur and can be a source of pain and frustration. The potential failure and complications must be discussed preoperatively. A problem of relatively minor consequence can be a source of great concern to the patient, if he or she is not informed before surgery. The patient better tolerates more significant postoperative complications if discussed preoperatively. About 80% of the patients have significant or complete pain relief after neuroma resection, which means that about

20% continue to have symptoms. Accurate diagnosis and preoperative counseling are essential.

*Recurrence* is a common complication after an interdigital neuroma excision. The cause of recurrence may be failure to resect the nerve far enough proximally, leaving a stump neuroma in a weight-bearing area. After interdigital neuroma resection, some may notice an annoying sensation in the toes or plantar forefoot close to where the neuroma was resected. This is more tolerable than the neuroma pain and, if discussed preoperatively, is well accepted. In patients with recurrent pain, failure to completely resect the nerve or recurrence may be partly responsible.

*Misdiagnosis before surgery* is another source of persistent pain after an interdigital neuroma resection. If there was a misdiagnosis, the patient will continue to have preoperative symptoms after an adequate excision of the nerve. In fact the symptoms may actually be worse than before surgery because of hypersensitivity of the stump of the common digital nerve or development of a painful scar. Accurate diagnosis of interdigital neuroma is essential.

*Tenderness of the dorsal incision* is usually temporary after interdigital neuroma excision as well as other foot and ankle procedures. This should be discussed before surgery.

*Toe ischemia* after interdigital neuroma surgery is rare but should be discussed with the patient who has had previous neuroma surgery and is anticipating surgery in an adjacent web space or in patients who have had or are anticipating multiple web space operations. Older patients with vascular disease are more at risk for this complication. Simultaneous dorsal exposure of adjacent web spaces, such as the second and third can potentially lead to injury or spasm to the multiple digital arteries and adversely affect the vascular supply to the third toe. Usually, if the artery is disrupted in a single web space, the other contributing arteries to the toe are sufficient to maintain viability.

Patients who experience failures or complications should be managed nonoperatively for a prolonged period before considering further operative treatment. It is not unusual for the aching, swelling, and difficulty with normal footwear to continue for weeks or months. Intervening with further surgery is usually not considered for a year or longer postoperatively.

## ACKNOWLEDGMENT

The authors gratefully acknowledge the contribution of James Amis, M.D.

## RECOMMENDED READING

1. Alexander I, Johnson KA, Parr JW: Morton's neuroma: a review of recent concepts. *Orthopedics* 10:103–106, 1987.
2. Amis JA, Siverhus SW, Liwnicz BH: An anatomic basis for recurrence after Morton's neuroma excision. *Foot Ankle* 13:153–156, 1992.
3. Bradley N, Miller WA, Evans JP: Plantar neuroma: analysis of results following surgical excision in 145 patients. *South Med J* 69:853–854, 1976.
4. Diebold PF, Daum B, Dang-Vu V, et al.: True epineural neurolysis in Morton's neuroma: a 5-year follow up. *Orthopedics* 19:397–400, 1996.
5. Friscia DA, Strom DE, Parr JW, et al.: Surgical treatment for primary digital neuroma. *Orthopedics* 14:669–672, 1991.
6. Johnson JE, Johnson KA, Unni KK: Persistent pain after excision of an interdigital neuroma. *J Bone Joint Surg Am* 70:651–657, 1988.
7. Mann RA, Reynolds JC: Interdigital neuroma critical clinical analysis. *Foot Ankle* 3:238–243, 1983.
8. Okafor B, Shergill G, Angel J: Treatment of Morton's neuroma by neurolysis. *Foot Ankle* 18:284–287, 1997.
9. Rasmussen MR, Kitaoka HB, Patzer GL: Nonoperative treatment of plantar interdigital neuroma with a single corticosteroid injection. *Clin Orthop* 326:188–193, 1996.

# 13

# Secondary Interdigital Neuroma Resection; Ankle Block Anesthesia

Jeffrey E. Johnson and Christopher B. Hirose

## INDICATIONS/CONTRAINDICATIONS

Pain is the primary indication for reoperation of an interdigital neuroma after failed primary resection. Recent reports have described continuing complaints of pain in the affected interspace by 10% to 20% of patients after the first attempt at excision of a primary interdigital neuroma (3,7). The location and quality of the pain are important determinants in deciding whether the presenting pain symptoms result from a surgically treatable cause such as an incompletely resected primary interdigital neuroma, amputation stump neuroma, or an unrelated cause. The most common cause of persistent pain after excision of an interdigital neuroma is incomplete initial excision (5). Other causes of persistent pain that should be considered are a painful amputation stump neuroma, a second neuroma in the same foot, surgery on the wrong web space, and surgery for pain due to some cause other than an interdigital neuroma (i.e., metatarsalgia, metatarsophalangeal [MTP] synovitis, flexor digitorum longus tenosynovitis, Freiberg's infraction, metatarsal neck stress fracture, neoplasm, or a diffuse peripheral neuropathy). Reoperation for persistent web space pain should only be undertaken when the surgeon is convinced that the persistent pain symptoms are secondary to a surgically treatable nerve lesion. This determination can only be made after a thorough history and physical examination accompanied by the appropriate supporting tests or imaging studies, as indicated by each individual case, to exclude other potential causes of web space pain.

The contraindications to reoperation for persistent pain after a primary interdigital neuroma excision include significant peripheral vascular disease, peripheral neuropathy, pain not characteristic of a recurrent neuroma of the interdigital nerve (i.e., pain at multiple areas, inconsistent physical findings), reflex sympathetic dystrophy syndrome, long history of chronic pain, and unrealistic patient expectations.

Friscia et al. (3), for a large series of primary interdigital neuroma excisions, reported that, if the preoperative symptoms could be localized to the second or the third web space,

J. E. Johnson, M.D. and C. B. Hirose, M.D.: Department of Orthopaedic Surgery, Washington University School of Medicine; and Barnes-Jewish Hospital, St. Louis, Missouri.

80% of the patients were either completely satisfied or satisfied with minor reservations after neuroma resection. When there were symptoms in both feet or when more than one web space in the same foot was symptomatic, the satisfaction rate dropped significantly. Therefore a relative contraindication to reoperation of a neuroma is pain at more than a single web space or pain at other than the second or third web space.

Reexploration for a neuroma is also contraindicated if the pain was not caused by a surgically treatable nerve lesion (i.e., diffuse peripheral neuritis, musculoskeletal pain, or neoplasm). Reflex sympathetic dystrophy syndrome is a relative contraindication to reoperation and is controversial. If it can be determined that there is a reflex sympathetic dystrophy syndrome superimposed on well-localized, characteristic symptoms of a recurrent interdigital neuroma at a previously operated web space, then it may be indicated to reexplore and excise the neuroma in the carefully selected patient in an attempt to remove this focus of irritation. However, this should not be undertaken without aggressive multidisciplinary treatment of the reflex sympathetic dystrophy during the preoperative, intraoperative, and postoperative periods.

Dorsal web space pain and hypersensitivity due to an incisional neuroma of the dorsal sensory branches of the superficial peroneal nerve do not respond to reexploration of the interdigital nerve for a neuroma. An incisional neuroma may respond to nerve exploration with neurolysis or neurectomy if initial nonsurgical treatment fails.

A relative contraindication to reoperation is the patient who has a chronic pain syndrome with abnormal personality traits or the patient who, despite appropriate counseling, has unrealistic expectations regarding the results of surgery. Both types of patients have a high rate of dissatisfaction despite a technically appropriate surgical procedure.

The patient with a multiply operated neuroma may have little to gain by a third or fourth nerve exploration unless they have all previously been done through the dorsal incision and there is a likelihood that an incompletely resected neuroma is the cause of the continued pain. In the absence of a discrete neuroma in the multiply operated foot, nonsurgical treatments are indicated. In recalcitrant cases, an implantable tibial nerve stimulator or spinal cord stimulator may provide significant relief from pain (4).

## PREOPERATIVE PLANNING

The history of the pain and the physical examination are the most helpful tools in distinguishing between the various sources of persistent pain after primary interdigital neuroma excision. Pain from an incomplete neuroma excision and an amputation stump neuroma can often be distinguished by the history. If the pain in the affected interspace was still present soon after the initial surgery (within a few days to weeks), then it is more likely that the neuroma was incompletely removed. If there was a pain-free interval after the initial surgery for at least several weeks to months, it is more likely that the neuroma was removed but that a painful amputation stump neuroma developed at the (proximal) cut end of the interdigital nerve. Approximately two thirds of patients with persistent pain after an interdigital neuroma excision have had an inadequate initial excision (5).

The quality of the pain caused by a recurrent neuroma is often different from the initial presenting pain of a primary neuroma. In addition to the web space pain and burning that radiates into the adjacent toes, there is often a significant hypersensitivity to the plantar skin in the metatarsal head region. Even light touch or stroking of the plantar skin in this area causes significant discomfort. This hypersensitivity is localized to the distribution of the operated nerve and should be distinguished from the more diffuse hypersensitivity that may accompany a peripheral neuropathy or reflex sympathetic dystrophy syndrome. There may be exquisite tenderness that is greater than the web space tenderness present preoperatively. The pain may be centered beneath the fourth metatarsal head after a third web space neuroma excision, especially if the communicating branch from the lateral plantar nerve (Fig. 13-1) courses close to the fourth metatarsal head rather than joining the medial plantar nerve branch more proximally. In this situation, transection of the third web space interdigital nerve allows the cut end of the communicating branch to retract into the area beneath

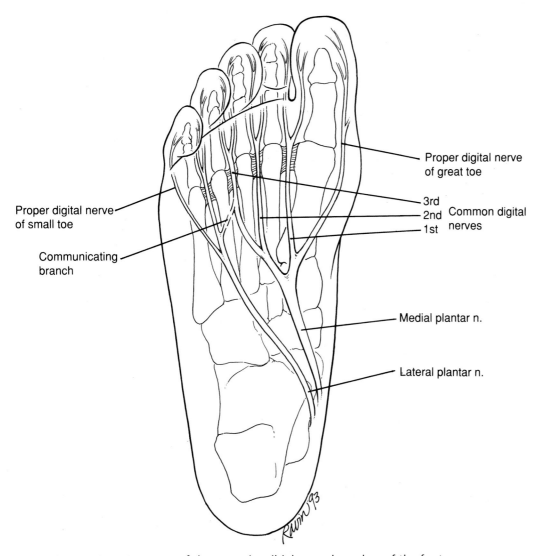

Proper digital nerve
of great toe

3rd
2nd  Common digital
1st  nerves

Proper digital nerve
of small toe

Communicating
branch

Medial plantar n.

Lateral plantar n.

**Figure 13-1.** Anatomy of the posterior tibial nerve branches of the foot.

the fourth metatarsal head and develop a painful amputation stump neuroma in a weight-bearing area (6).

If the persistent pain is localized to another interspace in the same foot and the symptoms are still characteristic of a primary neuroma, the wrong web space may have been operated on or a second neuroma in the same foot may be present. Thompson and Deland (10) reported that a second neuroma in the same foot was a rare entity, occurring in only 3 (3.4%) of 89 patients studied. However, they also reported that 2 (40%) of the 5 failed neuroma resections were caused by the initial surgery having been done on the wrong interspace.

Hypersensitivity of the dorsal scar usually results from an incisional neuroma of the cutaneous branch of the superficial peroneal nerve supplying the dorsal web space and may have no relation to a recurrence of the interdigital neuroma. If dorsal hypersensitivity and pain is the major symptom causing dissatisfaction after primary neuroma excision, web space reexploration would not provide relief, and treatment of the incisional neuroma would be indicated.

With normal radiographs of the foot, lack of a history of trauma, and absence of a palpable interspace mass, it may be necessary to obtain other diagnostic tests to rule out other causes of persistent pain if the history and physical examination findings are not characteristic for a recurrent neuroma. A bone scan is helpful to rule out an occult bone or joint abnormality in the foot, and a magnetic resonance imaging (MRI) scan may be necessary to rule out a neoplasm or other space-occupying lesion. However, an MRI scan is not very helpful in determining if a recurrent neuroma is present in the area of the previous surgery because of the difficulty in distinguishing neuroma from scar tissue. An MRI scan using a small forefoot surface coil might detect a neuroma at an adjacent web space, but correlation with clinical symptoms is needed to recommend reoperation.

## SURGERY

It is preferable to do the surgery under some type of regional blockade (i.e., spinal, epidural, femoral-sciatic block, knee block, or ankle block). The advantage of a regional block is that the dorsal horn of the spinal cord is protected from the noxious stimuli of manipulating the already excitable nerve lesion (i.e., preemptive analgesia).

If general anesthesia is chosen, there is good evidence to support the use of preoperative ankle block or other regional anesthetic (in addition to the general anesthetic) for use as analgesia. The ankle block has an advantage over the spinal or epidural for preemptive analgesia in that long-lasting postoperative anesthesia can be obtained by using bupivacaine as the anesthetic agent. The ankle block may last for 12 hours, allowing patients significant comfort until they are back at home. Other types of regional blocks must "wear off" for motor power to return to the lower extremities before the patient is allowed to return home. Some investigators (8) have reported a 95% success rate with the use of regional anesthesia. Because of the limited amount of local anesthesia used, it is possible to administer bilateral ankle blocks, as opposed to others such as the popliteal block.

### Ankle Block Anesthesia Technique

We routinely use an ankle block 20 minutes before surgery with 20 mL of 0.5% bupivacaine without epinephrine and a 1.25-inch, 25-gauge needle (Figs. 13-2 through 13-6). Knowledge of nerve anatomy is essential for successful blocks. Injecting a large amount of anesthetic in a ring around the ankle is commonly performed but always fails; the deep peroneal nerve and posterior tibial nerve lie deep to the retinaculum and are not anesthetized by a ring block, no matter how much agent is used. Iatrogenic neural injury is avoided with the use of a needle with a flatter bevel that is less likely to pierce the tibial nerve. The block is performed with the patient under conscious sedation to prevent inadvertent nerve injury from an intraneural injection.

First, we block the posterior tibial nerve with 10 mL of local anesthetic placed 3 cm above the tip of the medial malleolus and 1 cm anterior to the margin of the Achilles tendon. The needle is inserted from a posterior approach and advanced slowly and deliberately through the retinaculum until the tibial cortex is encountered and then it is withdrawn 3 mm. We aspirate first to avoid inadvertent intravenous or arterial injection. The posterior tibial is the most difficult to successfully block, and special techniques may be applied, such as the use of a nerve stimulator or paresthesia technique. A needle attached to a nerve stimulator is advanced until contractions in the intrinsic muscles are observed. The needle is withdrawn slightly, and then aspiration and injection are performed. In the paresthesia technique, the patient is warned that an electric shock sensation will occur. The needle is advanced until paresthesia occurs accompanied by an involuntary jerk when the nerve is contacted. The needle is withdrawn slightly, and the aspiration and injection are performed.

Second, the deep peroneal nerve is anesthetized with 2.5 to 5 mL of local anesthetic by identifying a point 1cm above the ankle joint line, between extensor hallucis longus and anterior tibial tendons. The needle is advanced through the skin and subcutaneous tissues, through the extensor retinaculum down to the tibia, and then withdrawn slightly. The syringe is aspirated, and the injection is given.

Third, the saphenous nerve is blocked. Usually, the greater saphenous vein is observed, which approximates the saphenous nerve and facilitates accurate placement of the local anesthetic anterior to the medial malleolus. This injection can be given through a separate

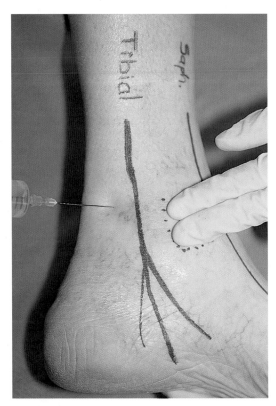

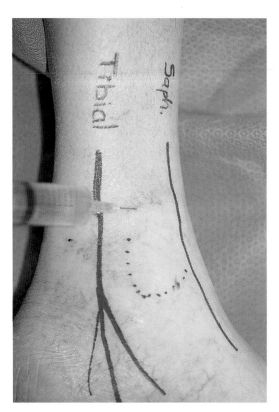

**Figure 13-2**. Ankle block being administered as preemptive analgesia before placing the patient in the prone position for plantar exposure of the recurrent neuroma. The tibial nerve is found two cm above the tip of the medial malleolus, deep to the flexor retinaculum. Positions of the posterior tibial nerve and its branches (medial calcaneal, lateral plantar, medial plantar) are shown.

**Figure 13-3.** A dorsal wheal of anesthetic is injected over the anterior aspect of the ankle with a 25-gauge needle. The saphenous nerve is being blocked superficial to the extensor retinaculum.

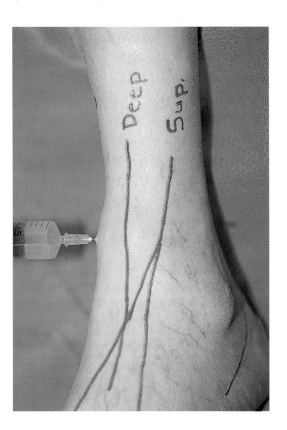

**Figure 13-4.** The subcutaneous tissue is infiltrated in a band-like pattern across the anterior ankle superficial to the extensor retinaculum to block the branches of the superficial peroneal nerve.

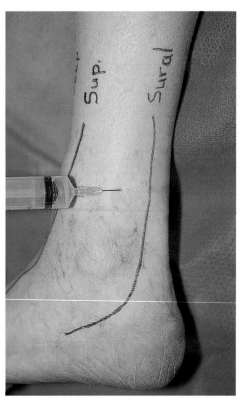

**Figure 13-5.** The sural nerve is anesthetized with 2.5 mL of 0.5% bupivacaine.

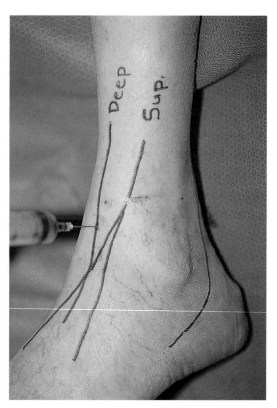

**Figure 13-6.** The deep peroneal nerve is found deep to the tendon of the extensor hallucis longus two cm above the ankle joint. Place the needle through the skin and extensor retinaculum until it contacts the anterior tibia, and then withdraw it 3 mm, aspirate, and inject the anesthetic.

needle stick or easily through the same entry point as the deep peroneal nerve block, directing the needle medially to the anterior margin of the malleolus; it must be superficial to the retinaculum. About 2.5 to 5 mL of local anesthetic is used.

The superficial peroneal nerve almost always divides into two branches proximal to the ankle joint level, both of which are effectively blocked by infiltrating 2.5 to 5 mL in the subcutaneous tissues in the anterior ankle; it must be given superficial to the retinaculum. This can be accomplished through the same needle stick as the deep peroneal nerve injection by directing the needle laterally toward the anterior margin of the lateral malleolus superficial to the retinaculum.

The sural nerve is blocked by identifying a point at the ankle joint level midway between the margins of the Achilles tendon and the lateral malleolus. The needle is placed in the subcutaneous tissue level, and 2.5 to 5 mL are injected.

Contraindications of ankle block anesthesia rarely occur. Intraneural injection can cause prolonged paraesthesia, pain, and permanent nerve injury. In bilateral ankle block anesthesias, the physician must be aware of the potential of overdose and systemic toxicity. There is a risk of intravascular injection that can cause systemic toxicity, involving seizures. This risk can be minimized by aspirating for blood before injecting the anesthetic. Patients tolerate application of an ankle Esmarch bandage for hemostasis very well in combination with ankle block anesthesia. It is useful to have systemic monitoring by an anesthesiologist or anesthetist and to use mild sedation.

## Surgical Technique

After the decision has been made to reoperate on a recurrent interdigital neuroma, the surgeon must decide whether to use the dorsal or plantar approach to the nerve. Reexploration of the nerve through the original dorsal approach may be useful when the initial incision was made very distal in the web space, the history is consistent with an inadequate primary excision of the neuroma, and the tenderness is at or distal to the metatarsal head level. In this case, the recurrent neuroma may be visible through a dorsal exposure. Proponents of the dorsal approach have reported good results using this technique, and it precludes the need for an incision on the weight-bearing surface of the foot (7). Nashi et al. (9) found a delay in return to weight-bearing status and a delay in returning to work after plantar incisions. In some cases, a hypertrophic callus may form. However, good results have also been reported by using the plantar approach without significant problems with the plantar incision (1,5). If there is doubt about being able to locate the neuroma from the dorsal approach, a plantar approach should be used.

The other role for a dorsal approach is the rare case when the "recurrent neuroma" is in an adjacent interspace. In this case the procedure is performed similarly to a primary neuroma excision. If the surgeon finds a completely normal-appearing nerve in the adjacent interspace, the transverse intermetatarsal ligament is divided and a section removed to decompress the nerve. The "normal" interdigital nerve may not be excised in this case, because it would needlessly denervate the third toe.

Plantar incisions (Fig. 13-7) are oblique/transverse (1) or longitudinal (5). The advantage of the oblique/transverse incision is that it is placed proximal to the weight-bearing area of the metatarsal heads and gives easy access to more than one interdigital nerve if necessary. The advantage of the longitudinal incision is the ability to extend it as far as necessary to locate the nerve lesion. Another major advantage of the longitudinal incision is the ability to find a "normal" plantar nerve trunk proximal to the site of the neuroma and to trace its path to the abnormal region (Fig. 13-8). If significant scarring is present around the cut end of the nerve, it may be difficult to identify a neuroma unless the dissection is begun proximal to the scarred portion of the nerve. In most cases, the (extensile) longitudinal plantar incision is the approach of choice and is the single incision with the most utility. The longitudinal incision also allows implantation into a proximal muscle belly in the arch of the foot if desired.

Preoperative antibiotics are given, and the patient is positioned prone on the operating table. We place a tourniquet at the thigh or ankle and use a bipolar cautery to limit potential injury to the nerve. Conventional electrocautery may injure a nerve by conduction of current through the nerve when a nearby blood vessel is cauterized. Loupe magnification is helpful in identifying nerve structures and distinguishing them from blood vessels.

A 3- to 4-cm longitudinal incision is made in the plantar surface of the forefoot between the metatarsal heads in the affected interspace (Fig. 13-9). Dissection is carried through the skin and plantar fat, and the digital nerve is identified (Fig. 13-10). The nerve is found just deep to, and often between, the distal extensions of the plantar fascia that fan out to attach to the plantar aspects of the MTP joints (Fig. 13-11). The digital nerve is identified proximally and traced distally to the site of the neuroma (Fig. 13-12). The intermetatarsal ligament is not routinely divided because the interdigital lies superficial to the ligament when viewing it from the plantar approach. The digital nerve is divided under gentle traction as far proximally as possible, so that it retracts from the weight-bearing areas of the fore part of the foot (Fig. 13-13). Only the skin is closed with interrupted vertical mattress sutures of 3-0 nylon (Fig. 13-14). No subcutaneous sutures are used. Great care is taken to approximate the edges of the skin evenly without inverting or overlapping the incision. A short-leg compressive dressing is applied (Fig. 13-15).

*(Text continues on page 193.)*

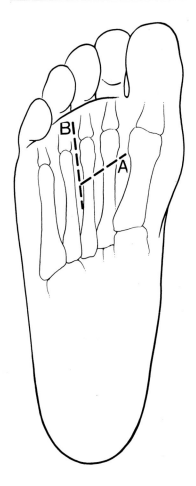

**Figure 13-7.** Examples of plantar incisions used for excision of a recurrent interdigital neuroma after a primary excision. *A,* Oblique/transverse incision to the 2-3 common interdigital nerve. *B,* Longitudinal (extensile) incision to the 3-4 common interdigital nerve.

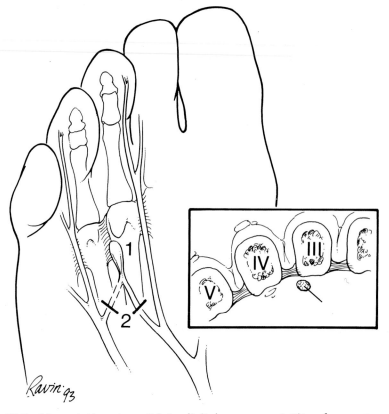

**Figure 13-8.** "Amputation stump" interdigital neuroma. *1,* Site of nerve transection following primary neuroma resection. Notice the location of the end bulb "stump" neuroma. *2,* Site of nerve transection for removal of a recurrent neuroma.

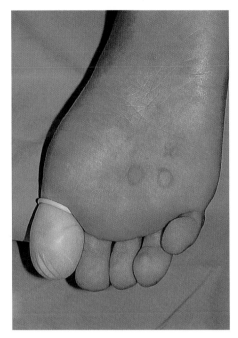

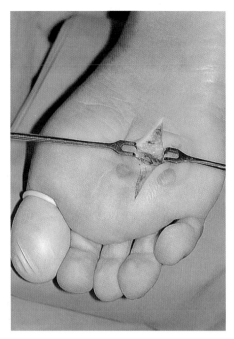

**Figure 13-9.** The third and fourth metatarsal heads are outlined.

**Figure 13-10.** Plantar dissection through the skin and subcutaneous tissue.

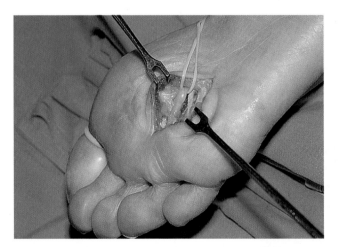

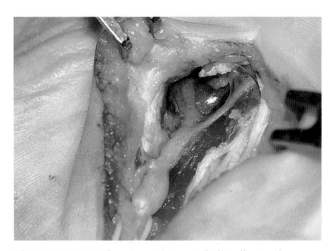

**Figure 13-11.** The third web space interdigital nerve is isolated proximally. (From Johnson JE, Johnson KA, Unni KK: Persistent pain after excision of an interdigital neuroma—results of reoperation. *J Bone Joint Surg Am* 70: 651–657, 1988, with permission.)

**Figure 13-12.** The nerve is traced distally to the neuroma. Notice the apparent incomplete initial excision. (From Johnson JE, Johnson KA, Unni KK: Persistent pain after excision of an interdigital neuroma—results of reoperation. *J Bone Joint Surg Am* 70: 651–657, 1988, with permission.)

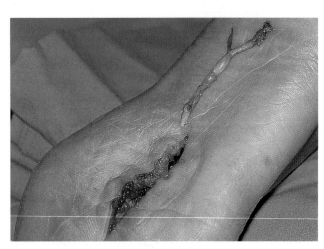

**Figure 13-13.** The nerve is divided distally and ready for proximal transection.

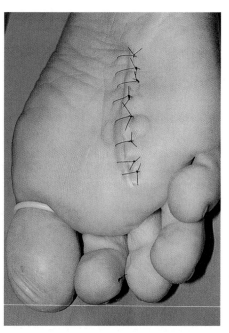

**Figure 13-14.** Skin edges are closely approximated with 3-0 nylon sutures. (From Johnson JE, Johnson KA, Unni KK: Persistent pain after excision of an interdigital neuroma—results of reoperation. *J Bone Joint Surg Am* 70: 651–657, 1988, with permission.)

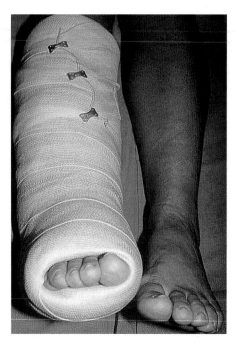

**Figure 13-15.** A short leg-compression splint is applied immediately postoperatively.

## Alternative Techniques

Symptomatic secondary interdigital neuromas can also be successfully treated by neuroma resection and muscle implantation (2). Histologic studies of cut nerve ends buried in muscle are notable for minimal neuroma formation with significantly less scar tissue. Suitable muscles are those with minimal excursion, such as the quadratus plantae and the adductor hallucis. The main goals of implantation are placement of the cut nerve end away from denervated skin, placement with little tension on the nerve, and stabilization of the nerve to muscle with a small 6-0 nonabsorbable suture.

## Pitfalls

We have learned that the proper preoperative diagnosis is essential for a successful result. A preoperative diagnostic injection is often helpful. If there is no improvement with the patient's symptoms, even temporarily, then we consider further workup to find the etiology of the patient's pain. Recurrent pain after neuroma excision can masquerade as a peripheral neuropathy and surgically removing the neuroma would not be expected to improve the pain. If the pain is not well localized to the web space or plantar forefoot, neuropathy should be ruled out. We examine the forefoot with Semmes-Weinstein monofilaments and maintain a low threshold for ordering an electromyogram and nerve conduction study or a neurology consultation.

Using the prone position for a plantar approach to the forefoot facilitates exposure of the nerve. We have discovered that the plantar nerves are much closer to the skin than expected, and they are easily missed by dissecting too deep. The neuroma should be found between the metatarsals just dorsal to the thin fibers of the plantar fascia as it fans out onto the weight-bearing surface of the forefoot. If the neuroma is not found at the site of tenderness, we continue our dissection proximal to find the trunk of the nerve and then trace the nerve distally to the neuroma.

Meticulous skin closure with nylon is essential to prevent plantar scar formation. The skin edges are reapproximated evenly and with slight eversion (Fig. 13-16).

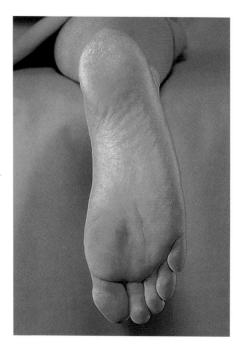

**Figure 13-16.** Appearance of the pain-free plantar scar at 2 years postoperatively. (From Johnson JE, Johnson KA, Unni KK: Persistent pain after excision of an interdigital neuroma—results of reoperation. *J Bone Joint Surg Am* 70: 651–657, 1988, with permission.)

## POSTOPERATIVE MANAGEMENT

We use the postoperative short-leg compression dressing with crutches, without bearing weight on the operated leg for 2 to 3 days. The dressing is then changed, and a short-leg cast is applied. Weight bearing as tolerated is allowed. The cast and sutures are removed at 3 weeks postoperatively, and walking is continued using a cushioned-soled shoe.

Reoperation for recurrent or persistent pain after primary interdigital neuroma excision is a worthwhile procedure in the carefully selected patient. However, the patient and the surgeon should understand that although a significant percentage of patients are satisfied, many patients continue to have some type of symptoms at the involved interspace. A small group of patients are either not improved or worse.

Johnson et al. (5) reported 66% "complete satisfaction or satisfaction with minor reservations" after reoperation of 37 feet in 34 patients using the technique described here. Beskin and Baxter (1) used a dorsal incision or an oblique/transverse plantar incision proximal to the metatarsal heads and reported approximately 80% of 30 patients with 39 recurrent neuromas were "satisfied." Fifty-eight percent of patients still had difficulty with certain types of footwear. They reported fewer failures using the plantar approach than the previous dorsal incision (8% versus 21%) (1). Mann and Reynolds (7), using the previous dorsal incision, reported 9 (82%) of 11 patients with recurrent neuromas were "significantly improved." However, 7 (64%) of 11 still had some plantar tenderness.

## REHABILITATION

If there is significant incisional pain or metatarsalgia, a custom-molded, total-contact insert is fabricated for an in-depth shoe. A rocker-bottom sole may be added if additional relief of metatarsal head loading is needed.

If there is a significant component of hypersensitivity to the incisional area at the time of cast removal, we prefer a manual desensitization program supervised by a physical therapist who is skilled in this technique. If pain and hypersensitivity do not respond within several weeks, oral medication and other nonsurgical treatments of neurogenic pain may be instituted. The surgeon must be watchful for the development of a pain syndrome and begin treatment early and aggressively if one develops.

## COMPLICATIONS

The most common complication after reoperation for a recurrent interdigital neuroma is failure to obtain relief in the preoperative *pain symptoms*. Johnson et al. (5) reported 47% residual pain in the interspace. The reasons for this are similar to the reasons why the initial procedure failed (i.e., wrong diagnosis, wrong web space operated, unrealistic patient expectations, or inadequate surgical excision). A more difficult complication is the development of a chronic localized pain syndrome or a reflex sympathetic dystrophy. Both of these problems can cause more pain and functional limitation than the isolated recurrent neuroma for which the surgery was performed. In general, the treatment for persistent pain after the second attempt at neuroma excision is nonsurgical and includes the modalities discussed previously including medication, physical therapy, local injections, and sympathetic blocks. In recalcitrant cases unresponsive to these modalities, a more proximal transection and implantation into muscle may be helpful. An implantable tibial nerve stimulator or spinal cord stimulator may also provide significant relief in pain as a salvage procedure (4).

A potential complication is development of a *painful plantar scar* because of hypertrophic changes and callus formation in the plantar incision. The series in the literature that used the plantar longitudinal incision, including primary and secondary neuroma excisions, have not reported problems other than rare instances (3%) of mild tenderness at the site of the scar (5). Most patients in one series stated they had difficulty finding the site of the previous plantar incision at the time of follow-up examination (5) (Fig. 13-16).

# RECOMMENDED READING

1. Beskin JL, Baxter DE: Recurrent pain following interdigital neurectomy—a plantar approach. *Foot Ankle* 9:34–39, 1988.
2. Dellon AL: Treatment of recurrent metatarsalgia by neuroma resection and muscle implantation: case report and proposed algorithm of management for Morton's "neuroma." *Microsurgery* 10:256–259, 1989.
3. Friscia DA, Strom DE, Parr JW, et al.: Surgical treatment for primary interdigital neuroma. *Orthopedics* 14:669–672, 1991.
4. Gould JS: Treatment of the painful nerve in-continuity. In: Gelberman RH, ed. *Inoperative nerve repair and reconstruction.* Philadelphia: JB Lippincott, 1991:1541–1550.
5. Johnson JE, Johnson KA, Unni KK: Persistent pain after excision of an interdigital neuroma—results of re-operation. *J Bone Joint Surg Am* 70:651–657, 1988.
6. Levitsky KA, Alman BA, Jevsevar DS, et al.: Digital nerves of the foot: anatomic variations and implications regarding the pathogenesis of interdigital neuroma. *Foot Ankle* 14:208–214, 1993.
7. Mann RA, Reynolds JC: Interdigital neuroma—a critical clinical analysis. *Foot Ankle* 3:238–243, 1983.
8. Myerson MS, Ruland CM, Allon SM: Regional anesthesia for foot and ankle surgery. *Foot Ankle* 13:282–288, 1992.
9. Nashi M, Venkatachalam AK, Muddu BN: Surgery of Morton's neuroma: dorsal or plantar approach? *R Coll Surgeons Edinburgh* 42:36–37, 1997.
10. Thompson FM, Deland JT: Occurrence of two interdigital neuromas in one foot. *Foot Ankle* 14:15–17, 1993.

# 14

# Osteotomy of the Fifth Metatarsal

Harold B. Kitaoka

## INDICATIONS/CONTRAINDICATIONS

Patients with bunionette (i.e., tailor's bunion) have pain over the lateral forefoot, corresponding to the lateral condylar process of the fifth metatarsal (1–2, 4–8, 10–12). There may be associated bursitis, intractable plantar keratosis of the fifth metatarsal head, and difficulty tolerating most footwear (1–2, 4–8, 10–12). The main indication for fifth metatarsal osteotomy is for pain relief. Although there is usually varus malalignment of the fifth toe associated with the bunionette, the malalignment alone is not a consistent source of symptoms. Patients with bunionettes often have significantly increased fifth metatarsophalangeal (MTP) and intermetatarsal 4-5 angles (9). The fifth metatarsal may be bowed laterally or splayed or the metatarsal head enlarged.

The distal chevron fifth metatarsal osteotomy has been successful for the treatment of hallux valgus (3), and a similar technique has been applied to the bunionette (6,8). It may be performed in patients with different types of bunionette deformities, including those with marked splaying (increased intermetatarsal 4-5 angle), lateral bowing of the metatarsal, and enlarged metatarsal head. Unlike the chevron first metatarsal osteotomy for hallux valgus, the operation may be successfully used even in patients that have more severe deformities, because there is no correlation between the degree of fifth metatarsal splaying and the clinical results (6). This operation may be successful in adults of all age groups. It is appropriate if there is satisfactory fifth MTP joint function. In some instances, this operation may be performed as a salvage procedure after failed lateral condylar process resection if most of the fifth metatarsal head remains.

Contraindications of distal fifth chevron metatarsal osteotomy are the absence of pain, and presence of stiffness and/or arthrosis of the fifth MTP joint. Another contraindication is skin ulceration or infection, which may occur in patients with bunionette and sensory neuropathy. Peripheral vascular disease is also a contraindication. When there are severe juxtaarticular erosions associated with an inflammatory disease, osteotomy at the distal level may not be possible.

H. B. Kitaoka, M.D.: Foot and Ankle Section, Department of Orthopaedics, Mayo Clinic and Mayo Foundation; and Mayo School of Medicine, Rochester, Minnesota.

## PREOPERATIVE PLANNING

It is important to carefully assess the patient's symptoms and signs to determine whether operative treatment is indicated. It should be considered in patients who have failed non-operative treatment such as use of footwear with a wider toe box, softer leather upper, and shoes in which the leather is stretched over the lateral forefoot prominence. Based on the patient's symptoms (e.g., pain, restricted activities, restricted footwear), medical evaluation, radiologic studies, and appropriate patient expectations, the decision regarding surgery can be made.

On physical examination, the alignment of the fifth toe should be assessed. Fifth MTP joint range of motion in the dorsiflexion-plantarflexion plane should be determined, as well as whether this motion is painful. The presence of intractable plantar keratosis beneath the fifth metatarsal head should be documented. The physician should also observe evidence of abnormal forefoot loading in other regions such as under the fourth metatarsal head and the presence of fat pad atrophy. The presence of other lesser toe or great toe deformities should be noted. Other associated fifth toe problems such as hammer toe with or without dorsal subluxation at the MTP level or corn formation at the interphalangeal level should be noted. A general medical examination is necessary to identify regional or general conditions that may be the source of problems such as peripheral vascular disease, diabetes mellitus, and systemic inflammatory diseases. Anteroposterior and lateral, weight-bearing radiographs of the standing patient and an oblique view of the foot should be obtained to assess the level of arthrosis at the MTP joint, juxtaarticular erosions, and alignment with respect to intermetatarsal 4-5, and MTP -5 angles. Fifth MTP subluxation also should be assessed on the radiographs.

Although this chevron-type metatarsal osteotomy has application for most bunionette problems, including those with severe deformities, there are alternative procedures that may be useful in specific situations. Removing the prominent lateral condyle is simple and has the advantages of preserving joint function and metatarsal length. Fixation and immo-

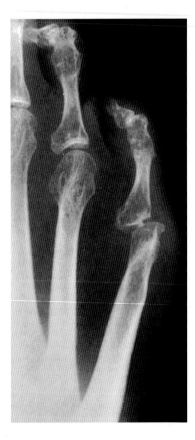

**Figure 14-1.** Anteroposterior radiograph of a patient with a painful recurrent bunionette 5 years after lateral condylar process section. The figure shows metatarsophalangeal joint subluxation.

bilization are not required. This operation has application in patients in which the simpler operation is preferred, but the physician must accept the possibility of residual pain in a higher percentage of patients than the distal chevron osteotomy (5), and late MTP joint subluxation or dislocation may occur (Fig. 14-1). The midshaft osteotomy with screw fixation proposed by Coughlin (1,2) has application, particularly in patients who have failed previous bunionette surgery. Although it has the potential of achieving a larger degree of correction of the intermetatarsal 4-5 angle, it requires more extensive exposure, fixation, and postoperative cast immobilization.

The fifth metatarsal head resection (4) is a useful procedure in patients who have significant juxtaarticular erosions in which the joint is not salvageable and an osteotomy operation is not possible at the distal level. It is useful in patients with marked stiffness or arthrosis of the fifth MTP joint, selected patients who have failed bunionette operations, and patients who have a neurotrophic ulcer with extension of the infection to the distal fifth metatarsal and MTP joint.

## SURGERY

This preferred chevron-type fifth metatarsal osteotomy can be done using ankle block, spinal block, or general anesthesia. It is usually performed as an outpatient procedure, and it is possible to perform the operation on both feet at the same time.

With the patient placed in the supine position, the foot and ankle are exsanguinated with a 4-inch rubber bandage. In most cases, when ankle block anesthesia is administered, the rubber bandage is then unwrapped at the foot level and wrapped several times at the ankle level for hemostasis. A sterile tourniquet may also be used at the distal leg level. In patients who have general or spinal anesthesia, a thigh tourniquet may be used.

### Technique

The skin incision is made in a dorsal lateral longitudinal fashion centered on the distal fifth metatarsal level and is 3 cm long (Fig. 14-2). The subcutaneous tissues are retracted.

An incisional neuroma may be avoided by identification of the small dorsal lateral sensory nerve after the skin incision and before the capsulotomy. Although hypesthesia in a

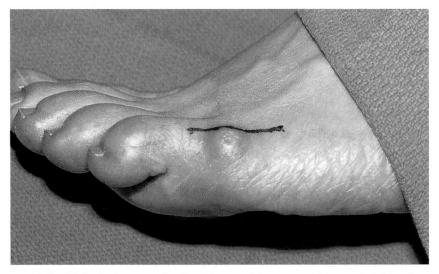

**Figure 14-2.** Clinical photograph of a 47-year-old woman with a painful bunionette. Notice the callus overlying the prominent lateral condylar process of the fifth metatarsal and the dorsolateral skin incision.

small area of the dorsal lateral aspect of the fifth toe may not be particularly bothersome, local irritation with footwear due to an incisional neuroma can be symptomatic.

A longitudinal incision of the MTP joint capsule is made. The dorsal lateral sensory nerve should be protected and care taken to avoid excessive removal of soft tissues about the distal fifth metatarsal, because this may have an effect on osteotomy union, the occurrence of osteonecrosis of the fifth metatarsal head, and stability of the osteotomy.

The lateral condylar process should be removed in a plane approximately parallel to the lateral border of the foot using a microsagittal saw with a small thin saw blade (Figs. 14-3 and 14-4). A chevron-shaped osteotomy is made at the metatarsal head level at an angle of 50°, with the apex facing distally (Figs. 14-5 and 14-6). Performing an osteotomy with an angle approaching 90° rather than 50° creates an osteotomy that is less stable. An osteotomy that is performed too proximally at the neck level may be less stable because the thicker cortical bone at the neck level may not impact to the same degree as the largely cancellous bone at the head level. If the lateral condylar process resection is excessive, it may affect the stability of the osteotomy as well.

The distal fragment is displaced medially 3 to 4 mm (Fig. 14-7). Care is taken to orient the plane of the osteotomy parallel to the plantar foot to avoid displacement of the osteotomy in the dorsal-plantar direction. Care is also taken to orient the plane of the osteotomy perpendicular to the long axis of the foot to avoid displacement of the osteotomy in the proximal-distal direction. The residual (proximal) lateral prominence of the metatarsal head and neck is resected in a plane parallel to the lateral border of the foot (Fig. 14-8). The osteotomy is gently impacted by axial compression of the phalanx on the metatarsal head (Figs. 14-9 and 14-10). Stability is tested by MTP joint motion. Usually, a percutaneous 0.045-inch Kirschner wire is directed obliquely from the proximal dorsal to the distal plantar aspect, spanning the osteotomy. The osteotomy is relatively stable, particularly if performed at an angle of 50°, and some surgeons do not apply fixation. The apex of the V-shaped bone cut could be made 1 to 2 mm distal to the usual level of the center of the metatarsal head, because the more distally placed osteotomy tends to be more stable. Care should be taken to avoid performing the osteotomy too far distally or impacting it too vigorously, which has the potential of splitting the distal fragment. It is unnecessary to perform a medial capsulotomy to adequately correct the toe alignment.

The distal chevron osteotomy has been modified since the clinical series reported earlier (5). The main modifications are performing an osteotomy at a 50° angle rather than 60° and more routine use of percutaneous pin fixation.

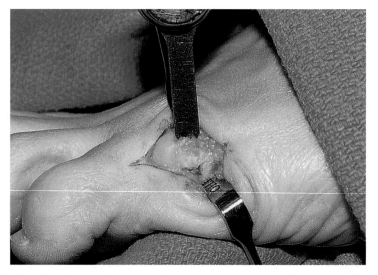

**Figure 14-3.** After longitudinal capsulotomy, the prominent lateral condylar process was resected with a microsagittal saw in a plane paralleling the lateral border of the foot.

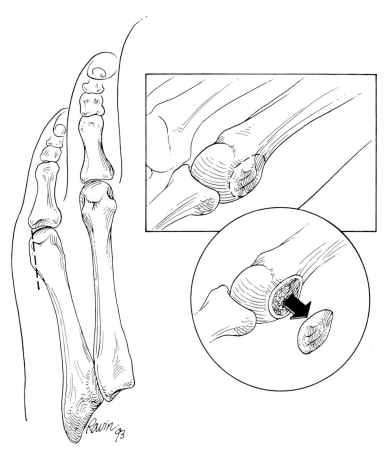

**Figure 14-4.** Through a dorsal lateral approach centered on the distal fifth metatarsal level, the lateral condylar process is resected at a level parallel to the lateral border of the foot.

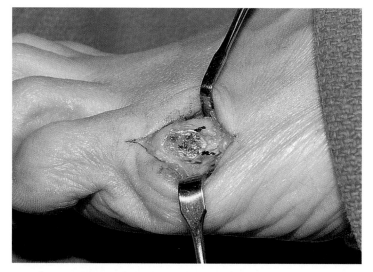

**Figure 14-5.** After resection of the lateral condylar process, the osteotomy is marked with the apex facing distally and centered 1 to 2 mm distal to the center of the metatarsal head, with the osteotomy angle of 50°.

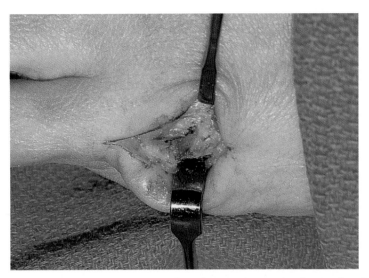

**Figure 14-6.** After the chevron osteotomy using a microsagittal saw, the distal fragment is displaced medially, as seen in this dorsolateral view. The remaining head and neck prominence is then removed with the microsagittal saw.

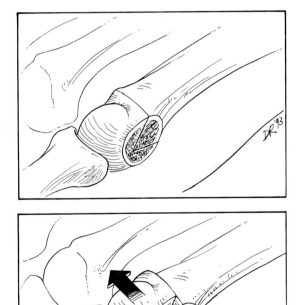

**Figure 14-7.** A chevron-shaped osteotomy is made with a microsagittal saw at an angle of 50°. Notice the apex of the osteotomy is 1 to 2 mm distal to the center of the metatarsal head. Displacement of the distal fragment is 3 to 4 mm. *Arrow* indicates displacement in the medial direction. Care is taken to avoid any dorsal displacement.

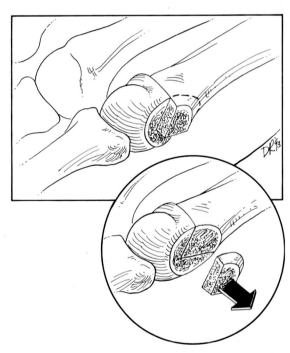

**Figure 14-8.** Removal of the remaining head and neck fragment with the microsagittal saw.

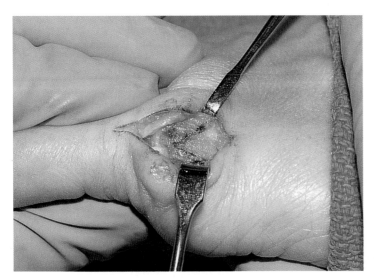

**Figure 14-9.** After removal of the remaining head and neck fragment, the osteotomy is gently impacted with longitudinal compression. A percutaneous, 0.045-inch pin may be inserted for fixation. A portion of the redundant capsule is excised, followed by skin closure.

The capsule is then closed tightly and a portion of the redundant capsule is excised. The skin is closed in the usual fashion in layers. During capsular and skin closure it is helpful to place a sponge between the fourth and fifth toes to assist in obtaining a tight capsular closure. After the wound is closed, the lateral prominence is reduced, and fifth toe alignment is improved. The wound is dressed with multiple 4 × 4 inch sponges and 2- or 3-inch Kling bandage. A stiff postoperative shoe may be applied and anteroposterior and lateral radiographs obtained in the recovery room. As an alternative, a Robert Jones dressing may be used for one day, followed by application of a short-leg cast for 3 weeks, then a postoperative shoe for an additional two to three weeks until union.

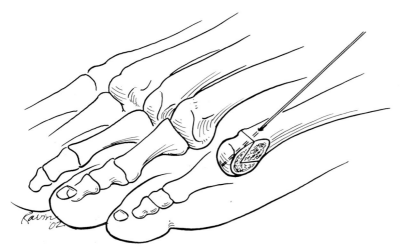

**Figure 14-10.** Drawing shows placement of a percutaneous pin to stabilize the osteotomy.

## POSTOPERATIVE MANAGEMENT

The soft dressing may be changed in several days and sutures and pin removed at 2 to 3 weeks postoperatively. It may be beneficial to immobilize the foot in a short-leg walking cast particularly when the operation is combined with other foot procedures. The patient is allowed to bear weight in the postsurgical shoe or cast; however, crutches are useful initially as an ambulatory aid. The stiff postoperative shoe is then worn for an additional 2 to 3 weeks, at which time anteroposterior and lateral radiographs are obtained to judge alignment and osteotomy union. If radiographs appear to be satisfactory, the patient can resume the use of a closed-toe shoe with a wide toe box. There is usually some degree of swelling for an additional month. To rehabilitate the foot, gentle range of motion exercises can be started at 3 weeks postoperatively and more vigorous exercises at 6 weeks, particularly at the fifth MTP joint.

The results are generally satisfactory for this operation. In a series of 19 procedures performed with a 7-year average follow-up, the overall results were considered good in 17 feet and fair in 2, and there were no failures. Complications such as transfer metatarsalgia occurred in one foot, and there was a wound infection in one foot (5). There was a high satisfaction rate, and pain over the lateral condylar process was usually relieved. A wider range of footwear was tolerated. The fifth toe varus malalignment was significantly improved.

## COMPLICATIONS

Various complications may occur after a fifth metatarsal chevron osteotomy for a bunionette deformity. *Displacement* of the osteotomy is a possibility that can be prevented by appropriate surgical technique. Avoiding excessive soft tissue dissection of the osteotomy site, making the angle of the osteotomy about 50°, supplemental fixation of the osteotomy with a percutaneous pin, and tight capsular closure all decrease the possibility of osteotomy displacement.

*Transfer metatarsalgia* to the fourth metatarsal head region is a possibility if the metatarsal head was displaced in a dorsal position or the metatarsal shortened. The stability of the osteotomy against dorsiflexion translation is an inherent advantage of this particular procedure, but if the axis of the V-shaped osteotomy is inadvertently angled dorsally or proximally, dorsal translation or shortening result. Being aware of these possibilities and exercising careful operative technique will minimize the occurrence of this complication.

*Nonunion or delayed union* of the osteotomy or rarely, avascular necrosis of the fifth metatarsal head may occur. A well-performed osteotomy with good bony apposition and minimal stripping of the soft tissues from the distal metatarsal should limit the chance of these problems occurring.

## ILLUSTRATIVE CASE

A 22-year-old woman presented with pain over the lateral condylar region of her fifth metatarsal in the left foot. She did not have satisfactory relief of symptoms with appropriate footwear. The appearance of the fifth toe was not particularly bothersome to her. Radiographs show some degree of splaying of the fifth metatarsal relative to the fourth (increase in intermetatarsal 4-5 angle) on the standing anteroposterior view (Fig. 14-11). A distal chevron osteotomy without fixation was performed. She was immobilized in a short-leg walking cast. Her cast and sutures were removed at 3 weeks postoperatively, and she was placed in a postsurgical shoe for an additional several weeks. Radiographs show the degree of correction of the prominent distal fifth metatarsal with medial displacement of the distal fragment (Fig. 14-12). The lateral border of the foot was no longer prominent distally, and the fifth toe alignment was improved. At follow-up 6 years later, the patient had

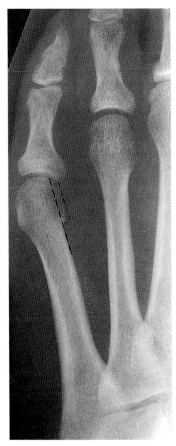

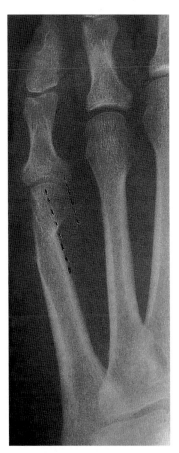

**Figure 14-11.** Preoperative radiograph of a 22-year-old woman with painful bunionette.

**Figure 14-12.** Six years after a successful distal chevron osteotomy. Notice the displacement of the metatarsal head medially *(dotted lines)*.

a good result with no pain, no restriction of activities, and no support requirement; some stylish shoes were tolerated, and there was no tenderness or painful callus, stiffness, or objectionable alignment.

## RECOMMENDED READING

1. Coughlin MJ: Treatment of bunionette deformity with longitudinal diaphyseal osteotomy with distal soft tissue repair. *Foot Ankle* 11:195–203, 1991.
2. Coughlin MJ: Etiology and treatment of the bunionette deformity. *Instr Course Lect* 39:37–48, 1990.
3. Johnson KA, Cofield RH, Morrey BF: Chevron osteotomy for hallux valgus. *Clin Orthop* 142:44–47, 1979.
4. Kitaoka HB, Holiday AD Jr: Metatarsal head resection for bunionette: long-term follow-up. *Foot Ankle,* 11:345–349, 1991.
5. Kitaoka HB, Holiday AD Jr: Lateral condylar resection for bunionette. *Clin Orthop* 278:183–192, 1992.
6. Kitaoka HB, Holiday AD Jr, Campbell DC II: Distal chevron metatarsal osteotomy for bunionette. *Foot Ankle* 12:80–85, 1991.
7. Kitaoka HB, Leventen EO: Medial displacement metatarsal osteotomy for treatment of painful bunionette. *Clin Orthop* 243:172–179, 1989.
8. Moran MM, Claridge RJ: Chevron osteotomy for bunionette. *Foot Ankle Int* 15:684–688, 1994.
9. Nestor BJ, Kitaoka HB, Ilstrup DM, et al.: Radiologic anatomy of the painful bunionette. *Foot Ankle* 11:6–11, 1990.
10. Sponsel KH: Bunionette correction by metatarsal osteotomy: preliminary report. *Orthop Clin North Am* 7:809–819, 1976.
11. Steinke MS, Boll KL: Hohmann-Thomasen metatarsal osteotomy for tailor's bunion (bunionette). *J Bone Joint Surg Am* 71:423–426, 1989.
12. Zvijac JE, Janecki CJ, Freeling RM: Distal oblique osteotomy for tailor's bunion. *Foot Ankle* 12:171–175, 1991.

# 15

# Rheumatoid Forefoot Reconstruction

Steven A. Herbst and Charles L. Saltzman

## INDICATIONS/CONTRAINDICATIONS

The indications for surgical reconstruction of the rheumatoid forefoot are pain unrelieved by nonoperative means and impending ulceration. The goals of surgery need to be considered in light of the natural history of rheumatoid arthritis. Although there may be temporary lulls in the progression of this devastating disease, it never truly "burns out." Consequently, the results of surgery naturally deteriorate over time. Factors that influence outcome include patient selection, surgical timing, and operative technique.

Virtually all patients with long-standing disease have metatarsophalangeal (MTP) joint involvement. Initially, these joints are swollen and painful. The swelling permanently stretches surrounding ligaments. When this acute phase of synovitis resolves, the residual joint laxity leads to subluxation and dislocation. Although any possible deformity can occur, the most common problems are hallux valgus and lesser toe clawing. Patients complain of pain under the central metatarsal heads, around the medial eminence, and on the dorsum of the toes.

Initial care includes the use of extra-depth shoes constructed from a soft, pliable, or temperature-moldable material. Custom inserts with metatarsal pads and a surface interface of medium-density Plastazote are frequently beneficial. If the patient develops severe metatarsalgia, a rocker bottom or metatarsal bar can be added to the sole of the shoe to unload the forefoot.

The primary indication for surgery is pain unrelieved by nonoperative means. Contraindications include vascular insufficiency and ongoing deep infection. Relative contraindications are cervical spine instability, gait unsteadiness, and severe soft tissue fragility.

S. A. Herbst, M.D.: Foot and Ankle Division, Central Indiana Orthopaedics, Muncie, Indiana.

C. L. Saltzman, M.D.: Departments of Orthopaedic Surgery and Biomedical Engineering, University of Iowa, Iowa City, Iowa.

## PREOPERATIVE PLANNING

A complete history and physical examination should be done on every rheumatoid arthritis patient before surgery. A history of increasing unsteadiness or the physical finding of lower extremity hyperreflexia can indicate cervical myelopathy and deserves prompt attention. Lateral flexion-extension radiographs of the cervical spine are routinely obtained. Patients with documented cervical instability should have a regional or spinal anesthetic. If general anesthesia is required, an awake fiberoptic intubation is recommended. Patients with significant instability or myelopathy may be advised to consider cervical spine stabilization before foot surgery. Patients on methotrexate are asked to discontinue its use 1 week before surgery and until 1 to 2 weeks after surgery. Prednisone-dependent patients may or may not be given a steroid burst in the perioperative period, depending on the preference of medical or rheumatologic consultation. Patients with upper extremity arthritic involvement benefit from preoperative instruction in the use of Canadian crutches or a walker with wheels. The ease of postoperative recovery can be enormously facilitated by arranging home care or physical therapy in advance of surgery.

The optimal timing of surgery for patients with bilateral problems is a matter of debate. Our preference is to stage procedures with a minimum of 6 months between operations.

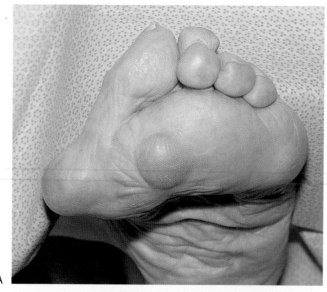

A

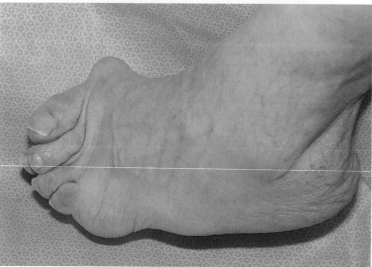

B

**Figure 15-1. A and B:** Typical rheumatoid forefoot appearance before surgery.

With this approach, the patient has the nonoperated foot on which to bear weight after surgery and, as a result, has less postoperative morbidity. Moreover, the patient is able to judge the true benefits of surgery before having both feet reconstructed. In rare circumstances (e.g., patients with bilateral plantar ulcerations or with significant anesthetic risks), it may be wiser to treat both feet simultaneously.

In addition to the general history and physical examination, a focused evaluation of the foot is necessary. The physical examination documents the condition of the peripheral vasculature, the severity and location of skin calluses, as well as the patient's locus of pain. The radiographs include a weight-bearing anteroposterior and lateral views and a non–weight-bearing oblique view. From these radiographs, the degree of osteoporosis, joint deformity (including subluxation or dislocation), and the amount of rheumatoid joint destruction is visualized. The typical clinical appearance of a rheumatoid forefoot before surgery is shown in Figure 15-1.

No single operative approach suffices for all patients. For example, consider derangements of the hallux in rheumatoid arthritis. The great toe can drift into valgus or varus at the MTP joint, have interphalangeal (IP) arthritis or dislocation, develop clawing from intrinsic imbalance or tendon attrition, and be endowed with either soft or hard bone stock. Although arthrodesis of the first MTP joint is generally preferred (3,8), a resection arthroplasty may be a better procedure for a patient with insufficient bone stock, extrinsic tendon rupture, or significant IP symptoms.

Similarly, treatment of the lesser toes should be individualized. Variable degrees of deformity can develop, ranging from mild MTP subluxation to fixed MTP dislocation with rigid clawing. The prevailing surgical approach to these problems is MTP resection arthroplasty (2). Synovectomy alone has been shown to be temporizing only (1). The approach and extent of resection, however, may be modified to accommodate each patient's particular problems. Mild deformities are treated with minimal resections, whereas severe deformities require more bone removal. We tend to remove more rather than less bone since attaining soft tissue relaxation through an adequate bony excision is fundamental to the procedure's success (2).

## SURGERY

The patient is positioned supine with the operative table inclined in mild, reverse Trendelenburg position. The foot is positioned with the heel within inches of the end of the table. This enables the surgeon to have full access to the forefoot from a seat at the end of the table.

A 12- or 18-inch inflatable tourniquet is wrapped above the ankle. The foot is prepped in a sterile fashion. For patients with marginal skin, the foot is exsanguinated by gravity; for all others, a 3-inch Esmarch bandage is used. The tourniquet pressure is set at 100 mm Hg greater than the systolic pressure. Complete reconstruction of the rheumatoid forefoot can be time consuming. After 2 hours, the tourniquet pressure is released to reduce the potential for neurovascular complications.

Meticulous, atraumatic technique is essential when performing rheumatoid forefoot surgery. This can be accomplished with single- and double-pronged skin hooks, Boyes-Goodfellow retractors, and Adson forceps. Self-retaining retractors are to be used only sparingly, because they can crush the fragile capillary networks of the rheumatoid forefoot.

### Technique: Hammer Toe Deformity

There are a variety of methods to address the hammer toe deformity that occurs in the rheumatoid forefoot. We prefer closed osteoclasis. We do this with direct extension manipulation and find that our deformity correction is usually adequate. We have not routinely found it necessary to do open hammer toe repair (i.e., proximal phalangeal condylectomy), but this is described in the literature (3).

### Technique: Lesser Metatarsophalangeal Resection Arthroplasties

Many different incisions have been advocated. These vary from transverse to longitudinal approaches, across plantar or dorsal surfaces, with or without soft tissue excision. We prefer to use two longitudinal dorsal incisions for the lesser resections and a third dorsal incision for the first MTP fusion. I place these directly over the first MTP joint and over the second and fourth intermetatarsal spaces (Fig. 15-2). When doing a first MTP fusion, the lesser toe procedures are completed first to protect the arthrodesis construct.

The initial incision is placed in the second web space and is approximately 3 cm long. Thick flaps are developed by sharp dissection directly down to bone with the neurovascular bundle remaining in the plantar flap. The second and third MTP joints are exposed through this incision. A 1-cm section of the short extensor is removed sharply (Fig. 15-3). A Z-shaped cut is made in the long extensor tendon of each toe (Fig. 15-4). These ends are later repaired in a Z-lengthening repair after the metatarsal head resection. The dorsal capsule is incised longitudinally and the collaterals, intrinsics, and plantar plate are dissected sharply from the distal metatarsal neck and head and proximal aspect of the proximal phalanx. Commonly, the proximal phalanx is in a dorsally dislocated position. Avoid transection of the neurovascular bundle. We prefer to use a Carroll or McGlamry elevator to deliver the metatarsal head out of the wound (Fig. 15-5). Oblique transection of the metatarsal neck is easily and safely accomplished with this retractor in place (Fig. 15-6A) and a small oscillating saw. The neurovascular bundle lies plantarward, and the surgeon should avoid overpenetration with the saw blade. The orientation of transection is slightly oblique in the coronal plane to avoid a sharp edge of distal metatarsal plantarly (Fig. 15-6B). A smooth arc of transection from distal medial to proximal lateral is preferred (Fig. 15-6C). Once the cut is made, a towel clip is used to grasp the distal fragment, and all soft tissue attachments are dissected sharply. Osteoporotic forefoot bones in patients with rheumatoid disease require delicate handling. Inadvertently leaving small pieces of bone behind may contribute to heterotopic ossification and/or symptomatic prominences. Removing as much investing soft tissue as possible facilitates bony excision.

We usually begin with the second toe and proceed laterally, but we sometimes begin with the most deformed toe first and then determine the level of resection of adjacent metatarsals

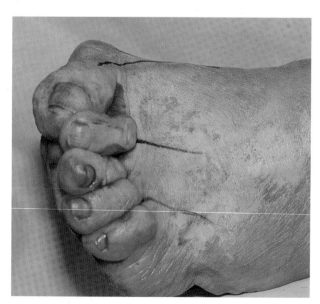

**Figure 15-2.** Typical incisions used for rheumatoid forefoot reconstruction.

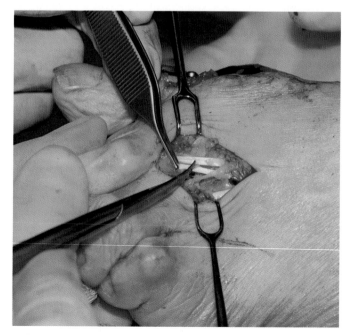

**Figure 15-3.** Removal of a 1-cm section of short extensor tendon.

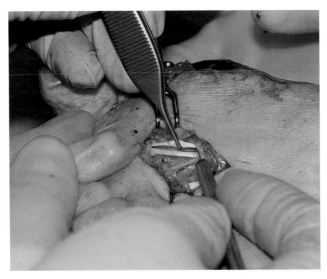

**Figure 15-4.** Z-cut of the long extensor.

from the most deformed toe. For mild deformities, this level of resection is the metatarsal head only; for moderate deformities, the level is more proximal into the neck/shaft region. We prefer to avoid removing any proximal phalanx. It may help to stabilize the resection and prevent dislocation (3,7). The fifth metatarsal is smoothed laterally to minimize the risk of skin irritation. At the completion of the lesser metatarsal head resections, there should be 1 to 1.5 cm of space between the metatarsals and the phalanges with gentle traction placed on the toes.

In summary, the three keys to metatarsal head resection are to recreate a natural arc or cascade from medial to lateral, to resect enough bone to allow for adequate deformity correction, and to leave no plantar bony prominences.

The lesser metatarsal resection arthroplasties are stabilized with 0.045- or 0.062-inch Kirschner wires. These are inserted in an antegrade fashion, beginning in the proximal phalanx and exiting the tip of the toe plantar to the nail bed and plate. The wire is then pulled distally so that its end is at the level of the articular surface of the proximal aspect of the proximal phalanx. The wire is then driven proximally in a retrograde fashion into the

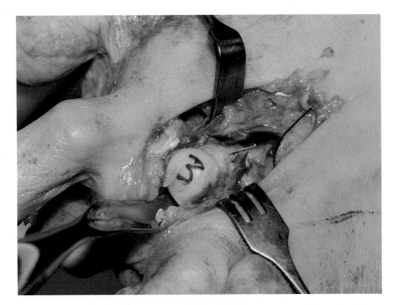

**Figure 15-5.** Presentation of the third metatarsal head with a McGlamry retractor.

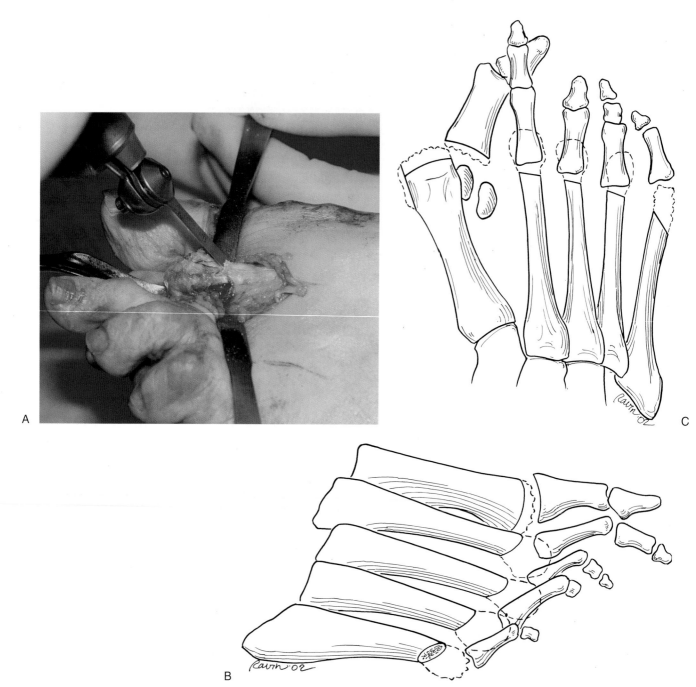

**Figure 15-6. A:** Transection of the metatarsal neck with an oscillating saw. **B:** The plane of metatarsal neck resection from distal-dorsal to proximal-plantar aspects. **C:** Typical amount of metatarsal head and neck resection. Notice the smooth arc from medial to lateral aspects.

metatarsal shaft (Fig. 15-7). The extensor digitorum longus tendons are then repaired in a Z-lengthening fashion (Fig. 15-8).

### Technique: First Metatarsophalangeal Arthrodesis

Arthrodesis of the first MTP joint is achieved using a modification of McKeever's cup-and-cone technique (10,11). Compared with other approaches, McKeever's method has several

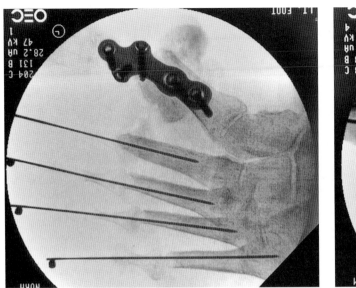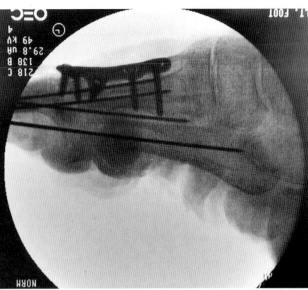

A                                                                                    B

**Figure 15-7.  A and B:** Kirschner wires are in place.

advantages. First, it is straightforward and reliable. Second, the IP joint becomes relatively protected as the hallux is shortened, functionally. Third, the IP joint is not violated by fixation hardware.

A 3- to 4-cm, longitudinal incision is placed along the medial aspect of the extensor hallucis longus tendon. The metatarsal head and most proximal aspect of the phalanx are exposed subperiosteally. The assistant presents the metatarsal head to the surgeon by holding the hallux in marked plantarflexion (Fig. 15-9). The metatarsal head is now ready to be shaped into a cone (Fig. 15-10). The particular type of reamer used is not important. The surgeon should, however, realize that the more conical the reamer is, the more directionality it has to it as opposed to a spherical reamer, which allows more adjustment or "fine-tuning" of alignment but somewhat less initial stability.

With the forefoot in neutral position, the surgeon determines the axis of the first metatarsal and places a mark approximately 3 mm superolateral to its projected intersection with the metatarsal head. This point becomes the tip of the cone and places the hallux

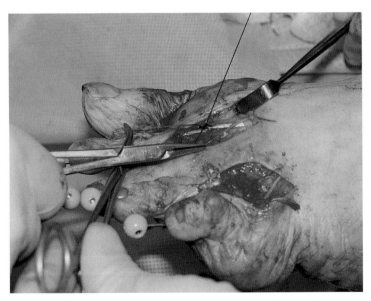

**Figure 15-8.** Z-lengthening extensor tendon repair.

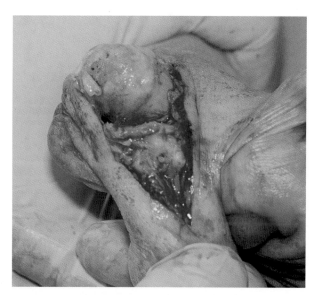

**Figure 15-9.** Presentation of the first metatarsal head.

in 15° of valgus and 25° of dorsiflexion in relation to the metatarsal shaft. Prepare the metatarsal head; take as little bone as possible. Do not ream beyond the point of subchondral cancellous bone of the head.

Next the proximal phalanx is flexed and presented into the surgical field. The cup is then excavated with the reamer. The reamer normally can be inserted so that its base is flush with the joint; however, in small bones, this is not feasible.

The cup of proximal phalanx is then opposed on the cone of the metatarsal. Typically, some adjustment around the base of the cone is needed to achieve close contact. To avoid further shortening of the metatarsal, we prefer to make these modifications with a small rongeur rather than with the reamer. The toe is positioned in approximately 15° of valgus and 25° of dorsiflexion. Temporarily, this alignment is maintained with 0.045-inch Kirschner wires placed from the superomedial proximal phalanx to the superolateral metatarsal. At this stage, hallux position is reassessed. The pulp of the great toe should be parallel to or slightly dorsiflexed from the sole of the foot. This should be checked by placing a flat surface (we use a basin turned upside-down) against the plantar foot. The pulp

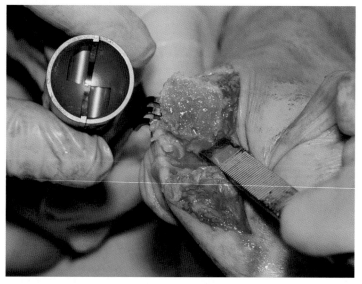

**Figure 15-10.** Shaping of the head into a cone.

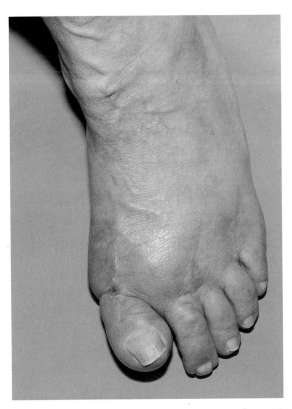

**Figure 15-13.** The follow-up photograph at 12 weeks shows the lesser toes are touching the ground without overlap, the great toe is well aligned, and the forefoot can now fit in a shoe with a standard toe box.

In a recent long-term follow-up, Coughlin felt that the keys to success are fusion of the first MTP to realign the first ray, increase weight bearing through the first ray, and protect the lesser toes; a smooth arc of resection and meticulous debridement to prevent recurrent plantar keratoses; Kirschner wire fixation to maintain alignment during healing; and correction of fixed hammer toe deformities, with fusion if possible (3).

Long-term functional results with the described procedure range from 84% to 96% good or excellent subjective results (3,7). In terms of pain relief, the results of surgery average 90% satisfactory at 2 years and 80% satisfactory at 5 years (4,6,14). Wound problems occur in approximately 10% of patients (5,9). Footwear rarely needs to be changed (4,9); the desire to wear more fashionable shoes is not a reasonable expectation or an indication for surgery. Gait unsteadiness can be exacerbated by procedures that shorten the functional length of the foot (6,12).

## COMPLICATIONS

Reconstructive surgery of the rheumatoid forefoot is palliative, not curative. Although there may be periods of relative inactivity, rheumatoid disease never truly goes away. Continued functional deterioration is expected.

The natural history of the disease needs to be considered when evaluating the results of surgery. Not all bad results are complications of surgery, and only the complications directly related to surgery are subsequently described.

*Incisional problems* may occur. Superficial and deep wound infections occur at a much higher rate than for most other forefoot surgeries. The key factors to minimizing the risks of developing wound problems are proper patient selection, meticulous handling of tissues (i.e., "hand surgery of the feet"), use of longitudinal dorsal incisions, and elevating the foot in a compressive postoperative dressing. Deep infections are treated with surgical debridement and intravenous antibiotics. Wound dehiscence is treated with various approaches, including soaks in lukewarm tap water, Silvadene or wet-to-dry dressing changes, and oral antibiotics, usually first-generation cephalosporins.

*Neurovascular problems* may complicate the procedure. Permanent hypoesthesia or vascular compromise can occur from inadvertent transection of a neurovascular bundle, usually during bony transection. Shielding all soft tissues from the oscillating saw blade can reduce this risk. After tourniquet reversal, it is not uncommon for the lesser toes to take a few minutes to regain full circulation. Toes with continued impaired vascular status should have all restrictive wrappings released or removed. A warm saline-soaked sponge should be wrapped around the toes. If this fails to improve capillary refill, the Kirschner wire to the affected toe should be removed. Venous engorgement is treated with elevation. Persistent and complete loss of arterial inflow to the great toe is an indication for immediate operative exploration and arterial repair. Marginal arterial inflow causing mild cyanosis and decreased turgor usually responds to strict bed rest with the foot maintained at or slightly below the level of the heart. A transcutaneous oxygen monitor can help with early surveillance of toes that may have vascular compromise.

*Calluses* may form. It is not uncommon for patients to develop plantar calluses or palpable bursae several years after surgery. The early return of these painful prominences, however, can be caused by technical problems. The most common error involves irregular bony resection. Sharp plantar spikes left under the metatarsals and an uneven cascade of metatarsal shaft lengths are the two major causes of recurrent callus formation. The offending bony prominences sometimes need to be surgically excised.

*Gait instability* may develop postoperatively. Resection of the metatarsal heads functionally shortens the foot. Some patients report difficulties with gait due to unreliable push-off. For patients with established instability, it is helpful to use a shoe with a full-length steel spring insert and slight rocker-bottom sole.

*First MTP nonunion* occurs infrequently in rheumatoid patients. Factors responsible for nonunion are insufficient bone stock, incomplete bone apposition, inadequate fixation, too short of a period of protected immobilization, and early, inadvertent weight bearing. If poor bone stock is encountered intraoperatively, we rarely perform a resection arthroplasty involving removal of the medial eminence and distal metatarsal head (i.e., modified Mayo procedure). Bony apposition should be evaluated at the time of surgery. Not uncommonly, a lip of cortical bone from the metatarsal is found to block full contact between the cup and cone. The stability of the arthrodesis construct should always be assessed intraoperatively. The options for improving stability depend on the quality of bone. With hard bone, the screw can be replaced with a slightly longer one or repositioned after reshaping the cup and cone. With moderately hard bone, placing an additional screw from the medial metatarsal neck to the lateral phalangeal base can strengthen the construct. For soft bone, we routinely apply a dorsal plate to enhance the stability. Radiographs should reveal trabecular bridging before resumption of unprotected weight bearing.

Established MTP nonunions are usually painless and need no treatment. A painful nonunion can sometimes be converted to a painless one by removing the hardware. Continued symptoms may necessitate an attempt at refusion. If, as a result of the initial procedure, first ray length has been shortened considerably, a corticocancellous interpositional graft is rarely necessary to restore function. Unfortunately, consolidation of these grafts can be slow and unpredictable. Non–weight-bearing immobilization averaging 3 months is required. This is extremely difficult for rheumatoid arthritis patients with polyarticular involvement. Those patients may be better served by conversion of the first MTP nonunion into a resection arthroplasty. Overall results tend to be worse with resection, but the options are limited for this group of patients (6).

## RECOMMENDED READING

1. Barton NJ: Arthroplasty of the forefoot in rheumatoid arthritis. *J Bone Joint Surg Br* 55:126–133, 1973.
2. Clayton ML: Surgery of the forefoot in rheumatoid arthritis. *Clin Orthop* 16:136–140, 1960. (Reprinted in Clin Orthop 349: 6–8, 1998.)
3. Coughlin MJ: Rheumatoid forefoot reconstruction: a long-term follow-up study. *J Bone Joint Surg Am* 82:322–341, 2000.
4. Craxford AD, Stevens J, Park C: Management of the deformed rheumatoid forefoot: a comparison of conservative and surgical methods. *Clin Orthop* 166:121–126, 1982.
5. Faithful DK, Savill DL: Review of the results of excision of metatarsal heads in patients with rheumatoid arthritis. *Ann Rheum Dis* 30:201–202, 1971.
6. Hasselo LG, Wilkens RF, Toomey HE, et al.: Forefoot surgery in rheumatoid arthritis: subjective assessment of outcome. *Foot Ankle* 8:148–151, 1987.
7. Mann RA, Schakel ME: Surgical correction of rheumatoid forefoot deformities. *Foot Ankle Int* 16: 1–6, 1995.
8. Mann RA, Thompson FM: Arthrodesis of the first metatarsophalangeal joint for hallux valgus in rheumatoid arthritis. *J Bone Joint Surg Am* 66:687–692, 1984.
9. McGarvey SR, Johnson KA: Keller arthroplasty in combination with resection arthroplasty of the lesser metatarsophalangeal joints in rheumatoid arthritis. *Foot Ankle* 9:75–80, 1988.
10. McKeever DC: Arthrodesis of the first metatarsophalangeal joint for hallux valgus, hallux rigidus, and metatarsus primus varus. *J Bone Joint Surg Am* 34:129–134, 1952.
11. Moynihan FJ: Arthrodesis of the metatarsophalangeal joint of the great toe. *J Bone Joint Surg Br* 49:544–551, 1967.
12. Newman RJ, Fitton JM: Conservation of metatarsal head in surgery of rheumatoid arthritis of the forefoot. *Acta Orthop Scand* 54:417–421, 1983.
13. Riggs SA, Johnson EW: McKeever arthrodesis for the painful hallux. *Foot Ankle* 3:248–253, 1983.
14. Saltzman CL, Johnson KA, Donnelly RE: Surgical treatment for mild deformities of the rheumatoid forefoot by partial phalangectomy and syndactylization. *Foot Ankle* 14:325–329, 1993.

# 16

# Transmetatarsal Amputation

James W. Brodsky

## INDICATIONS/CONTRAINDICATIONS

The primary indication for a transmetatarsal amputation is the presence of nonviable toes with or without loss of viability of the most distal forefoot. In practice, this usually translates into the clinical diagnosis of gangrene. Distal forefoot means involvement of tissue no more proximal than the distal one half of the metatarsals. The multiple or variable causes of the gangrene include, but are not limited to, diabetes, arteriosclerotic peripheral vascular disease, nondiabetic peripheral neuropathy, severe trauma, and embolic phenomena from sepsis or other causes.

The most common indications for transmetatarsal amputation, in decreasing order of frequency, are diabetic foot problems, vascular insufficiency in the absence of diabetes, and trauma. Because many of these procedures are done because of tissue death due to poor circulation, a special set of circumstances are presented with regard to the applicability of the operation. Patients who need the amputation because of trauma (e.g., from a boating accident) or because of embolism frequently do not have the problems with healing that the former group demonstrates.

Transmetatarsal amputation is the partial foot amputation that is most easily accommodated in footwear, requiring the least amount of special insoles and special footwear. It has the limitation of being applicable only for cases with the most distal level of trauma or dry or wet gangrene. Many patients with infection or local tissue death have involvement far too extensive to be treated with this procedure. Choosing this procedure inappropriately only condemns the patient to additional, possibly unnecessary operations. The choice of a transmetatarsal amputation should be made based on examination and diagnostic studies, but the presence of margins of bleeding and viable tissue at the time of closure is particularly important.

Transmetatarsal amputation is not indicated for the nonambulatory patient when the level of healing is doubtful. For a patient who cannot weight bear because of paralysis, de-

J. W. Brodsky, M.D.: Department of Orthopaedic Surgery, University of Texas Southwestern Medical School; and Foot and Ankle Surgery Fellowship, Baylor University Medical Center and University of Texas Southwestern Medical School, Dallas, Texas.

mentia, or severe debility, a more proximal amputation is indicated if the diminished circulation makes the prospect of healing questionable. One of the principal indications for the transmetatarsal amputation is to preserve the length of the foot so that the patient has maximum potential function and can wear an easily modified shoe rather than a prosthesis.

After the amputation is done through the tarsometatarsal joints themselves, rather than more distally at the transmetatarsal level, the nature of the amputation and the function of the residual foot are significantly altered. The loss of the attachments and thereby the functions of the peroneus brevis and longus and the anterior tibialis tendons creates a more dysfunctional foot with a notable muscle imbalance. The triceps surae, through the attachment of the Achilles tendon, gradually produce an equinus deformity of the ankle. If a transmetatarsal amputation is extended proximally and thus converted to a Lisfranc amputation or tarsometatarsal disarticulation, the surgeon should try to transfer the insertions of the midfoot tendons proximally to the residual skeletal structure. In addition, or even alternatively, it is usually necessary to do an Achilles tendon lengthening at the same time.

Transmetatarsal amputation may be a good procedure to salvage other, more distal procedures that have failed. Examples include failed toe amputations that have not healed because of inadequate circulation or persistent infections, and recurrent soft tissue breakdown, ulceration, or severe metatarsalgia after resection of two or more rays (e.g., metatarsal plus corresponding toe).

This operation is also indicated as a salvage procedure in selected diabetic or other patients with insensitive feet, who have recurrent neuropathic ulcerations, even in the absence of the other factors of infection, gangrene, or vascular insufficiency discussed earlier. These patients also may be candidates for a modified Hoffmann procedure to remove all of the lesser (and possibly the first) metatarsal heads. A candidate may be a patient who had two or three metatarsal heads resected for recalcitrant ulceration or localized infection, now resolved, who is experiencing yet another ulceration because of the concentration of loading on the remaining metatarsals. Although a modified Hoffmann procedure has the advantage of saving the toes, these toes are "floppy" and can be subjected to other recurrent infection and pressure in the shoe, especially if they are elevated by contraction of dorsal scars. The patient with a transmetatarsal amputation, especially if it is a proximal one, may have more difficulty in holding a shoe on, but the procedure obviates the risk of further recurrent toe lesions.

Age is not an important factor in patient selection for the procedure, provided that the general criteria of adequate perfusion and preexisting ambulatory function are met. Patients with an equinus contracture should not have a transmetatarsal amputation because of the excessive pressure applied to the end of the stump by the plantarflexed ankle, unless a concomitant Achilles lengthening is done. If the equinus deformity is of recent onset and is still relatively flexible (i.e., not yet a true fixed contracture), the procedure can be followed by stretching by placement of the limb in serial holding casts or by the use of a dorsiflexion ankle-foot orthosis. In contrast, a severe equinus contracture may require release of the posterior ankle and subtalar joint capsules as well. The surgeon should decide if it is worth performing extensive soft tissue releases to provide a plantigrade foot with a transmetatarsal amputation, especially if the release requires flexor tendon lengthening. In this case, it is usually better to do a more proximal amputation.

Another contraindication for a transmetatarsal amputation is extensive gangrene or infection of the plantar skin (i.e., more proximal plantar than dorsal soft tissue loss) because of the loss of the plantar flap, which is most often used to cover the end of the resected bones. It is relatively contraindicated in patients who have little or no function of the anterior compartment and lateral compartment muscles to oppose the pull of the triceps surae. In these patients, it is necessary to do lengthening of the Achilles tendon, and the permanent use of a polypropylene ankle-foot orthosis will probably be required. Even with these caveats, this procedure is still preferable to a proximal amputation, which requires the use of a prosthesis. It is relatively contraindicated in patients who have instability or deformity at Lisfranc's joint, especially diabetics with peripheral neuropathy who have had a Charcot midfoot joint.

## PREOPERATIVE PLANNING

In diabetic and in nondiabetic dysvascular patients, it is essential to evaluate the preoperative vascular status of the limb. As in all cases of amputation surgery, the foot should be carefully examined to determine adequacy of vascularity and integrity of the skin. The foot should be palpated to detect the presence of posterior tibial and dorsalis pedis pulses. Additional diagnostic studies are useful, particularly in the patient with nonpalpable pulses. Screening is most easily and most widely done using the Doppler ultrasound. The ankle-brachial index (ABI) is determined by measuring the ankle systolic pressure and dividing it by the brachial systolic pressure using Doppler detection of the pulse. The severity of arterial disease is relative to decreasing values of ABI, and a value less than 0.45 or 0.50 is considered abnormal in diabetics. However, this is only a screening test, and there are questions regarding the sensitivity and specificity of the test. It may underestimate the severity of the arterial insufficiency. The ABI is affected by upper extremity disease and stiff, calcified vessels, which are common in diabetics, and lead to falsely elevated values. When definitive evaluation is required in cases with marginal vascularity, a vascular surgery consultation is usually sought and other testing is performed, including arteriography. The vascular surgeon may also provide an opinion regarding the role of other procedures such as revascularization.

Transcutaneous oxygen tension measurement ($TcP_O_2$) is useful for evaluation of the viable level of amputation. The amputation is likely to heal at the level tested if the $TcP_O_2$ is greater than 20 mm Hg. For patients whose values fall into the range of 20 to 40 mm Hg, additional testing can be performed. Rather than a treadmill test, it is possible to "stress the system" by elevating the leg to an angle of 30° for 3 minutes before repeating measurements. If the $TcP_O_2$ falls more than 10 mm Hg with leg elevation, there is an 80% chance of the wound not healing. If it falls less than 10 mm Hg with leg elevation, there is an 80% chance of wound healing. The $TcP_O_2$ depends on the temperature, and an electrode surface temperature of 44°C to 45°C is considered a standard testing condition.

The absolute toe systolic pressure measurement is another noninvasive vascular study that has been used as a predictor for amputation in diabetics with foot ulcers. Values less than 40 mm Hg can be considered abnormal, but healing may occur with values between 30 to 40 mm Hg.

Radiographs are important in the preoperative routine planning to rule out the extension of osteomyelitis to a level that might preclude the use of this amputation. Other special studies are useful such as the technetium bone scan, indium scan, and magnetic resonance imaging to determine the presence and extent of deep infection.

It is important to examine the patient for a preoperative equinus contracture. This is frequently a subtle finding, and the testing needs to be done with the knee in flexion and extension positions. A tight Achilles tendon is suspected in patients who have been non–weight bearing for long periods, because the absence of walking and standing easily leads to a tight Achilles tendon. In severe cases of equinus deformity, it may be best to avoid this operation. However, even with moderate degrees of equinus, the transmetatarsal amputation may still be tenable; in these marginal cases, the deciding factor may be the presence of forefoot equinus that is in addition to and separate from the ankle equinus. Forefoot equinus is caused by plantarflexion contracture at Chopart's joint (i.e., calcaneocuboid and talonavicular joints), and this is frequently overlooked.

## SURGERY

The transmetatarsal amputation is not commonly performed, but it is not technically difficult. Like all operative procedures, proper attention to detail enhance the quality of the result. Gentle handling of the soft tissues, especially in diabetic and dysvascular patients, should be practiced. This translates into gentle retraction and minimal handling of the skin edges with the forceps.

Transmetatarsal amputations may be performed at different levels or length. In general, it is preferable to produce the longest possible stump that is likely to heal with primary closure of the soft tissue. It is not worthwhile to try to create a slightly longer stump if the skin and soft tissue will be closed under tension or if the edges are not viable.

## Technique

It is helpful to plan the flaps with a skin marker, designing a longer plantar flap to correspond to the length of the residual metatarsals. These are basically fish-mouth flaps, as illustrated in Figure 16-1. Although these can be of various lengths, the relative proportion is roughly the same. The plantar flap is generally longer, so that it can wrap up and around the end of the stump. The plantar flap should be long enough to bring the suture line to the dorsal-distal stump. It is also helpful to angle the contour of the flaps slightly from medial-distal to lateral-proximal, so that the lateral side of the soft tissue flaps is slightly shorter, corresponding to the pattern of bone resection described below.

Full-thickness flaps are developed with incisions extending from the skin level down to the bone (Fig. 16-2). The dorsal flap is fashioned first. Using a large blunt elevator, the soft tissue is elevated in a proximal direction beneath the flap (Fig. 16-3). The interosseous muscles are not yet divided because they are located between the metatarsals below the level of the dorsal cortices. At this point, the dorsalis pedis artery is usually ligated.

The plantar flap is fashioned next. In a long or more distal transmetatarsal amputation, the flap begins at the base of the toes on the plantar foot. The incision is carried down to the bone, and soft tissue dissection is performed with an elevator right on the level of the plantar cortices of the metatarsal shafts to create a full-thickness flap (Fig. 16-4). Hemostasis is usually achieved with electrocautery at this level.

Traction is placed on the exposed long flexor and long extensor tendons using a sturdy clamp such as a Kocher, and divided so that they retract proximally (Fig. 16-5). Attention should be paid to the condition of the tendons and adjacent soft tissues to confirm the absence of gross purulence within the tendon sheath. If there is evidence of infection tracking up the extensor or flexor tendon sheath, the technique is altered. First, dissection should be extended proximally along the course of the tendon to debride the infected tissue as far up

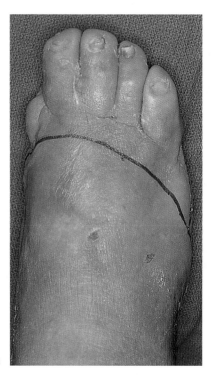
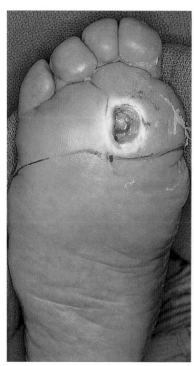
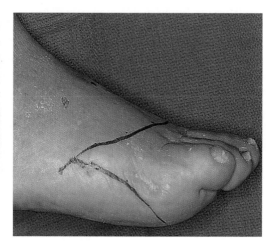

**Figure 16-1. A–C:** The skin is marked for the flaps for amputation. Notice that the plantar flap is longer whenever possible and that it has a fish-mouth junction on the medial and lateral sides. The flaps, especially the dorsal flap, are somewhat shorter on the lateral side, corresponding to the pattern of bone resection.

A, B

C

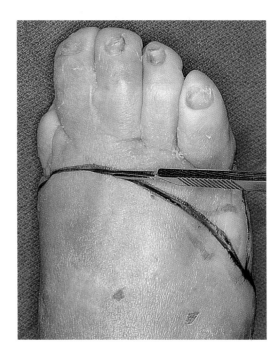

**Figure 16-2.** The dorsal flap is developed by cutting down to the bone.

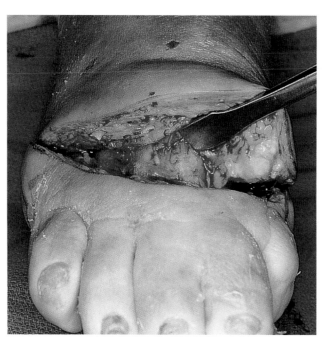

**Figure 16-3.** A full-thickness flap is developed with a broad elevator, taking care not to separate the skin and subcutaneous tissue from the deepest layer of the flap.

the leg as necessary to aggressively drain the infection. Second, it may be necessary to leave the amputation open and to perform local wound care until the wound is clean and covered with granulation tissue and then return the patient to the operating suite for a delayed primary closure at a later date.

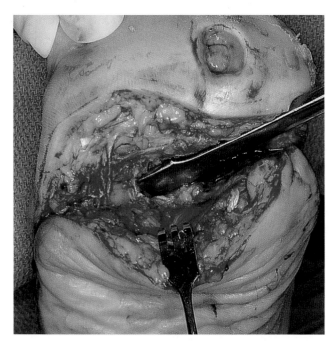

**Figure 16-4.** The plantar flap is developed by a similar incision down to the bone and then dissected as a single flap. Notice the greater thickness of the plantar flap compared with the dorsal flap, which usually requires thinning (see Fig. 16-9).

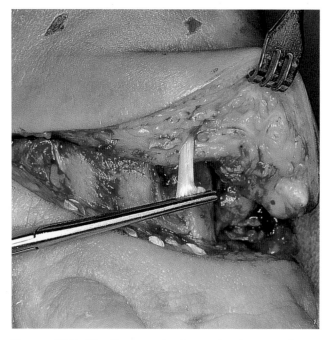

**Figure 16-5.** The flexor and extensor tendons are drawn down with a clamp and divided, allowing them to retract; the extensor tendons are shown here.

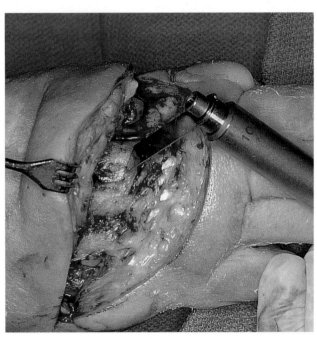

**Figure 16-6.** The metatarsals are divided using a small oscillating saw. Notice that the saw blade is angled in two planes.

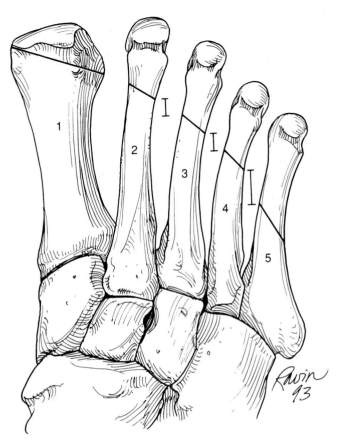

**Figure 16-7.** The "cascade" of length as each metatarsal is cut 2 to 3 mm more proximally than the one medial to it. Notice that the fifth metatarsal needs a greater increment of shortening. It usually should be at least 4 to 5 mm shorter than the fourth.

The metatarsals are then divided with a small oscillating saw (Fig. 16-6). Osteotomes are usually not used because of the risk of splintering the bone. The dorsal soft tissue flap is retracted with rakes or blunt retractors and protected while the bone is cut. The metatarsals are cut from medial to lateral. The angle at which the bones are cut and the length of each residual metatarsal are important. As the surgery progresses from medial to lateral, each metatarsal is cut in a "cascade" of lengths (i.e., each metatarsal is transected progressively shorter as the resections advance laterally). Specifically, each metatarsal should be cut 2 to 3 mm shorter than the metatarsal just medial to it, with the exception of the fifth metatarsal, which should be cut at least 4 to 5 mm shorter than the fourth, if not more (Fig. 16-7). The reason for this is the propensity to develop pressure-related problems under the end of the fifth metatarsal. In a patient with normal sensation, this would be a painful plantar keratosis. In a patient with peripheral neuropathy, such as a diabetic with an insensate foot, a neuropathic ulcer could develop.

In addition to the cascade of lengths, the saw blade orientation when the metatarsal is cut is important (Fig. 16-8). The blade should be angled from dorsal-distal to plantar-proximal to bevel the undersurface of the cut end of the metatarsal. This reduces the pressure under this sensitive area. The saw blade should simultaneously be angled slightly laterally, creating a line from distal-medial to proximal-lateral on the metatarsal. This approach reduces pressure on the end of the metatarsal at the toe-off phase of gait.

A small, straight osteotome, which is held against the cut edge of the metatarsal, serves as a simple and practical guide for marking the level of each successive metatarsal to be cut and improves the accuracy of the cuts. If the cut edges are rough, the surgeon must not hesitate to smooth them with a small rasp.

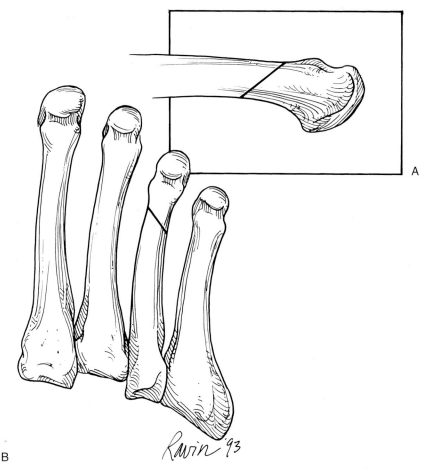

B

*Ravin '93*

**Figure 16-8.** The two planes in which each metatarsal cut is angled: first, from dorsal-distal to plantar-proximal **(A)**; second, mildly from distal-medial to proximal-lateral **(B)**.

After the metatarsals have been cut, the dorsal and plantar flaps must be evaluated for the closure. As in all amputations, it is essential to balance the length of residual bone to be covered with the length of viable soft tissue available to close over it. If less viable tissue is available (i.e., shorter flaps), the bone must be divided more proximally. It is essential to make every attempt to achieve a primary closure without tension on the skin. It is important to balance the amount of soft tissue with the amount of bone, and the shape and thickness of the flaps must be adjusted as well.

The plantar flap almost always needs to be trimmed to facilitate the closure. This should be a gradual, uniform reduction in the thickness of the flap from proximal to distal. Cut the tissue with a no. 10 blade, making smooth, even strokes to avoid leaving skin tags and bits of tissue. The purpose is to create an even surface and consistent thickness of the flap while avoiding the error of leaving bits of tissue behind that may necrose (Fig. 16-9).

The dorsal and plantar flaps are gently held together to estimate the necessary trimming for the proper closure (Fig. 16-10). The flaps may not approximate easily for three possible reasons: there is inadequate soft tissue to cover the bone, in which case all of the metatarsals need to be trimmed at a more proximal level; the flaps are shaped improperly (e.g., not longer medially than laterally) to match the contour of the underlying bone, in which case further trimming of the bone is required; or the plantar flap is too thick and is holding the edges of the skin apart, in which case the plantar flap needs to be trimmed further. This trimming often is done by additional "planing" of the intrinsic muscles in the flap, thinning the flap to a greater extent near the distal edge. Caution must be exercised not to trim the tissue excessively, thereby devascularizing the skin edge inadvertently (Fig. 16-9).

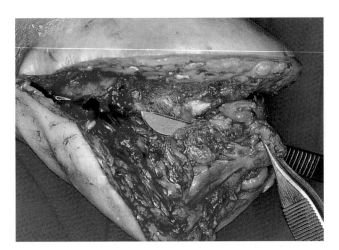

**Figure 16-9.** The plantar flap is trimmed to thin the flap. The flap is gently sloped toward the skin edge, taking care not to remove so much tissue distally as to devascularize the skin edge. The flap is smoothed uniformly so that tags and bits of tissue are not left behind.

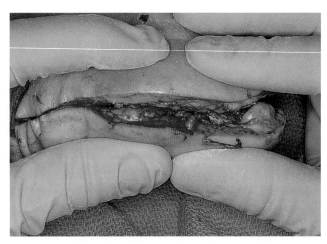

**Figure 16-10.** The flaps are gently held together to estimate the ease of closure. If the flaps do not readily approximate, then the flaps are too short relative to the length of the residual bones to cover, the flaps are improperly shaped, or the plantar flap is too thick and needs to be trimmed further.

After the flaps have been adequately shaped and trimmed and fit easily together while being held with gentle finger pressure, several minor steps are needed before suturing begins. When the amputation is being performed because of infection, a tissue sample should be taken from the wound just before closure. This more accurately reflects the risk of infection in the residual limb than a culture of the obviously infected and more distal part.

If a tourniquet has been used, it should be released to check the wound for hemostasis and to evaluate the perfusion of the skin and soft tissue edges. If good bleeding is present, hemostasis is achieved with the electrocautery; sutures can be used for the dorsalis pedis artery and accompanying veins. If there is poor bleeding or no bleeding from the skin edges, wait for 5 to 10 minutes, and if there is no change, the surgeon has the option to consider proceeding with a more proximal amputation. After release of the tourniquet, it may take 3 to 5 minutes for the bleeding to reach the edges of the wound.

If a drain is used, it is placed in the wound at this point in the operation. In grossly infected wounds, such as a distal forefoot abscess in a diabetic, the surgeon may elect to place an irrigation system instead of a suction drain in the wound. The irrigant usually does not require antibiotic. A liter of normal saline or Ringer's lactate solution is used to drip slowly through the wound. This is done by connecting a sterile intravenous extension tubing to a no. 8 pediatric feeding tube that is placed in the wound through a separate small stab incision proximal to the amputation site (Fig. 16-11). The solution is run into the wound at a rate of about 40 to 50 mL per hour. The fluid is allowed to exit the wound through the incision and between the loosely placed sutures. When this type of irrigation is used, I customarily do not use deep absorbable sutures, but rather use large mattress sutures of 2-0 monofilament. These mattress sutures are placed full thickness through the flap on the "far" side of the stitch and then very close to the skin edge on the "near" part of the stitch. These sutures usually are left in place for at least 1 month, and I do not hesitate to leave them in for 6 or 8 weeks if there is a slowly healing area of the incision line. If an irrigation system is used, a very large bulky wrap is applied around the foot for a dressing. All occlusive-type material (e.g., petrolatum gauze) is avoided so as not to impede the efflux of the irrigant through the incision line. The bulky wrap usually consists of 4 × 4 inch gauze squares, multiple gauze rolls, ABD pads, and an elastic wrap.

If the wound is not infected, then a suction drain is preferable. This is also placed through a small separate stab incision. It is preferable not to use Penrose drains unless they also exit

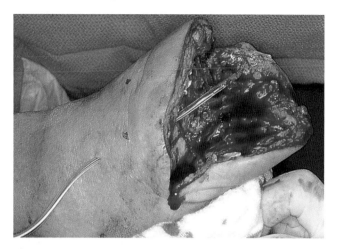

**Figure 16-11.** A suction drain is placed in the wound, right on the bone. It is brought out through a separate tiny stab incision proximally, avoiding the area of the dorsalis pedis artery.

through separate stab incisions. If Penrose drains are brought through the incision itself and in between the sutures, it tends to create a tract that stays open and continues to drain.

Closure is accomplished with 2-0 or 0 absorbable braided sutures placed through the deep fascia. Subcutaneous sutures usually are not used. Skin can be closed with skin staples or with interrupted vertical mattress sutures of 3-0 or 4-0 monofilament. Regardless of which skin closure is used, great care is taken to evert the skin edges. If skin staples are used, the edges are everted with two skin hooks or very gently with a pair of Adson forceps. If sutures are used, the trick is to place the near part of the mattress suture very close to the edge of the skin. A dressing is applied, beginning with a nonadherent material. I prefer the plastic portion of Telfa, otherwise called split Telfa dressing, because the material seldom sticks, and if it does, it simply tears and is not painful. It also has perforations to allow blood to pass through it. This is followed by gauze squares and gauze rolls and then an elastic wrap, applied as a covering but without much tension.

The most common pitfall is to resect too much skin. The surgeon should attempt to maximally conserve skin, cutting right up to the edge of necrotic skin in the case of gangrene. After the flap has been elevated, the soft tissue viability can be better discerned, and the flap can be shortened, if necessary. Sparing of the skin allows the maximal length of the amputation stump.

The next most common pitfall is failing to cut the metatarsals in the cascade of lengths described or failing to cut the metatarsals with the appropriate beveling. This can lead to painful bursae and pressure points in the patients with sensate limbs and to ulceration and infection in the patient with limb insensitivity.

Failure to maximally use the available skin and soft tissue for coverage forces the surgeon to cut the metatarsals at a more proximal level to produce more standard flaps. Very satisfactory results can be achieved with irregularly shaped flaps provided that the edges approximate well and there is no tension on the suture line.

## POSTOPERATIVE MANAGEMENT

After completion of the transmetatarsal amputation, the previously described soft compression dressing is applied. The foot is elevated postoperatively. It is best to elevate the foot in such a way that the heel hangs free in the air and is elevated off the bed at all times. This is easily accomplished with folded blankets stacked on top of each other or even taped together. The blankets provide a platform to support the calf and entire lower leg, and the foot hangs off the end. It is inexpensive, universally available, and preferable to pillows, which tend to shift around and require constant rearranging.

If an irrigation system is used, it is usually in place overnight and removed the following day. The irrigation tube is removed, and a fresh, dry dressing is applied. Although skin appears waterlogged, it quickly dries out.

If a suction drain is used, dressing changes in the early postoperative period are performed as needed, depending on the amount of drainage that appears on the bandage. If a concomitant Achilles tendon lengthening was done at surgery, the patient is placed in an extremely well-padded cotton wrap, on top of the regular dressing, that extends from toes to knee, over which is then applied plaster splints to hold the foot in dorsiflexion. I prefer the combination of a posterior splint with a "sugar-tong" or stirrup (U-shaped) splint. Posterior splints alone invariably break unless made of synthetic material, and the latter is to be avoided because of the cuts and scratches that its sharp edges can create rubbing against the contralateral limb in the bed. This double plaster splint is applied leaving a space along its entire length anteriorly, and it is wrapped with a moistened gauze roll (i.e., Kling bandage); this splint could be removed at any time if it is too tight simply by splitting the gauze anteriorly and spreading the splint apart with the hands.

The patient is kept from bearing weight until the incision is healed and no longer draining. If the patient is debilitated and unable to strictly observe the non–weight-bearing order, touch-down on the heel is allowed to mobilize the patient. If an Achilles tendon lengthening was performed, the period of immobilization is for a minimum of 8 weeks and for as long as 12 weeks.

Patients should be warned that some drainage or a small area of delayed healing is common. They should be warned that the exact interval between the operation and the time they are fitted in shoes is variable and unpredictable and depends on the rapidity of their healing. The time for removal of sutures is variable, but in amputation surgery, 3 to 4 weeks is a minimum interval before removal of sutures. In diabetic patients, it is often advisable to wait longer; in patients who have had an area of delayed healing, it is even longer, and it is not uncommon to leave at least some of the sutures in place for 6 to 8 weeks.

Patients must also be counseled regarding the types of shoes that they can wear later and the limitations in footwear that the amputation imposes. The primary problem for the transmetatarsal amputee in fitting shoes is that the shortened foot is less able to hold on a shoe because of the missing forefoot. A lace-up shoe is almost always necessary, because an open throat, slip-on shoe has inadequate ability to grasp the foot. Especially for very short transmetatarsal amputations, a high-top shoe may be required to provide the mechanical stability to hold the shoe on. Because of the ever-widening array of available leisure and athletic shoes, this is less of a cosmetic dilemma for patients than in years past.

It is generally advised that diabetic patients be professionally fitted with a shoe with additional depth. This allows fitting a custom-molded insole into the shoe that serves several purposes. The insole provides a cushioning and weight-distributing function to take pressure off of any residual pressure point on the plantar surface, as would be the case in any diabetic shoe insole. The insole is also modified to attach a toe filler to it to block out the area of the missing forefoot (Fig. 16-12). This toe filler can even be made to wrap around the forefoot. It reduces or eliminates the side-to-side and front-to-back movement of the foot inside of the shoe, which can cause friction that leads to further breakdown. This same type of shoe insole is generally used by almost all transmetatarsal amputees. In nondiabetic patients with normal sensation, the option exists to place the toe filler permanently within the shoe, and it does not need to be attached to an insole.

Patients, especially those with insensitive limbs, should be taught to regularly inspect their feet, especially the amputation sites, for evidence of ulceration or skin injury. This is the best way to monitor the durability of the amputated foot as the patient progressively increases the amount of walking and activity level. For patients with good sensation, the amount of walking they can do is a function of their vascular status and their tolerance. They are advised to increase their walking distance gradually and progressively. Consultation with a physical medicine specialist may be helpful in the rehabilitation process.

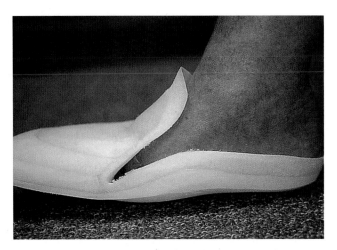

**Figure 16-12.** A shoe insole for the patient with a transmetatarsal amputation. The filler or block for the missing part of the forefoot reduces sliding of the foot inside the shoe.

After transmetatarsal or ray amputation in children, results were superior to more proximal amputations such as Syme amputations (4). Some investigators reported substantial rates of wound problems and reoperations, but these should be reduced when contemporary diagnostic modalities, operative indications, and techniques are used. Quigley et al. (9) found that 18 of 33 patients who underwent transmetatarsal amputation required revision to a major amputation, but this was offset by the significantly greater chance of preserving independent mobility in patients whose heels were preserved. Mueller et al. (8) found that 28% of patients required higher amputation in a review of 120 feet in 107 patients.

## COMPLICATIONS

Complications of the transmetatarsal amputation are similar to those of other amputations in that they concentrate problems of soft tissue healing or breakdown of the soft tissue, either of which eventually leads to superficial infection and ultimately to osteomyelitis and more proximal amputation. The four main complications—delayed primary healing, failed primary healing, recurrent plantar ulceration or pain, and ulceration or painful blisters on the distal stump—are considered along with preventive measures and suggestions for appropriate management strategies.

*Delayed primary healing* is so much a part of the natural history of the procedure that perhaps it should not even be considered a complication. It is often unavoidable. It is usually signified by a small amount of serous, noninfected drainage from a portion of the suture line. The likelihood may be reduced by gentle handling of tissue and by leaving a clean surface free of bits and tags of tissue on the flaps of the amputation. It is managed with local wound care in the area of the drainage, including moist-to-dry saline dressings and local debridement. Sometimes, one or two sutures need to be removed to pack the area gently with the gauze. The surgeon and the patient are counseled to be tolerant, especially because delayed healing is common in those who most often require amputation: dysvascular and diabetic patients. In a review of 120 feet with transmetatarsal amputation, Mueller et al. (8) found that 27% had skin breakdown.

*Failed primary healing* of the wound is usually a function of inadequate vascularity of the tissue, although it can occasionally be attributed to uncontrolled infection. Failure to heal is distinguished from delayed healing by the total absence of wound healing and/or persistent purulent drainage and recurring cellulitis. Management usually requires revision to a more proximal level of amputation. Repeat evaluation of the perfusion of the limb and repeat cultures for estimation of the adequacy of antibiotic coverage may also be advised.

*Ulceration or pain on the plantar surface of the stump* is caused by inordinate prominence of the end of one of the resected metatarsals. A metatarsal may shift position, especially after the destabilizing effect of the amputation on the midfoot tarsometatarsal joints. This can cause a gradually increasing pressure point that leads to pain or ulceration in sensate or insensitive patients, respectively. More frequently, it is caused by excessive pressure under a metatarsal that has been cut too long. Treatment can begin with conservative measures for nonoperative relief of pressure externally, but if it persists, surgical shortening of the metatarsal is performed. This may be caused by failing to produce the cascade of metatarsal lengths described previously.

*Ulceration of the distal stump* usually is a manifestation of pressure on the end of the stump that occurs from footwear, is exacerbated by walking, and is caused by an equinus position of the foot. The equinus most often occurs at the ankle, but some of the deformity can also occur at the midfoot transverse tarsal joint (i.e., talonavicular and calcaneocuboid joints). This is often the sequela of long periods of debilitation or bed rest. Garbalosa et al. (3) found altered kinematics and elevated plantar pressures in patients after transmetatarsal amputation, with less dynamic dorsiflexion in amputated feet. Initial management includes shoe modifications such as a rocker bottom and a stiff sole. If unsuccessful, Achilles lengthening is done. Rarely, posterior capsulotomies of the ankle and subtalar joints are required as well.

## ILLUSTRATIVE CASE

A 68-year-old, retired baker with a 20-year history of insulin-dependent diabetes mellitus had recurrent ulceration under multiple metatarsals over a period of almost 15 years. Despite conservative treatment with total contact casts and subsequent shoe and insole prescriptions, he developed recurrent ulcerations on both feet. He had been unable to work in his garden or walk in his neighborhood for many years because of these recurrent problems. Previous surgical procedures to resect isolated metatarsal heads, debride the ulcers, and amputate an osteomyelitic first ray provided transient improvement, always followed by recurrent ulceration at an adjacent metatarsal.

Examination of the feet showed recurrent neurotrophic ulceration (Fig. 16-13). There was no gross purulence or active infection. Severe claw toes accompanied the increased pressure under the metatarsal heads. Pulses, while somewhat diminished, were present, and preopera-

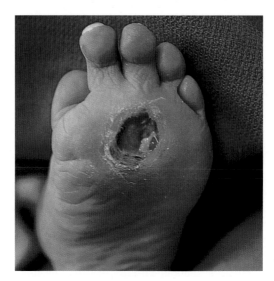

**Figure 16-13.** Preoperative appearance, demonstrating recurrent ulceration before transmetatarsal amputation.

tive Doppler studies showed satisfactory ankle indices and toe pressures bilaterally. Pulse volume recordings demonstrated pulsatile flow at the toe level on both feet. Radiographs demonstrated the previously resected first metatarsal (Fig. 16-14) and changes of neuroarthropathy at the second metatarsophalangeal joint, but no evidence of active osteomyelitis.

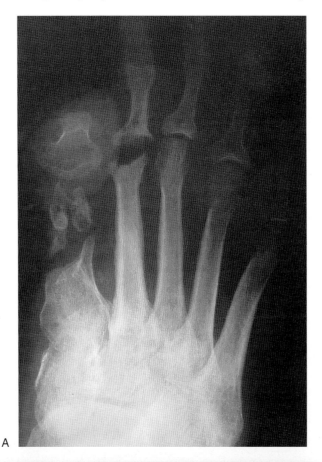

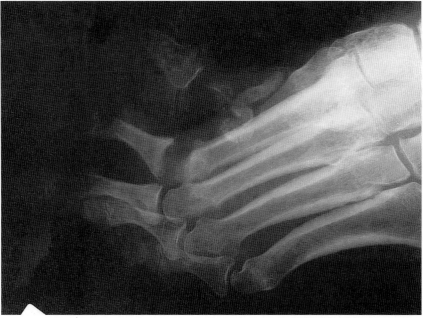

**Figure 16-14.** Preoperative radiographs show the previous resection of the first metatarsal and most of the second metatarsal head in anteroposterior **(A)** and oblique **(B)** views.

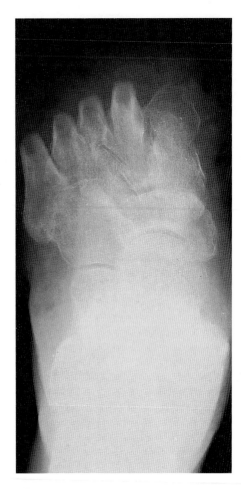

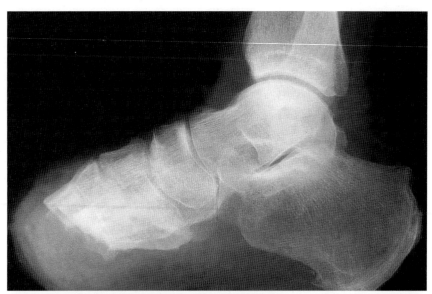

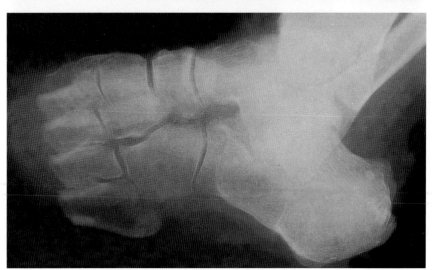

**Figure 16-15.** Postoperative radiographs of the transmetatarsal amputation.

A decision to proceed with transmetatarsal amputation was made. The procedure was done bilaterally, with the two feet being operated about 2 months apart (Fig. 16-15). The patient was hospitalized after each procedure and received a short course of intravenous antibiotics for 72 hours or less, and he was discharged with oral antibiotics for the following 10 days. He was kept non–weight bearing until the stumps healed, averaging 4 weeks. After each foot was healed, the patient was placed in high-top Extra Depth shoes (P. W. Minor and Son, Batavia, NY) with molded insoles that had attached toe fillers (Fig. 16-12).

The patient later began taking short walks in his neighborhood and was quite pleased with his newfound mobilization. No subsequent skin breakdown was experienced during the past 5 years. This case demonstrates the durability and utility of the transmetatarsal amputation for severe, recalcitrant problems of the forefoot.

## RECOMMENDED READING

1. Brodsky JW: Amputations of the foot. In: Mann RA, Coughlin M, eds. *Surgery of the foot and ankle.* St. Louis: Mosby, 1992.
2. Brodsky JW, Chambers RB: Effect of tourniquet use on amputation healing in diabetic and dysvascular patients. *Perspect Orthop Surg* 2:71–76, 1991.

3. Garbalosa JC, Cavanagh PR, Wu G, et al.: Foot function in diabetic patients after partial amputation. *Foot Ankle Int* 17:43–48, 1996.
4. Greene WB, Cary JM: Partial foot amputations in children: a comparison of the several types with the Syme amputation. *J Bone Joint Surg Am* 64:438–443, 1982.
5. Hodge MJ, Peters TG, Efird WG: Amputation of the distal portion of the foot. *South Med J* 82:1138–1142, 1989.
6. Larrson U, Andersson GBJ: Partial amputation of the foot for diabetic or arteriosclerotic gangrene. *J Bone Joint Surg Br* 60:126–130, 1978.
7. McKittrick LS, McKittrick JB, Risley TS: Transmetatarsal amputation for infection of gangrene in patients with diabetes mellitus. *Ann Surg* 130:826, 1949.
8. Mueller MJ, Allen BT, Sinacore DR: The incidence of skin breakdown and higher amputation after transmetatarsal amputation: implications for rehabilitation. *Arch Phys Med Rehab* 76:50–54, 1995.
9. Quigley FG, Fars IB, Xiouruppa H: Transmetatarsal amputation for advanced forefoot tissue loss in elderly patients. *Aust N Z J Surg* 65:339–341, 1995.

# Cuneiform-Metatarsal (Lisfranc) Arthrodesis

Bruce J. Sangeorzan and Sigvard T. Hansen, Jr.

## INDICATIONS/CONTRAINDICATIONS

The midfoot is the region of the foot that extends from the transverse tarsal (Chopart) joint to the tarsometatarsal (Lisfranc) joints. When clinically important instability or arthritis affects the midfoot joints, arthrodesis is the only established salvage procedure. The joints are too small, motion too limited, and the ligaments too complex to respond reliably to other reconstructive procedures. Primary osteoarthritis in the intertarsal or tarsometatarsal (TMT) joints is uncommon. Arthrosis of the TMT joint is usually secondary to trauma or to inflammatory arthritis. There are a limited number of patients with midfoot arthrosis and no history of trauma, inflammatory arthritis, or Charcot arthropathy. These patients may have other contributing factors, such as a tight heel cord with secondary midfoot breakdown, or tend to have a long second ray and a short first ray. Under the former circumstances, the inability of the ankle to dorsiflex leads to increasing motion and force in the midfoot and eventually to instability and secondary midfoot arthritis. In the second group, the increased bending force on the midfoot from the long second ray may be causative.

Preoperative complaints include pain, fatigue, and instability. Instability may occur during standing, but it is likely to be most noticeable during the propulsive part of gait, particularly while walking up hills. The patient usually notices that the foot is "turning outward." This tendency to abduct results from a combination of factors. The habitus of a normal limb is slightly externally rotated, and the center of mass of the body is in the midline, medial to the foot. During toe-off, the body weight acts medially to the foot to push the forefoot outward. Continued pressure on the forefoot leads to erosion of the dorsal and lateral aspects of the cuneiforms and progressive valgus deformity (Fig. 17-1). Although in some cases degenerative changes in these joints may occur in the absence of increasing joint instability, the degenerative changes are more often accompanied by increasing mechanical failure.

Nonoperative treatment may be effective in relieving short-term symptoms or an acute exacerbation of chronic symptoms. External support that diminishes bending forces across

B. J. Sangeorzan, M.D. and S. T. Hansen, Jr., M.D.: Department of Orthopaedics and Sports Medicine, University of Washington; and Harborview Medical Center, Seattle, Washington.

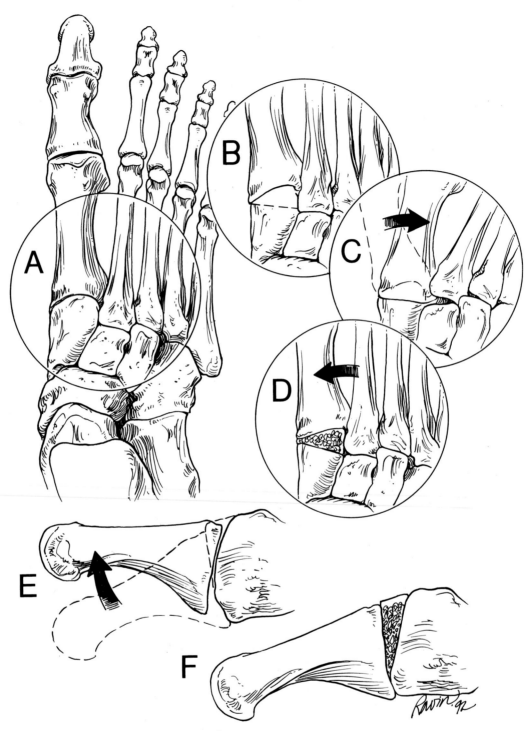

**Figure 17-1. A:** Diagrammatic representation of a dorsal view of a right foot. **B:** The *shaded area* of the first cuneiform is the part that becomes eroded. The first metatarsal angles into a valgus position and wears away the lateral aspect of the medial cuneiform *(shaded area).* Eventually, the medial cuneiform assumes a more flattened shape *(dashed line)* that makes the position of reduction uncertain. **C:** The entire forefoot has become abducted. The native position of the medial cuneiform is represented by a *dashed line.* The lesser metatarsals are subluxated laterally. **D:** Restoring the position of the first ray leaves the defect that must be filled with bone graft. The effect is generally wedge shaped and represents the normal contours of the unaffected medial cuneiform *(checkered area).* **E:** An exaggerated lateral view of the tarsometatarsal articulation of the first ray demonstrating a similar process. The dorsal edge becomes eroded from the repeated dorsiflexion of the first metatarsal. **F:** This up-and-down motion leaves a wedge-shaped defect that must be filled with bone graft. The defect is therefore a two-plane cuneiform shape.

the midfoot provides relief. A short period of cast immobilization is effective nonoperative treatment and ensures compliance. If this relieves the pain satisfactorily, a custom-made polypropylene clamshell orthosis may be an acceptable treatment solution. An alternative is a rocker-bottom sole or a custom-molded, full-length, total-contact insole. Although effective, rocker-bottom soles are not aesthetic, making compliance unpredictable. The height added to the treated limb may require a lift on the contralateral side. A less effective but more aesthetic orthotic option is a steel spring between the sole and the shank of the shoe. However, none of these orthotic methods of management is curative or seem to function adequately in the long term for an active person.

Contraindications to surgery include inadequate soft tissue envelope and inadequate arterial inflow.

## PREOPERATIVE PLANNING

The issues to address in preoperative planning include arterial and venous patency, selection of the joints to be fused, placement of surgical incisions, and extent of bony defect. Because the disease may occur in the elderly patient population and in patients with diabetes mellitus, both dorsalis pedis and posterior tibial pulses should be sought. If neither is palpable, preoperative consultation with a physician specializing in vascular disorders should be requested to clarify the question of the patency of the vessels and the blood flow into the forefoot. Duplex scanning is an effective noninvasive method of visualizing the vascular anatomy. It is also important to know whether the vascular anatomy is anomalous. The dorsalis pedis is at risk during the exposure and reduction of these joints and may be put under tension if substantial realignment has to be performed. There is much greater risk for a patient with an absent tibial pulse. As a rule, if both pulses are palpable, no further vascular evaluation is required. Because cigarette smoking has an adverse effect on wound healing, it is not permitted in the perioperative period, and an effort is made to prevent smoking completely during the period of healing.

Radiographic examination should include full-weight-bearing anteroposterior and lateral views, as well as an oblique view of the foot. Unless the patient is fully weight bearing, it is impossible to determine the severity of the midfoot breakdown and how much angular correction is required, particularly in the dorsoplantar direction. An oblique view provides a good perspective of the midfoot joints. The oblique view is particularly useful if the angle of the x-ray beam is aligned perpendicular to the lesser TMT joints. Sometimes, it is useful to obtain multiple oblique views. An anteroposterior and lateral radiograph of the contralateral foot should be obtained and a tracing performed of the talus and metatarsal. This tracing should be available in the operating room to superimpose on intraoperative radiographs to judge the reduction of the deformity. With erosion of the tarsal bones that occurs with advanced arthritis, it may be difficult to assess alignment without comparison to the other side. If instability is in question, stress view may be performed under fluoroscopic guidance. Computed tomography is generally not required, but it may be useful in sorting out problems in joints that are difficult to visualize with plain film radiography, such as the intercuneiform joints. There is indication for magnetic resonance imaging in the preoperative planning, although it may be helpful in rare cases for diagnostic purposes.

Preoperative diagrams are used to determine the degree of bony defect and therefore the size, shape, and location of corticocancellous bone graft needed. On weight-bearing anteroposterior and lateral radiographs, tracings are made of the first, second, and third metatarsals and cuneiform bones. The articulations are reduced on the paper tracings by cutting out the metatarsals and placing the bases back in the reduced position. By comparing the resulting diagram to the radiographs of the contralateral foot, it is possible to determine whether a block of corticocancellous bone graft will be needed to restore the metatarsals into anatomic position and length. It will also give the surgeon a good idea of the amount of reduction that will be required.

Preoperative planning should include providing an explanation of the procedure and obtaining a clear understanding of desired goals of the patient. Patients often complain of the medial bump on the foot. They are advised that the prominence will be significantly improved, although not always completely corrected. Metal implants on the medial side of the foot may make it appear as though there is still excess tissue remaining in this area postoperatively. It is important to explain the mechanical problems imposed by the incompetent medial column and the need for bone graft.

Although the first, second, and third TMT joints are almost always affected by the degenerative process, it is often difficult to determine the location of other painful joints in the midfoot. When deciding what joints require arthrodesis, particular attention should be paid to the joint between the medial and intermediate cuneiform. This joint has more motion than is generally recognized and is a frequent site of occult injury. Careful examination of this joint may reveal whether it is involved or not. To examine this joint, stabilize the midfoot with one hand, and grasp the first metatarsal head with the other. Passive plantarflexion and dorsiflexion of the first ray will cause pain in the midfoot if the intercuneiform joint is arthritic. If there is any question about the contribution of the intercuneiform joint with the symptoms, selective injection of lidocaine into the joint may be helpful. The use of a miniature fluoroscopy unit such as the Z Scan or HealthMate can help document that the needle is placed accurately in the joint. If there is still some uncertainty after selective injection, we generally fuse the joints we strongly suspect are related to the painful symptoms. The additional work required to fuse an extra joint is limited and the loss of motion negligible. Fusion of an additional intertarsal joint seems preferable to continuing pain or having to do a secondary fusion.

## SURGERY

The patient is placed supine on the operating table with a roll beneath the hip on the operative side. The roll is placed to support the pelvis and greater trochanter. This position helps to internally rotate the limb so that the lateral side of the foot is available for application of a small distractor. A pillow or bump is placed beneath the knee to allow the ankle to plantarflex. This allows a dorsal approach to the foot while viewing the foot as if it is in the standing position. The limb is prepped and draped to allow circumferential access. The anterior iliac crest is prepped to gain access to autogenous bone graft. The limb is exsanguinated with an Esmarch bandage before the tourniquet is inflated.

### Technique

The first dorsal incision is made over the second ray (Figs. 17-2 and 17-3). This incision is somewhat troublesome because it is located close to the neurovascular bundle and crosses the superficial peroneal nerve at its proximal end. However, it allows access to the first, second, and third rays and allows a longitudinal medial incision along the medial aspect of the foot if correcting the abduction deformity is problematic. The dorsalis pedis artery is located in this interval and sends a large branch (i.e., the first proximal perforating artery) to the plantar surface of the foot through the first web space. Care should be taken not to injure either artery. The second TMT joint is recessed in relation to the first, and both will be expected to be subluxated or dislocated under the circumstances of this operative procedure. The medial border of the medial cuneiform can be used as a guide to correctly align the first ray. Alternatively, a medial incision may be added, particularly if a plate is needed to hold the reduction.

The surgical approach may need to be altered if the soft tissue envelope is abnormal. Scars from the initial trauma or ulceration from pressure sores are the most likely to affect the approach. If the deformity has caused a weight-bearing ulcer, the most common area is the undersurface of the medial cuneiform. If this ulcer is healed, the placement of surgical incisions need not be altered. Every effort is made to ensure that the soft tissues are viable and intact before surgical intervention. Before the tourniquet is inflated, the dorsalis pedis pulse is again palpated, and its relationship to the first web space incision is documented.

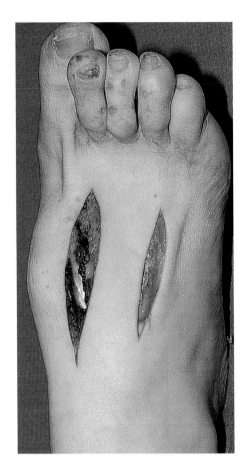

**Figure 17-2.** Intraoperative photograph of the surgical approach. The dorsal surface of a right foot is shown. Notice the medial dorsal deformity. The incisions allow access to two tarsometatarsal joints each.

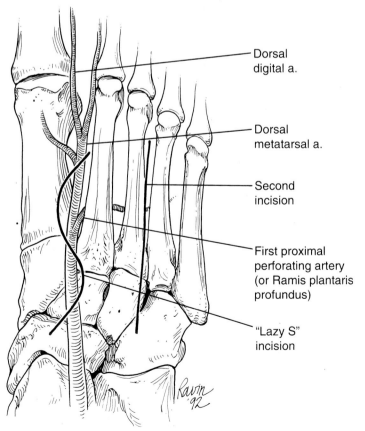

Dorsal
digital a.

Dorsal
metatarsal a.

Second
incision

First proximal
perforating artery
(or Ramis plantaris
profundus)

"Lazy S"
incision

**Figure 17-3.** A dorsal view representing the location of the skin incisions and perforating arteries. The lazy-S incision is represented by a *line* curving a little laterally at the level of the second tarsometatarsal joint and medially at the level of the first tarsometatarsal joint. Notice that the incision also exposes the intercuneiform joint. The same net effect can be accomplished by the long, straight incision that undermines the skin. The second incision is in the interval between the third and fourth ray. Notice the relationship of this incision to the perforating artery and dorsal digital artery. The perforating artery enters the plantar surface of the foot through the first web space.

After the first and second TMT joints are debrided of articular cartilage and subchondral bone, a second incision is made over the medial border of the fourth metatarsal for exposure of the third, fourth, and fifth TMT joints. After these joints are exposed, scar tissue and debris are removed carefully using a small rongeur, curette, or osteotome. Each joint is completely debrided of articular cartilage and subchondral bone so that reduction can be performed. Because ligaments connect the metatarsal bases, reduction cannot be performed until all of the displaced joints are mobilized. Sometimes, a third dorsal longitudinal incision is needed to completely prepare the fifth or fourth TMT joints for fusion.

If the first TMT joint is significantly subluxed and unstable and the disorder has been present for a long time, the position of reduction is critical. The medial cuneiform becomes eroded dorsally and laterally, which makes it difficult to appreciate the original position of the first TMT joint (Fig. 17-4). This joint is usually reduced before the second through fourth TMT joints. Because the forefoot is displaced laterally, the displaced first metatarsal may interfere with anatomic reduction of the second TMT joint. In addition, the first metatarsal is generally not rigidly bound to the other metatarsals and can be more freely manipulated. It helps to reduce and provisionally fix the first TMT joint, obtain radiographs, and compare them with those obtained of the opposite foot. The clinical appearance of the foot should guide the reduction.

The key to anatomic reduction is repositioning the first metatarsal in relation to the medial cuneiform medially and plantarward. Restoration of the proper relationship of the first metatarsal to the medial cuneiform should be confirmed in the anteroposterior and lateral radiographic views. Because the first cuneiform is often eroded in advanced arthritis, the usual cuneiform-metatarsal relationship can be deceptive in terms of judging appropriate reduction. There is a tendency toward accepting a slightly lateralized or valgus position in the first TMT joint in the intraoperative radiographs. It may be uncomfortable for the surgeon to deliberately place the first metatarsal into a position that seems to be in varus, but failure to achieve an anatomic varus position may result in residual malalignment. A small tension plate may be required along the medial side of the joint to maintain the native position if it has been dislocated for a long period (Figs. 17-5 and 17-6). A block of corticocancellous bone may also be required to help stabilize this joint. It is important to achieve plantarflexion and adduction alignment restored to the joint. A block of bone may be necessary to fill in a defect that remains when the first metatarsal is positioned appropriately.

After the first TMT joint alignment is restored, the entire forefoot needs to be reduced. This is accomplished by use of a laterally placed distractor. The distraction technique has several steps. First, a 2-mm Schanz pin is placed into the calcaneus, perpendicular to the long axis of the foot. A second pin is placed into the proximal fourth and fifth metatarsals. This pin is placed so as to diverge from the first pin inserted laterally in the calcaneus. The pin is closer to the proximal pin at its most lateral point rather than it is at its most medial point (Fig. 17-7A). The distractor is then placed on the end of these two pins and lengthened. As the distractor stretches the tissues, the forefoot adducts and, to some extent, restores the arch position (Fig. 17-7B). Sometimes, it is necessary to apply this tension in increments over a short time, with further debridement of each of the TMT joints as the position gradually improves. The forefoot is reduced to the extent that the base of the second metatarsal fits into its mortise (Fig. 17-8).

Provisional fixation of the first and second TMT joint is performed with 0.054-inch Kirschner wires. A lag screw is placed from the medial cuneiform to the base of the second metatarsal, from the base of the second metatarsal into the middle cuneiform, and from the base of the first metatarsal into the medial cuneiform. At this point, intraoperative radiographs are taken (Fig. 17-9).

The third TMT joint frequently becomes realigned passively as the first and second TMT joints are reduced. If not, a large Weber reduction clamp can be placed from the base of the third metatarsal to the medial cuneiform to apply compression force medially and proximally. A 3.5-mm cortical lag screw can then be placed across the base of the third metatarsal into the lateral cuneiform.

Under most circumstances, the fourth and fifth TMT joints are not fused because they are not as commonly affected by severe arthritis and because it is desirable to maintain

*(Text continues on page 247.)*

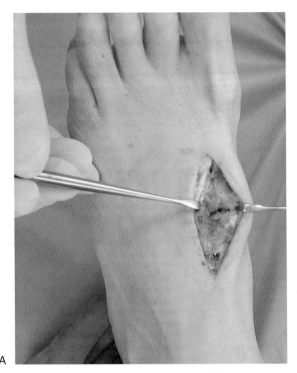
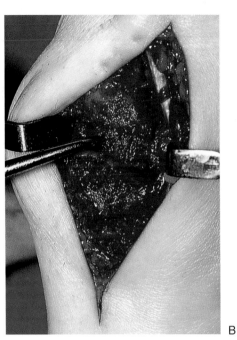

A                                                                                          B

**Figure 17-4. A:** The intraoperative photograph provides a dorsal view of the cuneiform-metatarsal joint after joint debridement and realignment, and it shows a bony deficiency. **B.** In the dorsal surgical exposure of a right foot, medial is to the left. The bone block is indicated by the Joker. The block of bone is in the dorsolateral tarsometatarsal joint.

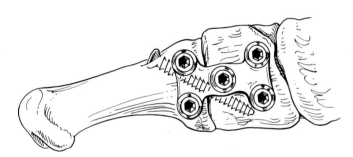

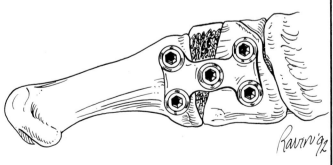

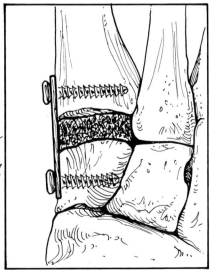

**Figure 17-5. Upper:** The arthrodesis technique used when there is limited or no erosion of the first tarsometatarsal joint; the joint surfaces are resected and fixed *in situ* with a plate and screw as shown, or with multiple screws (not shown). **Lower:** The technique used when substantial erosion has occurred in the first tarsometatarsal joint. The alignment of the first metatarsal is restored using a block of bone graft inserted dorsolaterally, then held with a combination of a medial tension plate (shown) and a 3.5-mm screw (not shown) across the tarsometatarsal joint. **Inset:** The dorsal view showing the bone graft and plate fixation.

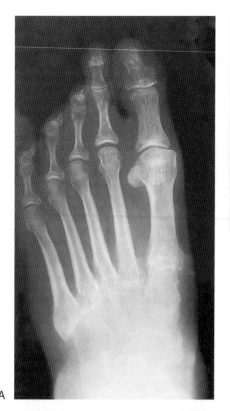

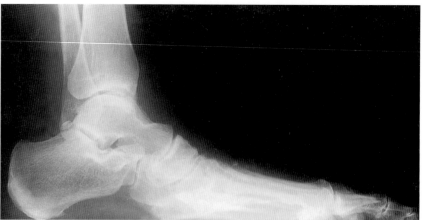

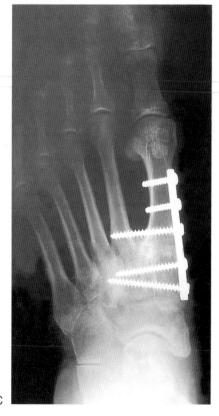

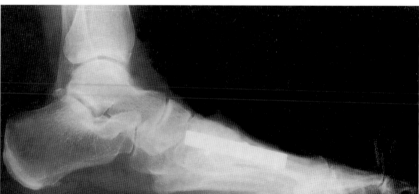

**Figure 17-6.** Preoperative anteroposterior **(A)** and lateral **(B)** radiographs of a patient with collapse through the midfoot. Notice the abduction of the foot through the Lisfranc joint. Postoperatively, the abduction is significantly improved, as is the midfoot sag, by use of a medially applied plate **(C and D)** . Notice that the intercuneiform articulations have been fused as well. (Case courtesy of Brad Olney, M.D., University of Kansas School of Medicine, Wichita, KS.)

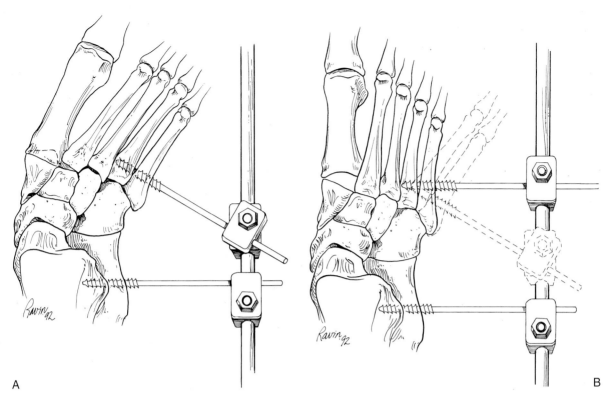

A                                                                                                B

**Figure 17-7. A and B:** Schematic representation of the use of a small distractor to reduce the forefoot. After all the tarsometatarsal joints have been debrided of scar and the forefoot appears mobile, a laterally placed small distractor is used. A 2-mm Schanz pin is placed into the calcaneus in a position perpendicular to the long axis of the foot. A second pin, angled distally, is placed into the base of metatarsal 5 and 4 and sometimes 3. This pin is inserted diverging medially relative to the calcaneal pin. The distractor is then placed across these two pins. As the two pins are distracted, the forefoot is forced out to length, out of abduction, and somewhat medially. When enough correction has been restored to get the second metatarsal into its mortise, provisional fixation is performed.

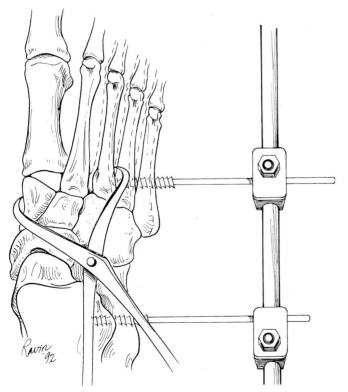

**Figure 17-8.** An additional reduction maneuver. Sometimes, the joint disruption is substantial, and the third, fourth, and fifth metatarsals do not stay secured when the second metatarsal is secured. Under these circumstances, additional reduction may be needed. Without removing the distractor, a large Weber reduction clamp may be placed from the medial cuneiform to the base of the third metatarsal. Closing the clamp reduces the base of the third metatarsal, where it may be secured to the cuneiform.

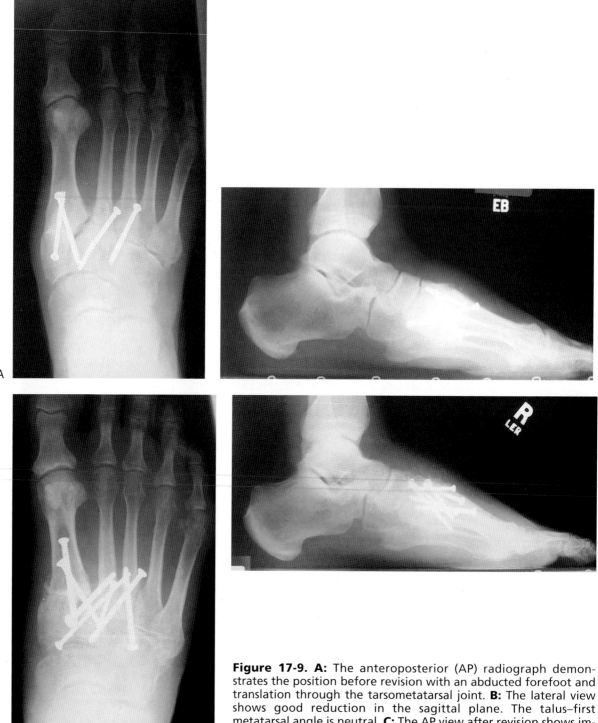

**Figure 17-9. A:** The anteroposterior (AP) radiograph demonstrates the position before revision with an abducted forefoot and translation through the tarsometatarsal joint. **B:** The lateral view shows good reduction in the sagittal plane. The talus–first metatarsal angle is neutral. **C:** The AP view after revision shows improved adduction of the metatarsals. The gap is closed by two lag screws crossing between the second metatarsal and the medial cuneiform. **D:** The lateral view after revision shows a normal talometatarsal angle.

some mobility on that part of the foot for more normal walking (Fig. 17-10). If these two joints have been subluxed or dislocated but the joint surfaces themselves are felt to be salvageable, we reduce them and hold the position with Kirschner wires that are maintained for 4 to 6 weeks. If the articular surfaces are clearly not salvageable, an "anchovy" procedure is performed, interposing soft tissue, and the joint is stabilized with Kirschner wires. These joints can be fused in certain instances, such as the neuropathic foot to prevent late recurrence of deformity and to provide improved stability for healing the medial part of the midfoot.

A newer screw design, called the Lisfranc screw (Synthes USA), is a small fragment screw that is stronger than the conventional 3.5- or 2.7-mm screw. It has a 4-mm outside diameter for added strength. This may be helpful, particularly in larger patients.

It may be necessary to apply a medial plate to maintain the alignment of the first ray. If needed, a 2.7-mm dynamic compression plate or a 2.7-mm reconstruction plate may be used. The plate can be positioned adjacent to the tibialis anterior tendon, but the tendon insertion should be respected. This medial plate should be preserved for those occasional in-

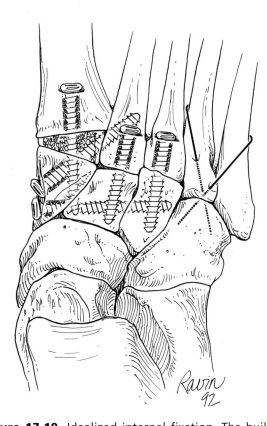

**Figure 17-10.** Idealized internal fixation. The building block of this fixation is the cortical lag screw. The near hole is overdrilled, which allows the screw to compress the two bones together. Conventional fixation includes a compression screw across the first, second, and third tarsometatarsal joints supplemented with a screw crossing from the second metatarsal into the medial cuneiform or the medial cuneiform into the second metatarsal. If intercuneiform fusion is required, another screw crosses the cuneiforms transversely. In feet fused for posttraumatic indications, the fourth and fifth tarsometatarsal joints are temporarily stabilized with Kirschner wires with the expectation of maintaining at least some motion at this level.

stances in which the position can otherwise not be maintained. The plate is applied in a sub-cutaneous location and often requires removal after the fusion process is complete. An alternative is to direct 3.5-mm lag screw or a 4.0-mm Lisfranc screw from the lateral side of the first metatarsal into the cuneiform.

If the intertarsal articulations are to be fused as well, they should be denuded of cartilage and fibrous tissue and fixation applied. A screw from the medial side of the medial cuneiform directed laterally across one or both intercuneiform joints will stabilize and compress these articulations. Cancellous bone graft is used in these joints to facilitate fusion. Bone graft may be obtained from the iliac crest, the proximal lateral tibia, or the distal medial tibia just above the medial malleolus. The anterior iliac crest yields the most bone with the highest density of cellular tissue. Lesser amounts of bone graft may be obtained from the distal tibia just above the medial malleolus or the proximal tibia just below Gerdy's tubercle.

When the bone is taken from the tibia, it should be taken through an elliptically shaped or round cortical window. The 2-mm drill is used to make a series of holes that form an ellipse, and the holes are connected using a 0.25-inch osteotome. The window is undermined at an angle with a 0.25-inch osteotome in such a way that the cortex is beveled, and the cortical window can be replaced without falling into the defect. Cancellous bone can then be removed from the tibia with curettes. The cortical window is then replaced and the soft tissues closed over the window. Patients experience essentially no morbidity from the tibial donor site, and no extra rehabilitation is required.

Except under unusual circumstances, the fourth and fifth TMT joints are not fused. Motion is desirable along the lateral border of the foot to progress from heel strike to toe-off in normal gait. There is limited normal motion of the calcaneocuboid joint. Much the motion along the lateral side of the foot occurs through the fourth and fifth TMT joints. These joints are difficult to fuse. However, if the fourth and fifth TMT joints are arthritic, there are two options for salvage. The first is a partial resection of the joint with interposition of soft tissue as mentioned previously. A small, longitudinal incision is made to expose the fourth and fifth TMT joints. A microsagittal saw is used to resect the dorsal 80% of the articular surface of the metatarsal while leaving the plantarmost aspect of the joint in contact. This leaves the plantar soft tissues intact to act as a hinge, allowing the fourth and fifth TMT joints to plantarflex and dorsiflex without placing pressure on the arthritic joint. This defect can be filled with extensor retinaculum or part of the extensor tendon to the fifth toe. The soft tissue is prepared by rolling it like an anchovy, placing it into the joint, and pinning the TMT joint with this soft tissue interposed. The pin is left in place for 6 weeks.

Another salvage procedure is arthrodesis of the fifth to the fourth metatarsal. It may be applicable in cases such as after a crush injury of the fifth TMT joint. The cuboid may not be available or may not provide adequate support for fifth TMT arthrodesis. Under these circumstances, the fifth metatarsal is fused to the fourth with two 2.7-mm cortical lag screws. It is performed by first reducing the position of the fifth metatarsal relative to the fourth. An osteotome is used to roughen the surfaces of both metatarsals at the their proximal metaphyses. The two lag screws are directed from lateral to medial aspects to prevent plantar and proximal migration of the fifth metatarsal, which disturbs normal weight-bearing balance.

In some instances, it is helpful to perform a heel cord lengthening in addition to the TMT arthrodesis. The indication for the addition of Achilles tendon lengthening is a fixed hindfoot equinus. The equinus may be primary or secondary. When midfoot collapse has been present for a long time, the heel cord may be contracted. Weakening the gastrocnemius by the tendon lengthening seems undesirable, but it has the effect of lessening the forces across the midfoot during walking. The gastrocnemius can be selectively released by a technique described by Vulpius (8). An appreciation of the midfoot collapse can be confirmed by obtaining a lateral radiograph of the foot in maximum dorsiflexion. It shows that some of the dorsiflexion is occurring through the midfoot. We prefer a closed tendon lengthening: a percutaneous three-level slide. It is often done before the fusion so that dorsiflexion can be applied across the foot without stressing the fixation.

## POSTOPERATIVE MANAGEMENT

At the conclusion of the surgical procedure, a bupivacaine ankle block provides postoperative pain relief. The patients are placed into a posterior plaster splint or a bivalved short-leg plaster cast. Non–weight-bearing ambulation is started on postoperative day 1. When patients are comfortable and able to walk safely on crutches, they are discharged from the hospital. Sutures are removed at 2 weeks postoperatively. If the indication for surgery was a neuropathic (Charcot) joint, a non–weight-bearing, short-leg cast is applied. This technique is also used if the surgery was done for other reasons, such as when the adequacy of fixation is less than satisfactory. If fixation is thought to be satisfactory, patients are placed in a removable splint, and ankle and toe motion exercises are initiated. Radiographs are performed 6 weeks postoperatively. If the healing appears to be progressing satisfactorily, patients can be allowed to bear weight. Fusions performed for Charcot midfoot collapse are immobilized in a cast for much longer, usually for approximately 16 weeks. Those done for degenerative or posttraumatic changes are not casted beyond 6 to 8 weeks unless there is evidence of delayed union.

About 80% of the patients heal with a solid arthrodesis within 3 months. All patients are told that healing of the arthrodesis usually takes 3 months, but that it will require 6 months or longer before they are comfortable walking on the foot because this is a major reconstructive procedure. Although some patients respond much faster, it is far easier to let them know ahead of time that 6 months is not an unreasonable expectation for the duration of recovery. The patient should be warned ahead of time that the procedure results in a stiff foot and that they will need to wear comfortable, supportive shoes after the operation. The desired footwear can range from a comfortable athletic shoe to a prescription-type extra-depth shoe. In most cases, standard, lace-up shoes are acceptable footwear after this operation. Routinely, we provide a custom-molded insole for the patient to use after immobilization is discontinued and for as long as the patient feels the need.

## COMPLICATIONS

*Injury to the superficial peroneal nerve* can occur. The incision crosses the course of the superficial peroneal nerve at several points during this operative procedure. The anatomy is also distorted in most patients. Care is taken to avoid cutting the nerve primarily by incising the skin sharply, identifying the nerve, and protecting it while completing the dissection. Patients are counseled preoperatively that they may be left with sensory deficits.

*Incomplete reduction* is common because of the long-standing nature of the deformity and the unusual anatomy. Attention to the overall shape of the foot rather than the appearance of the radiographs is often helpful in establishing a functional position for the foot. The position of the foot is what patients recognize, as well as an acceptable shape of the foot that allows them to fit into shoes.

A useful technique for estimating the correct position of the foot intraoperatively is to grasp the forefoot with one hand and the hindfoot with the other and passively reposition the forefoot relative to the hindfoot. Provisional fixation can be performed to maintain that position and definitive fixation performed after the adequacy of the alignment is confirmed radiographically.

*Nonunion* is common in neuropathic feet. The technique is altered, such as using more rigid fixation, in patients with neuropathic arthropathy. At least two screws are inserted across the first TMT joint, and screws across the second and third TMT joints are needed. Additional obliquely oriented screws often are added to maintain this position. In neuropathic feet, cast immobilization is performed until there is evidence that solid healing is underway (Fig. 17-11).

*Malunion* may occur. The most common position of deformity of the arthritic first TMT joint is dorsiflexion and abduction, and specific attention should be directed toward repositioning by plantarflexion and adduction of the metatarsal at the time of surgery (Fig. 17-12). In hallux valgus correction, one of the goals of surgery (e.g., metatarsal osteotomy,

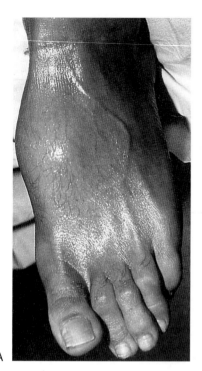
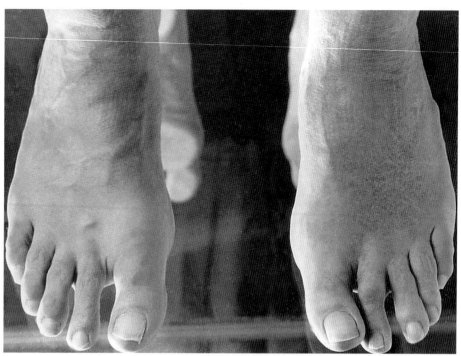

A                                                                                                                                      B

**Figure 17-11. A:** Photograph of a left foot shows a typical abducted position of the forefoot. Notice the convex medial border of the foot. This deformity is exaggerated during weight bearing. **B:** A clinical photograph of the same patient after reduction and fusion. Notice that the foot is moderately swollen but that its contours have been largely restored.

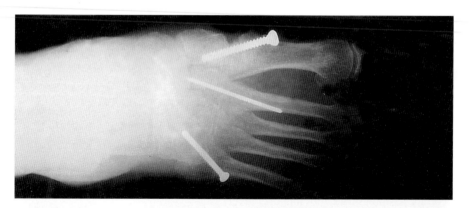

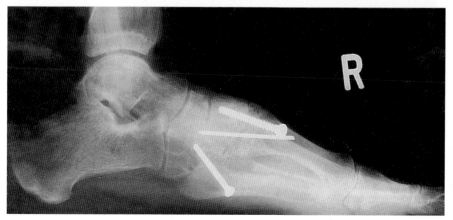

A

**Figure 17-12. A:** Anteroposterior and lateral views of a patient who underwent a tarsometatarsal fusion after failed treatment of a Lisfranc injury with Schanz pins. It improved from the initial position, but the first metatarsal is not sufficiently medialized. A screw could have been placed on the lateral side of the first metatarsal to bring it toward the cuneiform. Alternatively, a plate could have been placed medially. The second tarsometatarsal joint is incompletely reduced as well. *(continued)*

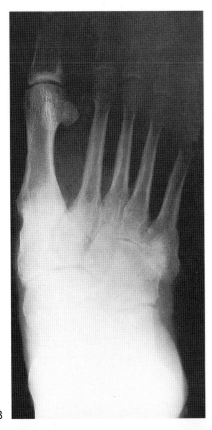

**Figure 17-12.** *Continued.* **B:** Five years later, the patient has pain in the talonavicular joint, and clinically, the forefoot is abducted. **C:** The lateral view shows no malalignment because the first metatarsal has been adequately plantar flexed. The metatarsals appear to have a normal relationship with the foot and are solidly fused to the cuneiforms. However, there is a slight talonavicular sag and some narrowing of the talonavicular joint.

B

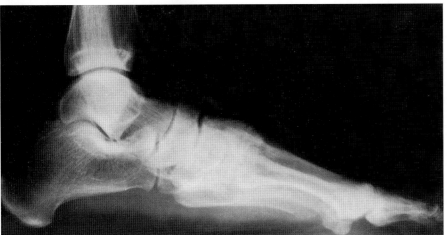

C

TMT arthrodesis) is to place the first metatarsal closer to a plane parallel to the second metatarsal. This is not the desired position in this midfoot fusion operation. The position should be established by placing the first metatarsal in an appropriate position with less emphasis on the radiographic appearance. If the first metatarsal appears to be too short relative to the second and third, an intercalated corticocancellous bone graft can be placed into the TMT joint. The joint can be distracted by placing a 0.062-inch Kirschner wire into the first metatarsal and cuneiform and distracting the pins. A structural corticocancellous graft is placed in the space created, with the cortical surface of the graft oriented dorsally. The bone graft can be shaped with increased thickness dorsally and laterally to provide plantarflexion and adduction of the first metatarsal.

## RECOMMENDED READING

1.  Ferris LR, Vargo R, Alexander IJ: Late reconstruction of the midfoot and transmetatarsal region after trauma. *Orthop Clin North Am* 26:393–406, 1995.
2.  Graham HK, Fixsen JA: Lengthening of the calcaneal tendon in spastic hemiplegia by the White slide technique: a long-term review. *J Bone Joint Surg Br* 70:742–745, 1988.
3.  Horton GA, Olney BW: Deformity correction and arthrodesis of the midfoot with a medial plate. *Foot Ankle* 14:493–499, 1993.
4.  Johnson JE, Johnson KA: Dowel arthrodesis for degenerative arthrodesis of the tarsometatarsal (Lisfranc) joints. *Foot Ankle* 5:243–253, 1986.
5.  Komenda GA, Myerson MS, Biddinger KR: Results of arthrodesis of the tarsometatarsal joint after trauma. *Orthop Clin North Am* 26:393–406, 1995.
6.  Mann RA, Prieskorn D, Sobel M: Mid-tarsal arthrodesis for primary degenerative osteoarthrosis or osteoarthrosis after trauma. *J Bone Joint Surg Am* 78:1376–1385, 1996.
7.  Sangeorzan BJ, Veith R, Hansen ST: Fusion of Lisfranc's joint for salvage of tarsometatarsal injuries. *Foot Ankle* 10:193–200, 1990.
8.  Vulpius O, Stoffel A. Tenotomie der end schren der mm. gastrocnemius el soleus mittels rutschenlassens nach vulpius. *Orthopadische Operationslehre*. Stuttgart: Ferdinand Enke, 1913:29–31.

# 18

# Talonavicular Arthrodesis

## G. James Sammarco and Laurette Chang

## INDICATIONS/CONTRAINDICATIONS

The talonavicular joint is similar to an elongated ball and socket joint (i.e., condyloid shape) that permits dorsiflexion-plantarflexion, external-internal rotation, and eversion-inversion. It works in concert with the subtalar and calcaneocuboid joints to allow the foot to accommodate to a variety of surfaces. Arthrodesis of this joint therefore affects motion of the hindfoot. Cadaveric studies revealed that simulated arthrodesis of the talonavicular joint significantly decreases motion of the subtalar and calcaneocuboid joints (2). Arthrodesis in hindfoot joints that included the talonavicular joint limited the motion of the remaining joints to less than 5°. It also limited the excursion of the posterior tibial tendon to 25% of normal. Anatomically, the talonavicular joint is continuous with the anterior facet of the subtalar joint.

Talonavicular arthrodesis is indicated when disease causes pain, disability, and alteration of motion, limiting function of the foot. Such indications include traumatic or inflammatory arthritis, septic arthritis, tibialis posterior tendon dysfunction with collapse of the medial longitudinal arches, and tumors (3,5,8,11,12,13). Posttraumatic arthritis may be caused by talar or navicular fractures or Chopart dislocation. Double arthrodesis of the talonavicular and calcaneocuboid joints has been reported to correct deformity in adult acquired flatfoot (15).

Triple arthrodesis is indicated for patients with arthrosis affecting multiple hindfoot joints and for fixed deformities of the hindfoot (9). Limited procedures such as talonavicular arthrodesis are attractive because they preserve more hindfoot function than does triple arthrodesis.

Techniques of talonavicular joint fixation include a single compression screw across the joint, two medial screws (12), one or more staples, staples with screws (13,15), and cylindrical dowel bone grafts (14). A lag screw is attractive because compression across the arthrodesis site encourages union. However, a single lag screw offers less torsional stability than multiple screws (16). The technique described includes a cannulated cancellous

G. J. Sammarco, M.D.: Department of Orthopaedic Surgery, University of Cincinnati School of Medicine; and Foot and Ankle Fellowship, The Center for Orthopaedic Care, Inc., Cincinnati, Ohio.

L. Chang, M.D.: The Center for Orthopaedic Care, Inc., Cincinnati, Ohio.

screw medially and a cannulated double-threaded (i.e., Herbert/Whipple) compression screw laterally.

A contraindication to talonavicular arthrodesis is arthrosis of multiple hindfoot joints. Advanced age is not a contraindication. The rationale for this single-joint arthrodesis is to address symptoms at this joint while preserving some of the shock absorbing capacity of the hindfoot compared with more extensive procedures such as triple arthrodesis, reducing the risk of arthritis in adjacent joints over time.

## PREOPERATIVE PLANNING

Before considering surgical correction of talonavicular disease, nonoperative treatment modalities such as orthotics, antiinflammatory medication, and shoe modifications should be tried. If these fail, the patient should be informed of the details of the operation, including postoperative expectations. The expected limitation in foot motion is discussed with the patient, although most patients have had restricted motion preoperatively. The foot is examined to confirm if localized tenderness is present at the talonavicular joint. Relief of pain after injection of 2 mL of 1% lidocaine into the joint is useful if there is some question of the diagnosis. A prominent talar head may be palpable medially with the collapse of the longitudinal arch. Preoperative evaluation of joint motion is important to determine painful motion, ease of reduction of the joint, and other factors such as the need for additional surgery to align the foot. Preoperative radiographic evaluation includes weight-bearing, anteroposterior and lateral views, and an oblique view of the foot. These radiographs define the nature of the arthritis, navicular and talar bony geometry, alignment, and bone quality, as well as the presence of other abnormalities that may require attention.

## SURGERY

Surgery is performed under general, spinal, or epidural anesthesia. In selected patients, an ankle block may be used, but this precludes the use of the supramalleolar tibia for bone graft. The procedure may be performed as an outpatient surgery. Instruments such as a set of osteotomes (2 to 15 mm), small surgical scalpels (Bard-Packer R no. 15 blades), small scissors, cervical lamina spreaders (Inge), and a mini-C-arm x-ray image are useful. Appropriate safety measures should be taken to protect against radiation exposure. A thigh tourniquet set at 300 mm Hg is used. Splint material should be available to immobilize the foot after surgery. Surgical screws such as the 4.0-mm, self-tapping, titanium, cannulated, compression-type screws (DepuyAce, Warsaw, IN), with or without a washer, are effective. Screw lengths of 40 to 46 mm and a 4.5-mm Herbert/Whipple cannulated titanium screw (e.g., Zimmer, Warsaw, IN) in lengths of 30 to 45 mm may be used.

The patient is position supine on the operating table. After adequate anesthesia, the lower extremity is prepped and draped, and the tourniquet is inflated. The C-arm is draped for sterile intraoperative use. A 5-cm, linear incision (Fig. 18-1) is made dorsal to the medial aspect of the navicular tuberosity and the head of the talus just above the insertion of the tibialis posterior tendon (Fig. 18-2). The soft tissues are dissected down to the joint capsule. About one half of the tibialis posterior tendon is elevated from the navicular (Fig. 18-3). The dorsal attachment of the capsule overlying the talonavicular joint is elevated from the navicular. The head of the talus is exposed, and a metatarsal head retractor placed. As dissection proceeds, a self-retaining cervical lamina spreader is carefully inserted to distract the joint surfaces (Fig. 18-4). After this, straight and curved, 10-mm osteotomes are used to remove the articular surface of the navicular and talar head (Fig. 18-5). Curved and straight curettes and a pituitary rongeur are used to remove the remaining articular cartilage and subchondral bone. It may be difficult to remove the central and lateral navicular joint surface because of the concavity and depth of the joint. Extra care must be taken to ensure that all articular cartilage is removed. The bony surfaces of the denuded joint are "feathered" with a small osteotome to increase the subchondral bone surface contact (Fig. 18-6).

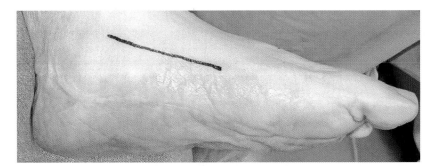

**Figure 18-1.** Medial skin incision is made longitudinally, dorsal to the navicular tuberosity.

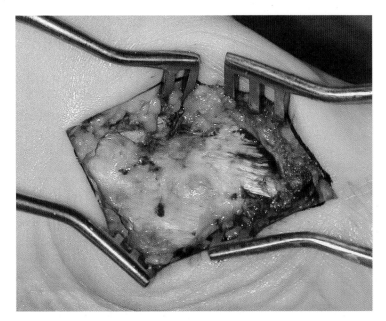

**Figure 18-2.** Tibialis posterior and joint capsule overlie the talonavicular joint.

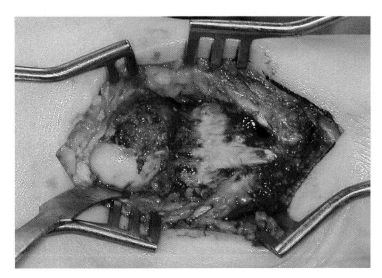

**Figure 18-3.** Exposure of the talonavicular joint. The heel is to the left. The talar head *(left)* and navicular tuberosity *(right)* are seen.

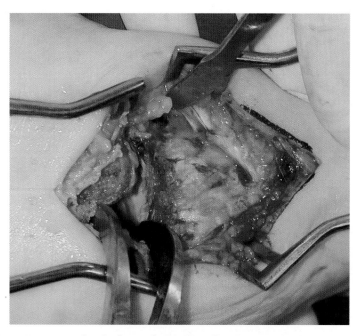

**Figure 18-4.** Exposure of articular surfaces. Visualization may be improved with a lamina spreader in the joint and a small metatarsal head retractor dorsally.

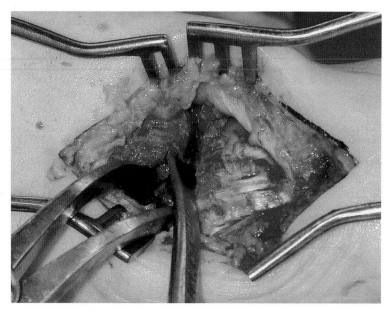

**Figure 18-5.** The articular surfaces of the talonavicular joint are decorticated with a sharp osteotome. The heel is to the left.

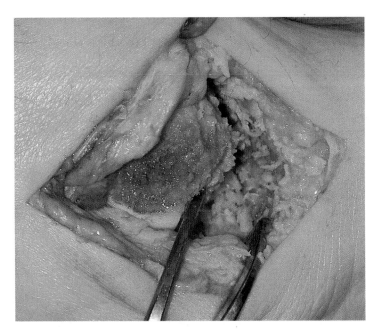

**Figure 18-6.** Decorticated articulated surfaces are "feathered." The heel is to the left.

Bone graft may be necessary to ensure adequate bony contact, depending on the degree of bony deficiency.

If bone graft is used, usually only a limited amount is needed; distal tibial graft is preferable to iliac crest bone graft. A 3-cm, longitudinal incision is made over the distal-medial aspect of the tibial metaphysis. The incision is carried down through the soft tissues to the periosteum, which is incised, and a 1 × 1 cm cortical bone window removed. Osteotomes and curettes are used to harvest cancellous bone graft. The bone window is replaced and incision closed with absorbable 3-0 suture in the subcutaneous tissue and a subcuticular 4-0 absorbable suture in the skin. The bone graft is placed into the talonavicular articulation and packed with 2- and 4-mm impactors.

The talonavicular joint is placed manually in the desired position, and a 1.6-mm guide pin is inserted through the tuberosity of the navicular medially, across the joint and into the talar neck (Fig. 18-7). The position of the guide pin is checked with an image intensifier. A

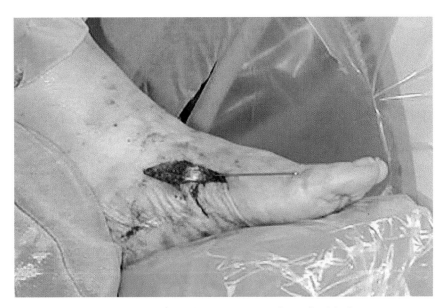

**Figure 18-7.** Guide wire placement is confirmed with the C-arm.

2.9-mm, cannulated drill is passed over the guide pin and through the navicular. A countersink is used to allow the screw head and washer to be seated in the navicular. A cannulated, 4.0-mm-diameter, cancellous, self-tapping, titanium screw with a washer is inserted (Fig. 18-8). A washer may be used to obtain better compression at the arthrodesis site (Fig. 18-9). An image intensifier is used to check fixation position and to ensure compression is achieved. Instrumentation for the lateral compression screw is shown in Figure 18-10.

Using C-arm imaging, a second guide wire (Fig. 18-10A) is passed percutaneously between middle and lateral cuneiforms into the navicular (Fig. 18-11). The guide pin traverses the navicular at the junction of the middle and lateral third and is driven through the navicular into the neck of the talus. C-arm images are obtained in anteroposterior, lateral, and oblique views to check the position of the guide pin in the talar neck. A cannulated, 4.6-mm drill (Fig. 18-10B) is used to drill through the distal navicular cortex and one half of its thickness (Fig. 18-12).

The proximal navicular subchondral bone is not breached by the 4.6-mm drill nor is the talar head. A cannulated, 3.1-mm drill (in the 4.5-mm Herbert/Whipple set) is placed over the guide

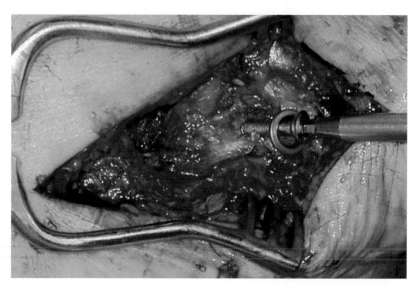

**Figure 18-8.** Insertion of cannulated lag compression screw with a washer.

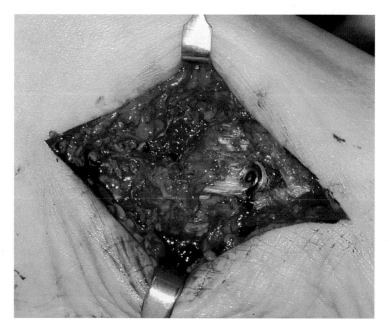

**Figure 18-9.** Medial lag compression screw with a washer. There is good bony apposition.

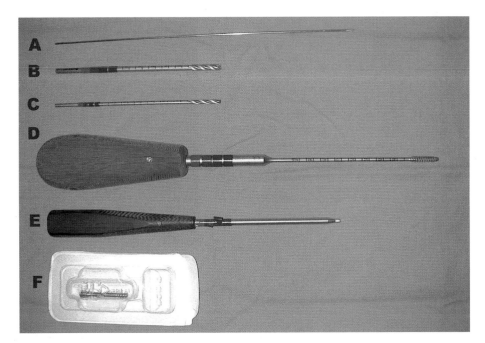

**Figure 18-10.** Instrumentation for Herbert/Whipple screw is placed in the lateral talonavicular joint. **A:** A 1.6-mm guide wire. **B:** Cannulated, 4.6-mm drill. **C:** Cannulated, 3.1-mm drill. **D:** Cannulated tap. **E:** Cannulated screwdriver for 4.5-mm Herbert/Whipple screws. **F:** Cannulated, 4.5-mm Herbert/Whipple screw.

wire (Figs.18-10C and 18-13) and used to drill through the remaining navicular and talus (Fig. 18-14). The 4.5-mm Herbert/Whipple tap (Figs. 18-10D and 18-15) is placed over the guide wire, and the drill hole is tapped in its entire length to allow the screw to properly compress the joint. The appropriate 4.5-mm-diameter Herbert/Whipple screw may be 30 to 45 mm long. It is inserted over the guide wire with C-arm imaging (Figs. 18-10E,F and 18-16). The proximal articular border of the navicular must not be traversed by the larger (more distal) head of the screw, because compression across the joint may be compromised (Figs.18-17 through 18-19).

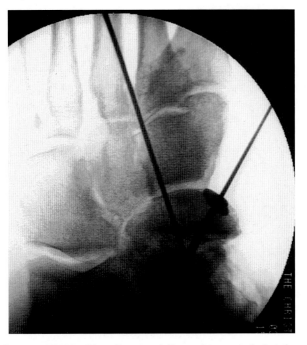

**Figure 18-11.** The C-arm oblique image of the foot shows a lateral guide wire traversing the navicular.

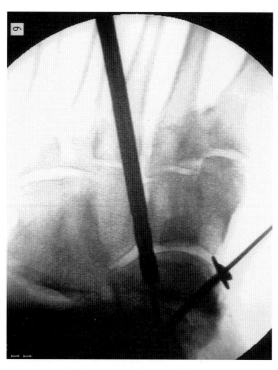

**Figure 18-12.** The C-arm image shows a 4.6-mm, cannulated drill (from the 6.5-mm Herbert/Whipple set) over a lateral guide wire through the distal cortex and one half of the thickness of the navicular.

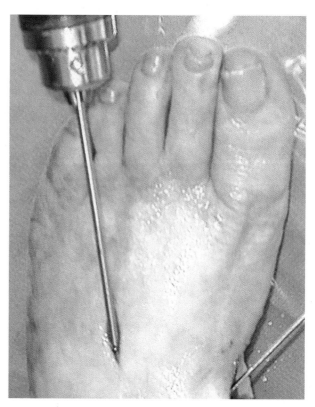

**Figure 18-13.** A 3.1-mm cannulated drill (from the 4.5-mm Herbert/Whipple set) over the lateral guide wire.

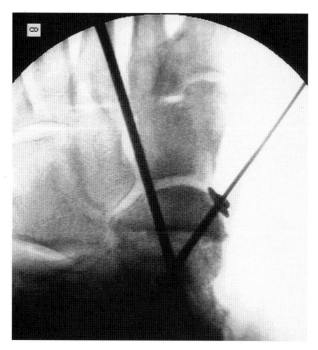

**Figure 18-14.** The C-arm image shows the 3.1-mm, cannulated drill traversing talonavicular joint into talar head.

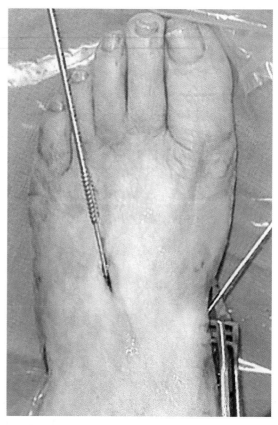

**Figure 18-15.** Insertion of the tap to traverse the talonavicular joint and talar head.

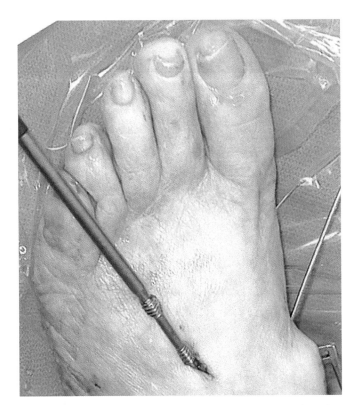

**Figure 18-16.** Insertion of a 4.5-mm Herbert/Whipple screw.

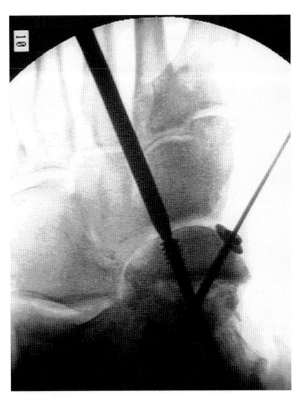

**Figure 18-17.** The C-arm image shows a 4.5-mm Herbert/Whipple screw insertion. The proximal articular border of the navicular is not traversed by the larger proximal head of the screw.

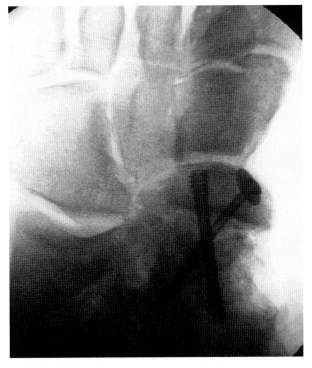

**Figure 18-18.** The C-arm image shows the medial and lateral compression screws across talonavicular joint.

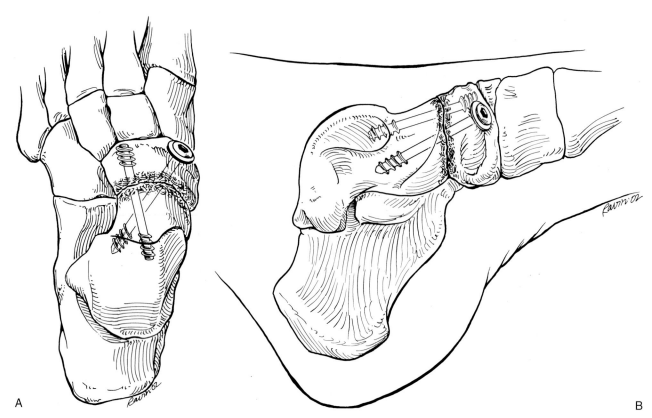

**Figure 18-19.** Preferred fixation placement. **A:** Dorsal view. **B:** Medial view.

The deep tissues are reapproximated with 3-0 absorbable suture, and the skin is closed with 4-0 subcuticular absorbable suture. Steri-Strips and a dressing of a 4 × 4 inch sponge folded once are placed over the wound. A compression dressing and a short-leg posterior splint are applied, after which the tourniquet is released, and the patient is transferred to the recovery room.

## POSTOPERATIVE MANAGEMENT

The patient may ambulate on crutches without bearing weight.. Follow-up includes an office visit 3 days postoperatively, at which time the splint and dressings are removed, the wound is checked, and radiographs may be taken to check bony alignment. The patient is placed in a short-leg, non–weight-bearing cast for 4 weeks, followed by a range of motion boot designed to allow ankle motion of 10° of plantarflexion and 10° of dorsiflexion. At 8 weeks postoperatively, an isometric exercise program is instituted, and 40% weight bearing is permitted. After 10 weeks, full weight bearing is permitted. After union is achieved, physical therapy is prescribed.

## COMPLICATIONS

*Nonunion* is the most common complication of talonavicular arthrodesis and may occur in up to 10% of cases. The relatively small size of the tarsal navicular and limited circulation of the bone may contribute to delay in healing. The high degree of normal forces across the joint or a noncompliant patient can also contribute to the occurrence of nonunion. Screw breakage can occur, usually at the screw-shaft junction. If nonunion occurs, painful pseudoarthrosis and collapse of the arch may result, which may require further surgery with revision talonavicular arthrodesis. It may also be necessary to extend the arthrodesis to other hindfoot joints, and the screws may be advanced or replaced with large-diameter screws to increase compression across the joint line. Additional bone graft may be harvested from the lateral calcaneus or proximal tibia and applied to the nonunion.

*Longitudinal arch collapse* may occur. In some conditions, such as chronic tear of the tibialis posterior tendon, the longitudinal arch may collapse despite successful arthrodesis. It is sometimes necessary to add a calcaneal osteotomy or subtalar arthrodesis to stabilize the hindfoot while reconstructing the tendon. The resulting double arthrodesis is quite functional.

*Malunion* is often the result of improper alignment of the initial surgery. Occasionally, it may be the ultimate position of a joint that had a delayed union after it healed. Treatment options include osteotomy at the malunion site, with or without extension of the arthrodesis to include the subtalar, calcaneocuboid, or both joints. The decision as to the extent of the arthrodesis depends on the conditions of the adjacent joints, the magnitude of the malalignment, and the ability to achieve a plantigrade position during revision surgery.

*Neuroma or infection* may occur after surgery. Incisional neuroma may be caused by excessive traction on the cutaneous branches of the superficial peroneal nerve. Injection with corticosteroid about the neuroma may be of benefit. However, care should be exercised so as not to create subcutaneous tissue atrophy, and the patient should be counseled before injection. If this fails, simple excision of the neuroma is suggested. Superficial infection is treated with appropriate antibiotics. If osteomyelitis occurs, one or more debridement operations, antibiotics, and if indicated, late reconstructions are preformed.

## RECOMMENDED READING

1. Adam W, Ranawat C: Arthrodesis of the hindfoot in rheumatoid arthritis. *Orthop Clin North Am* 7:827–840, 1976.
2. Astion DJ, Deland JT, Otis JC, et al.: Motion of the hindfoot after simulated arthrodesis. *J Bone J Surg Am* 79:241–246, 1997.
3. Chiodo CP, Martin T, Wilson MG: A technique for isolated arthrodesis for inflammatory arthritis of the talonavicular joint. *Foot Ankle* 21:307–310, 2000.
4. Clain MR, Baxter DE: Simultaneous calcaneocuboid and talonavicular fusion. *J Bone J Surg Br* 76:133–136, 1994.
5. Cracchiolo A: Surgical arthrodesis techniques for foot and ankle pathology. *Instr Course Lect* 39:49–63, 1990.
6. Dalziel R, Thornhill TS, Thomas WH: Isolated talonavicular fusion for hindfoot arthritis. *Orthop Trans* 6: 341, 1982.
7. Elbaor JE, Thomas WH, Weinfeld MS, et al.: Talonavicular arthrodesis for rheumatoid arthritis of the hindfoot. *Orthop Clin North Am* 7:821–826, 1976.
8. Fogel GR, Katoh Y, Rand JA, et al.: Talonavicular arthrodesis for isolated arthrosis: 9.5 year results and gait analysis. *Foot Ankle* 3:105–113, 1982.
9. Fortin PT, Walling AK: Triple arthrodesis. *Clin Orthop Rel Res* 365:91–99, 1999.
10. Gellman H, Lenihan M, Halikis N, et al.: Selective tarsal arthrodesis: an in vitro analysis of the effect on foot motion. *Foot Ankle* 8:127–133, 1987.
11. Harper M: Talonavicular arthrodesis for the acquired flatfoot in the adult. *Clin Orthop Rel Res* 365:65–69, 1999.
12. Harper MC, Tisdel CL: Talonavicular arthrodesis for the painful adult acquired flatfoot. *Foot Ankle* 17:658-661, 1996.
13. Kindsfater K, Wilson M, Thomas W: Management of the rheumatoid hindfoot with special reference to talonavicular arthrodesis. *Clin Orthop Rel Res* 340:69–74, 1997.
14. Ljung P, Kaij J, Knutson K, et al.: Talonavicular arthrodesis in the rheumatoid foot. *Foot Ankle* 13:313–316, 1992.
15. Mann RA, Beaman DN: Double arthrodesis in the adult. *Clin Orthop Rel Res* 365:74–80, 1999.
16. Mueller M, Allgower M, Schneider R: *Manual of internal fixation: techniques recommended by the AO-ASIF group*, 3rd ed. New York: Springer-Verlag, 1991:32–33.
17. Ruff ME, Turner RH: Selective hindfoot arthrodesis in rheumatoid arthritis. *Orthopedics* 7:49–54, 1984.

# 19

# Compartment Releases of the Foot

Arthur Manoli II and David J. Dixon

## INDICATIONS/CONTRAINDICATIONS

Many traumatic injuries of the foot result in severe pain and swelling. Multiple fractures or dislocations and fractures as a result of high-energy injuries (e.g., calcaneal fractures) may produce blood and interstitial fluid accumulation within the rigid, fascial confines of the compartments of the foot. As seen in compartment syndromes elsewhere in the body, the pressure built up in the compartments may result in muscle ischemia and necrosis, with subsequent scar formation and formation of contractures of the soft tissues. This often results in marked dysfunction of the foot with sequelae, including claw toes, chronic pain, stiffness, and nerve dysfunction. Early fasciotomy, performed emergently after the diagnosis of foot compartment syndrome is made, minimizes the chance of developing late contracture, nerve dysfunction, and disability.

Severe injuries of the foot, particularly those with multiple fractures or an element of crushing, are prone to develop foot compartment syndrome. Tense foot swelling that develops after an injury should alert the practitioner to the possibility of a compartment syndrome. Plantar foot ecchymosis is often present (Fig. 19-1). Severe pain, pain with passive stretch of the foot muscles (i.e., toe dorsiflexion stretches the plantar muscles), and nerve dysfunction (e.g., paresthesias, muscle paralysis) may be seen but are thought to be less diagnostic in the foot than elsewhere. To confirm the diagnosis, direct measurement of compartment pressures is suggested. There should be a low threshold for measuring the foot compartment pressures in clinically suspicious cases, particularly those associated with severe injury (e.g., crush injury) and in unconscious patients. The presence or absence of the peripheral pulses is of little use in diagnosing foot compartment syndrome.

---

A. Manoli II, M.D.: Michigan International Foot & Ankle Center, Pontiac, Michigan.

D. J. Dixon, M.D.: Private Practice, Foot and Ankle Surgery, Northeast Orthopaedics, and Albany Medical Center, Albany, New York.

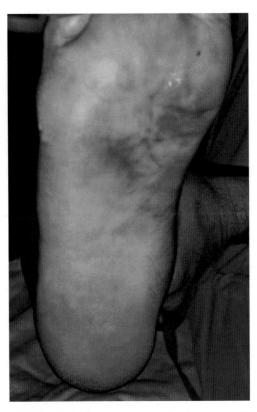

**Figure 19-1.** Clinical appearance of a tense, swollen foot with compartment syndrome after a calcaneal fracture with plantar ecchymosis.

## PREOPERATIVE PLANNING

Catheterization of the nine compartments of the foot can be done using any of the well-known established apparatuses. The development of portable pressure monitors (Pressure-Sense Monitor, Ace Medical Co., Los Angeles, CA, or Digital Quickset, Stryker Corp., Kalamazoo, MI) has made the measurement of pressures much easier. They may be performed almost anywhere with ease and accuracy.

The pressures within the compartments of the foot may be measured using local, infiltrative anesthesia (Fig. 19-2). In the hindfoot, the medial compartmental pressure is measured with needle placement approximately 4 cm inferior to the medial malleolus and over the abductor hallucis muscle (Fig. 19-3). After the pressure in the medial compartment is taken, the needle is advanced through the medial intermuscular septum of the foot into the deep hindfoot compartment, the calcaneal. Here, the pressure is often found to be the highest, especially in instances of calcaneal fractures.

The needle is removed and reinserted into the flexor digitorum brevis muscle in the arch, measuring the superficial compartment (Fig. 19-4). A third stick on the lateral aspect of the foot, just below the fifth metatarsal, measures the pressure in the lateral compartment (Fig. 19-5).

Any or all of the separate interosseous compartments can be sampled in the forefoot. It is recommended that at least one of the first and second interosseous compartments be measured (Fig. 19-6). If the needle is advanced deeply between the respective metatarsals, the pressure in the adductor compartment can also be measured.

Although the absolute pressure at which fasciotomy should be performed continues to be debated, normal pressures are known, and certain guidelines have been developed for abnormal pressures. Dayton et al. (4) reported that normal compartment pressures in the foot are less than 6 mm Hg. Others reported that the capillary vessel wall closing pressure is

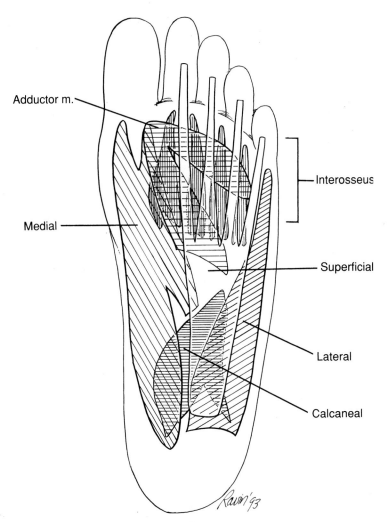

**Figure 19-2.** A plantar view of the nine compartments of the foot. The medial, superficial, and lateral compartments run the entire length of the foot. The adductor and four interosseous compartments are located in the forefoot only. The calcaneal compartment is in the hindfoot. (Adapted from Manoli A II, Fakhouri AJ, Weber TG: Compartment catheterization and fasciotomy of the foot. *Operative Tech Orthop* 2: 203–210, 1992, with permission.)

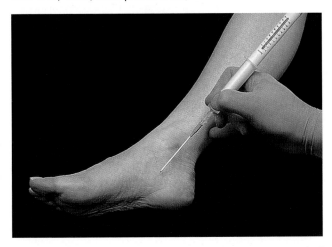

**Figure 19-3.** A medial stick, 4 cm below the medial malleolus, measures the pressure in the medial and calcaneal compartments.

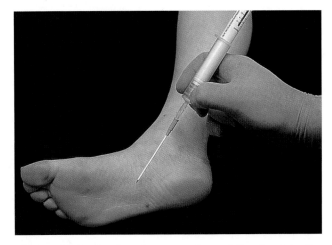

**Figure 19-4.** On the plantar surface of the foot, in the arch area, the superficial compartmental pressure is measured. This compartment contains the flexor digitorum brevis muscle.

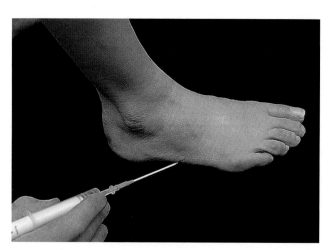

**Figure 19-5.** The lateral stick is just below the fifth metatarsal base. It measures the pressure in the lateral compartment.

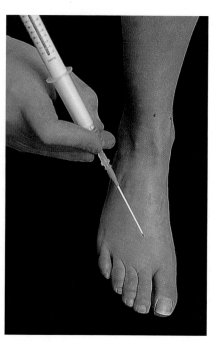

**Figure 19-6.** A stick in the first or second interspace measures the pressure in that space. Advancement of the needle deeper into the forefoot measures the pressure in the adductor compartment.

about 30 mm Hg (3). Some investigators recommended performing a fasciotomy for intracompartmental pressures exceeding 30 mm Hg. Whitesides et al. (18) suggested that they be performed for pressures greater than 30 mm Hg below diastolic blood pressure. A study by Schneck et al. (17) indicated that metabolic dysfunction is severe when the pressure exceeds 30 to 40 mm Hg below mean arterial pressure. The injury severity, overall metabolic status, circulatory status (i.e., blood pressure and pulse), and the clinical evaluation must also be considered. Hypotensive patients, usually from polytrauma, generally have a greater risk of developing compartmental syndromes at lower pressures. The duration of increased pressure and pressure trends may be helpful in decision making. Unconscious patients with foot injuries should also be observed closely; if the condition is suspicious, compartment pressures should be obtained.

Up to 10% of calcaneus fractures develop compartment syndrome of the foot (15). Of the nine compartments of the foot, the calcaneal compartment, which lies deepest in the foot adjacent to the calcaneus, is the most often affected compartment after calcaneus fractures (Fig. 19-7). Interosseous and adductor compartment syndromes can occur after Lisfranc's and Chopart's joint injuries and crush injuries to the forefoot (16). Isolated medial foot compartment syndrome (i.e., abductor hallucis muscle) has been reported as an exertional syndrome in athletes (1) and as an isolated syndrome occurring idiopathically without injury (14). Concurrent compartment syndromes of the leg and foot have been reported and are probably associated with communication between the deep posterior compartment of the leg and the deep compartments of the foot (9).

The antiquated notions that "foot compartment syndromes don't exist," that "the foot can tolerate higher pressures than other parts of the body," and that the late sequelae are "not too bad" should be abandoned. Mittlmeier et al. (12) showed that 11 of 16 feet that had measured pressures greater than 30 mm Hg after calcaneal fractures developed rigid toe clawing, plantar scarring, cavus, sensory disturbances, and significant disability. Michelson et al. (11) reported isolated calcaneal compartment syndrome after minimal incision surgery in the arch. Long-term disability secondary to rigid, claw toe deformities was re-

dorsal

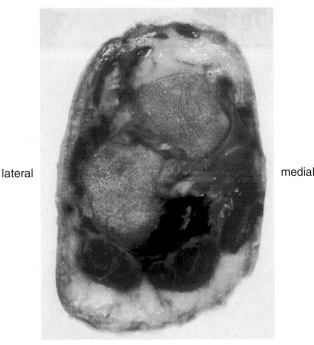

lateral                                                medial

plantar

**Figure 19-7.** An ink-injection study (coronal section of hindfoot) illustrates the fascial confines of the calcaneal compartment *(dark area)* superficial plantar compartment (plantar to calcaneal compartment), medial compartment, and lateral compartment. The neurovascular bundle is adjacent to medial fascia in calcaneal compartment. (From Manoli A II, Weber TG: Fasciotomy of the foot: an anatomical study with special reference to release of the calcaneal compartment. *Foot Ankle* 10: 267–275, 1990, with permission.)

ported as sequelae and related to interconnections in the calcaneal compartment between the quadratus plantae muscle and the long toe flexors of the leg.

## SURGERY

Foot fasciotomy may be performed under regional or general anesthesia. The patient is positioned supine on the operating table; a bump under the ipsilateral hip is usually not needed. In instances that require additional approaches, such as to the lateral hindfoot in patients with tongue-type fractures of the calcaneus or minimally displaced fractures of the talar neck, the lateral position on a bean-bag is preferable to facilitate percutaneous reduction and fixation of the fracture. This can be performed in conjunction with compartment release. In these cases, an assistant is required to hold the extremity in external rotation to access the medial foot during foot compartment release. A tourniquet is used to ensure a bloodless field. Either a thigh or a lower leg tourniquet may be used.

### Technique

A three-incision fasciotomy is used to decompress the nine compartments of the foot (Fig. 19-8). A medial hindfoot incision is used to decompress the deeply situated calcaneal compartment and the three compartments (medial, lateral, and superficial) that extend the en-

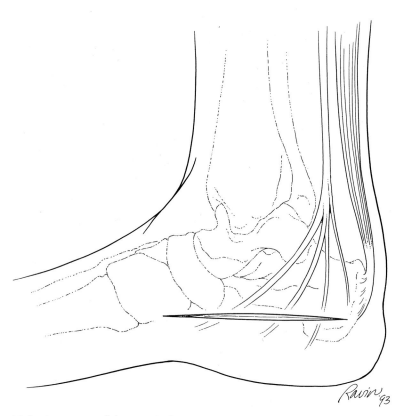

**Figure 19-8.** Summary of the surgical approach. Two dorsal forefoot incisions and one medial hindfoot incision are used to decompress the foot compartments. (Adapted from Manoli A II, Weber TG: Fasciotomy of the foot: an anatomical study with special reference to release of the calcaneal compartment. *Foot Ankle* 10: 267–275, 1990, with permission.)

tire length of the foot. This incision begins approximately 4 cm from the back of the heel and 3 cm. from the plantar surface. The abductor hallucis muscle bulge usually lies directly under the incision (Fig. 19-9A,B). The incision extends distally over the abductor hallucis muscle for a distance of approximately 6 cm. After the skin and subcutaneous tissues are divided, the very thin fascia over the abductor hallucis muscle is encountered (Fig. 19-9C). Before opening this thin fascial layer to decompress the medial compartment, the skin and subcutaneous tissue is dissected plantar to the medial compartment using the tension of the medial compartment fascia to facilitate dissection. This plane of dissection to the superficial plantar compartments is often obscured after opening the fascia overlying the medial compartment. The thin fascia overlying the abductor hallucis muscle is then opened the length of the incision (Fig. 19-9D). Undermining the skin slightly in the distal portion of the incision allows for most of the medial compartment to be released. After this, the inferior portion of the abductor hallucis muscle is defined. A small elevator is useful, and the muscle is lifted dorsally from the inferior portion of its investing fascia. On retracting the muscle upward with an Army-Navy, knee, or small Deaver retractor, the surgeon encounters the thick, glistening white, intermuscular septum of the foot (Fig. 19-10). This is the medial border of the deeper, calcaneal compartment. Occasionally, a headlamp may be useful during this part of the procedure to improve visualization.

The calcaneal compartment is released by opening the intermuscular septum. This is done by first perforating the septum bluntly with a hemostat and carefully enlarging it by spreading the hemostat. The length of the fascia is opened carefully with a small dissecting scissors, knife, or gloved finger. Great care is necessary at this point to avoid any injury to the lateral plantar nerve or blood vessels that lie immediately under the septum (Fig. 19-11A–C). The septum should be opened for the length of the skin incision. To open the septum more distally in the foot, the surgeon can use a gloved finger to "push" it open, sepa-

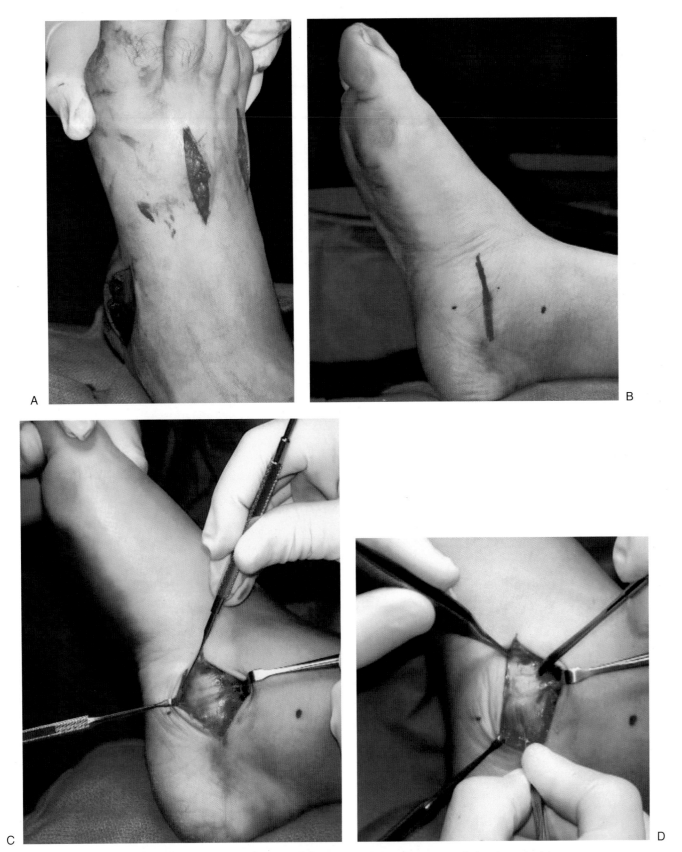

**Figure 19-9. A:** Clinical example of the appropriate placement of the three incisions for the foot compartment releases. **B:** The medial incision lies over the bulge of the abductor hallucis muscle, centered approximately 2 cm distal to the medial malleolus *(purple dot).* **C:** Dissection is carried out plantarward using the tension of the abductor hallucis fascia (along the path of the elevator in this example). **D:** Abductor hallucis muscle (medial) fascia release.

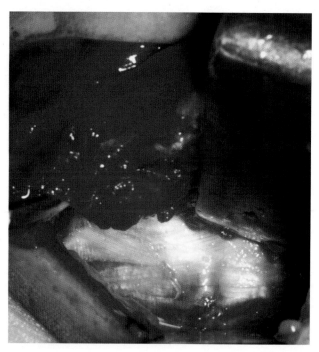

**Figure 19-10.** Fascial septum overlying the calcaneal compartment. The lateral plantar neurovascular bundle lies directly under this fascia.

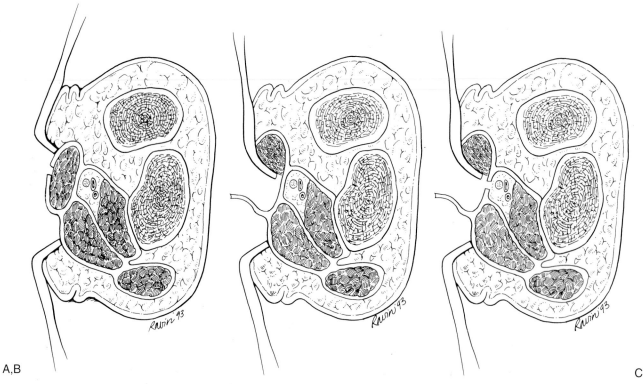

A,B                                                                                          C

**Figure 19-11.** **A:** This hindfoot section illustrates the release of the medial compartment. **B:** The abductor hallucis muscle is retracted superiorly. The medial intermuscular septum of the foot is then observed. **C:** The medial intermuscular septum is opened. The lateral plantar neurovascular bundle lies just deep to the septum in the calcaneal compartment. The quadratus plantae muscle may bulge considerably around these vessels as the calcaneal compartment is released. (Adapted from Manoli A II, Fakhouri AJ, Weber TG: Compartment catheterization and fasciotomy of the foot. *Operative Tech Orthop* 2: 203–210, 1992, with permission.)

rating the fibers. Because the medial plantar nerve and vessels run in the calcaneal compartment, superficial compartment, or in the septum itself in the middle of the foot, a blunt technique such as a gloved finger is suggested to avoid injury to these structures. Considerable bulging of the quadratus plantae muscle may occur when this fascia is opened. The muscles may bulge considerably around the lateral plantar nerve and artery (Fig. 19-12). If observed, this bulging suggests an adequate release of the calcaneal compartment. The retractors are removed, and the abductor muscle is allowed to return to its usual position.

Attention is then focused outside of the medial compartment in the plantarward direction. The investing fascia of the abductor hallucis muscle, which previously was dissected from the overlying skin and subcutaneous fat, is followed plantarward, retracting the fat from the medial side of the heel medially (Fig. 19-13A). On the plantar aspect of the foot, the superficial compartment is then encountered. This compartment is opened longitudinally with a blunt hemostat by perforating the septum and bluntly spreading, releasing the flexor digitorum brevis muscle (Fig. 19-13B). A gloved finger is then used to complete the release. The soft tissues may be undermined distally to ensure that the superficial compartment is opened completely.

The flexor digitorum brevis muscle is separated from the fascia overlying the dorsum of the compartment (i.e., the transverse septum of the hindfoot) and the flexor digitorum brevis muscle is retracted plantarward using an Army-Navy, knee, or small Deaver retractor (Fig. 19-14A). As the flexor digitorum brevis muscle is retracted, the medial aspect of the lateral compartment becomes accessible. This medial border of the lateral compartment is the lateral intermuscular septum of the foot. It is often difficult to visualize this septum clinically, but in the cadaver, it is possible to follow this septum posteriorly, and the lateral compartment sweeps medially in the posterior aspect of the heel.

The lateral compartment is best opened by using a blunt hemostat; a small dissecting scissors or a sharp elevator can also be used. The septum is opened beginning in the posterior aspect of the compartment and extending anteriorly to the middle of the foot (Fig. 19-14B). When the lateral compartment is released, the abductor digiti quinti muscle and flexor digiti minimi muscle are released.

The muscular compartments of the forefoot are then released. Generally, this is done through two separate longitudinal incisions located slightly medial to the second metatarsal and slightly lateral to the fourth metatarsal to ensure as wide a skin bridge as possible (Fig. 19-15). Although these incisions may theoretically compromise the skin on the dorsum of the foot, sloughing in this area has only been seen when the skin was already injured, as in

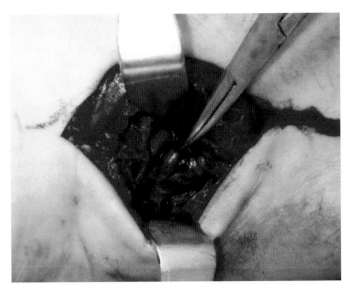

**Figure 19-12.** The quadratus plantae muscle is seen bulging proximally and distally to the lateral plantar neurovascular bundle (by hemostat).

**Figure 19-13. A:** The medial compartment is retracted dorsally and the skin and subcutaneous fat plantarward to facilitate the release of the superficial plantar compartment. **B:** It is opened longitudinally. The flexor digitorum brevis muscle can then be seen. (**A:** Adapted from Manoli A II, Fakhouri AJ, Weber TG: Compartment catheterization and fasciotomy of the foot. *Operative Tech Orthop* 2: 203–210, 1992, with permission.)

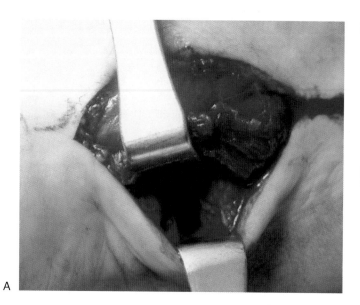

A

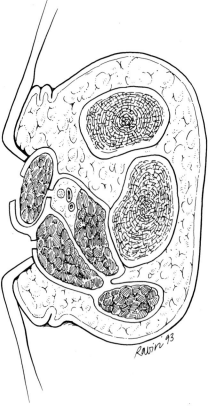

B

A

B

**Figure 19-14. A:** The flexor digitorum brevis muscle is retracted plantarward. **B:** The lateral intermuscular septum is opened bluntly and deeply in the plantar foot. (Adapted from Manoli A II, Fakhouri AJ, Weber TG: Compartment catheterization and fasciotomy of the foot. *Operative Tech Orthop* 2: 203–210, 1992, with permission.)

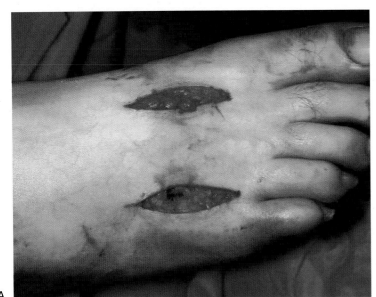

A

**Figure 19-15. A:** Clinical example of the appropriate position of the two dorsal incisions. **B:** They are made approximately over the second and fourth metatarsal shafts, which allows the individual interosseous compartments to be opened. **C:** The interosseous muscles are stripped from the medial surface of the second metatarsal shaft, and the fascia overlying the adductor muscle is accessible. The adductor fascia is then opened longitudinally. **D:** Cross section of **A**, **B**, and **C**.

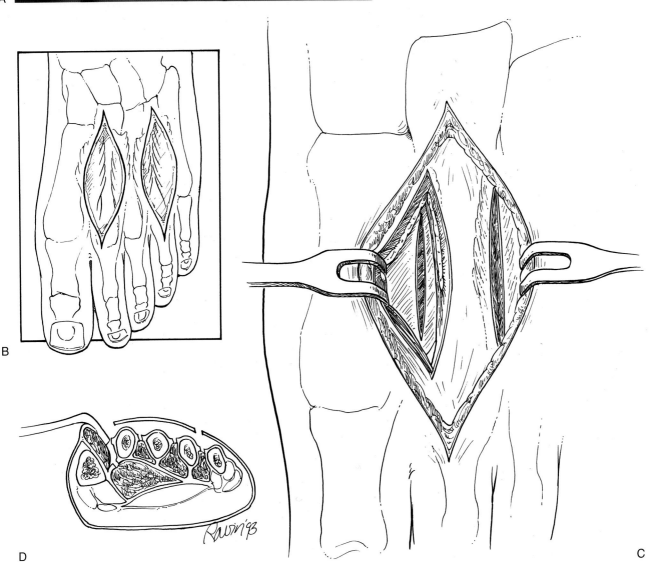

B

D

C

a crush injury. If the surgeon is concerned about the viability of the skin bridge in cases of crush injury of the forefoot, a lateral skin incision may be made as an alternative by making a small transverse incision over the distal one third of the fourth metatarsal. Undermining the skin proximally allows one to release the interosseous compartments in the third and fourth interspace without compromising the skin viability.

Through the medial incision, the dorsal interosseous muscles that lie in the first and second interspaces are identified. The thin dorsal fascia is opened using the blunt hemostat technique as described previously. Next, the muscles of the first interspace are stripped off of the medial portion of the second metatarsal, along the length of the metatarsal. As the interosseous muscles are retracted medially, the fascia of the adductor musculature become accessible deep in the interspace. This fascia is then opened longitudinally, preferably with a blunt hemostat. This is a safe technique because the vascular perforators and arch lie medial and proximal; return of fluid is often encountered and represents release of fluid accumulation in the plantar forefoot compartments. Through the lateral forefoot incision, the dorsal fascia of the third and fourth interosseous muscles are identified and these interosseous compartments are opened longitudinally.

After the fasciotomy is completed, any fractures of the forefoot or midfoot can be treated through the forefoot incisions. It may be necessary to extend them proximally or distally. Fractures of the talus or ankle may be approached through additional standard incisions.

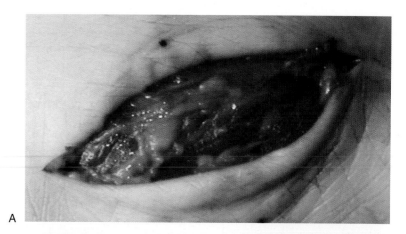

A

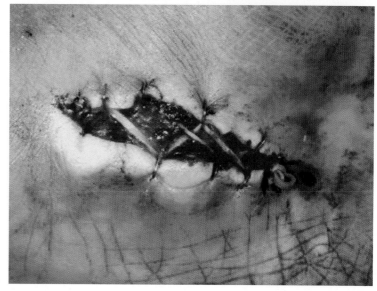

B

**Figure 19-16. A:** Clinical example of muscle bulging from the medial wound after the fasciotomy. **B:** Appearance of the wound 4 days later after using a rubber-band technique.

Percutaneous fixation of certain fractures of the calcaneus and talus can be performed at the same setting; however, it is important that preoperative planning be used because lateral positioning of the patient is often necessary. It is suggested that a comminuted, intraarticular, depression fracture of the calcaneus not be repaired at the time of fasciotomy. Although Rorabeck (3) recommends that the skeleton be fixed at the time of fasciotomy in other locations to provide stability, this is probably not necessary when dealing with a calcaneal fracture. Here, stability is not generally a problem, but restoration of the architecture of the calcaneus is usually the goal. The swelling associated with compartment syndrome of the foot can compromise the wound and skin flap of the extensile posterolateral approach to the calcaneus. We therefore recommend repairing an intraarticular, depressed, calcaneal fracture, if desired, later through an additional posterolateral incision after the fasciotomy wounds are healed.

## POSTOPERATIVE MANAGEMENT

The fasciotomy wounds are left open and dressed with a sterile dressing. If bulging of the wounds is excessive, we recommend using a small vessel-loop or rubber-band technique to approximate the skin edges and lessen the tension at delayed primary closure. This technique uses a rubber band and staples or nylon suture; the rubber band is "criss-crossed" between successive skin staples or nylon stitches and tied at both ends over the wound (Fig. 19-16).

The patients are generally returned to the operating room on the third through the fifth day postoperatively. In instances of isolated foot trauma, we often discharge patients home and have them return for delayed primary closure as an outpatient. The wounds are irrigated and debrided as necessary. The skin may be closed at that time if the wound conditions permit. Otherwise, it may be done at a later date. Split-thickness skin grafting should be used if the wound edges cannot be approximated without excessive tension. It is important to counsel patients preoperatively on the possibility of skin grafting, obtain consent, and prepare the ipsilateral thigh for donation. We have found it necessary to skin graft approximately one fifth of the cases.

## COMPLICATIONS

Complications from the procedure of foot fasciotomy are minimal. The major complications tend to result from not performing a fasciotomy or performing it too late. It is not uncommon to encounter compartment syndrome of the foot up to 24 to 36 hours after injury. Close observation in suspicious cases is recommended. Clawing of the lesser toes, paresthesias in the medial or lateral plantar nerve distribution, cavus deformity, stiffness, and residual pain are primarily seen after foot compartment syndrome without release.

The nerve damage can usually be avoided. There are three areas where nerves may be encountered and should be avoided. When making the initial skin incision, the surgeon should begin the incision at least 4 cm from the posterior aspect of the heel to avoid the medial calcaneal branches of the tibial nerve. When opening the medial intermuscular septum of the foot, the lateral plantar vessels and nerve lie immediately under this fascia. Care must be taken to avoid these structures. The medial plantar nerve and vessels lie just distal to the skin incision in the calcaneal or superficial compartments or in the medial intermuscular septum itself. It is practical to use the gloved finger to open the most distal part of the medial intermuscular septum, avoiding nerve damage.

Although these nerves are nearby during dissection, they appear to be consistently located and can be avoided or protected. With this approach, the surgeon can actually release the lateral side of the foot (i.e., lateral compartment) from the medial side. Using an approach through the superficial compartment, the medial and lateral plantar nerves are protected from the plane of dissection by the transverse hindfoot septum described by Martin (10).

## RECOMMENDED READING

1. Blacklidge DK, Kurek JB, Soto AD, et al.: Acute exertional compartment syndrome of the medial foot. *J Foot Ankle Surg* 35:19–22, 1996.
2. Bonutti PM, Bell GR: Compartment syndrome of the foot. *J Bone Joint Surg Am* 68: 1449–1451, 1986.
3. Bourne RB, Rorabeck CH: Compartment syndromes of the lower leg. *Clin Orthop* 240:97–104, 1989.
4. Dayton P, Goldman FD, Barton E: Compartment pressure in the foot: analysis of normal values and measurement technique. *J Am Podiatr Med Assoc* 80:521–525, 1990.
5. Fakhouri AJ, Manoli A II: Acute foot compartment syndromes. *J Orthop Trauma* 6:223–228, 1992.
6. Hargens AR, Akeson WH, Mubarak SJ, et al.: Tissue fluid pressures: from basic research tools to clinical applications. *J Orthop Res* 7:902–909, 1989.
7. Manoli A II: Compartment syndromes of the foot: current concepts. *Foot Ankle* 10:340–344, 1990.
8. Manoli A II, Fakhouri AJ, Weber TG: Compartment catheterization and fasciotomy of the foot. *Operative Tech Orthop* 2:203–210, 1992.
9. Manoli A II, Weber TG: Fasciotomy of the foot: an anatomical study with special reference to release of the calcaneal compartment. *Foot Ankle* 10:267–275, 1990.
10. Martin BF: Observations on the muscles and tendons of the medial aspect of the sole of the foot. *J Anat* 98: 437–453, 1964.
11. Michelson J: Isolated compartment syndrome of the calcaneal compartment secondary to minimal incision surgery. *Foot Ankle Int* 16:162–163, 1995.
12. Mittlmeier T, Machler G, Lob G, et al.: Compartment syndrome of the foot after intra-articular calcaneal fracture. *Clin Orthop* 269:241–248, 1991.
13. Myerson MS: Diagnosis and treatment of compartment syndrome of the foot. *Orthopedics* 13:711–717, 1990.
14. Myerson M, Berger BI: Isolated medial compartment syndrome of the foot: a case report. *Foot Ankle Int* 17: 183–185, 1996.
15. Myerson M, Manoli A II: Compartment syndromes of the foot after calcaneal fractures. *Clin Orthop* 290: 142–150, 1993.
16. Randt T, Dahlen C, Schikore H, et al.: Dislocation fractures in the area of the middle foot–injuries of the Chopart and Lisfranc joint. *Zentralbl Chir* 123:1257–1266, 1998.
17. Schneck S, Sapega A, Dobrasz J, et al.: The metabolic stages in an evolving compartment syndrome. *Trans Orthop Res Soc* 15:261, 1990.
18. Whitesides TE, Henry TC, Morimoto R, et al.: Tissue pressure measurements as a determinant for the need of fasciotomy. *Clin Orthop* 113: 4:3–51, 1975.
19. Ziv I, Mosheiff R, Zeligowski A, et al.: Crush injuries of the foot with compartment syndrome: immediate one-stage management. *Foot Ankle* 9:185–189, 1989.

# PART IV

# Hindfoot

# 20

# Posterior Tibial Tendon Release-Substitution

## Michael J. Shereff

## INDICATIONS/CONTRAINDICATIONS

Posterior tibial tendon dysfunction (PTTD) is a commonly occurring disorder in adults. Patients typically present with a unilateral painful flatfoot. In the past, the diagnosis was usually delayed, but with increased awareness of the condition, patients are now diagnosed and treated at earlier stages of the disease process. Several investigators, such as Kenneth A. Johnson, Melvin H. Jahss, and Roger A. Mann, can be credited for increasing the awareness of this problem in the early 1980s.

Abnormalities of the posterior tibial (PT) tendon have been classified as three stages (Table 20-1). Stage I denotes a tendon afflicted with a peritendinitis or tendinosis, but it remains at its normal length. In stage II, the PT tendon is elongated as a result of the inflammation and degeneration process. The hindfoot articulations in this second stage are still flexible, with no fixed hindfoot deformity. With weight bearing, the arch of the foot may be flattened, but in a non–weight-bearing situation, normal motion of the hindfoot usually exists. Stage III indicates the later development of a fixed hindfoot deformity in which the hindfoot is in eversion and forefoot in abduction as a result of PTTD.

Staging of PT tendon dysfunction can be useful in selecting proper treatment. For the initial symptoms of PT inflammation, conservative measures such as rest, arch supports, physical therapy, and oral antiinflammatory agents may be used. If necessary, immobilization in a brace or short-leg cast is effective. Corticosteroid injections about the PT tendon are usually not recommended. Many patients with stage I PTTD can be successfully managed nonoperatively. However, if the PT inflammation continues despite adequate conservative care over a few months, then the stage I situation could be treated with the PT tendon release, tenosynovectomy, and debridement. Persistent tenosynovitis can progress to stage II and III changes unless the inflammatory process is interrupted by nonoperative or operative measures.

M. J. Shereff, M.D.: Department of Orthopaedic Surgery, Medical University of South Carolina; and Foot and Ankle Center, Orthopaedic Specialists of Charleston, Charleston, South Carolina.

**Table 20-1.** *Stages of posterior tibial tendon disease and treatment*

| Stage | Abnormality | Tendon length | Hindfoot deformity | Treatment |
|-------|-------------|---------------|--------------------|-----------|
| I | Tendinosis—mild | Normal | No | Release, tenosynovectomy, debridement |
| II | Tendinosis—moderate | Elongated | Yes—flexible mild | Release, tenosynovectomy, debridement, FDL transfer |
| II | Tendinosis—moderate | Elongated | Yes—flexible moderate to severe | FDL transfer and medial displacement calcaneal osteotomy; limited hindfoot arthrodesis |
| III | Tendonesis—marked | Elongated | Yes—rigid ± hindfoot arthritis | Hindfoot arthrodesis |

FDL, flexor digitorum longus.

When the tendon has elongated and a flexible secondary deformity (stage II) has developed, a transfer of the flexor digitorum longus (FDL) tendon is suggested in addition to the tendon release and tenosynovectomy. This tendon transfer substitutes partially for the loss of the PT tendon function. It is useful for early-stage II PTTD in patients who have limited flatfoot deformity. Patients with stage II PTTD with severe but still flexible flatfoot deformity are more likely to be dissatisfied by the persistent flatfoot that commonly results from the isolated PT release or substitution operation. This operation has been combined with other procedures for stage II PTTD with severe deformity, such as medial displacement osteotomy of the calcaneus described in Chapter 27. We think there is no single procedure that is applicable for all patients with PTTD.

For a stage III fixed foot deformity, an arthrodesis procedure of the hindfoot is suggested. Various combinations of arthrodesis for the talonavicular, calcaneocuboid, and talocalcaneal joints have been used. The surgical technique for subtalar arthrodesis is described in Chapter 28.

Contraindications to the surgical care of the PT tendon difficulties center on the patient and the diagnosis. All patients should be treated with nonoperative measures initially. A physiologically older patient with limited symptoms could be treated with nonoperative measures. The use of corticosteroids and antimetabolic agents such as methotrexate are relative contraindications to surgical treatment, because tissue healing may be delayed with such medications. Marked obesity may place excessive stress on the transferred FDL tendon for stage II disease. Patients with stage II PTTD with severe flatfoot deformity may not be ideal candidates for the isolated soft tissue reconstruction.

The correct diagnosis is also important. Through appropriate history, physical examination, and radiologic valuation, the physician must exclude other causes of foot swelling and deformity, such as neuropathic arthropathy, tarsometatarsal degenerative arthritis (Lisfranc), or flexible flatfoot deformity.

## PREOPERATIVE PLANNING

Anticipating the correct surgical procedure before treatment is aided by the staging of PTTD. In general, the degree of tendon degeneration and tenosynovitis viewed at surgery is worse than suggested by the physical examination. Swelling and pain may be mild, although the tendon may show thickening, yellowish discoloration, longitudinal split tears, and a significant synovial proliferation. For stage I or early stage II PT tendon involvement, the patient usually is counseled that a FDL tendon transfer may be necessary in addition to tendon release and debridement.

The physical examination involves assessment of the location of pain symptoms, the associated swelling and hindfoot deformity, and the strength of the PT tendon. With involvement of the posterior tibialis tendon, tenderness is felt along the course of this tendon just posterior to the medial crest of the distal tibia. It can extend around the tip of the medial malleolus to the insertion of the tendon on the undersurface of the navicular. Swelling is most evident by viewing the standing patient from a posterior aspect (Fig. 20-1). Fullness in the medial malleolar region inferiorly is evident. The deformity of the foot is also assessed from a posterior view of the standing patient (Fig. 20-2). Increased hindfoot valgus occurs, and external rotation of the forefoot is evident by the "too many toes" sign; with loss of the tibial posterior tendon function, more lesser toes are evident than on the unaffected side.

Strength of the PT muscle and tendon can be assessed with manual muscle strength testing. The foot is placed in a plantarflexed and supinated position, and the patient is asked to maintain this position while the examiner attempts to pronate the foot. The examiner can readily pronate the foot against the patient's resistance in PTTD. Comparison is made with the opposite, unaffected side. Posterior tibial tendon and muscle function is also assessed with the single heel rise test (Fig. 20-3). This is done by asking the patient to rest his or her fingertips on a wall or examination table for support while the physician views the feet posteriorly. While the affected foot is raised in the air, the patient is first asked to raise the heel off the floor repeatedly on the normal foot, which should be easily accomplished. The heel rotates from eversion to inversion with the single heel rise test in the normal foot. When the same test is used on the affected foot with loss of the tibialis posterior function, the patient has difficulty raising the heel off the floor because of weakness and pain (Fig. 20-3C,D). The heel also fails to invert when the tendon is dysfunctional during the single heel rise test. With much effort, the patient with PTTD may be able to raise the heel of the affected foot off of the floor, but it is judged by the patient to be more difficult than the unaffected foot. It is common for PTTD patients to accomplish heel rise with both feet simultaneously but not be able to do a single heel rise.

When secondary deformity has occurred, there may be tenderness laterally in the region of the lateral malleolus as calcaneofibular impingement occurs. With time, the hindfoot motion may become restricted as well. Painful hindfoot motion and rigid forefoot supination may also occur in stage III PTTD.

Routine preoperative radiographs should include weight-bearing, lateral and anteroposterior views of the feet (Fig. 20-4). The flatfoot deformity that develops if the tendon lengthens or ruptures is a rotation outward of the calcaneus from beneath the talus, especially in eversion and external rotation. As the head and neck of the talus is left unsupported, the talus deviates, especially in plantarflexion and internal rotation. These changes

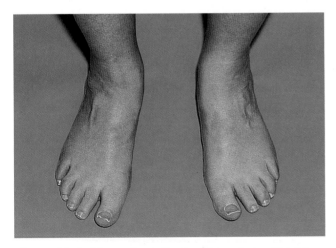

**Figure 20-1.** View of a patient with posterior tibial tendon dysfunction while standing. Patient has loss of right posterior tibial tendon function.

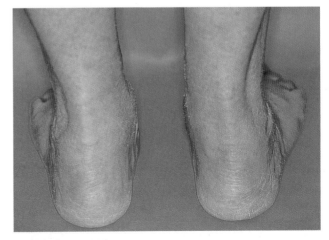

**Figure 20-2.** Posterior view of the patient in Figure 20-1 shows forefoot abduction with more toes seen on the affected right side than on the left.

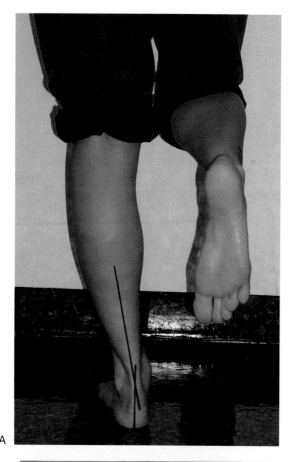

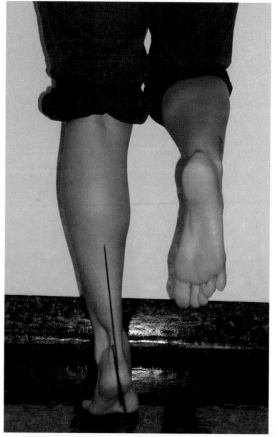

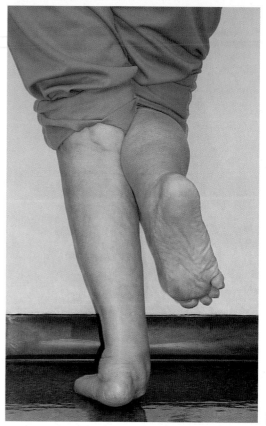

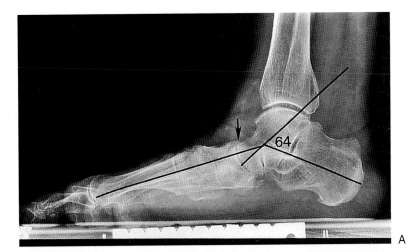

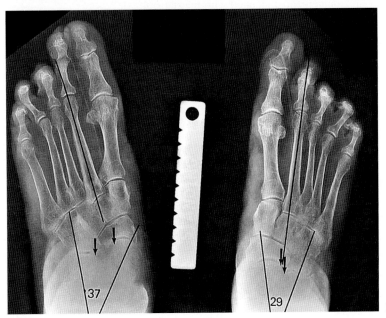

**Figure 20-4. A:** Lateral, weight-bearing radiograph of a typical patient with posterior tibial tendon dysfunction (PTTD) and flatfoot. The arch height *(arrow)* is decreased. The lines representing the talar axis and first metatarsal form a negative angle rather than a straight line. The angle formed between the calcaneal axis and the floor (i.e., calcaneal pitch angle) is decreased in flatfoot. The talar head is plantarflexed. **B:** Weight-bearing, anteroposterior radiograph of patient with PTTD on the left side. The peritalar subluxation is evident by the increase in the talocalcaneal angle, seen as a separation between lateral margin of talar head and medial margin of anterior calcaneus *(arrows)*. Abduction of the forefoot, represented by the second metatarsal axis, is seen. The talar head is uncovered medially (i.e., increased talonavicular coverage angle).

**Figure 20-3. A:** This normal subject is being tested for strength of the posterior tibial tendon and muscle with a single heel rise test. The subject is standing with the left foot plantigrade, while the right foot is raised off the floor by flexing the knee. Notice the valgus position of the heel. **B:** The normal subject is easily able to raise the right heel off the floor. Notice the left heel position is in varus. **C:** The patient with posterior tibial tendon dysfunction with flatfoot on the left is being tested for strength of the posterior tibial tendon and muscle with a single heel rise test. Notice the valgus deformity of the left heel. **D:** The patient has difficulty raising the left heel off the floor. The lifted heel position remains in valgus. (**A–D** courtesy of H. B. Kitaoka, M.D., Mayo School of Medicine, Rochester, Minnesota.)

can be seen on the routine weight-bearing radiographs but not consistently in non–weight-bearing views. On the anteroposterior foot view, an increase in the angle (i.e., divergence) between the longitudinal axis of the talus and calcaneus is seen (Fig. 20-4B). In the anteroposterior view, the magnitude of deformity can be also be assessed by the degree of abduction of the navicular relative to the talus and the amount of talar head that is "uncovered" by the navicular.

A lateral view of a flatfoot deformity shows a decrease or negative angle between the axis of the talus and the first metatarsal; this angle should normally be close to a straight line. An increased angle between the longitudinal axis of the talus and calcaneus is seen (Fig. 20-4A).

A weight-bearing, anteroposterior view of the ankle is helpful to determine the presence of ankle pathology, which can easily be missed until after surgery. Ankle arthritis, valgus tilting of talus in the mortise, and even lateral malleolare stress fracture may be seen. Typically, the ankle height is decreased in the flatfoot deformity on the anteroposterior ankle view compared with the opposite, unaffected side. It can also show calcaneofibular impingement associated with the flatfoot.

By the physical examination and routine radiographs, staging of the tendon involvement is possible. Occasionally, magnetic resonance examination is useful. Such a technique is most helpful early, when the cause of the medial ankle pain is uncertain and the possibility of PT tendon involvement is being considered. It is usually not routinely performed.

## SURGERY

The procedure is carried out with the patient supine and under general or spinal anesthetic. A pneumatic thigh tourniquet is used.

### Technique

The incision starts about 10 cm proximal to the tip of the medial malleolus and about 1 cm posterior to the medial border of the tibia (Fig. 20-5). The incision is then extended distally along the tibia margin to just behind the tip of the medial malleolus (Fig. 20-6). From the tip of the medial malleolus, the incision gently curves along the medial aspect of the foot to the PT insertion at the lower aspect of the navicular tuberosity.

The deep fascia is exposed, and the medial tendons can usually be seen through the partially translucent fascia (Fig. 20-7). At the upper end of the skin incision, the deep fascia is incised and the PT exposed. The large PT tendon lies very close to the posterior margin of

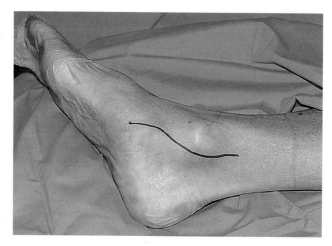

**Figure 20-5.** Position of the foot at the time of surgery is seen with the skin incision marked.

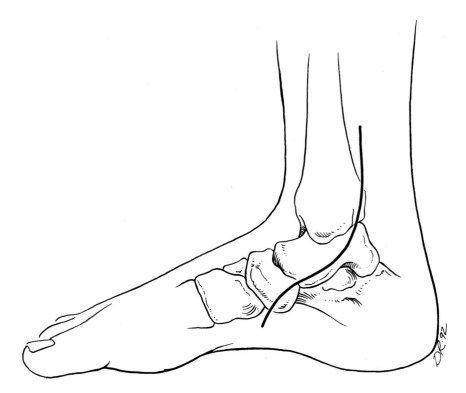

**Figure 20-6.** Relation of the skin incision to the underlying bone structure.

the tibia. The tendon is then traced distally to its insertion while leaving a 2-cm wide pulley just posterior to the medial malleolus at the level of the tibial plafond. At this juncture, a decision is made about whether the tendon is of a normal length or elongated. This decision dictates the subsequent operative treatment. If the tendon is of normal length (stage I), tendon debridement, tenosynovectomy, and sheath resection are done, and the wound is closed. If the tendon is elongated (stage II), a tendon transfer of the FDL is added to the procedure.

Debridement of the tendon depends on the surgical findings. If there is some fraying of the tendon, the tags of tendon tissue are smoothly excised, leaving the major portion of the tendon intact. In some instances, there is bulbous enlargement of the tendon just distal to the tip of the medial malleolus. With such an abnormality, an ellipse is removed from the bulb, and

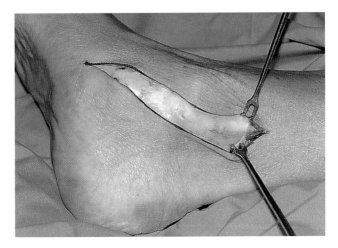

**Figure 20-7.** The posterior tibial tendon lies beneath the superior flexor retinaculum.

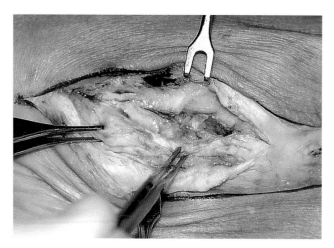

**Figure 20-8.** This tendon shows marked degeneration with loss of the normal tendon architecture.

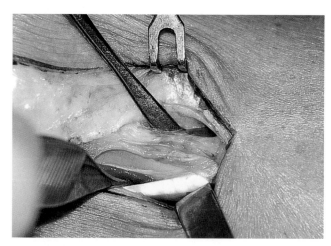

**Figure 20-9.** Posterior tibial tendon proximal from its distal tear.

the tendon is sutured, burying the knots to leave the tendon a normal size. Occasionally, a prominent longitudinal split of the tendon exists, in which case the inner sides of the tear are cleared of scar tissue and the sides apposed with a buried-knot technique. A tenosynovectomy can vary from removing a minimal amount of tissue for mild involvement to a large amount of tissue when the synovium is more severe. The outer portion of the tendon sheath distal to the pulley is removed to prevent possible reformation of a stenotic tendon sheath.

If, on close inspection of the PT tendon, there is evidence of elongation, a transfer of the FDL into the undersurface of the navicular tuberosity is done in addition to debridement, tenosynovectomy, and partial tendon sheath resection. The tendon may show degeneration over several centimeters with enlargement, multiple longitudinal tears, and adhesions to the tendon sheath (Fig. 20-8). Proximal to the region that is directly involved, the tendon has a dull white appearance if the tear is old and tension has not been transmitted through the tendon for some time (Fig. 20-9). In other cases, there is a single, complete transverse tear, with rounding off of the tendon ends.

The transfer of the FDL entails detaching the FDL distally and reinserting it into the undersurface of the navicular through a drill hole (Fig. 20-10). The skin incision is the same as for a stage I PT problem. When it is evident that an FDL transfer is necessary, the incision is extended distally to the crossover area of the FDL and flexor hallucis longus (Fig. 20-11). The FDL is cut under direct vision, giving as much length as possible for transfer.

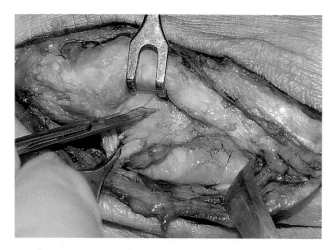

**Figure 20-10.** Tuberosity of navicular is identified.

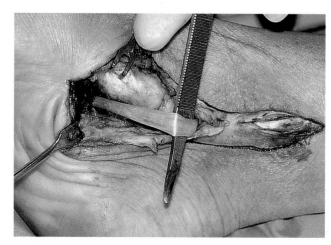

**Figure 20-11.** The flexor digitorum longus tendon is exposed, leaving the pulley of flexor retinaculum intact just posterior to the medial malleolus.

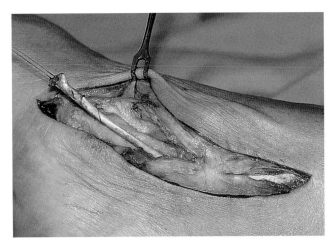

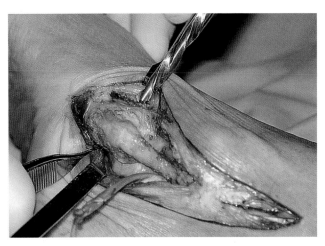

**Figure 20-12.** Zigzag suture has been placed through the flexor digitorum longus tendon after it has been cut distally at the "knot of Henry" area.

**Figure 20-13.** Drill entering superior aspect of navicular tuberosity.

The distal portion of the FDL can be, but does not have to be, sutured to the adjacent flexor hallucis longus tendon. The intrinsic toe flexors are so strong that leaving the distal portion of the FDL alone causes no functional loss of lesser toe function later. Avoiding the tenodesis to the flexor hallucis longus allows a greater length of FDL to be used for transfer. A zig-zag suture of a strong, nonabsorbable material is then placed through the end of the FDL, and the tendon is elevated from its sheath (Fig. 20-12).

The tuberosity of the navicular is identified by supinating and pronating the foot and feeling the joint movement. A longitudinal incision is made in the joint capsule at the inferior surface of the navicular and in the superior surface (Fig. 20-10). Usually, a 0.25- or 0.375-inch drill bit is passed through the tuberosity from superior to inferior (Fig. 20-13). This drill hole should come out inferior to the main insertion of the PT (Fig. 20-14).

The FDL is left in its own sheath and is not rerouted through the diseased PT sheath. Using a bent wire or suture passer, the FDL is brought through the drill hole from inferior to the superior (Fig. 20-15). It is pulled as tight as reasonably possible with the ankle plantarflexed and the forefoot supinated (Fig. 20-16). The zigzag suture can be placed through soft tissue capsule dorsally to hold the tendon in place. A line of nonabsorbable sutures is

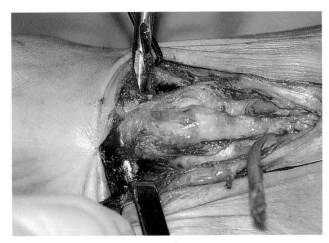

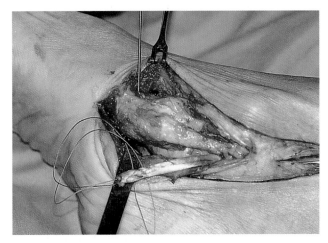

**Figure 20-14.** Drill protruding out through the inferior aspect of the tuberosity of the navicular.

**Figure 20-15.** A folded wire is placed through the drill hole from dorsal to plantar to assist in passing the suture in the end of the flexor digitorum longus tendon from plantar to dorsal.

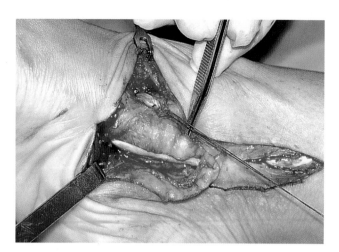

**Figure 20-16.** The flexor digitorum longus tendon has been passed through the drill hole in the tuberosity of the navicular and will be sutured to the surrounding soft tissues.

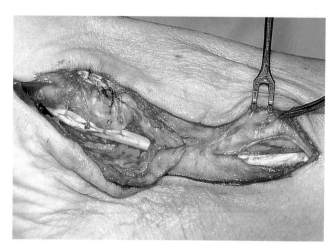

**Figure 20-17.** The tendon has been sutured dorsally to the soft tissues and to the remaining portion of the posterior tibial tendon adjacent to the flexor digitorum longus.

also placed along the transferred FDL tendon to the PT distal portion before the tendon enters the drill hole (Fig. 20-17). This provides a secure soft tissue and bony attachment for the transferred FDL.

The advisability of doing a proximal tenodesis of the PT muscle power to the FDL is assessed next (Fig. 20-18). With disuse, the muscle becomes fibrotic and stiff. By pulling on the proximal portion of the PT tendon, the pliability of the muscle can be determined. If there is some elasticity suggesting a functional muscle, a tenodesis of the PT to the transferred FDL is completed with side-to-side technique using multiple buried sutures. With a fibrotic stiff muscle, the PT is left unattached proximally. A substitution for the PT has been accomplished by the FDL transfer (Figs. 20-19 and 2-20).

Reefing of the talonavicular capsule and calcaneonavicular (spring) ligament can be performed to provide static stability of the arch. Suturing of the FDL to the undersurface of the talonavicular joint may accomplish this to some degree. Historically, static ligament-capsular repair alone has not been successful in maintaining the arch of the foot but may be a useful adjunct to the soft tissue reconstruction.

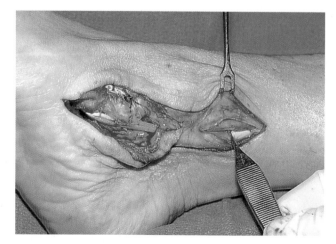

**Figure 20-18.** Because the fibrotic muscle-tendon unit of the posterior tibia is nonfunctional, it will not be tenodesed to the transferred flexor digitorum longus tendon.

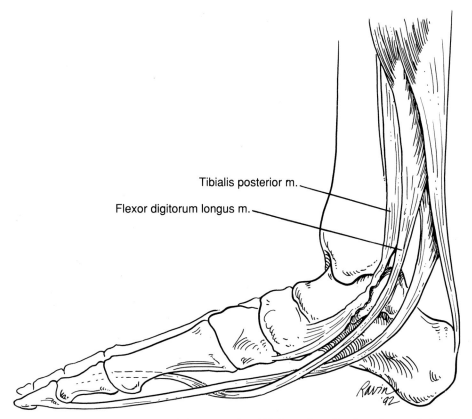

Tibialis posterior m.

Flexor digitorum longus m.

**Figure 20-19.** Degeneration of the posterior tibial tendon distal to the medial malle-olus.

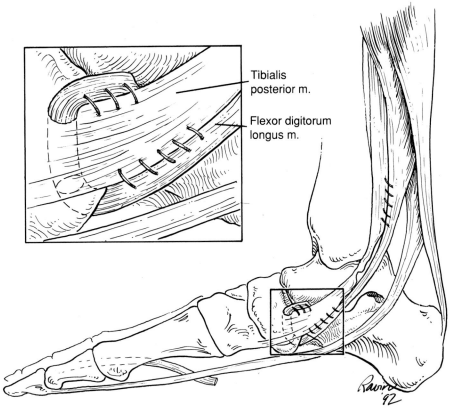

Tibialis posterior m.

Flexor digitorum longus m.

**Figure 20-20.** Transection of the flexor digitorum longus tendon distal to the level where it crosses the flexor hallucis longus and subsequent transfer to the tuberosity of the navicular with suturing. A proximal tenodesis of the muscle of the tibialis posterior to the flexor digitorum longus is also shown.

It is typical that the operative findings are more impressive than what was suspected clinically. It is necessary to carry the surgical exploration all the way to the PT insertion, where the tearing and elongation may be located. Closure is secured with absorbable subcutaneous suture and nylon mattress suture for the skin.

### Posterior Tibial Tendon Substitution with Side-to-Side Flexor Digitorum Brevis Repair

An alternate technique of PT reconstruction involves identification and resection of the diseased section of the PT tendon. This segment usually is proximal to its navicular insertion

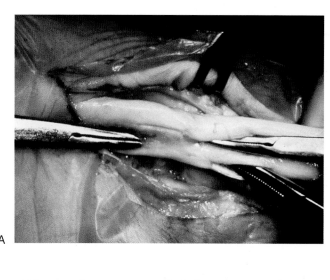

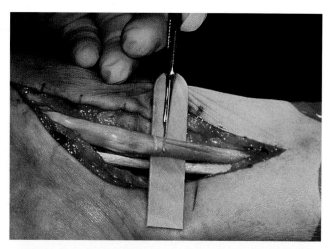

A                                                                                    B

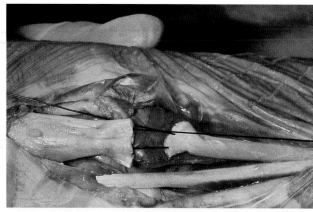

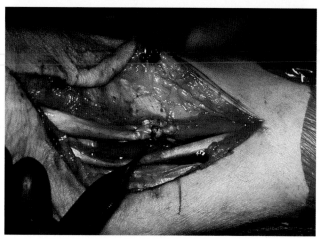

C                                                                                    D

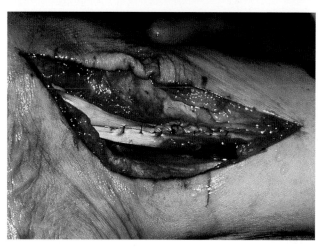

E

**Figure 20-21.** Posterior tibial tendon substitution with side-to-side repair. **A:** Example of a patient with posterior tibial tendon dysfunction. Notice the longitudinal tears and enlargement in the tendon segment proximal to the navicular attachment. **B:** Resection of a portion of degenerated posterior tibial tendon. The flexor digitorum longus tendon is adjacent to the posterior tibial tendon. **C:** End-to-end repair of the posterior tibial tendon using nonabsorbable suture. **D:** The posterior tibial tendon after repair. **E:** The adjacent flexor digitorum longus tendon is sutured side to side of the posterior tibial tendon using nonabsorbable suture.

and extends proximal to the medial malleolus. This technique is applicable in selected patients with PTTD accompanied by a limited flatfoot deformity, such as early stage II disease. The tendon is then reconstructed by a side-to-side repair to the adjacent FDL tendon, because the FDL tendon is usually normal in appearance and function. This reconstruction has some limitations; it cannot restore a significant flatfoot deformity to normal alignment, but pain relief and improved function is expected. This technique has been applied to patients with stage II disease with very favorable results (Fig 20-21). As with the PT tendon substitution with FDL transfer through the navicular, the procedure can be combined with other operations, such as medial displacement calcaneal osteotomy.

## POSTOPERATIVE MANAGEMENT

When the PT tendon sheath release, debridement, and tenosynovectomy are done with or without an FDL transfer, a compressive dressing with plaster splints is applied immediately postoperatively to hold the ankle in plantarflexion and inversion. After about 1 or 2 days, a short-leg cast is applied.

Without the FDL transfer, a walking cast holds the hindfoot in a neutral dorsiflexion-plantarflexion position for about 3 weeks. The cast is then removed, and walking is encouraged, initially in a postoperative shoe. Gradual progression is advised from the postoperative shoe to a spacious, lace-up, low-heeled shoe to usual footwear. Resolution of pain and postoperative swelling is gradual, occurring over several months after immobilization is discontinued.

With the FDL transfer, the postoperative recuperation is more prolonged. The initial cast is applied 1 to 2 days after surgery and is a non–weight-bearing, short-leg cast that holds the foot in adduction and hindfoot in inversion. After 3 weeks, sutures are removed. The foot and ankle are brought to neutral flexion-extension position, and a second short-leg, non–weight-bearing cast is applied for an additional 3 weeks. At 6 weeks postoperatively, immobilization is discontinued, and the patient is instructed to begin bearing weight as tolerated. Patients should be instructed about a foot and ankle rehabilitation program and encouraged to gradually advance activities.

Formal physical therapy to facilitate weight bearing and strength development are occasionally necessary. Crutches or a walker are necessary during the non–weight-bearing period. A compression stocking after cast removal helps control postoperative swelling. The patient is instructed to use the compression stocking during the waking hours only and as long as necessary for swelling. The duration of appreciable swelling is usually about as long as the period of cast immobilization.

The expectations for recovery depend on the tendon changes seen at surgery and the specific surgical procedure. When the procedure just involves sheath release, debridement, and tenosynovectomy without FDL transfer, the outlook is excellent. Usually, the sequence of inflammation and tendon degeneration is halted, and pain relief is obtained. These patients have not had recurrence of their tendon disease at a later time.

With transfer of the FDL, the patient can expect pain relief. Restitution, however, of PT function by the transferred FDL usually does not occur. The patient will still have a pes planus deformity, and the single heel rise test will indicate loss of heel inversion, but the hindfoot deformity will not progress, and recurrent pain has not been a problem after FDL transfer.

## COMPLICATIONS

The difficulties associated with surgery for PT tendon inflammation include delayed wound healing, stiffness, persistent deformity, pain, and prolonged recuperation.

*Wound healing* can be a problem if wound closure is not secure and if corticosteroid is administered locally or systemically. Previously, it was felt that a corticosteroid applied (i.e., "bathing" the tendon) at the conclusion of the operation would help decrease inflammation. Wound healing, however, was significantly impaired and, in a few instances, led to wide dehiscence; this practice is no longer performed. The incision used for the tendon surgery is under tension with swelling and ankle motion. Using multiple mattress sutures with nylon for the skin closure and leaving them in place for 3 weeks has improved wound healing.

*Stiffness* may occur after the FDL transfer procedure. Instead of holding the ankle and foot in equinus and adduction for a full 6 weeks, the advised postoperative plan is to bring the ankle and foot to neutral position after 3 weeks at the time of the first cast change. This practice has decreased the stiffness.

*Continued pes planus deformity* is a common result after FDL transfer. If the patients are advised before treatment of such an expectation, they can adjust to the abnormal foot position. This operation is less appealing for stage II disease with severe deformity. If normal alignment of the foot is important, an alternate procedure may be preferred, such as combining the procedure with a calcaneal osteotomy or a limited hindfoot arthrodesis (i.e., subtalar or distraction calcaneocuboid arthrodesis). Although PT tendon substitution with FDL transfer as an isolated procedure used to be the most commonly performed operation for PTTD, its indications have become more focused in the past decade as some of its limitations were recognized.

*Pain* that persists after FDL transfer is probably related to the abnormal hindfoot position. If the deformity preoperatively is moderate to severe, there may be persistent calcaneofibular impingement. This problem can be anticipated if the deformity is advanced and preoperative pain is located laterally. In such a situation, alternate procedures should be considered.

*Prolonged recovery* after a PT release with or without FDL transfer is not unusual. Swelling in the incision area and about the ankle can be controlled with compressive stockings. If the patients understand that they will not be able to resume all desired activities immediately after the final cast is removed, it is easier for them and for the surgeon. Allowing a few months for recuperation is appropriate.

## RECOMMENDED READING

1. Alexander IJ, Johnson KA, Berquist TH: Magnetic resonance imaging in the diagnosis of disruption of the posterior tibial tendon. *Foot Ankle* 8: 144–147, 1987.
2. Chao W, Wapner KL, Lee TH, et al.: Nonoperative management of posterior tibial tendon dysfunction. *Foot Ankle Int* 17: 736–741, 1996.
3. Churchill RS, Sferra JJ: Posterior tibial tendon insufficiency: its diagnosis, management, and treatment. *Am J Orthop* 27: 339–347, 1998.
4. Crates JM, Richardson EG: Treatment of stage I posterior tibial tendon dysfunction with medial soft tissue procedures. *Clin Orthop* 365: 46–49, 1999.
5. Funk DA, Cass JR, Johnson KA: Acquired flat foot secondary to posterior tibial tendon pathology. *J Bone Joint Surg Am* 68: 95–102, 1986.
6. Gazdag AR, Cracchiolo A 3rd: Rupture of the posterior tibial tendon: evaluation of injury of the spring ligament and clinical assessment of tendon transfer and ligament repair. *J Bone Joint Surg Am* 79: 675–681, 1997.
7. Jahss MH: Spontaneous rupture of the tibialis posterior tendon: clinical findings, tenographic studies, and a new technique of repair. *Foot Ankle* 3:158–166, 1982.
8. Johnson KA: Tibialis posterior tendon rupture. *Clin Orthop* 177:140–147, 1983.
9. Johnson KA, Strom DE: Tibialis posterior tendon dysfunction. *Clin Orthop* 239:196–206, 1989.
10. Kaye RA, Jahss MH: Tibialis posterior: a review of anatomy and biomechanics in relation to support of the medial longitudinal arch. *Foot Ankle* 11:241–247, 1991.
11. Mann RA, Thompson FM: Rupture of the posterior tibial tendon causing flat foot. *J Bone Joint Surg Am* 67: 556–561, 1985.
12. Pomeroy GC, Pike RH, Beals TC, et al.: Acquired flatfoot in adults due to dysfunction of the posterior tibial tendon. *J Bone Joint Surg Am* 81:1173–1182, 1999.
13. Teasdall RD, Johnson KA: Surgical treatment of stage I posterior tibial tendon dysfunction. *Foot Ankle Int* 15:646–648, 1994.

# 21

# Peroneal Tendon Repair and Reconstruction

Diane L. Dahm and Harold B. Kitaoka

## INDICATIONS/CONTRAINDICATIONS

The peroneus longus and peroneus brevis tendons originate in the lateral compartment of the leg and course distally, posterior to the lateral malleolus toward their insertions in the foot. The peroneus longus courses posterior to the peroneus brevis tendon, and both tendons pass through a common peroneal synovial sheath approximately 4 cm proximal to the lateral malleolus. Within this synovial sheath, the tendons pass through a fibro-osseous tunnel at the level of the lateral malleolus. This tunnel is formed by the fibula anteriorly, the superior peroneal retinaculum posterolaterally, and the calcaneofibular and posterior talofibular ligaments medially (Fig. 21-1A). An indentation in the posterior surface of the distal fibula is known as the retromalleolar sulcus. The sulcus is 6 to 7 mm wide and is concave in 82% of fibula specimens (5). At the posterolateral border of the fibula, a 3- to 4-cm-long fibrocartilaginous ridge is typically present, augmenting stability of the tendons within the tunnel.

The superior peroneal retinaculum is formed as a confluence of superficial fascia, peroneal tendon sheath, and distal fibula periosteum, approximately 2 cm proximal to the fibula tip. It is approximately 2 cm wide and is important in maintaining stability of the peroneal tendons. Peroneal tendon dislocation involves stripping of the superior peroneal retinaculum and periosteum from the lateral malleolus, creating a false pouch into which the tendons dislocate. This often occurs from trauma in which there is a sudden dorsiflexion to stress with forceful contraction of the peroneals (2). Other factors, such as a congenitally shallow retromalleolar sulcus, may contribute to peroneal tendon instability. Chronic peroneal dislocation is often associated with recurrent ankle sprains, which can contribute to incompetence of the superior peroneal retinaculum (6,7).

Longitudinal tears of the peroneus brevis may occur at the level of the distal fibula (Fig. 21-1B). These tears are often associated with ankle sprains and typically occur with per-

D. L. Dahm, M.D. and H. B. Kitaoka, M.D.: Foot and Ankle Section, Department of Orthopaedics, Mayo Clinic and Mayo Foundation; and Mayo School of Medicine, Rochester, Minnesota.

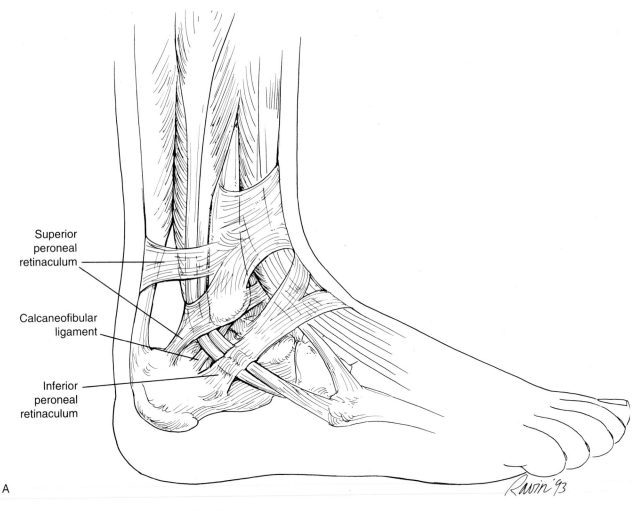

Superior peroneal retinaculum

Calcaneofibular ligament

Inferior peroneal retinaculum

A

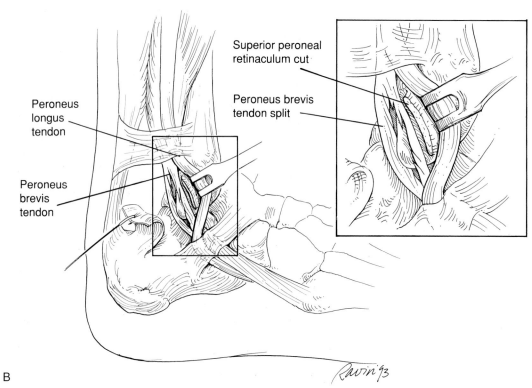

Superior peroneal retinaculum cut

Peroneus brevis tendon split

Peroneus longus tendon

Peroneus brevis tendon

B

oneal subluxation over the fibrocartilaginous ridge of the posterolateral aspect of the distal fibula (3). Other pathologic conditions include peroneal tendinitis or tenosynovitis, which involves inflammation of the tendon and surrounding synovial lining. Complete peroneal tendon rupture is commonly associated with peroneal tenosynovitis and often occurs in locations such as at the level of the retromalleolar sulcus, the peroneal tubercle, and the cuboid groove, where stenosing tenosynovitis is observed (4). A low-lying peroneus brevis muscle belly or an anomalous peroneus quartus tendon may contribute to stenosis within the sheath and subsequent tendon irritation.

Nonoperative management of acute peroneal tendon subluxation or dislocation includes treatment in a short-leg cast with the ankle in neutral to slight inversion for 6 weeks, but this treatment is associated with a 30% to 40% rate of redislocation (8). Nonoperative treatment of patients with tendinitis or tenosynovitis includes a period of immobilization in a brace such as a walking boot or in a cast, antiinflammatory medications, activity modifications, and occasionally, a corticosteroid injection.

Indications for surgery include an active patient with significant pain and impairment localized to the peroneal tendons. Contraindications to surgery include infection, severe peripheral vascular disease, and limited symptoms.

## PREOPERATIVE PLANNING

Patients with peroneal tendon subluxation or dislocation often present with a history of a traumatic event involving dorsiflexion and eversion of the ankle but may also report a history of recurrent inversion type of ankle sprain and lateral ankle instability. The clinical course may initially be similar to that of an acute lateral ankle ligament sprain, but with time, it may be possible to distinguish ligament from tendon injury. The symptoms and signs of ligament instability are localized to the anterolateral and lateral ankle, whereas with peroneal tendon injuries, they are localized to the posterolateral ankle. There may be obvious ankle instability seen with anterior drawer and inversion stress testing of the ankle in the case of ligament sprains. Patients with dislocating peroneal tendons may be able to voluntarily dislocate the tendons. In some cases, both problems coexist.

On examination, swelling is often observed in the posterolateral ankle and hindfoot along the peroneal tendon sheath. There is tenderness posterior to the lateral malleolus along the peroneal tendons. Subluxation or dislocation of the peroneal tendons may be provoked by active dorsiflexion and eversion. There may be weakness to resisted eversion strength testing, particularly in the setting of significant tendinitis, tenosynovitis, and partial or complete peroneal rupture. Ankle stability should be examined with anterior drawer and inversion stress testing. A diagnostic lidocaine injection into the peroneal tendon sheath can be helpful in confirming the source of pain.

Plain film radiographs of the ankle should include anteroposterior, lateral, and mortise views, as well as anteroposterior and oblique views of the foot. The mortise view of the ankle may show a shell-like avulsion fracture of the lateral malleolus, indicating disruption of the superior peroneal retinaculum. A fracture of the os peroneum may indicate peroneus longus rupture. Stress radiographs of the ankle (e.g., anterior drawer, talar tilt) can confirm the presence of lateral ligamentous instability.

If the diagnosis is uncertain, magnetic resonance imaging (MRI) examination can be helpful (Figs. 21-2 and 21-3). It provides information about the specific tendons affected and the extent of injury. MRI allows visualization of disorders such as tendinitis or tenosynovitis, partial tendon tears, and peroneal tendon ruptures (Figs. 21-2 and 21-3). T1-weighted spin echo and T2-weighted fast spin echo images in axial and coronal cuts are ob-

**Figure 21-1. A:** Normal anatomy of the tendons and ligaments of lateral ankle and hindfoot. **B:** Course of the peroneal tendons along the lateral aspect of the ankle and foot. Retraction of the peroneus longus shows the split tear of the peroneus brevis tendon.

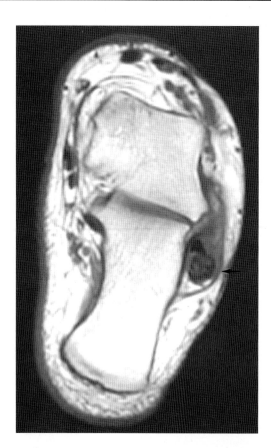

**Figure 21-2.** Coronal MRI scan of a patient who sustained a twisting injury to the ankle and had persistent lateral ankle pain and swelling. Plain film radiographs were normal. MRI shows marked enlargement of the peroneus brevis tendon *(arrow)* and increased signal intensity in the brevis tendon.

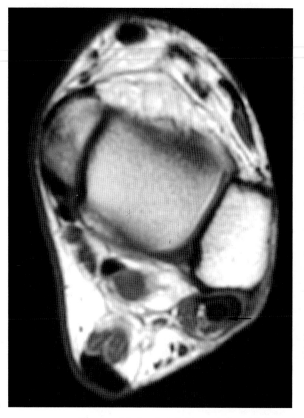

A

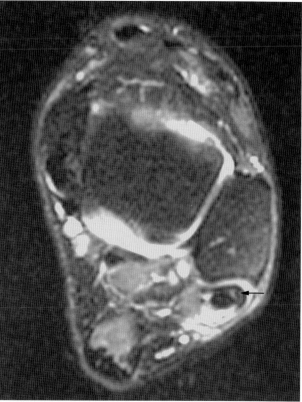

B

**Figure 21-3.** Axial, T1-weighted **(A)** and T2-weighted **(B)** magnetic resonance scans of the ankle show a partial tear of the peroneus brevis at the level of the lateral malleolus *(arrow)*. Abnormal signal around tendons within the peroneal sheath is consistent with fluid associated with tendonitis.

tained. Some advocate sagittal and oblique axial views. Increased intrasubstance signal intensity in T1- and T2-weighted images is seen in cases of partial tears. Tendon distortion, bisected tendon, tendon enlargement, complete tendon rupture, increased fluid in the tendon sheath, and a convex or flat fibular groove may be observed (Figs. 21-2 and 21-3). It is common for the peroneus longus tendon to appear normal and the brevis tendon to be enlarged and distorted. It is possible to visualize the superior peroneal retinaculum and the muscle belly of the peroneus brevis with MRI. An anomalous tendon, such as a peroneus quartus, can also be observed with MRI.

Other studies such as ultrasound, tendon sheath endoscopy, computed tomography, tenography, and kinematic MRI can aid in the diagnosis of peroneal tendon pathology, but they are not widely used.

## SURGERY

The patient is positioned supine, with a sandbag under the ipsilateral hip or, alternatively, in the lateral decubitus position. Spinal or general anesthesia may be used. A thigh tourniquet is typically used.

### Technique

A curvilinear, 5- to 7-cm incision is made along the posterolateral fibula in line with the peroneal tendons (Fig. 21-4). Full-thickness flaps are developed, and the superior peroneal retinaculum is identified. In the cases of tendon dislocation, the outpouching of the retinaculum away from the posterior margin of the lateral malleolus is observed. The peroneal sheath and superior peroneal retinaculum are incised close to the posterolateral border of the fibula (Figs. 21-5 and 21-6). The peroneal tendons are inspected, specifically looking for subluxation, partial or complete tears, and tenosynovitis. Retraction of the peroneus longus tendon anteriorly allows for visualization of the peroneus brevis tendon and often

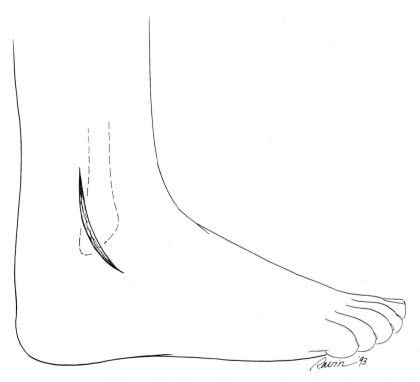

**Figure 21-4.** A lateral skin incision is used for peroneal repair and reconstruction.

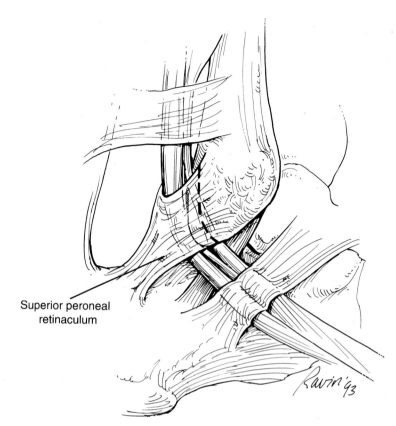

**Figure 21-5.** The retinaculum is incised close to the border of the fibula.

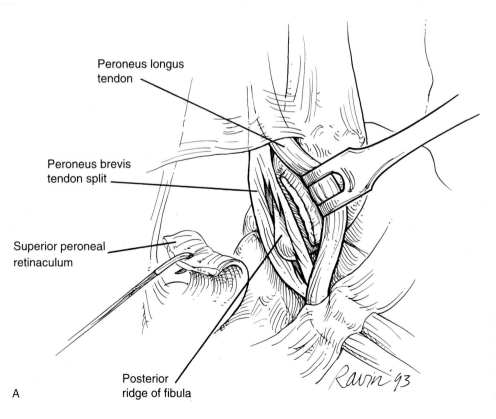

A

**Figure 21-6. A:** Exposure of the peroneus brevis tendon tear is achieved by retraction of the superior peroneal retinaculum posteriorly and the peroneus longus tendon anteriorly. *(continued)*

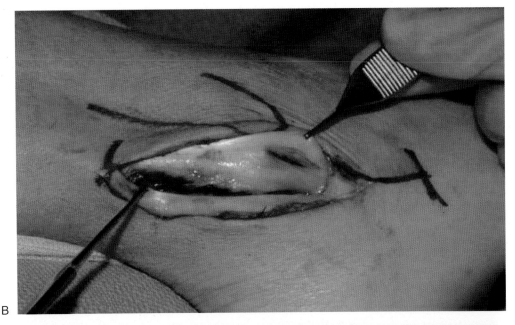

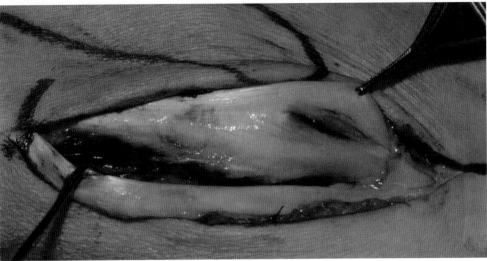

**Figure 21-6.** *Continued.* **B:** Through a posterolateral incision, the retinaculum is incised at the posterior margin of the malleolus, revealing a partial tear of the flattened brevis tendon. **C:** A closer view shows dislocation of the anterior third of the brevis tendon over the fibro-osseous ridge of the lateral malleolus.

reveals a central split and subluxation over the posterior ridge of the fibula (Figs. 21-5 and 21-6). If a peroneus brevis tear is found and the degenerated portion of the tendon constitutes 50% or less of the tendon, the degenerative tissue is debrided. The more normal-appearing portion of the tendon is tubularized, using a running, absorbable suture to allow for smooth excursion within the fibular groove (Figs. 21-6 and 21-7). If an anomalous peroneus quartus tendon or a low-lying peroneus brevis muscle belly or a discrete thickening in the tendon is encountered, it should be excised (Figs. 21-8 through 21-10).

In the patient with lateral instability of the ankle, reconstruction with the Gould modification of the Broström procedure may be performed (see Chapter 33). Alternatively, when ligament repair is not possible, a portion of the split peroneus brevis tendon may be used for reconstruction of the lateral collateral ligament to the ankle in a tenodesis-type repair, such as the Chrisman-Snook procedure (Fig. 21-11).

The superior peroneal retinaculum is then reattached through drill holes in the lateral ridge of the fibula after preparing a fresh-bleeding bed using a curette or rongeur

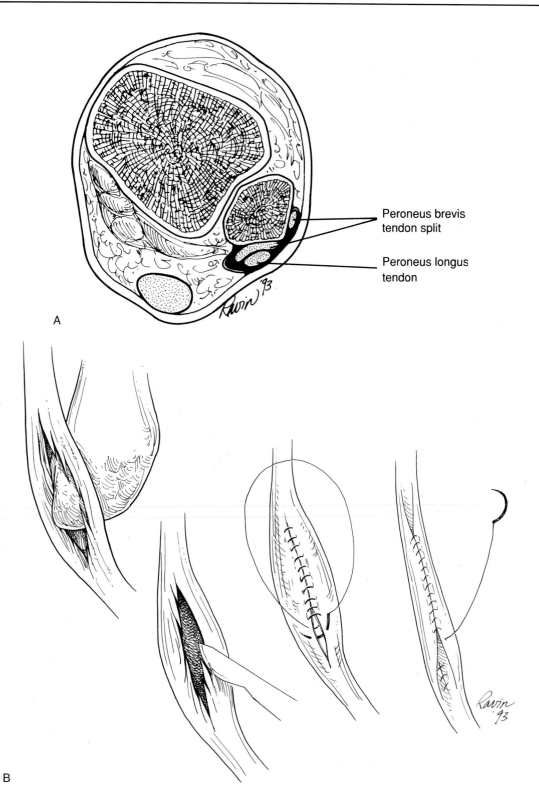

Peroneus brevis
tendon split

Peroneus longus
tendon

A

B

**Figure 21-7.  A:** Cross-sectional view at the level of the fibular groove shows that the lateral part of the split peroneus brevis tendon is dislocated over the posterior ridge of the fibula. **B:** Debridement and repair of the peroneus brevis tendon and tubulation. Approximately one half of the anterior portion of the peroneus brevis tendon can be resected. *(continued)*

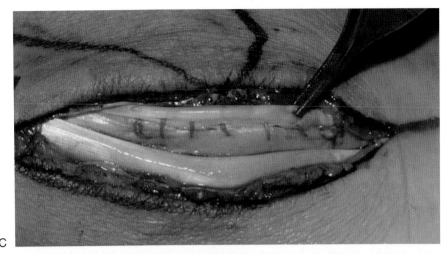

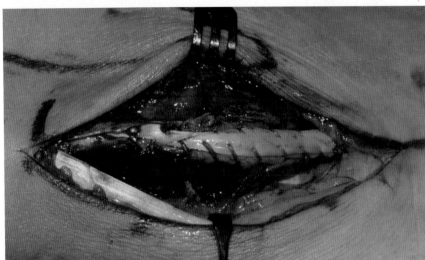

**Figure 21-7.** *Continued.* **C:** Intraoperative photograph after resection of the degenerated one third of the tendon and tubulation with running suture. **D:** Closer view of the repaired tendon.

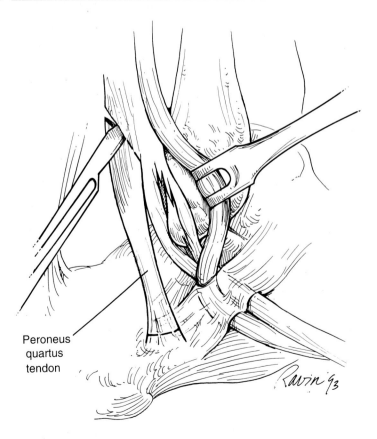

Peroneus quartus tendon

**Figure 21-8.** An anomalous peroneus quartus tendon in the peroneal tendon sheath should be removed.

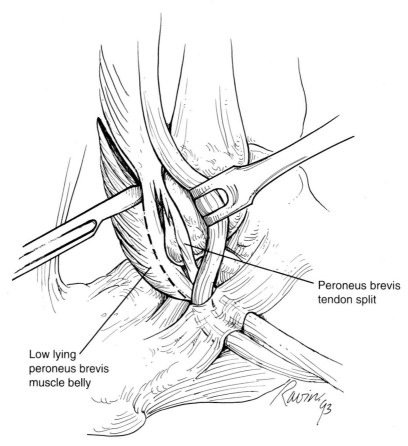

**Figure 21-9.** An abnormally low-lying portion of the muscle belly of the peroneus brevis should be resected.

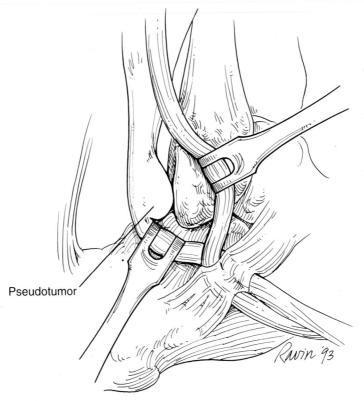

**Figure 21-10:** A thickened area of the peroneus brevis tendon is resected, leaving the tendon in continuity.

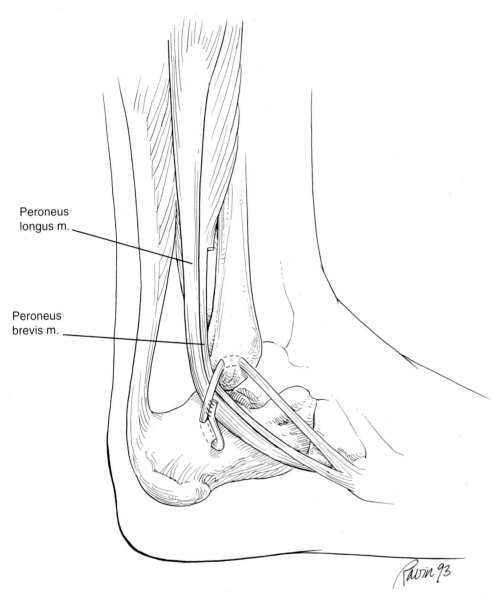

Peroneus
longus m.

Peroneus
brevis m.

*Ravin 93*

**Figure 21-11.** In the patient, who also has lateral instability of the ankle, one half of the split peroneus brevis tendon may be used for a reconstruction of the lateral collateral ligaments of the ankle in a tenodesis-type repair (i.e., Chrisman-Snook ankle procedure). This procedure is applicable when ligament repair and reconstruction with extensor retinaculum (i.e., Gould modification of the Broström procedure) is not possible.

(Figs. 21-12 and 21-13). Rather than excision of the excess retinacular tissue, this tissue is used to reinforce the repair in a pants-over-vest fashion, sutured over the superior peroneal retinaculum. If the peroneus brevis shows signs of extensive degeneration, the diseased segment may be excised, and the proximal and distal stumps may be sutured to the peroneus longus tendon (Fig. 21-13).

The floor of the fibro-osseous groove is inspected, and if deemed shallow or deficient, a groove-deepening procedure can be performed (Fig. 21-14). This involves creating a longitudinal, 3-cm, cortical, osteoperiosteal flap that is about 2 mm thick using a sharp osteotome. The osteotome is advanced until it penetrates the medial cortex. The flap is hinged open, and a portion of the underlying cancellous bone is removed from the posterior fibula with a burr and curette. The flap is then replaced and tamped in position creating a trough effect. The retinaculum is secured to the fibula with sutures passed through bone. The anterior margin of the retinaculum is overlapped and sutured to reinforce the repair.

*(Text continues on page 309.)*

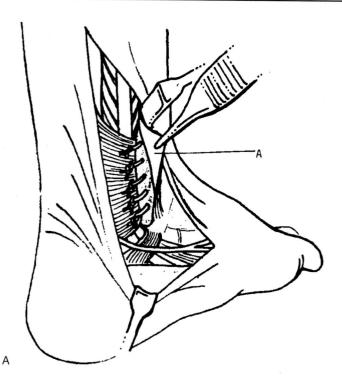

A

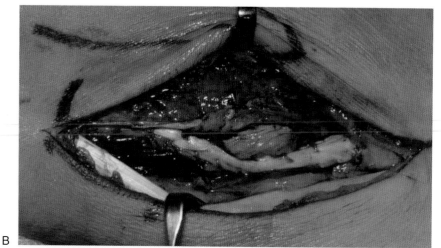

B

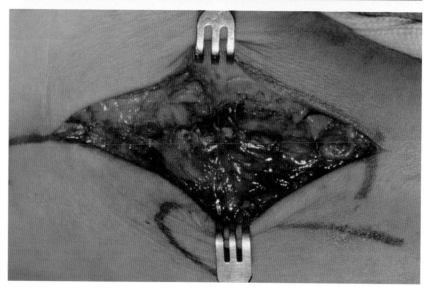

C

**Figure 21-12. A:** Retinacular repair. The retinaculum, which was incised at the posterior margin of the malleolus, is sutured through drill holes in the malleolus and prevents tendon subluxation. The redundant retinaculum *(A)* is sutured over this repair for further reinforcement. **B:** An intraoperative photograph shows the repaired brevis tendon replaced in the fibular groove and a redundant retinaculum anteriorly. **C:** The retinaculum has been sutured to the fibula, and the redundant retinaculum has been sutured over this repair. (**A** from Krause JO, Brodsky JW: Peroneus brevis tendon tears: pathophysiology, surgical reconstruction, and clinical results. *Foot Ankle Int* 19:271–279, 1998, with permission.)

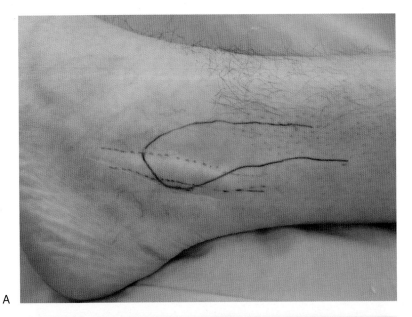

A

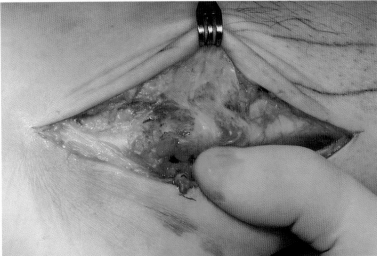

B

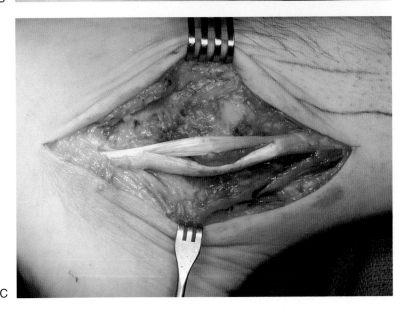

C

**Figure 21-13. A:** Lateral view of the ankle shows the outline of a dislocated peroneus brevis tendon *(dotted lines)* and the fibula *(solid line)*. **B:** The skin incision exposes the retinaculum. Notice the anterior dislocation of the grossly enlarged brevis tendon over the malleolus, as seen through the retinaculum. **C:** The retinaculum is incised, exposing the enlarged, degenerated brevis tendon with dislocation of the anterior one half. *(continued)*

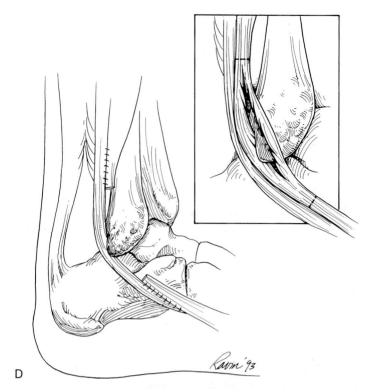

D

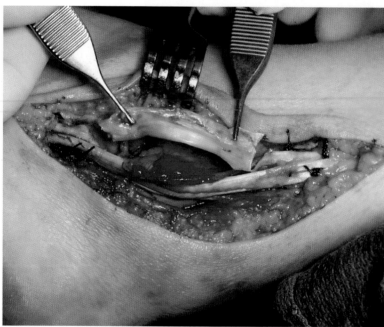

E

**Figure 21-13.** *Continued.* **D:** If a severely degenerated segment of the peroneus bre-vis tendon is found to constitute most of the tendon, the diseased area is resected, and the proximal and distal ends of the tendon are sutured to the peroneus longus tendon. **E:** The degenerated segment of the brevis tendon is resected, and side-to-side repair to the peroneus longus tendon is performed proximally and distally. *(continued)*

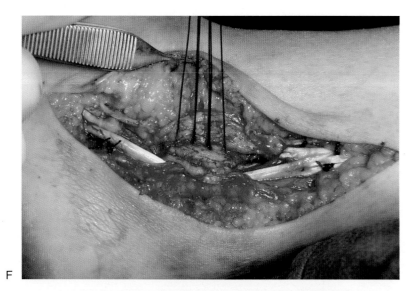

F

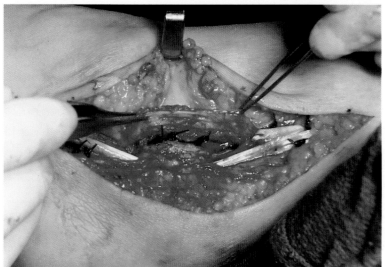

G

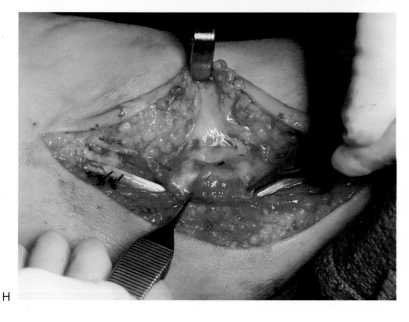

H

**Figure 21-13.** *Continued.* **F:** Intraoperative view of the retinaculum sutured through drill holes to the lateral malleolus. **G:** The anterior "outpouched" retinacular tissue is shown. **H:** Rather than excising this redundant tissue, it is used to reinforce the repair. (**A–H** courtesy of James W. Brodsky, University of Texas Southwestern Medical School, Dallas, Texas.).

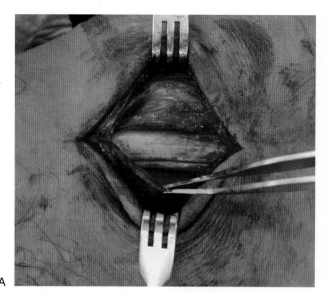
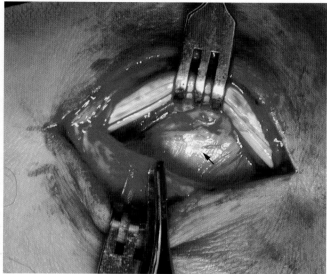

**Figure 21-14. A:** Lateral view of the right ankle shows the peroneal tendons reduced in shallow fibular groove. The retinaculum has a false pouch anteriorly where tendons are dislocating. The posterior retinaculum is held in the forceps. **B:** The peroneal tendons are retracted anteriorly, and the shallow groove is observed *(arrow)*. **C:** The groove-deepening procedure involves retracting the peroneal tendons posteriorly and dissecting periosteum off the lateral malleolus, starting at the fibrocartilaginous ridge of the posterolateral aspect of the distal fibula. A chisel or osteotome is placed on the edge of the shallow fibular groove to raise an osteoperiosteal flap that is approximately 2 mm thick. *(continued)*

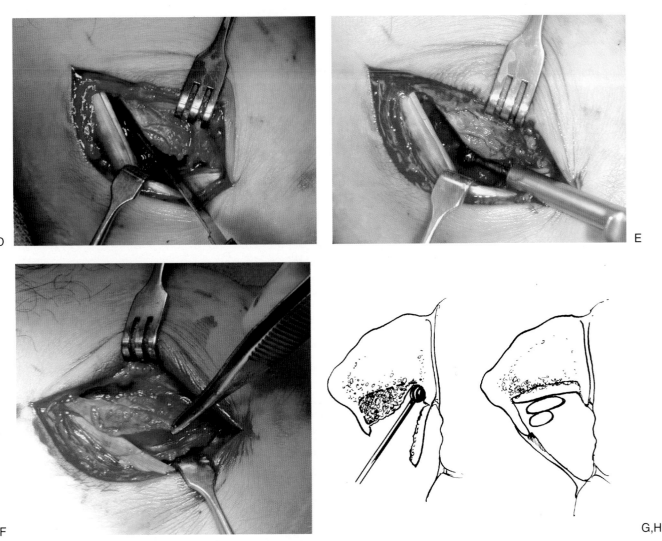

**Figure 21-14.** *Continued.* **D:** An osteotome or chisel is used to raise a flap. **E:** The flap is retracted, and the bone beneath it is removed with a burr. **F:** The flap is replaced and tamped into place. Notice the deepened groove. **G:** Cross-sectioned view shows burr removing bone beneath flap. **H:** View shows deepened groove and repaired retinaculum. (**C** from Schon LC: Decision-making for the athlete: the leg, ankle, and foot in sports. In: Myerson MS, ed. *Foot and ankle disorders.* Philadelphia: WB Saunders, 2000, with permission. **G,H** courtesy of Leland McCluskey, McCluskey Orthopaedic Surgery, P.C., and Hughston Foundation, Columbus, GA.)

## POSTOPERATIVE MANAGEMENT

The patient is placed in a non–weight-bearing splint for up to 1 week. A short-leg walking cast is then applied for 4 to 6 weeks. A rehabilitation program, including range of motion, progressive strengthening, and proprioceptive training, is then instituted. Patients typically resume sports participation at 4 to 6 months after surgery.

Results of surgical treatment of peroneal tendon injuries have been good or excellent in 80% to 90% of reported cases (1,10). Studies comparing the benefits of each type of operation have not been performed, but investigators who have reported small individual series have described uniformly good results (9,12).

## COMPLICATIONS

Potential surgical complications include sensitivity of the incision, sural nerve paresthesias or hypesthesia, recurrent peroneal tendon instability, stiffness, and infection. With careful attention to surgical technique and proper rehabilitation, complications after peroneal tendon repair and reconstruction are infrequent.

## ACKNOWLEDGMENTS

The authors acknowledge the contribution of Dr. Walther H. Bohne, for his insightful work related to peroneal tendon anatomy and disorders, and gratefully acknowledge the illustrations provided by James W. Brodsky, Lew C. Schon, and Leland McCluskey.

## RECOMMENDED READING

1. Alanen J, Orava S, Heinonen OJ, et al.: Peroneal tendon injuries: report of 38 operative cases. *Ann Chir Gynecol* 90:43–46, 2001.
2. Arrowsmith SR, Fleming LL, Allman FL: Traumatic dislocations of the peroneal tendons. *Am J Sports Med* 11:142–146, 1983.
3. Bassett FH III, Speer KP: Longitudinal rupture of the peroneal tendons. *Am J Sports Med* 21:354–357, 1993.
4. Clark HD, Kitaoka HB, Ehman RL: Peroneal tendon injuries. *Foot Ankle Int* 19:280–288, 1998.
5. Edwards ME: Relations of peroneal tendons to fibula, calcaneus and cuboideum. *Am J Anat* 42:213–253, 1928.
6. Geppert MJ, Sobel M, Bohne WH: Lateral ankle instability as a cause of superior peroneal retinacular laxity: an anatomic and biomechanical study of cadaver feet. *Foot Ankle* 14:330–334, 1993.
7. Sobel M, Geppert MJ, Warren RS: Chronic ankle instability as a cause of peroneal tendon injury. *Clin Orthop* 296:187–191, 1993.
8. Stover CN, Bryan DR: Traumatic dislocation of the peroneal tendons. *Am J Surg* 103:180–186, 1962.
9. Kollias SL, Ferkel RD: Fibular grooving for recurrent peroneal tendon subluxation. *Am J Sports Med* 25:329–335, 1997.
10. Krause JO, Brodsky JW: Peroneus brevis tendon tears: pathophysiology, surgical reconstruction, and clinical results. *Foot Ankle Int* 19:271–279, 1998.
11. Schon LC: Decision-making for the athlete: the leg, ankle, and foot in sports. In: Myerson MS, ed. *Foot and ankle disorders.* Philadelphia: WB Saunders, 2000:1435–1476.
12. Zoellner G, Clancy W Jr: Recurrent dislocation of the peroneal tendon. *J Bone Joint Surg Am* 61:292–294, 1979.

# 22

# Acute Repair of the Achilles Tendon

Jason H. Calhoun

## INDICATIONS/CONTRAINDICATIONS

Acute Achilles tendon ruptures usually occur in less-active, male patients between the ages of 30 and 50 years old while they are engaged in an occasional sporting activity (1). Although many etiologies have been suggested as predisposing factors, most theories suggest that decreased vascularity of the tendon places it at risk for rupture (8). Relatively minor injury from an abrupt push-off or sudden fall may cause an acute contracture of the powerful triceps surae muscle complex or forced dorsiflexion of the ankle that can produce a rupture. Rupture may also occur in "weekend" athletes during high-demand sporting activities such as tennis or basketball. Some surgeons believe that acute rupture is preceded by peritendinitis or tendinosis and is caused by a combination of mechanical and degenerative injury (7).

The diagnosis of an acute rupture of the Achilles tendon is usually made by a history of a pop or snap in the posterior aspect of the ankle along with acute onset of pain. Physical examination reveals a swollen, painful ankle with ecchymosis posteriorly. Swelling and hematoma within the paratenon may obscure a palpable gap within the tendon itself, but tenderness is generally present. Many patients can still actively plantarflex the ankle against mild resistance because of the pull of the posterior tibial tendon and the long flexor tendons (1,21). Inability to rise onto the toes or a heel resistance test, performed by grasping the heel and resisting plantarflexion, showing absence of plantarflexion power, are consistent with an Achilles tendon rupture. The Thompson test (24) has proved to be a reliable indicator of Achilles tendon rupture (Fig. 22-1). During this test, the calf muscle is squeezed with the patient prone and the feet extending over the end of the examination table. If the tendon is intact, the foot can plantarflex. If it is ruptured, the foot cannot move much or at all. This is diagnostic of Achilles tendon rupture.

Some controversy exists regarding open versus closed treatment of acute tendon ruptures. Proponents of open treatment cite many factors such as the ability to use a short-leg cast

J. H. Calhoun, M.D.: Department of Orthopaedics and Rehabilitation, University of Texas Medical Branch, Galveston, Texas.

311

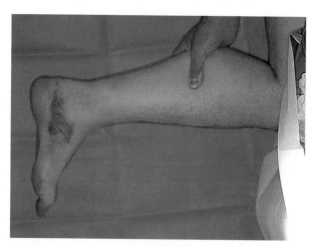

**Figure 22-1.** In a demonstration of the Thompson test, the foot does not plantarflex as the calf is squeezed.

postoperatively, lower rerupture rates, greater strength, and greater endurance after open treatment (5,6,9,12,19,23). In older or lower-demand patients, nonoperative treatment may be appropriate. I recommend open surgical treatment for younger or more active patients.

The general health of the patient and any associated systemic diseases may influence the decision process regarding open versus closed treatment. Frank discussion of the risk and benefits of closed and open treatments should be undertaken with the patient, and an informed mutual decision about treatment should be reached.

Contraindications to surgical care, in addition to a low-demand, older patient, are associated with wound healing. Systemic cortisone and methotrexate, insulin-dependent diabetes mellitus, and vascular compromise of the lower extremity are relative contraindications to open surgical treatment.

## PREOPERATIVE PLANNING

If operative treatment is planned, the foot should be maintained in a compressive Jones-type dressing in mild plantarflexion before surgery. This prevents the formation of fracture blisters and diminishes swelling, which can otherwise compromise wound healing.

Ruptures may occur at the myotendinous junction but more commonly occur in the midsubstance of the tendon. Avulsion off of the calcaneal insertion may also occur. The level of rupture can usually be determined by physical examination through the identification of the level of the gap within the substance of the tendon. Plain lateral radiographs may reveal a defect in the shadow of the Achilles tendon, and the triangular lucency of the fat pad anterior to the Achilles tendon is generally obliterated. Magnetic resonance imaging (MRI) can also confirm the level and the extent of rupture. However, the diagnosis of rupture is generally based on clinical examination, and MRI, although instructional for educational purposes, should be reserved for when the diagnosis is in doubt.

## SURGERY

The patient is placed in a prone position, with axillary rolls under the chest and adequate padding of the upper extremities to avoid any possible neurovascular injury during surgery. General or spinal anesthesia is satisfactory. A pneumatic tourniquet is applied at the level of the thigh on the affected extremity, which is then prepped and draped in sterile fashion. After the blood is evacuated with an Esmarch wrap, the tourniquet is inflated. The incision is made along the posteromedial aspect of the leg, starting just above the level of the my-otendinous junction and extending to the level of the tendinous insertion on the calcaneus (17) (Fig. 22-2). When avulsion of the tendon from its calcaneal insertion is suspected, the incision is extended plantarward to give better exposure. The incision is deepened to the level of the paratenon. The paratenon is then opened to give exposure to the Achilles tendon (Fig. 22-3). It is critical that no flaps are raised until this level is reached so the blood supply to the overlying skin can be protected.

A careful review and understanding of the anatomy of the Achilles tendon and its surrounding paratenon are essential to avoid postoperative wound complications. The tendon rotates 90° externally from its muscular origin to its insertion on the calcaneus (15). The sural nerve perforates the crural fascia at the myotendinous junction and passes subcutaneously distally on the lateral aspect of the Achilles tendon. A medial incision avoids injury to this nerve. It also allows easier access to the plantaris tendon, which, if present, passes deep to the crural fascia along the medial aspect of the Achilles tendon. The plantaris may be used to augment primary surgical repair of the tendon.

The Achilles tendon is not covered by a tendon sheath, but by a paratenon composed of areolar connective tissue and elastic fibers (7). During surgical repair, the tendon should be exposed to the layer of the paratenon. The paratenon should be reflected as part of the full-thickness flap with the overlying subcutaneous tissue and skin to avoid disruption of the vascular supply to the skin.

If the plantaris tendon is present, it is easily identified within the substance of the wound. The paratenon can then be elevated as part of a full-thickness flap off of the Achilles tendon, and inspection of the level of the rupture can be performed. Any hematoma is removed with irrigation. Ruptures are generally mop-handle–type tears (Fig. 22-4), which prevent easy repair. The frayed ends of the tendon are debrided by placing the torn end of the tendon over a tongue depressor and using a wide blade to trim the ruptured portion of the tendon (Fig. 22-5).

A tear at the level of the myotendinous junction is often difficult to repair because of inadequate purchase of suture material into the proximal tissues. Lindholm's (13) technique can be modified to allow repair. Rather than inverted tendon strips being raised from the proximal portion of the tendon and reflected distally, the tendon strips are raised from the long distal portion of the tendon and inverted proximally. These strips can be woven into place to allow continuity of tendon material to augment the repair. Primary suturing of the tendon is carried out in an identical fashion to that for midsubstance tendon ruptures as described below.

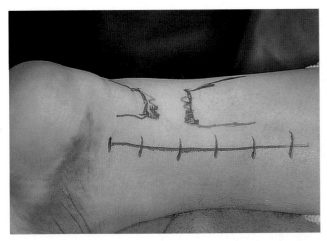

**Figure 22-2.** Site of the incision for the posterior medial approach.

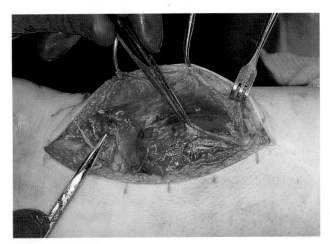

**Figure 22-3.** The paratenon is opened, giving exposure to the Achilles tendon. The paratenon is grasped by the hemostats. The posterior flap of skin should be a full-thickness flap, including skin and subcutaneous fat, extending down to this level of the paratenon.

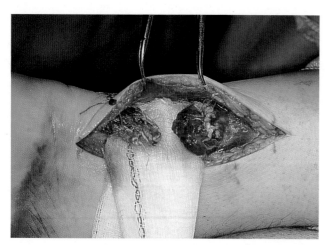

**Figure 22-4.** Mop-handled tear of the midsubstance of the Achilles tendon.

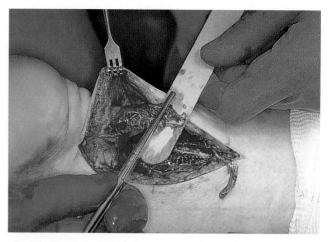

**Figure 22-5.** Debridement of the torn end of the tendon using a tongue depressor and a wide blade.

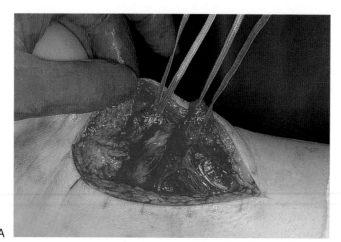

**Figure 22-6. A:** A heavy, nonabsorbable suture, such as no. 3 Dacron, is placed in the proximal and distal stumps using a Bunnell-type stitch. **B:** Suture placement.

A

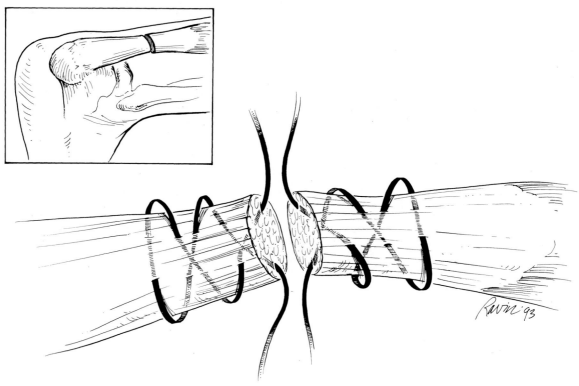

B

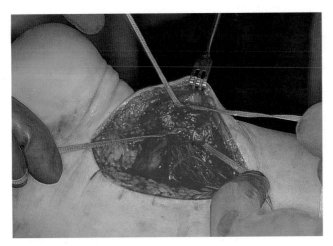

**Figure 22-7.** With the knee flexed and the foot plantarflexed, the torn end of the tendon can be opposed without tension.

For a midsubstance tear of the Achilles tendon, after debridement of the tendon edges, a heavy, nonabsorbable suture such as no. 3 Dacron is placed using a Bunnell technique in the proximal stump. A second suture is then placed in the distal stump (Fig. 22-6). The knee is then flexed, and the foot is plantarflexed, allowing the ends of the suture to be tied without tension (Figs. 22-7 and 22-8). The repair is then augmented using an absorbable suture such as no. 1 Vicryl in a vertical circumferential stitch (Fig. 22-9).

The wound is then copiously irrigated and the edges of the paratenon approximated (Fig. 22-10). The paratenon is then closed with a 3-0 absorbable suture. Paratenon closure prevents scarring of the tendon to the overlying soft tissues and skin. The skin is closed with an interrupted 3-0 nylon skin stitch. The foot should be in plantarflexion, so the repair is not under tension, while the paratenon and overlying skin are closed. For acute repair of Achilles tendon rupture, other types of stitches may be used with success besides the Bunnell type, such as the modified Kessler (Fig. 22-11) and Krackow (Fig. 22-12).

When the tendon has been avulsed off of the insertion of the calcaneus, it is repaired by drilling holes in the calcaneus where the tendon avulsed (Figs. 22-13 through 22-17). The calcaneus is curetted to remove overlying fibrous tissue down to cancellous bone. A no. 3

*(Text continues on page 319.)*

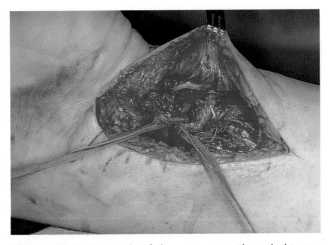

**Figure 22-8.** The ends of the suture are then tied to secure repair and opposition of the tendon ends.

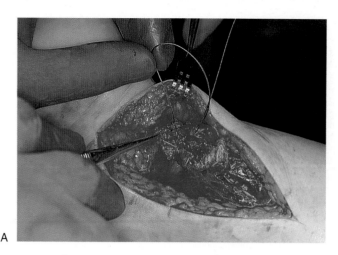

A

**Figure 22-9.  A:** Repairs are augmented using no. 1 Vicryl in a vertical circumferential stitch. **B:** Suture placement.

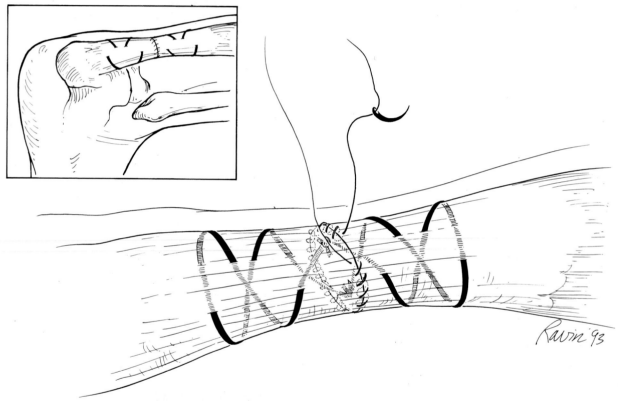

B

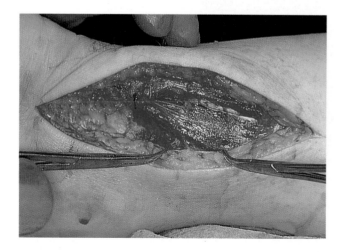

**Figure 22-10.**  Anterior margin of the paratenon. The anterior and posterior margins should be closed before skin closure.

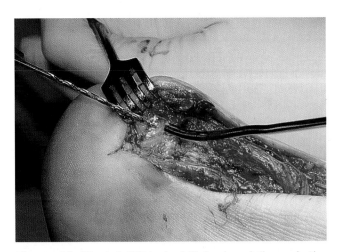

**Figure 22-16.** A 0.125-inch drill is placed through the tuberosity of the os calcis up to the defect where the bone fragment was avulsed. Two drill holes are placed.

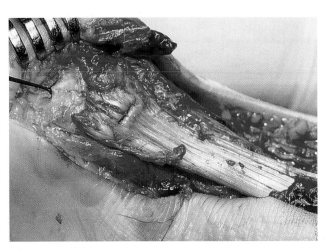

**Figure 22-17.** The end of the Achilles tendon is brought down into the cancellous area of the calcaneal tuberosity, and the suture is tied over the bone island between the drill holes distally.

Dacron suture is placed through the stump of the tendon as previously described, and the ends of the suture are brought through the drill holes within the substance of the bone. They are then tied securely to the bone. If the plantaris tendon is present, it can be woven through the repaired Achilles to make the repair stronger.

After closure, the foot is placed in a below-knee, bulky compressive dressing with plaster splints holding the foot in about 20° of plantarflexion (Fig. 22-18). When a very proximal rupture occurs at the level of the myotendinous junction or if the repair is tenuous, the patient can be placed in a long-leg splint with the knee and ankle flexed.

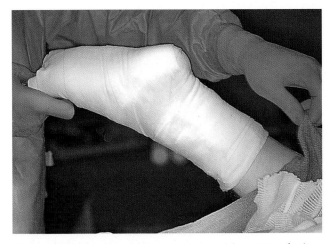

**Figure 22-18.** The foot is maintained in 20° of plantarflexion. The initial soft dressing seen here is covered with a bulky compressive dressing and plaster splints to maintain the foot in this plantarflexed position.

## POSTOPERATIVE MANAGEMENT

The patient is usually discharged home on the day of surgery. The bulky compressive dressing is left on for 7 to 10 days postoperatively, until the first clinic visit. The dressings are then removed and the wound inspected. The sutures are generally removed 10 to 14 days after surgery. The high incidence of dehiscence requires that the sutures be left in the skin until the wound is well healed. The sutures are removed when there is good skin bridging between them; this may be at 7 to 10 days for the young patient and 2 to 3 weeks for the older patient. After the sutures are removed, Steri-Strips are applied to the wound. The foot is maintained in its plantarflexed position during the cast change. The patient is then recast, maintained in 20° of plantarflexion, and continued on a non–weight-bearing program for an additional 2.5 weeks.

Four weeks after surgery, the patient is taken out of the cast and placed in a sitting position on the side of an examination table. A footrest is then placed under the ball of the foot and elevated so that the hip and knee are flexed (Fig. 22-19). The patient is placed in this position and allowed to sit for approximately 15 to 20 minutes. This allows gradual reduction of the foot to a more neutral posture by gravity rather than active motion or passive manipulation. Most patients at this point reach a neutral position and are then recast in a short-leg walking cast for an additional 2 to 4 weeks. We frequently use a brace instead of a cast that can be removed for bathing and active range of motion exercises three times each day. This allows for early mobilization, which has proven to be beneficial in many studies (3,16,18,22). If a neutral posture is not obtained, the patient is brought back to the office after 1 week and again sits in the same position to allow achievement of neutral position.

The patient is taken out of the cast or brace 6 to 8 weeks after surgery and placed into a shoe with a 1-inch heel lift. Active physical therapy is started. Although the incidence of rerupture of the Achilles tendon in most reports is lower after surgical repair than nonoperative repair (2,9,11), prevention of rerupture is helped by a gradual but continual program

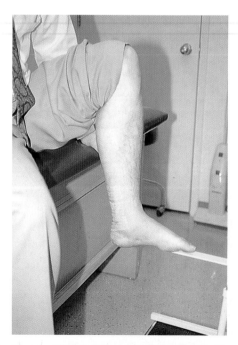

**Figure 22-19.** The patient is placed sitting, with the hip and knee flexed and the forefoot resting on a footrest. The patient stays in this position until gravity allows the foot to achieve a plantigrade posture. At this point, a short-leg walking cast or a removable brace is applied.

of stretching. Attempts should be made to regain full dorsiflexion of the involved ankle, but the patient should be cautioned that this is a very slow process that can take 3 to 6 months after the injury. Similarly, physical therapists should be cautioned about overenthusiasm regarding passive stretching of the repaired tendon. Instructing patients about the importance of compliance of long-term stretching, especially before engaging in any sporting events, can also diminish the incidence of rerupture of the tendon.

Initial therapy involves general passive stretching and active use of Thera-Band to return strength to the gastrosoleus complex and to the other muscles about the foot and ankle. The heel lift is continued until 10° of dorsiflexion are obtained. A physical therapy program should incorporate retraining of all the muscles about the foot and ankle, as well as proprioceptive training. This is critical to avoid further injury to the ankle. Most of the therapy can be done as a home program if the patient is well motivated. The patient is allowed to resume normal activities after he or she has achieved full motor strength equal to the uninvolved extremity. Patients are instructed to continue on a long-term stretching program for at least 1 year after surgery. They are also instructed to perform stretching exercises before commencing any type of sporting activity on a permanent basis.

## COMPLICATIONS

Most complications of operative Achilles tendon repair can be avoided by meticulous technique. The most significant complication is skin *necrosis*, which can be avoided by carrying out the dissection to the level of the paratenon and avoiding separation of the paratenon from the overlying subcutaneous tissues and skin. Adequate immobilization with compressive dressings before surgery also contributes to the avoidance of this complication. When skin necrosis occurs, the size of the defect determines what options are available. For a small area, local wound care allows granulation closure. However, larger areas require local myocutaneous gastrocnemius Y-V slides or medial plantar artery flaps. It may be necessary to incorporate a free flap using a radial forearm, scapular flap, or any larger flap if the area of necrosis is extensive.

Other possible complications are *dehiscence* and *infection*. Dehiscence can be avoided by leaving the sutures in until the wound is well healed. Antibiotics may be necessary if cellulitis develops. Usually, Keflex is adequate, but the regimen should be modified if the patient is allergic, if the cellulitis does not resolve, or if cultures indicate that other antibiotics should be used.

*Painful scar tissue* may be a long-term complication of surgical repair. The location of the incision may contribute to this problem. Placing the incision posteromedially rather than using a direct posterior incision avoids the sural nerve and keeps the scar from being irritated by shoe wear.

## RECOMMENDED READING

1. Arner O, Lindholm A: Subcutaneous rupture of the Achilles tendon. *Acta Chir Scand Suppl* 239:1–51, 1959.
2. Beskin JL, Sanders RA, Hunter SC, et al.: Surgical repair of Achilles tendon ruptures. *Am J Sports Med* 15:1–8, 1987.
3. Carter TR, Fowler PJ, Blokker C: Functional postoperative treatment of Achilles tendon repair. *Am. J Sports Med* 20:459–462, 1992.
4. Elstrom JA, Pankovich AM: Muscle and tendon surgery of the leg. In: Evarts CM, ed. *Surgery of musculoskeletal system,* vol 3. New York: Churchill Livingstone, 1983:197.
5. Gillies H, Chalmers J: The management of fresh ruptures of the tendoachilles. *J Bone Joint Surg Am* 52:337–343, 1970.
6. Haggmark T, Liedberg H, Eriksson E, et al.: Calf muscle atrophy and muscle function after nonoperative vs. operative treatment of Achilles tendon ruptures. *Orthopedics* 9:160–164, 1986.
7. Hansen ST: Trauma to the calcaneus and its tendon: trauma to the heel cord. In: Jahss MH, ed. *Disorders of the foot and ankle: medical and surgical management.* Philadelphia: WB Saunders, 1991.
8. Hatrup SJ, Johnson KA: A review of ruptures of the Achilles tendon. *Foot Ankle* 6:34–38, 1985.
9. Inglis AE, Scott WN, Sculco TP, et al.: Ruptures of the tendoachilles. *J Bone Joint Surg Am* 58:990–993, 1976.
10. Inglis AE, Sculco TP: Surgical repair of ruptures of the tendoachilles. *Clin Orthop* 156:160–169, 1981.

11. Jacobs D, Marteus M, Van Audekercke R, et al.: Comparison of conservative and operative treatment of Achilles tendon rupture. *Am J Sports Med* 6:107–111, 1978.

12. Lea RB, Smith L: Non-surgical treatment of tendoachilles rupture. *Bone Joint Surg Am* 54:1398–1407, 1972.

13. Lindholm A: A new method of operation in subcutaneous rupture of the Achilles tendon. *Acta Chir Scand* 117:261, 1959.

14. Lynn TA: Repair of the torn Achilles tendon using plantaris tendon as a reinforcing membrane. *J Bone Joint Surg Am* 48:268–272, 1966.

15. Maffulli N: Rupture of the Achilles tendon. *J Bone Joint Surg Am* 81:1019–1036, 1999.

16. Mandelbaum BR, Myerson MS, Forster R: Achilles tendon ruptures: a new method of repair, early range of motion, and functional rehabilitation. *Am J Sports Med* 23:392–395, 1995.

17. Mann RA: Traumatic injuries to the soft tissues of the foot and ankle. In: Mann RA, ed. *Surgery of the foot,* 5th ed. St. Louis: CV Mosby, 1985:480.

18. Motta P, Errichiello C, Pontini I: Achilles tendon rupture: a new technique for easy surgical repair and immediate movement of the ankle and foot. *Am J Sports Med* 25:172–176, 1997.

19. Nistor L: Surgical and non-surgical treatment of Achilles tendon rupture. *J Bone Joint Surg Am* 63:394–399, 1981.

20. Phillips BB: Traumatic disorders. In: Crenshaw AH, ed. *Campbell's operative orthopedics,* 8th ed. St. Louis: CV Mosby, 1991:1905.

21. Ralston EL, Schmidt ER: Repair of the ruptured Achilles tendon. *J Trauma* 11:15–21, 1971.

22. Solveborn SA, Moberg A: Immediate free ankle motion after surgical repair of acute Achilles tendon ruptures. *Am J Sports Med* 22:607–610, 1994.

23. Stein SR, Leukens CA: Closed treatment of Achilles tendon ruptures. *Orthop Clin North Am* 5:89, 1974.

24. Thompson TC, Doherty JH: Spontaneous rupture of tendon of Achilles: a new clinical diagnostic test. *J Trauma* 2:126, 1962.

# 23

# Delayed Repair of the Achilles Tendon

Keith L. Wapner

## INDICATIONS/CONTRAINDICATIONS

Patients with an old or missed Achilles rupture present with complaints of plantarflexion weakness of the ankle during ambulation, climbing, or carrying objects and during other activities of daily life that require push-off power in gait (5).

Nonsurgical management with footwear modifications, including heel lifts, can alleviate pain but not improve function. Laced-up high-top shoes, boots, or braces, such as a molded ankle-foot orthosis, may improve gait in addition to controlling pain. Work or activity modifications may also be attempted to decrease the demands to plantarflex the foot. These modalities do not restore push-off strength.

Surgery is indicated to restore normal push-off power. Selection of the specific surgical procedure used is determined by analyzing the mechanism of injury, duration of time from the initial injury, and the quality of the tissues. The longer the duration from the initial injury, the less likely a primary end-to-end repair can be performed. In my experience, primary end-to-end repair can be successfully achieved up to 3 months after injury. Connective tissue disease such as rheumatoid arthritis, diabetes mellitus, obesity, autoimmune disorders, and malnutrition may adversely affect the success of end-to-end repair and may necessitate augmentation. Local factors that make the repair weaker or contribute to postoperative wound problems include ischemia due to peripheral vascular disease, scarring, and foot infections.

## PREOPERATIVE PLANNING

The diagnosis is made by reviewing the patient's history and performing a physical examination. The usual history of an acute rupture is acute onset of pain and inability to rise onto

K. L. Wapner, M.D.: Department of Orthopaedic Surgery, University of Pennsylvania; Department of Orthopaedic Surgery, MCP Hahnemann University; and Orthopaedic Foot & Ankle Surgery, Pennsylvania Hospital, Philadelphia, Pennsylvania.

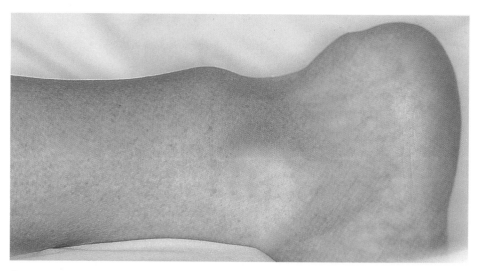

**Figure 23-1.** Appearance of the depression of the shin overlying the Achilles tendon with an untreated rupture.

the toes. At the time of rupture, patients often report the sensation of being struck in the calf from behind and experience immediate pain and weakness. The pain may increase as hematoma formation occurs. Patients with systemic connective tissue disorders such as rheumatoid arthritis may relate a more gradual onset, with Achilles tendinosis pain and eventual loss of the ability to rise onto the toes. Tendon rupture from progressive degener-

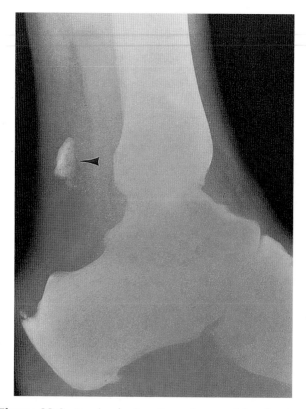

**Figure 23-2.** Proximal migration of an avulsion fracture fragment (*arrow*) from the Achilles tendon insertion.

ative tendinosis also presents with an insidious course. On examination, active but weak plantarflexion is maintained because of the extrinsic toe flexors, posterior tibial, and peroneal muscles. Misdiagnosis of the time of the rupture can occur in up to 20% of cases (2). Initially, there may not be an obvious tendon defect, but with time, the ends of the ruptured tendon separate, and the overlying skin conforms to the posterior leg, appearing as a hatchet-type defect. It may appear that there is an overgrowth of the posterior calcaneus (Fig. 23-1). The Thompson test (i.e., calf squeeze test) result is positive but does not cause as much pain as an acute injury.

Tendon rupture from progressive degenerative tendinosis presents with an insidious course. There is progressive thickening of the tendon and lengthening, with loss of function and increased pain. In these cases, a defect is not evident unless an acute or chronic traumatic rupture occurs. In general, the tendon is markedly thickened and tender to palpation.

Radiographs should be obtained to exclude avulsion of the posterior tuberosity of the calcaneus (Fig. 23-2), bony deformities, and calcification of the tendon. Magnetic resonance imaging (MRI) may be helpful in the uncertain diagnosis of an Achilles tendon rupture and chronic tendinosis (Fig. 23-3). It is most helpful in the sagittal plane to determine the length of tendon injured and to anticipate the type of surgical procedure needed (6).

The rupture usually occurs 2 to 6 cm from the calcaneal insertion, which is the most avascular region of the tendon. If clinical examination or MRI finds the defect is less than about 3 cm and if the injury has occurred within the past 3 months, direct end-to-end repair is often possible. If the gap is larger than 3 cm after scar tissue debridement, then V-Y lengthening to close the gap or Lindholm turn-down procedure may be considered if the remaining tendon tissue is healthy. If the remaining tendon tissue is not healthy and has chronic tendinosis, augmentation with transfer of the flexor hallucis longus (FHL) tendon can be used.

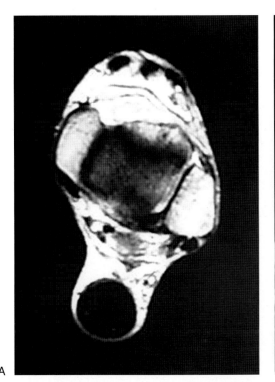
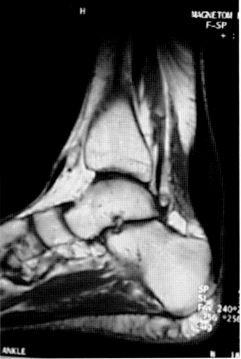

A
B

**Figure 23-3. A:** Axial MRI demonstrates chronic tendinosis of the Achilles with marked fusiform swelling of the tendon. **B:** Sagittal MRI demonstrates chronic tendinosis of the Achilles with marked fusiform swelling of the tendon.

## SURGERY

### Technique

Most procedures are carried out under spinal anesthesia. The patient is positioned supine, with the foot externally rotated. This allows for easy access to the midfoot if augmentation with tendon graft is indicated. It may also be performed in the prone position. An incision is made over the medial distal leg, along the anterior border of the Achilles tendon (Fig. 23-4). This approach avoids irritation of the resulting scar with footwear postoperatively and avoids trauma to the sural nerve. Dissection is carried through full thickness down to the level of the paratenon. The surgeon opens the paratenon and dissects deep to the paratenon to avoid compromising of the skin flaps. The tendon is inspected, and any adhesions are mobilized proximally and distally. In the case of a neglected complete rupture, the surgeon assesses the size of the gap.

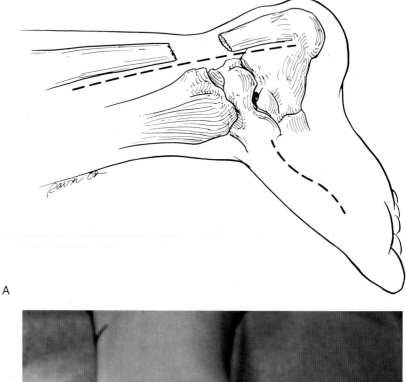

A

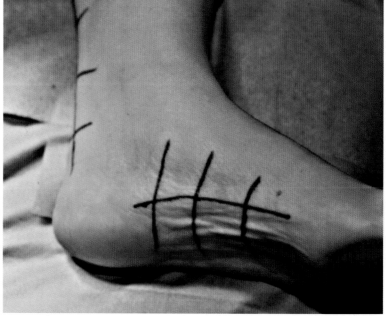

B

**Figure 23-4. A:** Incisions used for flexor hallucis longus reconstruction of Achilles. **B:** Photograph of incision placement.

It is often possible to free the proximal adhesions within the tendon sheath up to the level of the muscles of the gastrocnemius-soleus complex. By placing a suture on the proximal stump of the Achilles and supplying tension for 5 to 10 minutes, the size of the gap between the tendon ends can be significantly narrowed. If the gap can be closed, direct repair can be accomplished end to end if the tendon margins ends have viable tissue.

If the tendon ends are viable and the gap is less than 3 cm, a V-Y slide or advancement can be used to close the deficiency and lengthen the Achilles tendon to allow end-to-end repair (Fig. 23-5). The paratenon of the gastrocnemius is opened to the proximal end of the myotendinous junction. An inverted V incision is made, leaving the underlying muscle attached to the anterior paratenon. The flap is then advanced distally, and the rupture is repaired as described previously for an end-to-end repair (Fig. 23-6). The proximal portion is repaired by closing the inverted V to a Y. This V-Y technique is most helpful when a defect of more than 3 cm is present after the Achilles tendon is debrided to more healthy tissue. If the gap is large, a very long V with a more acute angle is necessary to provide the proper degree of tendon advancement. Up to about 7 cm can be advanced, but the width of

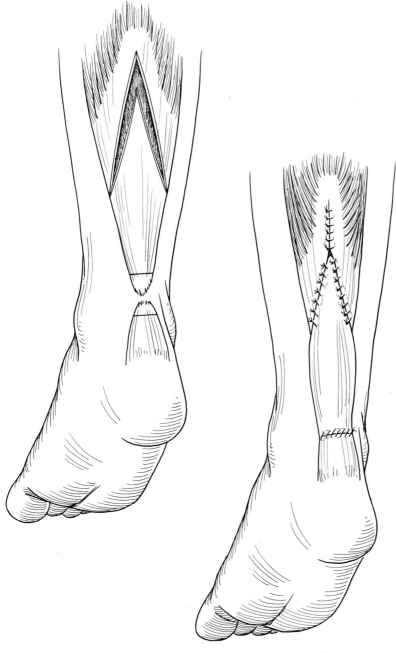

**Figure 23-5.** V-Y lengthening to close a gap in the Achilles tendon.

the remaining tendon tissue will be less and its tensile strength diminished. Augmentation should be considered in these instances.

Most frequently, the tendon ends are not viable in neglected tears, and significant debridement is necessary to get to the level of more healthy tissue. The remaining gap is too large to close, or the remaining tissue cannot withstand tensile loads and rupture may recur. Augmentation with tendon transfer facilitates repair in this instance (8,9). Augmentation is also useful when there is chronic tendinosis and a significant degenerative part of the Achilles must be debrided.

With the patient in a supine position, a medial incision is used to expose the Achilles tendon. The surgeon carries dissection down to the level of the paratenon, opens the paratenon, and debrides the tendon.

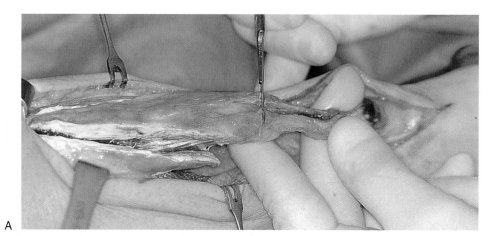

A

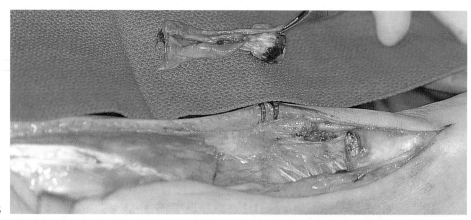

B

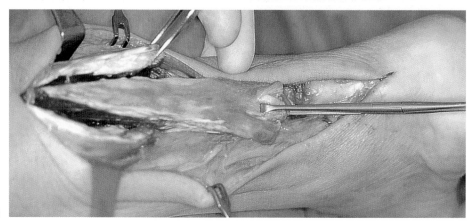

C

**Figure 23-6.  A:** The tendon is sectioned at the level of more normal tendon tissue. **B:** A 7-cm gap was present after resection of the scar tissue. **C:** A proximal V was made in the gastrocnemius-soleus aponeurosis. *(continued)*

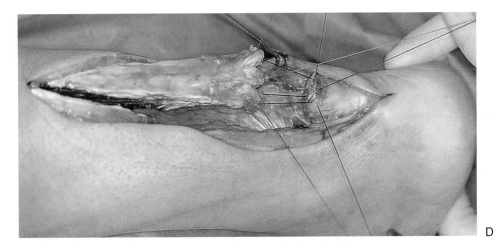

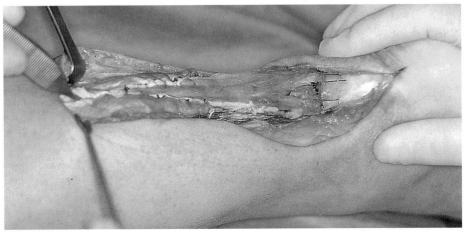

**Figure 23-6.** *Continued.* **D:** A zigzag (Bunnell) suture was placed in each end of the sectioned Achilles tendon. **E:** The advanced tendon ends are tied to close the gap of resected fibrous tissue. The proximal limb of the Y is closed.

The FHL tendon is harvested from an incision along the medial border of the midfoot, just above the level of the abductor muscle, from the navicular to the head of the first metatarsal (Fig. 23-4). The skin and subcutaneous tissues are sharply divided down to the level of the abductor hallucis fascia. The abductor is then reflected plantarward, and a small Weitlaner retractor is placed in the wound. The flexor hallucis brevis is then reflected plantarward, and the origin is released, exposing the deep midfoot anatomy.

The FHL and flexor digitorum longus tendons are identified within the midfoot. They usually are covered by a layer of fatty tissue. Identification of the tendons is accomplished by placing a finger over the lateral margin of the short flexor and manually plantarflexing and dorsiflexing the hallux interphalangeal joint. Motion of the tendon can be palpated and dissection carried down to identify tendons of the FHL medially and the flexor digitorum longus laterally. The FHL is sectioned as far distally as possible, generally at the level of the midshaft of the first metatarsal, but the surgeon should leave an adequate distal stump to be sutured to the flexor digitorum longus (Fig. 23-7). The proximal portion of the FHL tendon is tagged with a suture. The distal limb of the FHL tendon is sutured to the flexor digitorum longus tendon with all five toes in a neutral posture, providing flexion to all five toes through the flexor digitorum longus (Fig. 23-8).

In the posterior medial incision, the fascia overlying the posterior compartment of the leg is incised longitudinally directly over the muscle belly of the FHL. Applying traction to the suture attached to the FHL tendon in the midfoot assists in identifying the level of the muscle belly and indicates where to open the fascia. The tendon is then retracted into the posterior incision from the midfoot (Fig. 23-9).

A transverse drill hole is made just distal to the insertion of the Achilles tendon halfway

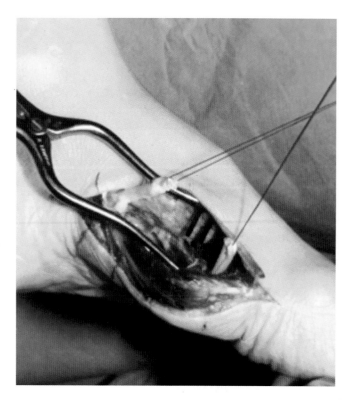

**Figure 23-7.** The abductor hallucis and flexor hallucis brevis muscles are reflected plantarward, and the flexor hallucis longus (FHL) tendon identified. The FHL tendon has been tagged and sectioned at the level of the proximal third of the first metatarsal.

through the bone from medial to lateral. A second vertical drill hole is made just anterior to attachment of the Achilles tendon to intersect the first hole (Fig. 23-10). A large towel clip is used to connect the holes. A suture passer is placed through the tunnel from distal-medial to proximal aspects. The suture is then pulled through the tunnel, drawing the FHL tendon through the drill hole (Fig. 23-11).

**Figure 23-8. A:** Diagram of a flexor hallucis longus (FHL) and flexor digitorum longus (FDL) anastomosis. **B:** The FDL tendon is identified and tagged, and the distal FHL tendon is sutured to the FHL tendon with all the toes held in neutral.

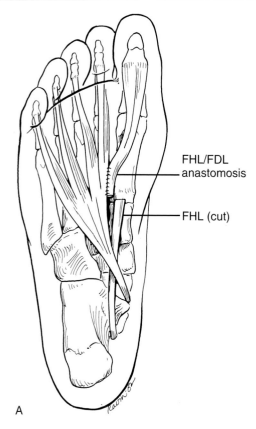

FHL/FDL anastomosis

FHL (cut)

A

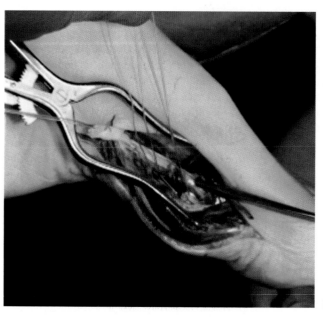

B

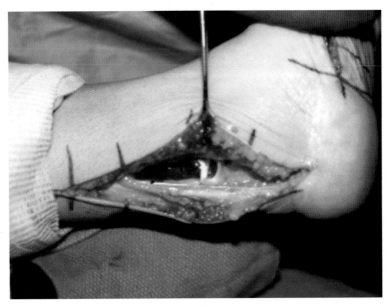

**Figure 23-9.** A posterior incision is made, and the posterior fascia of the leg is opened to allow transfer of the flexor hallucis longus tendon into the wound.

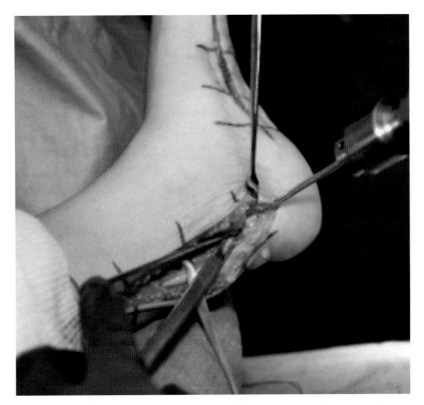

**Figure 23-10.** Two drill holes are made in the calcaneus, with one starting superior and the other starting medial to intersect in the posterior body of the calcaneus to create a tunnel for tendon transfer.

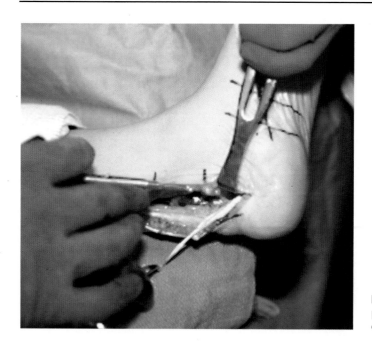

**Figure 23-11.** The flexor hallucis longus tendon is passed into the superior hole and out of the medial side of the tunnel.

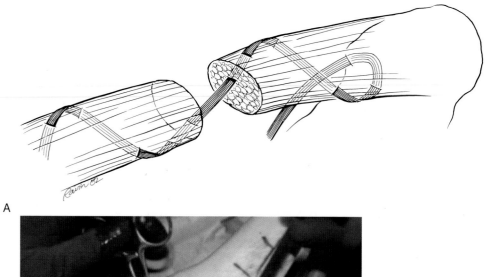

A

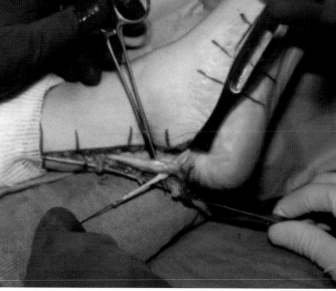

B

**Figure 23-12. A:** Completed weaving of the flexor hallucis longus (FHL) tendon through the Achilles tendon. Notice the orientation of the tunnel through the posterior calcaneus. **B:** The FHL tendon is woven through the Achilles tendon using a tendon weaver.

The FHL is woven from distal to proximal through the Achilles tendon using a tendon weaver (Fig. 23-12). The tendon weaver is passed through the Achilles, creating a "tunnel" in the tendon. The tag suture on the flexor hallucis is then grasped and pulled back through the tunnel, bringing the flexor tendon through the Achilles. This process is repeated to use the full length of tendon harvested. The tendon is secured with multiple sutures of no. 1 cottony Dacron. After completion of the reconstruction, the paratenon is repaired. The subcutaneous tissue and skin are closed. Compressive dressings and plaster splints are applied to maintain 15° of ankle plantarflexion.

## POSTOPERATIVE MANAGEMENT

The patient is placed in a short-leg, non–weight-bearing cast at 15° of equinus for 4 weeks. Remove the sutures 2 weeks after surgery. At 4 weeks postoperatively, the cast is removed, and the forefoot is placed on a foot rest with the patient seated with the hip flexed. This position is maintained until the foot reaches neutral flexion-extension. The foot is then placed into a short-leg walking cast or removable cast walker with the ankle at neutral for an additional 4 weeks and range of motion and weight bearing are begun. A rehabilitation program for strengthening and range of motion is begun 8 weeks postoperatively. The patient is maintained in a removable cast walker for community ambulation until 10° of dorsiflexion is obtained and grade 4/5 plantarflexion strength is demonstrated. Home ambulation is allowed with a $^7/_{16}$″ heel lift during this time. The patients are then advanced to regular footwear and continued on a home strengthening program with an elastic band. Athletic activity is restricted for 6 months after surgery.

## COMPLICATIONS

The main complications are wound necrosis, infection, rerupture, ankle stiffness, and sural neuroma formation.

*Wound edge necrosis* is prevented by maintaining the posterior skin flap as thick as possible by performing all dissection deep to the paratenon, avoiding excessive flap retraction, by careful wound closure, and by an adequate period of wound compression and immobilization postoperatively. If skin necrosis occurs, debridement procedures, soaks, and antibiotics should be provided to allow healing by secondary intention. In instances of large soft tissue deficiencies, skin grafting may be necessary after the wound granulates. If the defect is extensive and there is a large portion of exposed tendon, a free flap may be required.

*Infection* is closely related to wound necrosis. If the infection occurs deep to a wound that was closed primarily, it needs to be debrided, antibiotics administered, and in some instances, left open to heal by secondary intention.

*Rerupture* is unusual if reconstruction is adequate and the rehabilitation program is followed. It is important that healthy tissue be used to span the site of rupture. Rerupture has not been a problem with augmentation with FHL tendon transfer.

*Sural neuroma* formation is possible if a lateral approach is used. Leaving the fatty tissue around the nerve after identification is important. If the nerve is injured, a more proximal nerve transection in a relatively undisturbed subcutaneous level can decrease the sensitivity of the resulting end-bulb neuroma.

## ILLUSTRATIVE CASE

A 56-year-old lawyer suffered an injury to his left ankle playing tennis at a company outing. He felt immediate pain and swelling of the ankle and was unable to walk without pain. He did not seek medical attention until a week later. He was found to have a swollen ankle with ecchymosis. A Thompson test was not performed, and he was diagnosed by his primary care physician as having an ankle sprain and sent for rehabilitation. At 3 months post

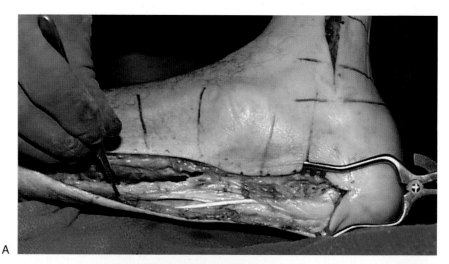

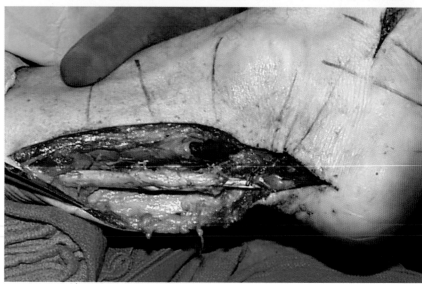

**Figure 23-13. A:** Intraoperative picture of a neglected Achilles rupture 6 months after the initial injury. **B:** Intraoperative picture after flexor hallucis longus transfer.

injury, he was still experiencing weakness. His primary care physician ordered an MRI, which was not performed until 4 months after injury, and he was diagnosed as having a partial tear of his Achilles tendon. Additional physical therapy was ordered.

Six months after injury, the patient had continued complaints of weakness in push-off and stair walking. On examination, he had a palpable gap in his Achilles tendon and a positive Thompson test result. At the time of surgery, he was found to have a complete tendon tear and a 5-cm gap between the tendon ends. This was narrowed to a 2-cm gap with traction on the tendon using sutures as described previously. The gap was then bridged by a FHL tendon transfer (Fig. 23-13). At 1 year postoperatively, he has regained full range of motion and plantarflexion strength and returned to playing tennis.

## RECOMMENDED READING

1. Abraham E, Pankovich AM: Neglected rupture of the Achilles tendon: treatment by V-Y tendinous flap. *J Bone Joint Surg Am* 57:253–255, 1975.
2. Calhoun JH: Delayed repair of the Achilles tendon. In: Johnson KA, ed. *Master techniques in orthopaedic surgery,* 1st ed. New York: Raven Press, 1994.
3. Hattrup SJ, Johnson KA: A review of ruptures of the Achilles tendon. *Foot Ankle* 6:34–38, 1985.

4. Inglis AE, Scott WN, Sculco TP, et al.: Ruptures of the tendon Achilles. *J Bone Joint Surg Am* 58:990–993, 1976.
5. Justis EJ Jr: Traumatic disorders. In: Crenshaw AH, ed. *Campbell's operative orthopaedics*, 7th ed, vol 3. St. Louis: CV Mosby, 1987:2226–2233.
6. Schweitzer ME, Karasick D: MR imaging of disorders of the Achilles tendon. *AJR Am J Roentgenol* 175: 613–625, 2000.
7. Serafin SK: *Anatomy of the foot and ankle: descriptive, topographic, functional.* Philadelphia: JB Lippincott, 1983:313–316.
8. Wapner KL, Hecht JP, Mills RH Jr: Reconstruction of neglected Achilles tendon injury. *Ortho Clin North Am* 26:249–263, 1995.
9. Wapner KL, Padlock GS, Hecht JP, et al.: Repair of chronic Achilles tendon rupture with flexor hallucis longus tendon transfer. *Foot Ankle* 14:443–449, 1993.

# 24

# Plantar Fascia Release

W. Grant Braly

Plantar fascia release has application for several conditions; usually for intractable plantar fasciitis. There is no consensus of opinion regarding some aspects of the procedure, including specific indications, technical points such as incision placement, and the use of open versus endoscopic methods.

Complete fasciotomy is an important component for correction of the cavus foot. This procedure was previously performed with regularity in patients with heel pain. Investigators demonstrated the adverse effects of complete fasciotomy on arch stability, which led to modifications of the technique, such as partial fasciotomy. Complete fasciotomy and partial fasciotomy techniques are described.

## INDICATIONS/CONTRAINDICATIONS

Complete fasciotomy is performed for cavus deformities with operations such as triple arthrodesis or calcaneal osteotomy. Partial fasciotomy is usually performed for heel pain due to intractable plantar fasciitis.

The cause of heel pain is multifactorial, and treatment can be frustrating for the patient and practitioner alike. It usually has a self-limiting course, but conservative treatment may be quite helpful in alleviating symptoms.

Typically, the patient is middle-aged, often overweight, and usually not able to recall any precipitating traumatic event. However, there may be a history of overuse or sudden change in activity level temporally related to the onset of symptoms.

It is generally accepted that the cause of heel pain, or *heel pain syndrome*, is plantar fasciitis. This condition may represent a degenerative attritional or fatigue interstitial tear of the plantar fascia in the proximity of its calcaneal insertion with associated chronic inflamma-

W. G. Braly, M.D.: Department of Orthopaedic Surgery, University of Texas Health Science Center–Houston; Fondren Orthopedic Group, Foot and Ankle Section, Texas Orthopedic Hospital, Houston, Texas.

tion and eventual fibrosis. Other possible causes of heel pain are nerve entrapment, inflammatory arthritis with enthesitis, subtalar arthritis, stress fractures, chronic infection, and tumors. The significance of the calcaneal heel spur is controversial and probably is a normal variant that is not directly related to the heel pain itself.

Conservative treatment modalities are numerous and varied. They include restriction of activities, especially repetitive impact loading sports, along with weight reduction, heel cord or plantar fascia stretching exercises, heel pads or cups, arch supports, nonsteroidal antiinflammatory medications, steroid injections, physical therapy, night splinting, and immobilization. In most patients, these measures are successful but may require months of such treatment and patient reassurance.

Another approach to noninvasive management is extracorporeal shock wave treatment (ESWT). Early trial investigations are encouraging, with minimal patient morbidity. ESWT may represent a viable treatment alternative, especially in the patient who has failed previously described conservative treatment and has reached the point of seeking operative treatment with its associated significant risks and complications.

Surgical treatment (partial plantar fascia release) is only considered after a diligent effort of conservative management for at least 6 months in the patient with intractable heel pain. The heel pain must be of such severity that it has significantly altered the patient's lifestyle or ability to participate in desired conditioning activities.

Contraindications include a dysvascular foot, localized infection, and dermatologic disorders that could compromise wound healing. Other contraindications are conditions for which surgical treatment may not be effective, such as an occult autoimmune disease, calcaneal stress fracture, senile heel pad atrophy, tendon disorders, subtalar joint arthritis, tarsal tunnel syndrome, and lumbar disk disease.

The astute diagnostician must be keenly aware of the patient with bilateral heel pain, particularly the younger man with no other predisposing factors. Such a patient profile may herald the onset of Reiter's syndrome. A thorough history investigating other signs and symptoms of this syndrome and screening laboratory serum tests often suggest this diagnosis.

Morbid obesity may be a relative contraindication. Weight loss should be encouraged as a conservative treatment measure.

## PREOPERATIVE PLANNING

The patient with heel pain usually cannot recall any precipitating traumatic event, but an overuse pattern may be elicited while obtaining the history. The pain usually begins gradually and may wax and wane in its intensity. It may resolve for an extended period, only to return just as inexplicably as it first began. Typically, the pain is worse on rising in the morning or after significant periods of recumbency or sitting (i.e., "start-up" pain). The first few steps are often bothersome, but as the foot "warms up," the pain gradually resolves or diminishes. It often returns or intensifies later in the day, especially with prolonged periods of standing or walking. Such a history is almost pathognomonic for heel pain secondary to plantar fasciitis.

The patient may present with an antalgic gait and localizes the pain in the central heel or plantar medial heel. Occasionally, the discomfort extends distally into the arch along the course of the plantar fascia. The patient's pain is reliably reproduced by deep palpation in the central or plantar medial heel. It may be increased by passively dorsiflexing the toes, which stretches the inflamed plantar fascia. Swelling is rarely encountered. A tight or contracted heel cord is a common finding. Some patients, especially women, experience relief with use of higher-heel shoes, presumably related to heel cord contracture.

Weight-bearing foot radiographs (i.e., anteroposterior, lateral, and oblique) and an axial heel view are recommended. If bony pathology is suspected and not readily evident on plain films, other studies such as a bone scan may be helpful. Computed tomography or magnetic resonance imaging may be indicated in selected cases.

## SURGERY

The rationale for the plantar fascia release procedure is to decrease the tension on the often tight and fibrotic plantar fascia. This may also decompress anatomic structures deep to it, particularly the intrinsic muscles and various nerves in the plantar heel region. Release of the conjoined ligament of the forearm extensor muscles for chronic lateral epicondylitis or "tennis elbow" is perhaps an analogous procedure.

Most cases can be accomplished in an outpatient setting unless significant medical problems dictate otherwise. The patient is placed in the supine position, and a local anesthetic is administered in the plantar medial heel or an ankle block is administered with a mixture of equal amounts of 1% or 2% lidocaine and 0.5% bupivacaine without epinephrine; 10 to 25 mL usually suffice. Intravenous sedation is administered. General anesthesia is an alternative, but it is usually unnecessary. A pneumatic proximal thigh tourniquet is preferred for general anesthesia and a supramalleolar ankle tourniquet for local anesthesia (Fig. 24-1).

The foot and ankle are prepped and draped in a sterile manner. To exsanguinate the foot, the extremity may be elevated, or an elastic bandage (sterile Ace wrap or Esmarch) may be used. The pneumatic tourniquet is then inflated (250 to 300 mm Hg for ankle and 300 to 350 mm Hg for thigh tourniquets) after administration of a broad-spectrum prophylactic antibiotic; I prefer cephazolin.

The foot is left suspended over a well-padded foam wedge or block. An assistant is essential to keep the foot in a dorsiflexed or neutral position to enhance exposure and to keep the plantar fascia taut during the procedure (Fig. 24-2).

### Technique: Complete Fasciotomy

An oblique incision 3 to 4 cm long is made just distal and medial to the heel pad near the junction of the thicker plantar heel pad and the thinner skin of the proximal medial arch (Fig. 24-3). The oblique incision is important to avoid transection of the medial calcaneal nerve branches, which can result in a postoperative neuroma. Dissection proceeds through

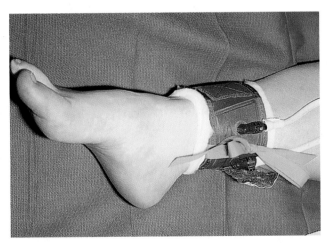

**Figure 24-1.** The patient is placed in the supine position, with a supramalleolar pneumatic ankle tourniquet applied for ankle block or local anesthesia with intravenous sedation. I prefer an injection be given before prepping and draping.

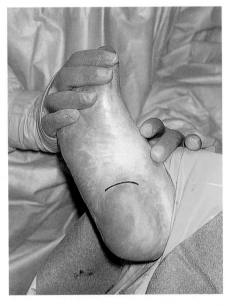

**Figure 24-2.** After prepping, draping, and inflation of the tourniquet, the foot is left suspended over a padded wedge. An assistant keeps the foot in a neutral or dorsiflexed position to enhance exposure and keep the plantar fascia taut.

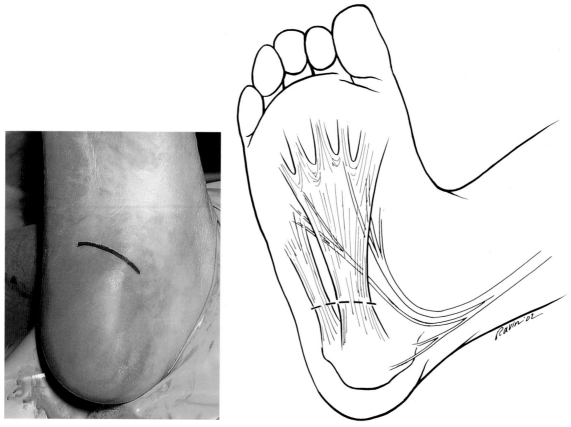

A    B

**Figure 24-3.  A and B:** A 3- to 4-cm, oblique incision is made just distal and medial to the heel pad in the proximal arch region. The oblique orientation of the incision reduces the potential of injury to the medial calcaneal nerve.

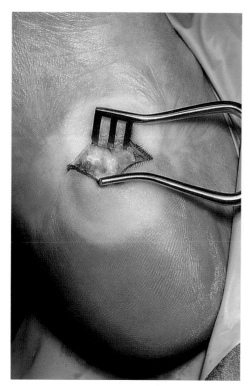

**Figure 24-4.** A self-retracting or small hand-held retractor displaces the billowing subcutaneous and heel pad tissue.

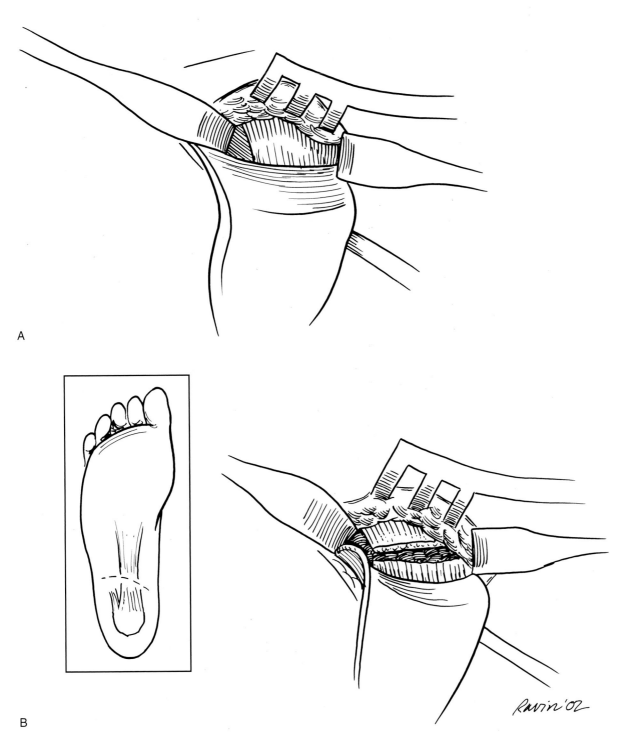

A

B

**Figure 24-5.  A:** The medial and lateral borders of the proximal plantar fascia are identified 1 to 2 cm distal to its attachment to the calcaneus. **B:** The complete plantar fascia release is shown.

the subcutaneous tissue, coagulating bleeders as they are encountered. A self-retaining or small, hand-held retractor for the billowing subcutaneous and heel pad tissue is recommended (Fig. 24-4). The medial and lateral borders of the proximal plantar fascia are identified 1 to 2 cm distal to its attachment to the calcaneus (Fig. 24-5). The plantar fascia is then cut sharply in this area, taking care not to violate the intimately associated intrinsic musculature (Fig. 24-6).

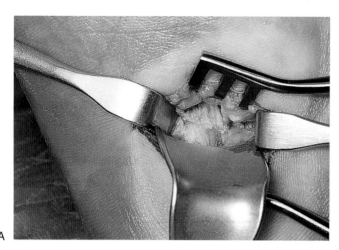

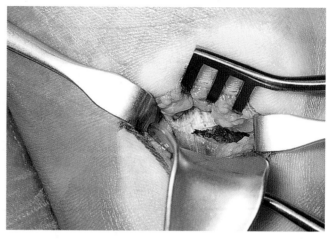

A

B

**Figure 24-6. A:** This intraoperative view shows the surgical exposure of the plantar fascia. **B:** The plantar fascia is cut sharply, taking care not to violate the underlying intrinsic muscles. The intraoperative view shows the fasciotomy before complete transection.

The wound is then thoroughly irrigated, the tourniquet released, hemostasis achieved, and the skin closed with nonabsorbable, monofilament-type (3-0 Prolene), interrupted vertical mattress sutures (Fig. 24-7). A bulky compressive dressing is then applied; it is made of Xeroform, 4 × 4 inch gauze pads, ABD pad, Kerlix, 3-inch Kling bandage, and a 3-inch Ace wrap, in that order (Fig. 24-8).

### Technique: Partial Fasciotomy

Under loupe magnification, a 2- to 3-cm, vertically oriented incision is made over the medial foot hindfoot, roughly in line with the posterior margin of the medial malleolus (Fig. 24-9).The inferior or plantar edge of the incision should not violate the thicker epidermis of the heel pad. The longitudinal alignment of this incision is important to avoid transec-

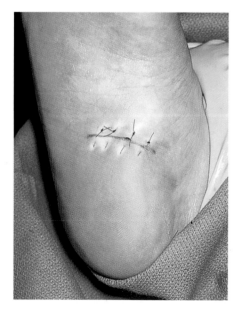

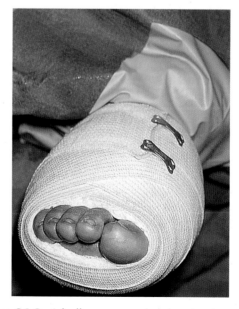

**Figure 24-7.** Hemostasis is achieved after the release of the tourniquet, and the skin is closed with nonabsorbable, monofilament-type, interrupted, vertical mattress sutures.

**Figure 24-8.** A bulky compressive dressing is applied.

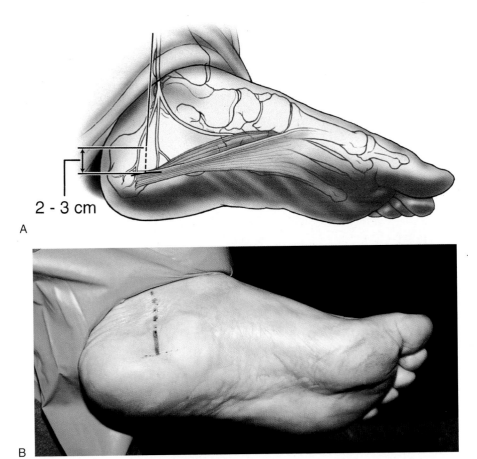

**Figure 24-9. A:** A 2- to 3-cm, longitudinal incision *(dotted line)*, which is in line with the posterior edge of the medial malleolus and parallel to the medial calcaneal nerve, is made avoiding the thicker plantar heel pad skin. **B:** Clinical photograph shows the incision.

tion of the medial calcaneal nerve branches, which can result in a painful postoperative neuroma. Dissection proceeds through the subcutaneous tissue, coagulating bleeders as they are encountered. A self-retaining retractor is recommended for the subcutaneous tissue (Fig. 24-10). The medial and lateral borders of the proximal plantar fascia are then identified 1 to 2 cm distal to their origin from the calcaneus. To protect the soft tissue lateral and plantar to the fascia, a Swanson or similar type of retractor is placed. The medial one half to two thirds of the plantar fascia is then cut sharply, taking care to not violate the intimately underlying intrinsic musculature (Figs. 24-10 and 24-11). The superficial and deep abductor fascia are identified and released. Preserving the lateral one third of the plantar fascia is recommended, because releasing the entire structure may result in a soft tissue flatfoot deformity or the so-called lateral column syndrome, which is thought to result from instability of the longitudinal arch. The medial part of the fascia is usually thicker and corresponds to the area of maximal tenderness in most patients.

If a heel spur is to be removed, dissection proceeds from the cut edge of the plantar fascia posteriorly to the calcaneus at a level between the fascia and intrinsic muscles. The spur is then removed with a rongeur under direct visualization, and all rough edges are smoothed. Surgical removal of a heel spur may be performed but is usually unnecessary.

The wound is then thoroughly irrigated, the tourniquet released, hemostasis achieved, and the skin closed with nonabsorbable, monofilament-type (3-0 Prolene), interrupted vertical mattress sutures (Fig. 24-12). A bulky compressive dressing is then applied; it is made of Xeroform, 4 × 4 inch gauze pads, ABD pad, Kerlix, 3-inch Kling, and a 3-inch Ace wrap, in that order.

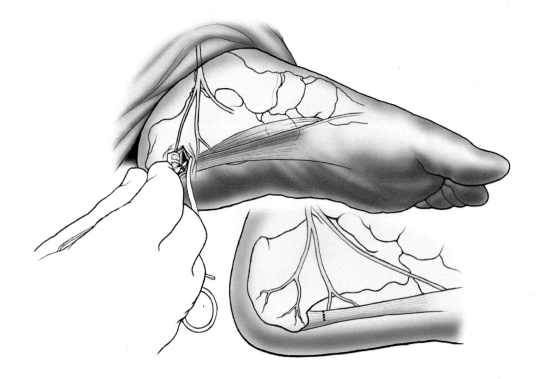

A

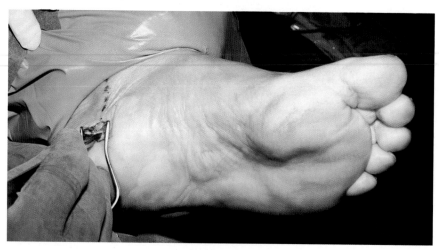

B

**Figure 24-10. A:** A self-retaining retractor displaces the subcutaneous tissue and enhances visualization. **B:** Clinical photograph.

Plantar fasciotomy may also be performed endoscopically, and favorable results have been reported. As with other endoscopic or arthroscopic surgical procedures that have smaller incisions and less soft tissue dissection, the potential for reduced morbidity may provide an advantage over the traditional open techniques. However, complications of endoscopy have been described, some of which are the same as for the open method. We think that some of these complications may be the result of more limited endoscopic visualization, and the relatively modest 2- to 3-cm incision in an open technique, compared with a 1-cm incision in endoscopy, may allow superior definition of important anatomic structures, diminishing the likelihood of complications.

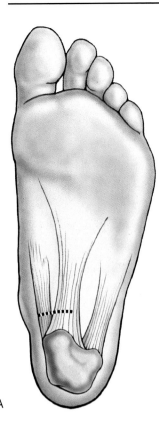

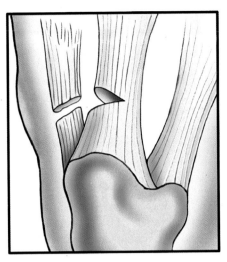

A

B

**Figure 24-11. A:** The medial and lateral borders of the proximal plantar fascia are identified 1 to 2 cm distal to its origin from the calcaneus. **B:** The extent of the plantar fascia release is shown. The abductor fascia and medial one half to two thirds of the plantar fascia are cut sharply, taking care not to violate the underlying intrinsic muscles. The lateral one third to one half of the plantar fascia is preserved.

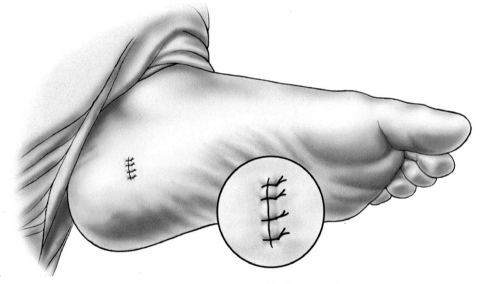

A

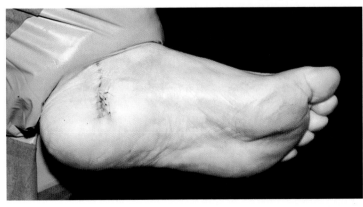

B

**Figure 24-12. A:** Hemostasis is achieved after release of the tourniquet, and the skin is closed with nonabsorbable, monofilament-type, interrupted, vertical mattress sutures. A bulky compressive dressing is applied. **B:** Clinical photograph.

## POSTOPERATIVE MANAGEMENT

After leaving the recovery room following partial fasciectomy, the patient is instructed in the use of crutches or a walker and is not allowed to bear weight on the operated heel (Table 24-1). Some balance or touchdown weight bearing with a postoperative shoe is permitted on the forefoot.

The dressing is usually changed in 3 to 5 days. The patient is then given instructions on local wound care with daily hydrogen peroxide cleaning of the wound and Kerlix or a similar dressing. The patient is allowed to shower, but tub bathing or soaking is not permitted until suture removal.

At approximately 2 weeks postoperatively, progressive heel weight bearing is allowed as tolerated in the postoperative shoe. The patient is encouraged to wean from the crutches or walker and begin a normal gait pattern at this time. Sutures are removed 10 to 14 days after surgery.

Supportive, soft-sole footwear such as athletic shoes is encouraged at the point when sutures are removed and heel weight bearing is consistently tolerated (generally 2 weeks postoperatively). No repetitive impact loading conditioning activities or sports are allowed until at least 6 weeks postoperatively. Alternative, nonimpact forms of exercise before this time may include cycling or swimming.

Most patients are able to return to all desired activities by 6 to 12 weeks postoperatively. Patients must be counseled preoperatively about the anticipated recovery time, because some patients may require a much longer period to recover. The surgeon should allow a generous amount of time for resolution of symptoms. Complete recovery may occasionally require more than 6 months. Prolonged swelling postoperatively is common after foot surgery, and plantar fascia release is no exception.

Beyond crutch or walker training, formalized physical therapy is not usually prescribed. At the time of suture removal with a well-healed incision (10 to 14 days postoperatively), patients are given instructions on warm soaks, gentle massage, and foot and ankle range of motion exercises.

For the patient who has persistent heel pain with weight bearing at 6 weeks postoperatively, formalized physical therapy may be indicated. It may include whirlpool, massage, and ultrasound modalities. Such treatment is generally recommended for the patient who has an unusual level of swelling and incisional fibrosis.

## COMPLICATIONS

*Infection* is a rare problem. If it occurs, it is usually superficial and responds readily to local wound care and oral antibiotics. Deep infection requiring inpatient care, surgical debridement, or parenteral antibiotics is exceptionally rare. Meticulous aseptic technique is essential, and preoperative antibiotics are recommended to avoid this complication.

**Table 24-1.** *Postoperative care for partial plantar fascia release*

| Time postoperative | Care |
| --- | --- |
| Day of surgery | Soft, bulky dressing |
| | Crutch or walker training; no weight bearing on operated heel with postoperative shoe |
| 3–5 days | Dressing changed |
| | Local wound care begins |
| 10–14 days | Heel weight bearing permitted |
| | Wean from crutches or walker |
| | Sutures removed |
| | Supportive, soft-sole footwear encouraged |
| | Home program of physical therapy |
| 2–4 weeks | Low-impact sports and activities prescribed (e.g., swimming, cycling) |
| 6–12 weeks | Formalized physical therapy, if necessary |
| | Resumption of all activities as tolerated |

*Flatfoot* may theoretically be prevented by avoiding complete release of the plantar fascia and perhaps by limiting early postoperative heel weight bearing. When it occurs, the soft tissue support of the arch is lost to some degree, and this may ultimately lead to measurable radiographic changes in the bony arch. When complete release of the plantar fascia was avoided, the incidence of this complication decreased.

In addition to a subtle radiologic change in the arch height, the patient may also complain of dorsal and lateral midfoot pain. This is referred to as *lateral column syndrome* or *settling phenomena*, and it may be the result of strain of the calcaneocuboid and tarsometatarsal joint capsules that are subjected to greater weight-bearing forces because of loss of the support provided by the intact plantar fascia. The symptoms associated with this complication eventually resolve but may require a prolonged period. The patient is encouraged to wear supportive shoes with prefabricated or prescribed arch supports if this complication occurs.

Major *nerve damage* is rare in this procedure. The vertically oriented heel incision avoids the medial calcaneal nerve that is often damaged with other approaches such as the traditional, horizontally oriented DuVries incision. Theoretically, the medial calcaneal and the lateral plantar are the deep nerves most vulnerable to surgical damage. To avoid deep nerve damage, familiarity with the nerve anatomy is essential, and loupe magnification is recommended.

*Plantar intrinsic muscle damage* may occur. With time, the foot may develop a mild intrinsic minus foot with the possible development of hammer toes, and this condition is thought to be caused by insertional detachment or severance of the plantar intrinsic muscles. I discourage heel spur excision associated with a plantar fascia release to avoid this complication. If the heel spur is removed, meticulous dissection under magnification can minimize damage to the intrinsic muscles.

## RECOMMENDED READING

1. Anderson RB, Foster MD: Operative treatment of subcalcaneal pain. *Foot Ankle* 9:317–323, 1989.
2. Baxter DE, Thigpen CM: Heel pain—operative results. *Foot Ankle* 5:16–25, 1984.
3. Bordelon RL: Subscalcaneal pain: a method of evaluation and plan for treatment. *Clin Orthop* 177:49–53, 1983.
4. Furey JG: Plantar fasciitis: the painful heel syndrome. *J Bone Joint Surg Am* 57:672–673, 1975.
5. Heller KA, Niethold FA: The use of extracorporeal shock wave therapy in orthopedics: a review of the literature and meta-analysis. *Z Orthop* 136:390–401, 1998.
6. Hofineister EP, Elliott MJ, Juliano PJ: Endoscopic plantar fascia release: an anatomical study. *Foot Ankle Int* 16:719–723, 1995.
7. Kahn C, Bishop JO, Tullos HS: Plantar fascia release and heel spur excision via plantar route. *Orthop Rev* 14: 222–225, 1985.
8. Kitaoka HB, Luo ZP: Mechanical behavior of the foot and ankle after plantar fascia release in the unstable foot. *Foot Ankle Int* 18:8–15, 1997.
9. Leach RE, Seavey MS, Salter DK: Results of surgery in athletes with plantar fasciitis. *Foot Ankle* 7:156–161, 1986.
10. Lester DK, Buchanan JR: Surgical treatment of plantar fasciitis. *Clin Orthop* 186:202–204, 1984.
11. Michetti ML, Jacobs SA: Calcaneal heel spurs: etiology, treatment, and a new surgical approach. *J Foot Surg* 22:234–239, 1984.
12. Ogilvie-Harris DJ, Lobo J: Endoscopic plantar fascia release. *Arthroscopy* 16:290–298, 2000.
13. Rompe JB, Hopf C, Nafe B, et al.: Low-energy extracorporeal shock wave therapy for painful heel: a prospective controlled single-blind study. *Arch Orthop Trauma Surg* 115:75–79, 1996.
14. Snider MP, Clancy WG, McBeath AA: Plantar fascia release for chronic plantar fasciitis in runners. *Am J Sports Med* 11:215–219, 1983.
15. Sundberg SB, Johnson KA: Painful conditions of the heel. In: Jahss MH, ed. *Disorders of the foot and ankle: medical and surgical management.* Philadelphia: WB Saunders, 1991.
16. Ward WG, Clippinger FW: Proximal medial longitudinal arch incision for plantar fascia release. *Foot Ankle* 8:152–155, 1987.

# 25

# Release of the Nerve to the Abductor Digiti Quinti

## Donald E. Baxter

## INDICATIONS/CONTRAINDICATIONS

Entrapment neuropathy, affecting the nerve to the abductor digiti quinti, is one of the many causes of chronic heel pain. This small nerve is consistently the first branch off the lateral plantar nerve. The course of this nerve was defined by Rondhuis et al. (11) in fetal and adult cadaveric feet. The nerve appears to be at risk of injury in retrograde intramedullary nailing, but there is less risk with procedures such as intrascopic fasciotomy. Abnormalities were observed in the electrodiagnostic studies of patients with chronic heel pain in 23 of 38 symptomatic heels in the medial and/or lateral plantar nerve (14), supporting the concept that plantar nerve disorders can be underlying causes of chronic heel pain.

The indication for release of the nerve to the abductor digiti quinti or the first branch of the lateral plantar nerve is chronic neuritic pain that does not resolve with conservative care. This neuritic pain is localized to the medial aspect of the heel underneath the inferior aspect of the abductor hallucis muscle. The pain often radiates proximally up into the ankle and may migrate across the foot on the plantar surface. After all other causes of heel pain have been ruled out and pain persists for an extended period (preferably 1 year), nerve release may be indicated. Nonoperative management includes orthoses, footwear modifications, physical therapy, antiinflammatory medications, and rarely, corticosteroid injections.

Contraindications to this procedure include the presence of other causes of heel pain. Other contraindications are a local injection or blister or dysvascular extremity. A relative contraindication is a patient who refuses to comply with nonoperative treatment measures such as activity modifications.

D. E. Baxter, M.D.: Fondren, Houston, Texas.

## PREOPERATIVE PLANNING

The diagnosis of entrapment of the first branch of the lateral plantar nerve or the nerve to the abductor digiti quinti is made on a clinical basis. Clinical expertise is an important factor in determining which patient with a painful heel may benefit from operative decompression of the first branch of the lateral plantar nerve. The examiner must differentiate first nerve branch entrapment from the other common causes of heel pain, which include plantar fasciitis, retrocalcaneal bursitis, heel pad atrophy, various arthritides (e.g., Reiter's syndrome, ankylosing spondylitis, psoriatic arthritis), chronic infection, calcaneal stress fracture, heel contusion, plantar fascia rupture, tarsal tunnel syndrome, radiculopathy, peripheral neuropathy, tumors, and vascular disease.

The pathognomonic sign of entrapment of the first branch of the lateral plantar nerve is the consistent finding of maximal tenderness where the nerve is compressed between the taut deep fascia of the abductor hallucis muscle and the medial caudal margin of the quadratus plantae muscle. Chronic inflammation of the plantar fascia may predispose to entrapment of the first branch of the lateral plantar nerve. The patient may have some tenderness over the proximal plantar fascia at its medial calcaneal tuberosity attachment. However, without maximal tenderness over the course in the nerve of the plantar medial aspect of the foot, the diagnosis of entrapment is not established. Some patients may have paresthesias elicited with pressure over the nerve entrapment site (i.e., positive Tinel's sign). Patients should not have tenderness in the heel pad, retrocalcaneal bursa, Achilles tendon insertion, body of calcaneus, sinus tarsi, or posterior tibial region. There is typically no swelling, increased warmth, erythema, or malalignment. Radiographs are negative for fractures or arthrosis or bony lesions.

Electromyographic and nerve conduction studies are not always helpful, but these electrodiagnostic studies occasionally show abnormalities consistent with chronic nerve compression. The preoperative evaluation of the patient should include electrodiagnostic studies to determine the point of entrapment and to exclude more proximal disorders such as lumbar radiculopathy tarsal tunnel syndrome. A technetium bone scan may be helpful to detect occult pathology such as stress fractures or bone tumors. A rheumatologic workup should be considered for any patient who has any symptoms suggestive of systemic rheumatic disease.

## SURGERY

The patient is placed in the supine position on the operating table. The hip and knee are flexed at 90° and externally rotated. The foot is palpated and the site of maximal tenderness is marked (Fig. 25-1). Ankle block anesthesia is used most frequently. No tourniquet is required, although an ankle tourniquet may be used. A 4-cm, oblique incision is made (Fig. 25-2) on the medial heel over the proximal abductor hallucis muscle. The incision is centered over the course of the first branch of the lateral plantar nerve (Figs. 25-2 and 25-3). The sensory branches of the medial calcaneal nerve are not encountered as they course posterior to the incision. Care is taken, however, to preserve any aberrant nerve branches.

The interval between the fascia overlying the abductor hallucis and the medial border of the plantar fascia is identified (Fig. 25-4). A small portion of the medial plantar fascia may be removed to facilitate exposure and clearly define the plane between the deep abductor fascia and the plantar fascia (Fig. 25-5). The superficial fascia of the abductor hallucis muscle is divided with a no. 15 blade scalpel, and the muscle is retracted superiorly or released (Fig. 25-6). A section of the deep fascia of the inferior abductor hallucis is removed directly over the area where the nerve is compressed between the taut fascia and the medial border of the quadratus plantae muscle (Figs. 25-7 and 25-8). The deep fascia of the abductor hallucis is then divided from the inferior to superior direction to sufficiently free the nerve from the entrapment (Fig. 25-9). Avoid injury to the first branch of the lateral plantar nerve coursing underneath the deep fascia. A heel spur, if present, can be removed, taking care to protect the nerve that runs superiorly (Fig. 25-10). The abductor hallucis muscle and most

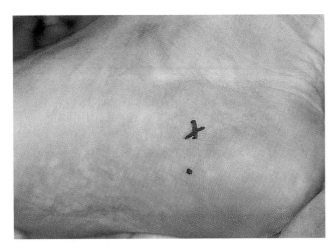

**Figure 25-1.** Medial heel. The point of maximum tenderness is marked on the skin.

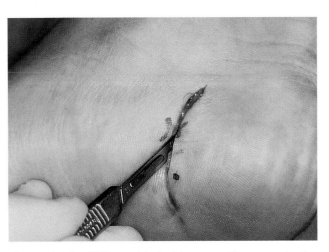

**Figure 25-2.** Oblique skin incision over the nerve to the abductor digiti quinti.

of its superficial fascia are left intact. The posterior tibial nerve more proximally in the tarsal tunnel is not explored.

If the plantar fascia is chronically inflamed and thickened, more of the proximal plantar fascia can be released or preferably resected if the patient has a component of plantar fasciitis. Partial fasciotomy of one third to one half of the fascia is generally preferred over complete fasciotomy. The recovery is longer with complete release of the fascia, and there is greater potential for arch instability. Even though the heel spur is not usually the cause of pain, it can be readily removed at the time of nerve and fascia release.

Patients with heel pain due to nerve compression benefit from releasing the nerve. In patients who have heel pain primarily from intractable plantar fasciitis rather than nerve compression, I usually release fascia and release the nerve to avoid a nerve compression that may occur as the fascia migrates distally.

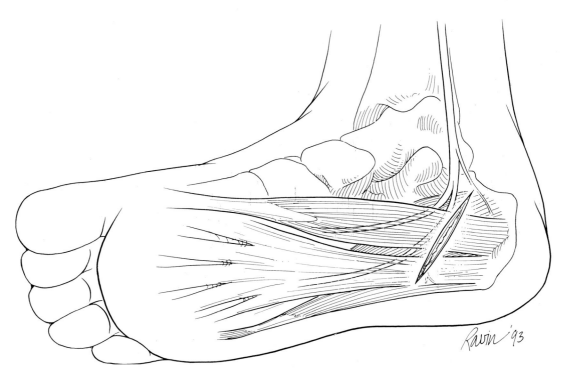

**Figure 25-3.** The relationship of the skin incision to the underlying bony structures.

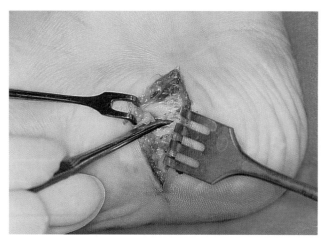

**Figure 25-4.** The interval between the plantar fascia and the investing fascia of the abductor hallucis muscle belly is developed.

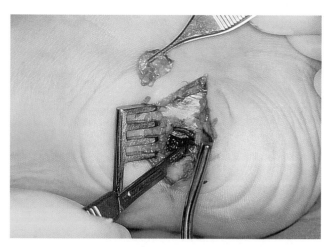

**Figure 25-5.** A portion of the plantar fascia is removed, exposing the quadratus plantae muscle deep to this structure.

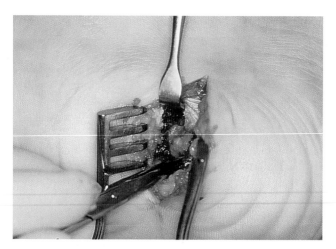

**Figure 25-6.** Retraction of the quadratus plantae muscle to the lateral aspect of the foot and the abductor hallucis muscle superiorly allows exposure of the nerve to the abductor digiti quinti.

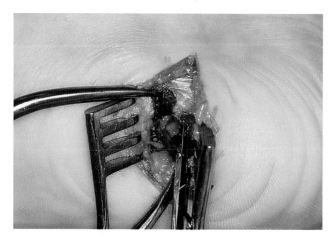

**Figure 25-7.** The undersurface of the abductor hallucis fascia tethers the nerve. The nerve to the abductor digiti quinti is released by removing a section of the deep fascia.

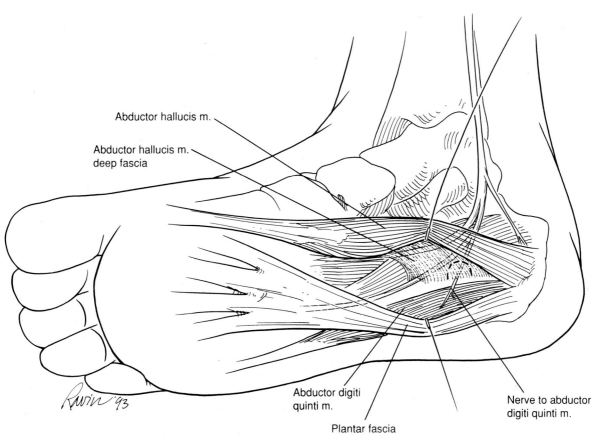

Abductor hallucis m.

Abductor hallucis m.
deep fascia

Abductor digiti
quinti m.

Plantar fascia

Nerve to abductor
digiti quinti m.

**Figure 25-8.** Removal of the fascia that tethers the nerve to the abductor digiti quinti.

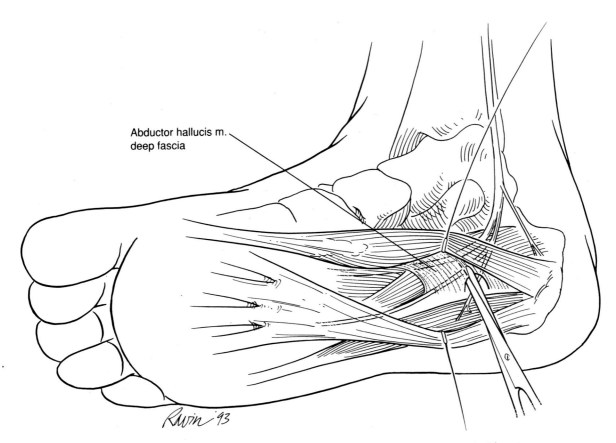

Abductor hallucis m.
deep fascia

**Figure 25-9.** The investing fascia on the undersurface of the abductor hallucis is released.

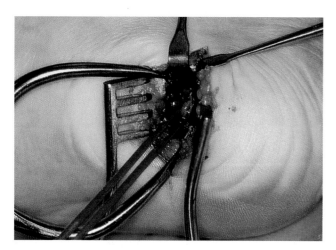

**Figure 25-10.** The nerve to the abductor digiti quinti is shown with the red retraction rubber. Care is taken to ensure this nerve is adequately released at the end of the procedure.

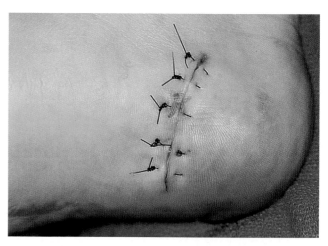

**Figure 25-11.** Careful skin closure, coapting the skin edges with nylon interrupted mattress sutures.

At the end of the operation, a small hemostat is used to palpate along the course of the nerve to confirm that it is free from any adhesions proximally or distally. The wound is closed with 4-0 nylon interrupted horizontal mattress sutures (Fig. 25-11). A bulky compressive dressing is applied to the foot and ankle.

## POSTOPERATIVE MANAGEMENT

Postoperatively, a bandage is maintained on the patient for 3 days. The patient is asked to elevate the foot for 2 days as much as possible, ambulating only for short periods. Crutches are generally used for 4 to 5 days. A postoperative shoe is used over the bandage for 2 weeks.

When the bandage is changed at 3 days, a smaller bandage is applied to the foot and ankle. Compression is continued for 2 weeks until the stitches are removed. At that time, the patient gradually discontinues the use of the bandage and progresses to a jogging shoe with a soft heel pad. At 3 weeks postoperatively, stationary bicycling is allowed. At 4 weeks, the patient is allowed to run or walk as tolerated. The average length of recovery is about 3 months. The recovery can extend as long as 6 months or be as short as 1 month; 3 months is a reasonable estimate.

The operative results of releasing the nerve to the abductor digiti quinti along with the associated aspects of this operation were reported by Baxter and Thigpen (2). In 34 operated heels, good results were obtained in 32 and poor results in 2. The patients with good results reported relief of the preoperative symptoms of pain. Those with poor results had continued difficulties with pain. Only 26 patients had this operative procedure performed over a 6-year period in which the senior author (D.E.B.) had a very busy practice, specializing in foot surgery.

Other investigators had favorable results of release of the nerve to the abductor digiti quinti. Sammarco et al. (12) reported results of neurolysis of the nerve to the abductor digiti quinti muscle combined with partial fasciotomy in patients who had failed nonoperative treatment for an average of 21 months. For 35 feet, results were excellent or good in 32 and fair in 3, and there were no failures. Baxter and Thigpen (2) updated his results of nerve release operations in 1992, and 61 (89%) of 69 feet had excellent or good results. Goecker and Banks (7) performed neurolysis in 18 feet, and all were considered successful. One half of the patients continued to have mild pain with extended activity. Over the past 15 years, this procedure has had a success rate of 92%. The procedure is used only when the diagnosis is compression of the nerve by the abductor digiti quinti.

## COMPLICATIONS

There are several notable complications of operative treatment of heel pain by release of the abductor digiti quinti nerve. Inadvertent transection of the medial calcaneal nerve branch to the medial aspect of the heel results in numbness along the medial and plantar aspect of the heel and hypersensitivity of the neuroma. This complication can be avoided by making the incision parallel to the course of these medial calcaneal nerve branches and by keen awareness of their location. Excessive dissection and bleeding in the wound may cause scarring about the nerve or in the skin. Meticulous hemostasis with or without the use of the tourniquet at the time of the operation is important. Using an adequate postoperative compression dressing and limiting the early weight bearing can lessen the potential of this complication occurring. Other branches from the lateral plantar nerve may be injured at the time of this surgical procedure, and being aware of nerve anatomy should obviate such a situation.

A potential complication from releasing too much of the plantar fascia and abductor muscle fascia is the development of a flatfoot. Theoretically, the soft tissues adjacent to the tibial nerve could compress the nerve when deformity develops, creating an iatrogenic tarsal tunnel syndrome. If this occurs, immobilization during the postoperative period in a short-leg walking cast can hold the foot in the proper position while the wound heals. Being careful to release only the proper amount of fascia about the abductor hallucis and just the medial portion of the plantar fascia limits the possibility of such a complication.

## RECOMMENDED READING

1. Baxter DE, Pfeffer GB: Treatment of chronic heel pain by surgical release of the first branch of the lateral plantar nerve. *Clin Orthop* 279:229–236, 1992.
2. Baxter DE, Thigpen CM: Heel pain—operative results. *Foot Ankle* 5:16–25, 1984.
3. Bordelon RL: Subcalcaneal pain: a method of evaluation and plan for treatment. *Clin Orthop* 177:49–53, 1983.
4. Davis PF, Severud E, Baxter DE: Painful heel syndrome: results of nonoperative treatment. *Foot Ankle* 15: 531–535, 1994.
5. Davis TJ, Schon LC: Branches of the tibial nerve: anatomic variations. *Foot Ankle* 16:21–29, 1995.
6. Flock TJ, Ishikawa S, Hecht PJ, et al.: Heel anatomy for retrograde tibiotalocalcaneal roddings: a roentgenographic and anatomic analysis. *Foot Ankle Int* 18:233–235, 1997.
7. Goecker RM, Banks AS: Analysis of release of first branch of the lateral plantar nerve. *J Am Podiatr Med Assoc* 90:281–286, 2000.
8. Graham CE: Painful heel syndrome: rationale of diagnosis and treatment. *Foot Ankle* 3:261–267, 1983.
9. Henricson AS, Westlin NE: Chronic calcaneal pain in athletes: entrapment of the calcaneal nerve? *Am J Sports Med* 12:152–154, 1984.
10. Lutter LD: Surgical decisions in athletes' subcalcaneal pain. *Am J Sports Med* 14:481–485, 1986.
11. Rondhuis JJ, Huson A: The first branch of the lateral plantar nerve and heel pain. *Acta Morphol Neerl Scand* 24:269–279, 1986.
12. Sammarco GJ, Helfrey RB: Surgical treatment of recalcitrant plantar fasciitis. *Foot Ankle Int* 17:520–526, 1996.
13. Schon LC, Baxter DE: Neuropathies of the foot and ankle in athletes. *Clin Sports Med* 9:489–509, 1990.
14. Schon LC, Glennan TP, Baxter DE: Heel pain syndrome: electrodiagnostic support for nerve entrapment. *Foot Ankle* 14:129–135, 1993.

# 26

# Calcaneal Prominence Resection

Carol Frey

## INDICATIONS/CONTRAINDICATIONS

In 1928, Patrick Haglund reported the clinical condition of retrocalcaneal bursitis and described a calcaneus with a prominent posterior-superior border that compressed the Achilles tendon and its surrounding bursa against the posterior shoe counter, causing irritation. Retrocalcaneal bursitis can be the result of a prominent or sharply angled posterior-superior margin of the calcaneus.

The main indication for surgery is a painful bony prominence in the retrocalcaneal region that is not adequately relieved by 6 months of nonoperative management. The goal of surgery is to eliminate pain by relieving pressure from the underlying prominent bone.

Contraindications are a prominence with an infection, open wound, blister, and a dysvascular extremity. Surgery is not indicated in a patient with minimum symptoms or whose main concern is addressing the cosmetic appearance of the foot.

## PREOPERATIVE PLANNING

With the patient in a prone position on the examining table and resting the foot in the examiner's hand, the index finger and thumb are used to palpate the medial and lateral aspects of the posterior-superior tuberosity of the calcaneus. When inflammation of the retrocalcaneal bursa is present, a soft mass is felt bulging on both sides of the Achilles tendon that is painful when palpated. Dorsiflexion of the foot, which compresses the bursa between the tendon and the bone, also causes pain. On external inspection, loss of the skin lines due to distension of the retrocalcaneal bursa may be evident. In severe cases, erythema and warmth may also be present. Signs of retrocalcaneal bursitis differ from insertional Achilles tendonitis, in which there is tenderness several centimeters proximal to the tendon attachment.

C. Frey, M.D.: Department of Orthopaedic Surgery, University of California, Los Angeles; Foot and Ankle Surgery, West Coast Sports Performance, Manhattan Beach, California.

On a standing, lateral radiograph of the heel, a thin strip of fat can be identified between the tendon and the bone proximal to the insertion of the Achilles tendon. The anterior aspect of the Achilles tendon is sharply outlined throughout its extent by the pre-Achilles fat pad (PAFP). Retrocalcaneal bursitis is indicated when the sharp definition of the retrocalcaneal recess is lost and the lucency of the PAFP in this region is replaced by soft tissue density. The distended fluid-filled bursa often projects above the calcaneus and into the PAFP. Erosion of the cortex of posterior-superior aspect of the calcaneus may be evident with retrocalcaneal bursitis. A thickening of the tendon and a loss of its sharp anterior interface with the PAFP denotes Achilles tendonitis.

Plain, weight-bearing radiographs of the foot (i.e., anteroposterior, lateral, and oblique views) are important to rule out other causes of hindfoot pain such as a stress fracture, chronic infection, or tumor. Numerous radiologic measurements can be made on plain radiographs, such as the total angle of Ruch, parallel pitch lines, calcaneal inclination angle, Fowler and Philip angle (i.e., posterior calcaneal angle). No radiologic criteria used for the diagnosis of Haglund's disease has been absolutely reliable. Schneider et al. (9) found that formerly published angular threshold of radiologic calcaneal angles could not be confirmed to be predictors for the preoperative symptoms or the postoperative outcome. The patient's history and physical symptoms are most important in surgical decision making.

The anatomy of the retrocalcaneal bursa (Fig. 26-1) can be demonstrated with bursogra-

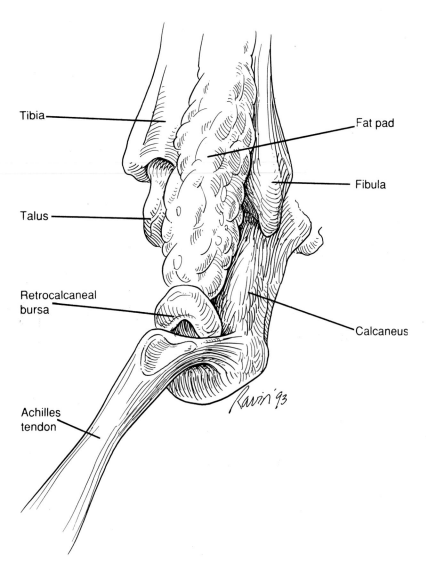

**Figure 26-1.** The Achilles tendon has been turned down, and the horseshoe-shaped retrocalcaneal bursa and the fat pad anterior to the Achilles tendon are seen.

phy, but magnetic resonance imaging (MRI) is more helpful in demonstrating anatomy and in differentiating retrocalcaneal bursitis from Achilles tendinitis. Accurate recognition of these entities is necessary for proper management. On the MRI scan, the retrocalcaneal bursa is a potential space that is most clearly demarcated when inflamed. MRI is recommended only for cases in which making a definitive diagnosis is difficult.

Initial treatment for "Haglund's syndrome" is nonoperative and includes nonsteroidal antiinflammatory medications, heel lifts, soft heel counters, and a backless shoe. A running athlete with this problem is instructed to decrease mileage and to stop training on hills and hard surfaces. Because the problem can be aggravated if the heel counter irritates the posterior heel, external pressure should be decreased. This can be done by removing or softening the heel counter or by adding a small internal heel lift to elevate the heel away from the shoe counter. Alternatively, a heel cup can be used to pad the area. Tight calf muscles, tight hamstrings, or a cavus foot may be associated with a symptomatic Haglund's deformity. Achilles tendon stretching is encouraged. If a problem such as a cavus foot is seen on physical examination, appropriate orthotic devices can be prescribed.

If the above measures are not successful, immobilization in a short-leg walking cast often reduces acute symptoms. Corticosteroid injections are not routinely performed because fluid can leak out of an inflamed bursa into the paratendonous structures of the Achilles tendon, even if placed into the bursa under image control.

Most patients respond to nonoperative treatment within 6 months. After this period, surgery can be considered.

## SURGERY

Operations such as calcaneal osteotomy have been described, but the preferred approach is resection of the superior prominence of the calcaneus along with associated bursal tissue. A medial and lateral incision along the Achilles tendon can be used for resection of the superior prominence, although complete resection can usually be carried out using just a lateral incision. A single lateral incision decreases the incidence of wound problems as well as the possibility of injury to the medial calcaneal sensory nerve.

### Open Technique

The patient is placed in the prone position, with a bolster placed under the distal leg (Fig. 26-2). An 8-cm, longitudinal incision is made just anterior to the Achilles tendon on the lat-

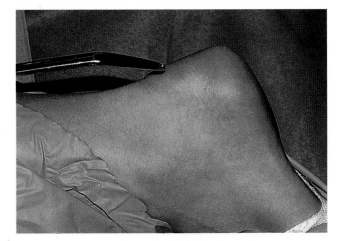

**Figure 26-2.** At the time of operation, with the patient in a prone position, the prominence of the posterior aspect of the calcaneus is at the end of the surgical instrument.

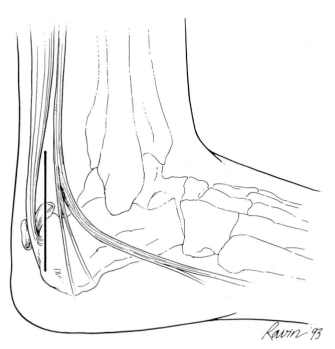

**Figure 26-3.** An incision is made along the lateral aspect of the heel, centered over the posterior-superior tuberosity of the calcaneus. The Achilles tendon bursa is superficial to the tendon incision, and the retrocalcaneal bursa is deep to the tendon.

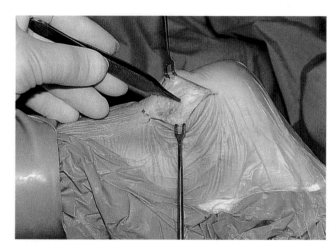

**Figure 26-4.** The thumb forceps shows the prominent posterolateral aspect of the superior calcaneus.

eral side of the heel (Fig. 26-3). The retrocalcaneal area and the superior aspect of the calcaneus (Fig. 26-4) are exposed by a combination of blunt and sharp dissection, being careful to avoid the sural nerve, which lies approximately 6 mm anterior to the lateral border of the Achilles tendon. Retracting it anteriorly with the subcutaneous tissues should protect the sural nerve. The incision is carried down to the bone, making sure that the insertion site is adequately exposed (Fig. 26-5). If there is extensive inflammation of the retrocalcaneal bursa, the bursal tissue should be removed. Removal of the bursal tissue is not as important as adequate decompression of the posterior calcaneal prominence. This decompression is carried out using an oblique osteotomy of the superior angle of the calcaneus starting approximately 1.5 cm anterior to the posterior border of the calcaneus and angling downward

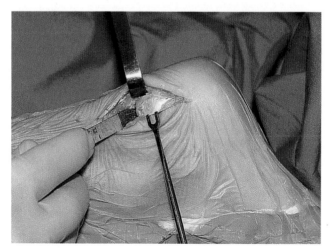

**Figure 26-5.** Subperiosteal dissection of the tuberosity of the calcaneus is done all the way to its medial side.

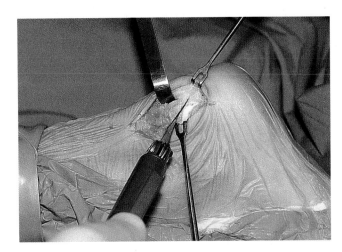

**Figure 26-6.** A saw is used to resect the posterior aspect of the calcaneus from the insertion of the Achilles tendon at about a 45° oblique angle to the superior aspect of the posterior calcaneus.

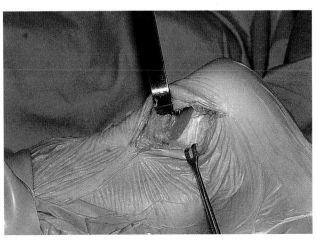

**Figure 26-7.** The amount of bone resected can be seen in the depths of the wound.

to the insertion of the Achilles tendon (approximately 2 cm distal to the superior margin of the calcaneus) (Fig. 26-5). The osteotomy is performed with a power saw, approximately perpendicular to the longitudinal axis of the calcaneus (Fig. 26-6). A ridge of bone is always left at the insertion site of the Achilles tendon and must be carefully removed with a small curette and microreciprocating rasp.

To successfully decompress the retrocalcaneal space, adequate bone must be removed. Bone can be removed up to the insertion site of the Achilles tendon. Do not leave a ledge or spike of bone near the insertion site of the Achilles tendon, because it may become painful and a source of irritation to the Achilles tendon.

The microreciprocating rasp is also helpful in rounding off the margins of the calcaneus in all directions, especially on the medial side. If the medial ridge still cannot be reached adequately, a medial incision could be added, but this is rarely necessary.

The area of the calcaneal prominence is repeatedly palpated through the overlying skin to make certain that all ridges and prominences are removed. The wedge of bone removed must be of adequate size to ensure thorough decompression of the retrocalcaneal area (Fig. 26-7). The Achilles tendon does not insert at the superior aspect of the calcaneus but significantly more inferior in the apophyseal portion of the calcaneus. The Achilles tendon sweeps backward and away from the tibia to meet the inclined calcaneus obliquely, with the bone and the tendon forming an acute angle. By resecting bone down to the insertion site of the Achilles tendon, adequate decompression of the retrocalcaneal space can usually be obtained (Fig. 26-8).

It is possible to remove too much distal bone and cut into the insertion of the Achilles tendon. This could allow the tendon to avulse later. Careful exposure of the insertion site of the Achilles tendon at the time of surgery should help the surgeon avoid this pitfall. In the case of a markedly enlarged calcaneal prominence, the lateral margin of the Achilles tendon may be raised to allow for the prominence to be removed. The margin of the tendon attachment can be repaired with nonabsorbable suture passed through drill holes in the calcaneus. Some surgeons feel it is safe to raise as much as 2 cm of the tendon insertion to resect the appropriate amount of bone.

The Achilles tendon should be inspected for tendinosis. A longitudinal incision is carefully made with a scalpel in the anterior 50% of the tendon and often reveals necrotic areas of tendon that require debridement. After the tendon is debrided, it is repaired with buried 3-0 nonabsorbable suture such as Ethibond.

Inspection of the resected portion of the posterior-superior process of the calcaneus (Figs. 26-9 and 26-10) sometimes shows the eburnation of the posterior-superior aspect of the calcaneus caused by the Achilles tendon. This aspect of the calcaneal tuberosity almost has a cartilaginous appearance to it, particularly with prolonged inflammation. The wound is closed routinely in layers.

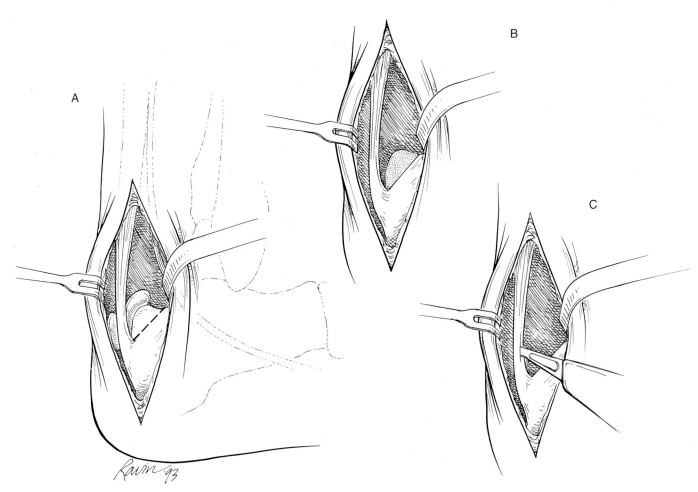

**Figure 26-8. A-C:** The amount of bone resected along with the associated retrocalcaneal bursa is illustrated. An incision in the Achilles tendon can be made to remove heterotopic calcification if this is a significant source of symptoms.

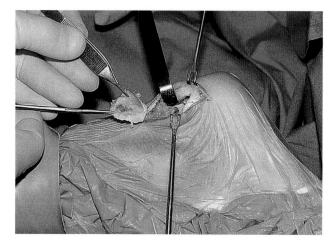

**Figure 26-9.** The excised tuberosity of the calcaneus is shown beside the surgical wound.

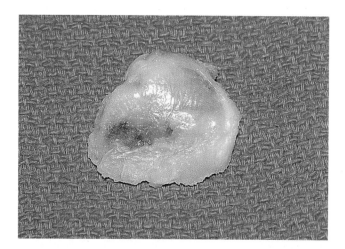

**Figure 26-10.** A close-up view of the excised tuberosity shows the result of chronic irritation of the calcaneus. Eburnation and hemorrhage of the bone is seen.

## Endoscopic Technique

The retrocalcaneal space may be approached endoscopically. As with the open procedures, to perform the endoscopic procedure well, the anatomy of the retrocalcaneal space should be understood. The superficial anatomy of the posterior aspect of the hindfoot is not complex. The medial and lateral borders of the Achilles tendon are easily palpated. The posterior-superior aspect of the calcaneus is also readily located. The Achilles tendon inserts on the posterior margin of the calcaneus, approximately 2 cm distal to its posterior-superior margin. The sural nerve runs, on average, 7 mm anterior to the anterior margin of the Achilles tendon. Care must be taken when making a portal medially, because the calcaneal branches of the lateral plantar nerve are at risk for injury in this region. The location of even a small portal in this area can cause a long period of postoperative tenderness aggravated by a firm heel counter when the patient returns to footwear.

Endoscopic calcaneoplasty is undertaken with the patient in a prone position, with a "bump" under the ankle, or in the lateral decubitus position. Medial and lateral portals are created just above the superior aspect of the calcaneus, medial and lateral to the Achilles tendon (Fig. 26-11). A 2.7-mm arthroscope and small joint instrumentation are used inter-

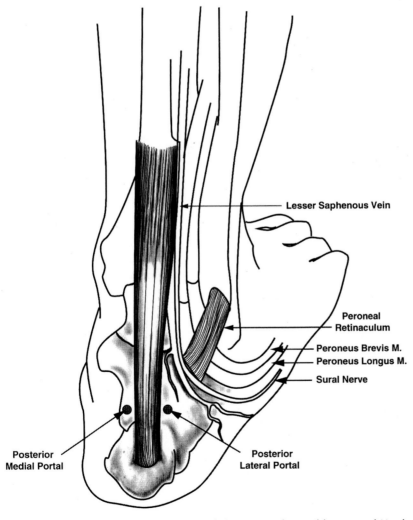

Lesser Saphenous Vein

Peroneal Retinaculum

Peroneus Brevis M.

Peroneus Longus M.

Sural Nerve

Posterior Medial Portal

Posterior Lateral Portal

A

**Figure 26-11. A:** Endoscopic debridement of the retrocalcaneal bursa and Haglund's deformity. *(continued)*

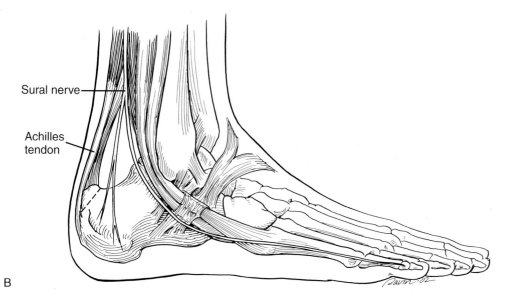

Sural nerve

Achilles tendon

B

**Figure 26-11.** *Continued.* **B:** Endoscopic debridement of the retrocalcaneal bursa and Haglund's deformity.

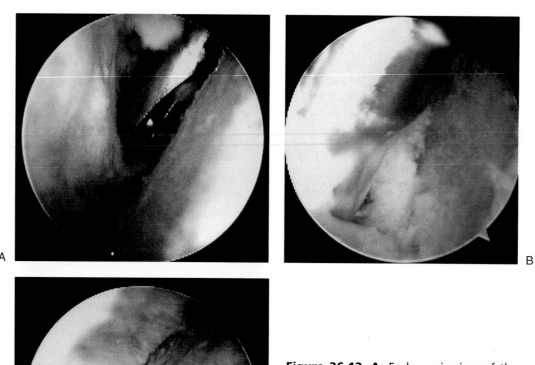

A

B

C

**Figure 26-12. A:** Endoscopic view of the calcaneal prominences *(right)* and Achilles tendon attachment *(left)*. The shaver and arthroscope are inserted into retrocalcaneal bursa using portals created just medial and lateral to the Achilles tendon and just above the superior aspect of the calcaneus. **B:** The posterior cortex of the calcaneus is removed starting posterosuperiorly and moving inferiorly 2 to 4 cm toward the superior attachment of the tendon. **C:** View after endoscopic calcaneoplasty shows reduction in the calcaneal prominence *(right)*.

changeably through these portals. A full-radius synovial shaver is used to remove the bursa. The endoscopic procedure allows removal of the posterior cortex of the calcaneus with a small acromionizer or abrader starting at the posterior-superior aspect of the calcaneus and progressing inferiorly 2 to 4 cm toward the superior attachment of the Achilles tendon (Fig. 26-12). Some surgeons continue to remove the prominence as much as 2 cm beyond the superior insertion of the tendon. It is important to dorsiflex the ankle to check for further impingement. No complications have been reported with these incisions.

## POSTOPERATIVE MANAGEMENT

The patient is placed into a short-leg, non–weight-bearing cast with the foot in mild plantarflexion for the first 1 to 2 weeks, depending on the amount of involvement of the Achilles tendon. He or she is then placed into the short-leg walking cast with the foot gradually repositioned up to neutral position for the next 2 weeks. When the cast is removed, the patient is placed into a shoe with a $^7/_{16}$-inch, tapered internal heel lift that is gradually reduced to $^3/_{16}$ of an inch, and this is worn for 3 months. General muscle conditioning is begun when the cast is removed.

The recovery period for the open operative procedure can be 3 to 6 months. After that period, full activity may be resumed.

## COMPLICATIONS

Possible *nerve damage* includes injury to the sural nerve laterally or the posterior tibial nerve or its branches medially. This can be avoided by incision placement, using careful dissection technique, and controlling the position of the saw blade.

*Wound problems* are a source of worry around the Achilles tendon and great care should be taken when handling the soft tissues and posterior skin. Maintaining full-thickness skin flaps is recommended. Ankle stiffness and pain and persistent heel pain have been reported.

Removing too much bone at the insertion of the Achilles tendon may result in avulsion of the tendon. Removing insufficient bone from the posterior-superior aspect of the calcaneus may result in inadequate decompression of the retrocalcaneal bursa and persistent pain. In an effort to provide guidelines for how much tendon may be detached without risking rupture, Kolodziej et al. (7) performed a cadaver study and concluded that as much as 50% of the Achilles tendon may be resected safely.

The protracted recovery period may be a source of dissatisfaction. Patients should be advised preoperatively. Residual symptoms may also be concerning.

Sammarco and Taylor (8) reported results of 39 feet that underwent excision of the posterior calcaneal tuberosity and reattachment of the Achilles tendon with bone anchors. The investigators reported a rate of 97% excellent or good results with an average of 3 years follow-up. Complications included one recurrence of painful prominence, one wound infection, and one incisional neuroma. After 2 years of follow-up, Jarde et al. (5) reported the results of resection in 74 feet, with excellent or good results in 73%, fair in 16%, and poor in 11%. Schneider et al. (9) found that complete relief of symptoms after resection was achieved in 34 (69%) of 49 feet and that the course of rehabilitation averaged 6 months.

## ILLUSTRATIVE CASE

A 22-year-old woman described pain in the posterior-lateral aspect of her heel. Although high-heeled shoes tended to be the most aggravating, she had pain even with low-heeled, lace-up shoes because of the irritation of the posterior aspect of the lateral calcaneus (Fig.

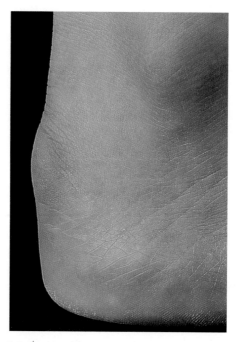

**Figure 26-13.** Profile view of the posterior calcaneus shows the bony prominence posterior and lateral to the Achilles tendon.

26-13). This restricted her work and recreational activities, and she sought permanent relief.

Resection of the posterior-superior tuberosity of the calcaneus along with associated bursal inflammation was done (Fig. 26-14). Two years later, she was asymptomatic on this side, but was starting to develop pain in the opposite heel region and thought she would have a similar procedure done on that side.

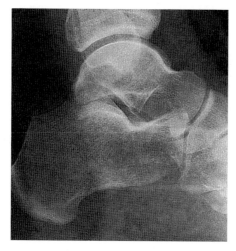

**Figure 26-14.** Appearance of the posterior calcaneus after excision of the posterior-superior aspect.

## RECOMMENDED READING

1. Fiamengo S, Warren RF, Marshall JL, et al.: Posterior heel pain associated with a calcaneal step and Achilles tendon calcification. *Clin Orthop* 167:203–211, 1982.
2. Fowler A, Philip JF: Abnormality of the calcaneus as a cause of painful heel. *Br J Surg* 32:494, 1945.
3. Frey C, Rosenberg Z, Shereff MJ, et al.: The retrocalcaneal bursa: anatomy and bursography. *Foot Ankle* 13: 203–207, 1992.
4. Heneghan MA, Pavlov H: The Haglund painful heel syndrome: experimental investigation of cause and therapeutic implications. *Clin Orthop* 187:228–234, 1984.
5. Jarde O, Quenot P, Trinquier-Lautard JL, et al.: Haglund disease treated by simple resection of calcaneal tuberosity: an angular and therapeutic study, apropos of 74 cases with 2 year follow-up. *Rev Chir Orthop Reparatrice Appar Mot* 83:566–573, 1997.
6. Keck S, Kelley P: Bursitis of the posterior part of the heel. *J Bone Joint Surg Am* 47:267, 1965.
7. Kolodziej P, Glisson R, Nunley JA: Risk of avulsion of the Achilles tendon after partial excision for treatment of insertional tendonitis and Haglund's deformity: a biomechanical study. *Foot Ankle Int* 20:433–437, 1999.
8. Sammarco GJ, Taylor AL: Operative management of Haglund's deformity in the non-athlete: a retrospective study. *Foot Ankle Int* 19:724–729, 1998.
9. Schneider W, Niehus W, Knahr W: Haglund's syndrome: disappointing results following surgery—a clinical and radiological analysis. *Foot Ankle Int* 21:26–30, 2000.

# 27

# Medial Displacement Osteotomy of the Calcaneus and Flexor Digitorum Longus Transfer

Roger A. Mann and Gregory P. Guyton

## INDICATIONS/CONTRAINDICATIONS

The indication for a medial displacement calcaneal osteotomy with a flexor digitorum longus (FDL) transfer is a patient with painful posterior tibial tendon dysfunction (PTTD) with a flexible flatfoot deformity. The osteotomy is designed to enhance the correction of the deformity and improve the longevity of a simultaneously performed FDL tendon transfer (4). The indications for operative intervention are identical to those for the FDL tendon transfer alone, but the osteotomy can be used to improve the posture of the foot in patients with a flexible deformity and increased hindfoot valgus (i.e., PTTD stage II deformity) (4,7,11,12).

The FDL transfer alone can have a satisfactory clinical result over the short term, but it rarely results in a significant change in the posture of the longitudinal arch (2,5,10). There have also been concerns about the longevity of the FDL transfer alone when the arch remains uncorrected. As an isolated procedure, the FDL transfer continues to be useful in the management of recalcitrant posterior tibial tendinosis that has not progressed to a pes planus deformity (i.e., PTTD stage I). For patients with any detectable degree of deformity, adding a calcaneal osteotomy to the procedure confers a degree of mechanical protection to the tendon transfer while incurring little operative morbidity or additional recovery time.

The medial displacement osteotomy functions through static and dynamic mechanisms. Simplistically, a flatfoot can be viewed as a tripod in which one leg is collapsed: the hind leg of the tripod corresponds to the heel, and the two medial/lateral legs correspond to each border of the forefoot. If the hind leg of the tripod has fallen too far to the lateral side, the entire construct will sag medially. The medial displacement calcaneal osteotomy is analo-

---

R. A. Mann, M.D.: Foot Fellowship Program, Private Practice, Oakland, California.

G. P. Guyton, M.D.: Departments of Orthopaedic Surgery and Orthopaedics, University of North Carolina at Chapel Hill, Chapel Hill, North Carolina.

gous to restoring this posterior leg back into position, thereby raising the arch on the medial side. This is an old concept, first proposed in 1893 by Gleich (3) and later extended to the adolescent flatfoot in the modern literature by Koutsogiannis (6).

A dynamic mechanism for the function of the medial displacement osteotomy has also been proposed (11,12). When the hindfoot sags into valgus, the line of pull of the Achilles tendon moves laterally, which tends to pull the calcaneus further into valgus and accentuate the deformity. The osteotomy brings the Achilles insertion back toward the midline. Although this mechanism is not responsible for the radiographic improvement in the arch, it may play a role in reducing the forces on the transferred FDL tendon.

The contraindications for the procedure are identical to those for the FDL tendon transfer alone (4,11,12) and include a rigid flatfoot, hindfoot arthritis, peripheral neuropathy, infection, and dysvascular foot. The foot must be flexible for the procedure to succeed. The subtalar joint must be at least able to invert 15° to 20°, and there must not be a fixed varus deformity of more than 10° to 15° of the forefoot relative to the hindfoot. Forefoot varus is a fixed torsional deformity through the midfoot that occurs with long-standing deformity; the forefoot accommodates to balance the valgus malalignment of the hindfoot to maintain the foot in a plantigrade position (8). In a fixed varus deformity, the lateral border of the foot is more plantarflexed than the medial border when the heel is manually corrected to neutral by the examiner.

Other surgical options for the treatment of the adult flatfoot exist and may be more appropriate for a given patient. Rigid deformities of the hindfoot or forefoot must be addressed with a triple arthrodesis; by taking down the transverse tarsal joint, the forefoot can be derotated relative to the position of the hindfoot. Even in flexible deformities, a subtalar arthrodesis combined with debridement of the tendon can be used to bypass the posterior tibial tendon and control the hindfoot (9). Although much of the ability of the foot to accommodate to uneven ground is lost, an isolated subtalar arthrodesis is very durable and does not incur a major risk of causing symptomatic arthritis in the adjacent joints. More importantly, subtalar fusion is a very reliable procedure in the nonsmoking patient, and the length of time to maximum recovery is much shorter than that of the FDL transfer with or without calcaneal osteotomy (1). The durability and dramatically shortened rehabilitation period make subtalar fusion an attractive option for patients older than 70 years of age or who are morbidly obese.

Lateral column lengthening represents another conceptual approach to the correction of the adult flatfoot. Over the middle term, the results of flatfoot correction by performing a distraction arthrodesis through the calcaneocuboid joint in conjunction with an FDL transfer have been satisfactory and roughly equivalent to those reported for FDL transfer with a medial displacement calcaneal osteotomy (13). The appropriate indications for choosing one approach over another remain controversial, and long-term follow-up data are not yet available. No factors have been identified that can clearly delineate a group of patients who would benefit from one procedure over another. Distraction arthrodesis of the calcaneocuboid joint does have some disadvantages in the early perioperative period, including the partial loss of hindfoot motion, the necessity for bone graft, a relatively high rate of nonunion and hardware prominence, and a tendency to exacerbate mild degrees of fixed forefoot varus during the correction. By comparison, the minimal morbidity associated with a medial displacement calcaneal osteotomy makes it more attractive as an adjunct to FDL transfer based on the available data. Not all cases of PTTD are identical, and future work may identify patients in whom lateral column lengthening is more appropriate.

## PREOPERATIVE PLANNING

The physical examination is important for the patient who presents with a painful flatfoot. The medial displacement calcaneal osteotomy with FDL transfer will fail in the presence of limited subtalar inversion or a fixed forefoot varus of more than 15°. Conversely, a patient without any significant deformity who has isolated PTTD may be well served by an FDL transfer alone.

PTTD is not the only cause of the pes planus deformity in the adult. Arthrosis of the medial tarsometatarsal joints is often accompanied by collapse of the longitudinal arch, and special attention should be paid to determine that the deformity originates at the hindfoot level rather than the midfoot. Neurologic dysfunction and peroneal spasticity should be ruled out, and the vascular status of the foot should be examined.

Obtaining a thorough history from the patient regarding the nature of the problem and the impairment of activities can help determine what type of treatment is optimal. Symptoms can be dramatically improved in some patients using an ankle-foot orthosis or a reinforced, leather ankle lacer. Other nonoperative treatments that should be considered for PTTD include nonsteroidal antiinflammatory medications, activity modifications, and cast immobilization. Corticosteroid injection is generally not recommended.

The decision to undertake surgery should not be taken lightly. Recovery from FDL transfer is remarkably slow; our data indicate the median time to (self-reported) maximal medical improvement is 10 months.

Radiographic evaluation consists of weight-bearing radiographs of the foot, including anteroposterior, lateral, and oblique views. In cases of PTTD, the anteroposterior radiograph reveals increased abduction of the foot with increased exposure of the talar head (uncovered talar head) as the axes of the talus and calcaneus diverge. On the lateral view, the talonavicular joint sags and can be measured by the angle between the axis of the talus and the axis of the first metatarsal (i.e., talometatarsal angle).

## SURGERY

Surgery consists of two separate procedures: a medial displacement osteotomy and a FDL transfer. The osteotomy is routinely done first to allow the foot to be immediately immobilized on completion of the FDL transfer.

### Technique: Medial Displacement Calcaneal Osteotomy

The patient is placed on the operating table, with a large "bump" under the ipsilateral hip to facilitate access to the lateral side of the foot. A thigh tourniquet is used to avoid compressing the muscle belly of the FDL, which must be transferred in the second stage of the procedure. The skin incision begins 1 cm posterior to the fibular border at the level of the superior border of the calcaneus. It is carried distally in line with the fibula to the plantar surface of the calcaneus. It usually ends just above the beginning of the glabrous skin (Fig. 27-1). The incision is deepened through the subcutaneous tissue, taking care to identify the

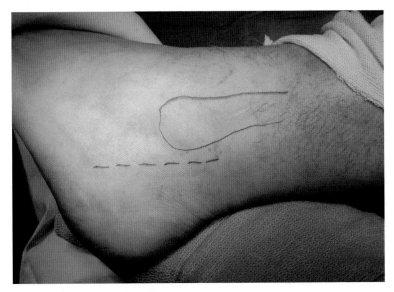

**Figure 27-1.** Lateral view of the lower extremity shows a hindfoot skin incision for calcaneal osteotomy.

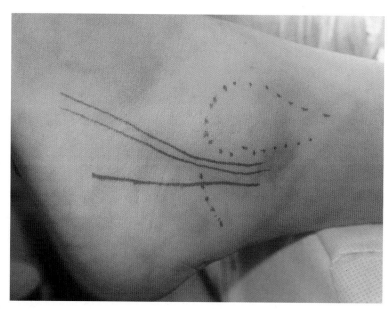

**Figure 27-2.** The sural nerve *(outlined)* usually lies anterior to the skin incision.

sural nerve and its branches, which are usually mobilized anteriorly (Figs. 27-2 through 27-3). Occasionally, the entire nerve lies just above the incision, but this finding is not consistent, and caution should be exercised when making the incision. The peroneal sheath may be encountered and should be left *in situ*.

The osteotomy is carried out posterior to the peroneal tubercle. The incision is deepened to bone using a periosteal elevator. Only 2 to 3 mm on each side of the line of the proposed osteotomy needs to be dissected, which is considerably less than that required for a Dwyer closing wedge osteotomy because no bone is removed (Fig. 27-4).

A microsagittal saw is used to scribe a line on the calcaneus from a location roughly 1 cm posterior to the posterior facet of the subtalar joint, vertically to the inferior border of the tuberosity. The osteotomy is carried down through the bone using the saw. Extreme

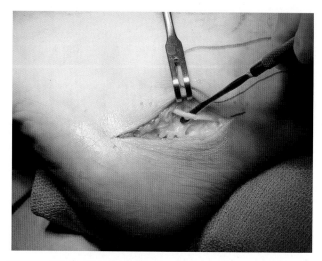

**Figure 27-3.** The incision is deepened, retracting the sural nerve anteriorly and leaving peroneal sheath *in situ*. The osteotomy is typically posterior to the peroneal tubercle.

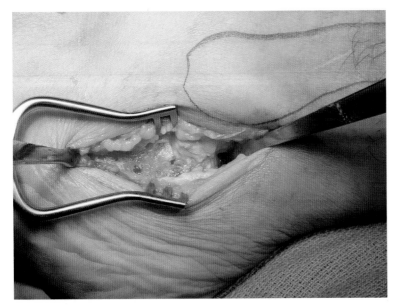

**Figure 27-4.** The incision is carried down to bone, and then a periosteal elevator is used to carefully dissect only 3 mm on each side of the line of the proposed osteotomy.

caution should be taken to avoid overpenetration of the medial side to avoid injuring the neurovascular bundle (Figs. 27-5 and 27-6). A 25-mm osteotome is inserted into the osteotomy site to gently pry it apart. A smooth lamina spreader is then inserted and left in a distracted position for at least a minute to further loosen the tissues about the osteotomy (Fig. 27-7). A Cobb elevator can be used to carefully reach through to the medial side and further free the soft tissue attachments.

The calcaneus is then displaced medially by approximately 1 cm. To accomplish this, the foot is plantarflexed to relieve tension across the osteotomy site. After the tuberosity is displaced medially, the foot is dorsiflexed. The pull of the Achilles tendon and plantar fascia tends to "lock" the fragment in place. Usually, approximately 1 cm of displacement

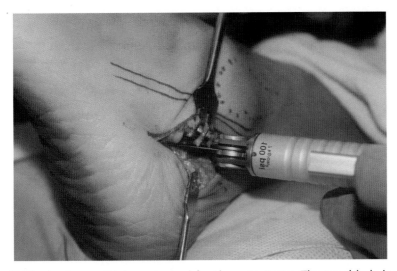

**Figure 27-5.** A microsagittal saw is used for the osteotomy. The saw blade is used to scribe a line on the calcaneus 1 cm posterior to the margin of the posterior facet in the same orientation as the original skin incision.

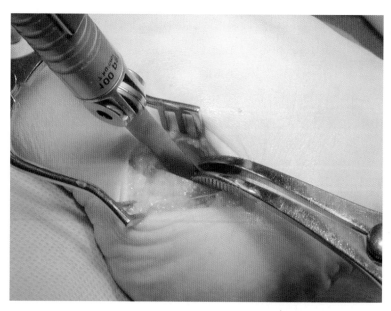

**Figure 27-6.** The osteotomy is performed with caution to avoid overpenetration of the medial cortex to avert injuring the neurovascular bundle.

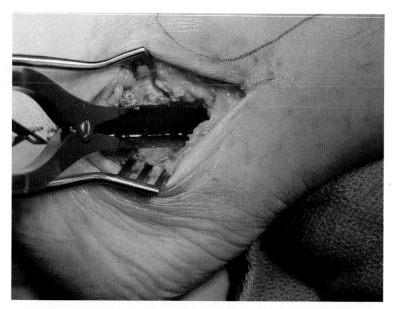

**Figure 27-7.** The osteotomy can be gently "sprung" open using a smooth laminar spreader to visualize the completion of the cut on the medial wall of the calcaneus. The osteotomy is gently distracted to mobilize the soft tissue attachment with a 25-mm osteotome, smooth lamina spreader, and Cobb elevator. Holding the osteotomy distracted for 1 to 2 minutes with the laminar spreader can facilitate mobilization of the tuberosity fragment.

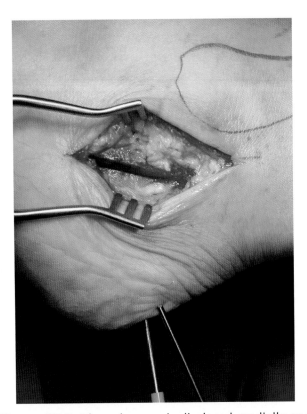

**Figure 27-8.** The calcaneus is displaced medially and temporarily fixed with a 0.062-inch Kirschner wire from posterior to anterior. The typical displacement is about 1 cm; it is difficult to overdisplace the fragment. Posteriorly, a 1-cm, longitudinal incision is made lateral to the Achilles tendon, and a guide pin for a cannulated screw is placed across the osteotomy into the anterior process of the calcaneus midway between the plantar and dorsal bony surfaces.

can be achieved. It is essentially impossible to overdisplace the osteotomy (Figs. 27-8 and 27-9).

The osteotomy position is temporarily maintained with a 0.062-inch or larger Kirschner wire driven from posterior to anterior, just medial to the Achilles tendon. A 1-cm, longitudinal incision is made just lateral to the Achilles tendon, approximately 2 cm above the plantar surface of the calcaneus. A hemostat is used to spread longitudinally down to bone, and the guide pin for a 6.5- to 7.3-mm cannulated screw is advanced across the osteotomy site toward the lateral portion of the calcaneus. Optimal placement of the pin is in the anterior process of the calcaneus, midway between the plantar and dorsal surfaces. A 6.5- to 7.3-mm, cannulated screw is inserted across the osteotomy site. The osteotomy position, fixation placement, and bony apposition are checked radiographically. A partially threaded screw is typically used, but because the large surface area of the osteotomy does not require a perfect lag technique to heal, a fully threaded screw may also be used if additional stability is desired (Fig. 27-10 and 27-11). In most patients, the bone on the posterior aspect of the tuberosity is dense enough to support the head of the screw, and a washer is not required. If additional stabilization is required, a 0.125-inch Steinmann pin can be added.

The wound is then irrigated and closed in layers using a 3-0 absorbable suture for the subcutaneous tissues and staples or nylon on the skin (Fig. 27-12).

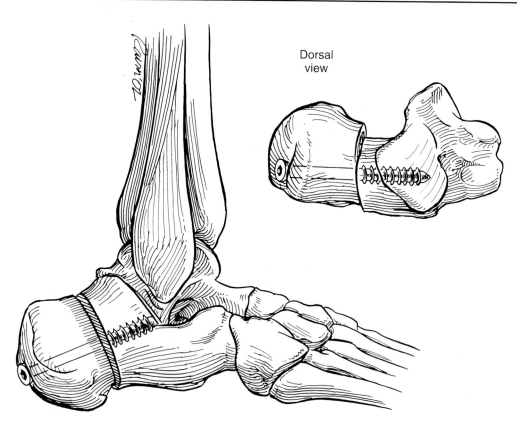

Dorsal
view

**Figure 27-9.** Displacement of the osteotomy and proper screw placement are illustrated.

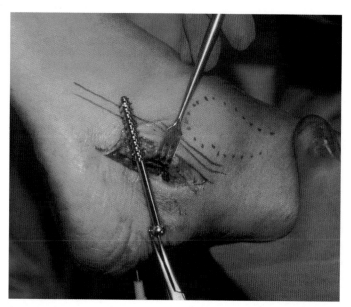

**Figure 27-10.** A 7.0-mm, partially threaded, cannulated screw is inserted across the osteotomy in the orientation shown.

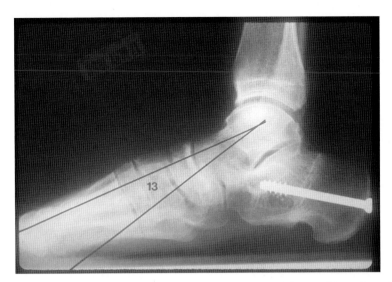

**Figure 27-11.** Radiograph demonstrates proper screw position and location of the osteotomy.

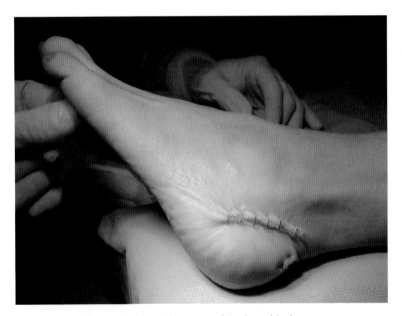

**Figure 27-12.** The wound is closed in layers.

## Technique: Flexor Digitorum Longus Transfer

The bump is removed from the ipsilateral hip, allowing the patient to become supine on the operating table. The foot externally rotates, which enhances the approach to the medial aspect of the foot (Fig. 27-13). An incision is made from the tip of the medial malleolus and is carried distally approximately 1 cm distal to the insertion of the posterior tibial tendon into the medial aspect of the navicular and along the dorsal aspect of the posterior tibial tendon. The posterior tibial tendon sheath is opened and the tendon inspected. The surgeon usually observes increased fluid and an area of tendinosis and fissuring, often associated with proliferative synovitis (Fig. 27-14).

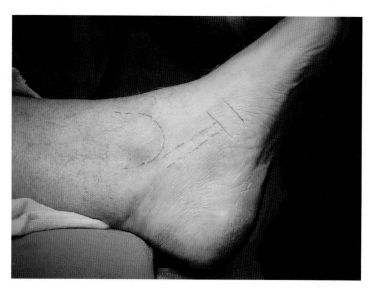

**Figure 27-13.** Medial view of the foot demonstrates the distal course of the posterior tibial tendon.

After carefully evaluating the tendon to confirm the pathology, the incision is extended distally along the dorsal aspect of the abductor hallucis muscle to about 2 cm proximal to the first MTP joint.

The incision is deepened through the subcutaneous tissue and fat through this relatively avascular plane, displacing the tissues in a plantar direction by sharp and blunt dissection. At the distal portion, a Weitlaner retractor is inserted that pulls the abductor plantar along with the flexor hallucis brevis (FHB) muscle (Fig. 27-15). The tendinous origin of the FHB is identified and carefully detached in a medial-to-lateral direction. As this is carried out, a fatty area is identified just deep to the FHB origin, through which the FDL and flexor hallucis longus (FHL) tendons pass. After the plane of the two tendons is identified, the surgeon dissects proximally through the master knot of Henry up to the area just proximal to the talonavicular joint (Fig. 27-16). This is a relatively avascular area, although occasionally some large veins cross it and require ligating. After the FHL and FDL tendons are iden-

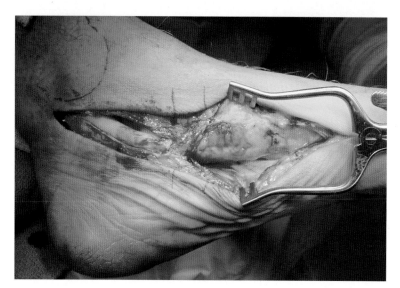

**Figure 27-14.** An incision is made from the tip of the medial malleolus distally along the dorsal aspect of the abductor hallucis muscle to about 2 cm proximal to the first MTP joint.

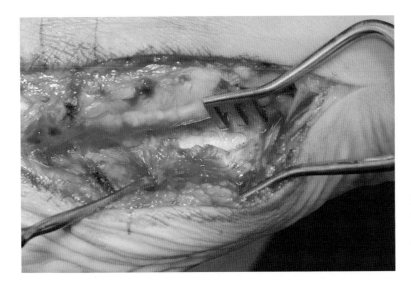

**Figure 27-15.** The distal end of the incision is created in the interval between the superior border of the abductor hallucis and the plantar aspect of the first ray. A Weitlaner retractor is used to retract the abductor hallucis and flexor hallucis brevis (FHB) plantarward.

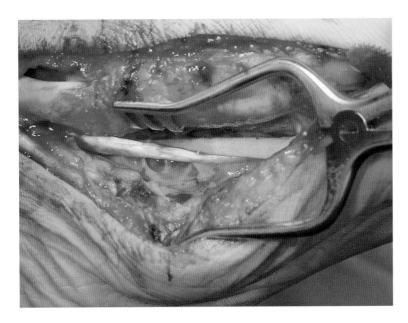

**Figure 27-16.** A portion of the tendinous origin of the flexor hallucis brevis (FHB) is detached from the plantar surface of the first ray to gain access to the flexor digitorum longus (FDL) and flexor hallucis longus (FHL) at the level of the master knot of Henry. A significant venous plexus must often be taken down during this portion of the approach.

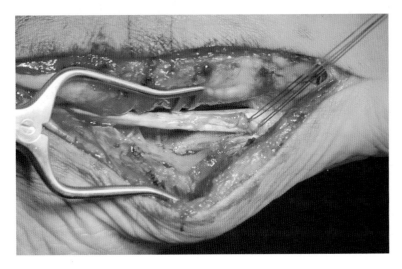

**Figure 27-17.** The flexor digitorum longus and flexor hallucis longus tendons are sutured together distally, after which the flexor digitorum longus tendon is sectioned.

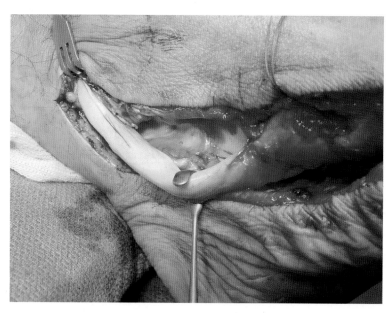

**Figure 27-18.** The degenerated posterior tibial tendon is pulled distally as far as possible. The incision is extended proximally if necessary to ensure access to the entire pathologic segment of the tendon.

tified, the adherent soft tissues are then removed using scissors. The two tendons are then sutured together distally, after which the FDL tendon is detached (Fig. 27-17). This detached tendon can be used to substitute for the dysfunctional posterior tibial tendon.

Attention is redirected to the area of the posterior tibial tendon, where it is removed from its insertion into the navicular, leaving a 1 cm cuff of tendon still attached distally. The proximal portion of the tendon is pulled as far distally as possible and transected proximally to allow the tendon to retract above the medial malleolus. (Figs. 27-18 and 27-19). If significant tendinosis is identified in the area behind the medial malleolus, the surgeon may extend the incision proximally to remove as much of the diseased tendon as possible.

The deltoid ligament is carefully inspected, as is the spring ligament. If there is abnormal synovial tissue invading these structures, it is removed by sharp dissection. Occasionally, the spring ligament is attenuated or stretched; if so, a 3- to 5-mm segment is removed and the ligament plicated (Fig. 27-20).

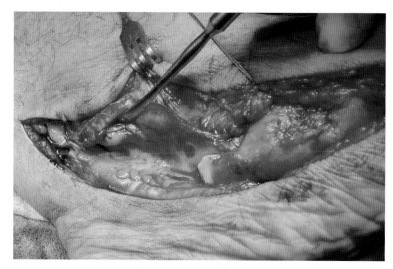

**Figure 27-19.** The degenerated portion of the posterior tibial tendon is excised, leaving a 1-cm cuff of tendon attached to the navicular tuberosity.

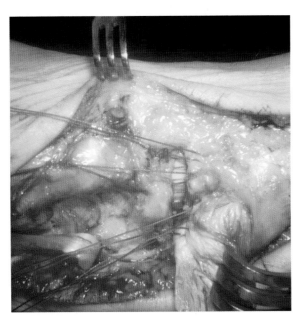

**Figure 27-20.** If the spring ligament is attenuated, a 3- to 5-mm segment is removed and plication performed.

The navicular is exposed dorsally, and its proximal and distal extents are identified. A vertical hole is drilled through the midsubstance of the navicular (i.e., in the navicular body midway between proximal and distal margins). The hole is drilled so as to exit as far medial as possible, and the surgeon must be sure that sufficient bone stock is present medially so the tendon will not fracture through the navicular (Fig. 27-21). A ligature is placed on the end of the FDL tendon and is passed from plantar to dorsal through the hole in the navicular (Fig. 27-22). The foot is then positioned into maximum inversion, and as this occurs, it aligns into about 20° of plantarflexion. The tendon is then sutured into the periosteum (Fig. 27-23). The wound is thoroughly irrigated and closed in layers. The abductor hallucis muscle is reapproximated to the inferomedial border of the first metatarsal.

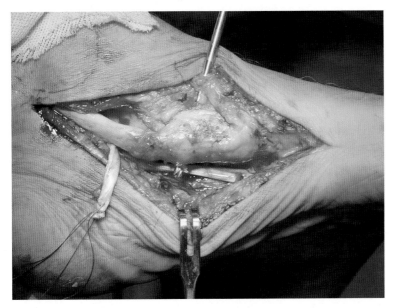

**Figure 27-21.** The navicular is exposed, and a vertical hole is drilled through the middle substance of the navicular. For demonstration purposes, the posterior tibial tendon has been left intact to show the position of the navicular tunnel relative to the original insertion of the tendon. It has usually been resected by this point.

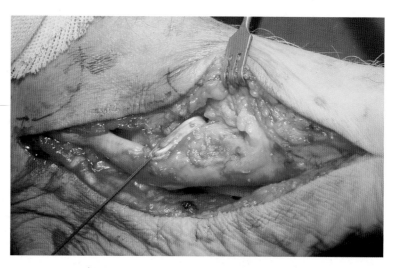

**Figure 27-22.** A ligature is placed on the end of the flexor digitorum longus tendon and is passed from plantar to dorsal through the hole in the navicular. A suture passer can help to accomplish this.

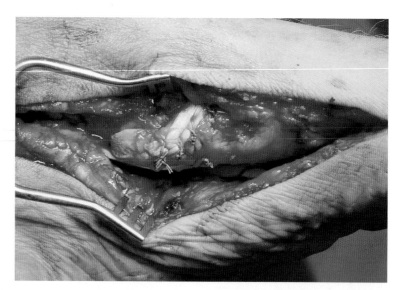

**Figure 27-23.** The foot is placed into maximum inversion and 20° of plantarflexion. This tendon is sutured into the periosteum. The abductor hallucis muscle is reapproximated to the inferomedial border of the first metatarsal, and the wound is then closed in layers.

### Additional Procedure: Tendo-Achilles Lengthening

In a subset of patients, the heel cord is contracted as a result of the chronic positioning of the heel in a valgus position. When the heel is realigned into varus, the Achilles becomes functionally tighter, and a tight heel cord may be unmasked after a corrective osteotomy. Although a minor amount of heel cord tightness can be expected to stretch out postoperatively, a percutaneous heel cord lengthening should be added to the procedure if the foot cannot be brought up to neutral after the hindfoot valgus has been corrected.

## POSTOPERATIVE MANAGEMENT

Immediately after surgery, the patient is held in a short-leg compressive dressing consisting of a wound dressing, a bulky cotton roll, plaster splints, and an overwrap of gauze or Coban, with the foot held in full inversion and approximately 20° to 25° of plantarflexion to protect the tendon transfer. The sutures are removed after approximately 2 weeks, and a standard, short-leg, non–weight-bearing cast is applied to keep the foot in full inversion and 20° to 25° of plantarflexion.

Five weeks after surgery, the cast is removed, and radiographs are obtained to verify adequate union of the osteotomy site. The osteotomy typically heals rapidly and with minimal callous. The absence of displacement or detectable loosening of the screw at this point is sufficient to proceed with weight bearing. The patient is placed in a removable short-leg boot and allowed to initiate weight bearing.

Eight weeks after surgery, active open chain range of motion exercises are begun. The patient is allowed to gradually discontinue the boot after 10 weeks and gradually begin unprotected ambulation. At this point, they are encouraged to continue working on range of motion exercises and are instructed in resistive inversion exercises using a Thera-Band to strengthen the transferred FDL.

Most patients are able to accomplish their own rehabilitation. We caution patients that a median of 10 months is needed for the maximum benefit of the surgery to be realized, and this is almost certainly from the prolonged period required for the transferred FDL motor unit to recover from the atrophy related to the procedure.

A few patients request or require supervised physical therapy to work on inversion strengthening and range of motion. We do not discourage this, but the patient and the ther-

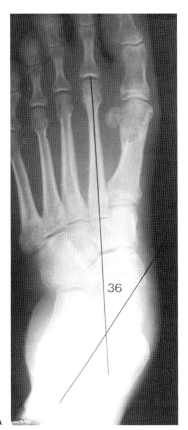

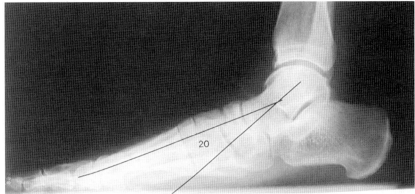

**Figure 27-24.** Preoperative anteroposterior **(A)** and lateral **(B)** radiographs of a 55-year-old woman with posterior tibial tendon dysfunction. Notice the dorsolateral subluxation of the foot relative to the talar head and the increased talus–first metatarsal angles measured in both planes.

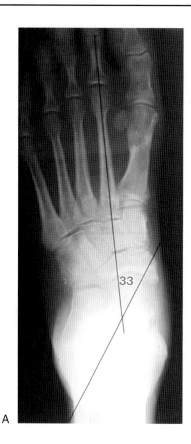

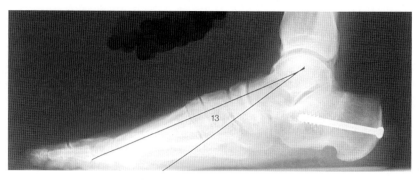

**Figure 27-25.** Postoperative anteroposterior **(A)** and lateral **(B)** radiographs from the same patient as in Figure 27-24. The static radiographic parameters are all improved.

apist should be cautioned not to initiate rising or walking on the tiptoes until at least several months after removal of the cast.

It takes several months after unrestricted ambulation is allowed for the transferred FDL motor unit to hypertrophy and become fully functional in its new role. For this reason, the time required to achieve the eventual end result is prolonged. Our patients have indicated that it took a median of 10 months to reach the maximum improvement in symptoms, but individual patients have reported periods as long as 2 years (4). Patients are often underwhelmed about their perceived change in the appearance of the foot despite improved function and diminished pain. Although the medial displacement osteotomy reliably leads to radiographic improvement in the height of the arch and alignment of the hindfoot, the effect is less easily noticed visually by the untrained eye. It is vital to counsel patients about the length of time expected for full recovery and the often subtle visual changes in the arch. Radiographically, the coverage of the navicular and the talus–first metatarsal angle, as measured on lateral and anteroposterior radiographs, should improve (Figs. 27-24 and 27-25).

It is reasonable to expect patients with a functioning FDL transfer to regain the ability to perform a single-leg toe rise within the first year after surgery. The functional results of the operation appear to be quite durable, at least over the midterm. Late failures of the transferred FDL tendon are rare. In our series of FDL transfers combined with medial displacement calcaneal osteotomies, only 1 of 26 patients suffered a loss of function occurring outside the initial postoperative year. There is no evidence to indicate that additional orthotic management after surgery modifies the quality or durability of the ultimate result. Custom orthotics do not need to be routinely used postoperatively.

## COMPLICATIONS

Complications from FDL transfer are relatively few. Significant complaints referent to motion of the lesser toes have not been reported, nor has the development of lesser toe deformities. The most notable complication is early rupture or pull-out of the transferred FDL tendon itself. In our series, this occurred in 2 of 26 cases (4). Reexploring the wound and reinserting the tendon should be attempted, but unless the problem occurs within the immediate postoperative period, the FDL will become retracted and scarred; the chances of obtaining a good result are then relatively dismal. Subtalar fusion should be offered as a salvage procedure sooner rather than later in these cases.

Complications from the medial displacement osteotomy are rare. Occasionally, the sural nerve may become injured or disrupted, leading to numbness or a sural neuralgia. These usually resolve without complication, and in our recent series, no patients required surgical exploration for neuritic symptoms. The posterior-to-anterior screw can become prominent in the heel, and it requires eventual removal in approximately 10% of patients. It is theoretically possible to injure the medial neurovascular bundle at the time of osteotomy, but careful surgical technique should minimize the risk of this complication from occurring. This complication has not been reported in the literature. The osteotomy heals quite reliably; nonunion has not been reported.

## RECOMMENDED READING

 1. Easley ME, Trnka HJ, Schon LC, et al.: Isolated subtalar arthrodesis. *J Bone Joint Surg Am* 82:613–624, 2000.
 2. Funk DA, Cass JR, Johnson KA: Acquired adult flat foot secondary to posterior tibial tendon pathology. *J Bone Joint Surg Am* 68:95–102, 1986.
 3. Gleich A: Beitrag zur operativen plattfussbehandlung. *Arch Klin Chir* 46:358–362, 1893.
 4. Guyton GP, Jeng C, Krieger LE, et al.: Flexor digitorum longus transfer and medial displacement osteotomy for posterior tibial tendon dysfunction, a middle-term clinical follow-up. *Foot Ankle Int* 22:627–632, 2001.
 5. Johnson KA, Strom DE: Tibialis posterior tendon dysfunction. *Clin Orthop* 239:196–206, 1989.
 6. Koutsogiannis E: Treatment of mobile flat foot by displacement osteotomy of the calcaneus. *J Bone Joint Surg Br* 53:96–100, 1971.
 7. Mann RA: Flatfoot in adults. In: Coughlin MJ, Mann RA, eds. *Surgery of the foot and ankle.* St. Louis: Mosby, 1999:745–762.
 8. Mann RA: Biomechanics of the foot and ankle. In: Coughlin MJ, Mann RA, eds. *Surgery of the foot and ankle.* St. Louis: Mosby, 1999:21.
 9. Mann RA, Beaman DN, Horton GA: Isolated subtalar arthrodesis. *Foot Ankle Int* 19:511–519, 1998.
10. Mann RA, Thompson FM: Rupture of the posterior tibial tendon causing flat foot. Surgical treatment. *J Bone Joint Surg Am* 67:556–561, 1985.
11. Myerson MS, Corrigan J, Thompson F, et al.: Tendon transfer combined with calcaneal osteotomy for treatment of posterior tibial tendon insufficiency: a radiological investigation. *Foot Ankle Int* 16:712–718, 1995.
12. Myerson MS, Corrigan J: Treatment of posterior tibial tendon dysfunction with flexor digitorum longus tendon transfer and calcaneal osteotomy. *Orthopedics* 19:383–388, 1996.
13. Toolan BC, Sangeorzan BJ, Hansen ST Jr: Complex reconstruction for the treatment of dorsolateral peritalar subluxation of the foot: early results after distraction arthrodesis of the calcaneocuboid joint in conjunction with stabilization of, and transfer of the flexor digitorum longus tendon to, the midfoot to treat acquired pes planovalgus in adults. *J Bone Joint Surg Am* 81:1545–1560, 1999.

# 28

# Talocalcaneal (Subtalar) Arthrodesis

## Harold B. Kitaoka

## INDICATIONS/CONTRAINDICATIONS

The primary indication for subtalar or talocalcaneal arthrodesis is pain due to arthritis or instability of the joint. Isolated subtalar arthrodesis is used for correction of posttraumatic arthritis of the subtalar joint, as is typically seen after fractures of the talus or the calcaneus. Degenerative arthritis, rheumatoid and other inflammatory arthritides, infectious arthritis, and metabolic disorders are other indications. It is useful for selected patients who have instability due to posterior tibial tendon dysfunction and flatfoot. It is applicable for failed hindfoot reconstruction operations such as failed medial calcaneal osteotomy, posterior tibial tendon reconstruction with flexor digitorum longus transfer, or failed spring ligament repair. It is also applicable for talocalcaneal coalition or failed talocalcaneal coalition resection operation. Selected comminuted fractures, such as comminuted intraarticular calcaneal fractures, may be effectively treated with primary subtalar arthrodesis. Hindfoot malalignment may also be corrected, such as valgus or varus related to congenital abnormalities, neurologic disorders, or other acquired disorders.

Contraindications include patients who have multilevel disease, such as ankle and subtalar joint arthritis. An unrecognized coexisting ankle disorder may be a source of patient dissatisfaction and persistent symptoms. Arthritis of multiple hindfoot joints is common, such as posttraumatic arthritis of subtalar and calcaneocuboid joints after an intraarticular calcaneal fracture. Widespread arthritis affecting the hindfoot and midfoot is unlikely to be successfully addressed with subtalar arthrodesis. Other contraindications are local or general medical conditions, which may preclude a successful result such as dysvascular extremity, local or remote infection, or a patient who cannot comply with or tolerate the required postoperative management of cast immobilization and no weight bearing. A relative contraindication is a significant sensory neuropathy or neuropathic arthropathy and neuropathic fractures. Only rarely is arthrodesis indicated in severely deformed, unbraceable hindfoot with recurrent neuropathic ulceration. Another relative contraindication is advanced age. Some experts feel that tobacco use is a relative contraindication.

H. B. Kitaoka, M.D.: Foot and Ankle Section, Department of Orthopaedics, Mayo Clinic and Mayo Foundation; and Mayo School of Medicine, Rochester, Minnesota.

The limitations of the technique include more rigid, severe hindfoot deformities. Pathologic disorders involving the talonavicular and calcaneocuboid joint may require extension to a triple arthrodesis. Patients who sustain severe trauma to the hindfoot resulting in late posttraumatic arthritis of the subtalar joint frequently have other problems not addressed by subtalar arthrodesis, such as a compartment syndrome and its sequelae, smashed heel pad syndrome, nerve injury, and trauma to the adjacent hindfoot or midfoot or ankle joints. A severe bony deficiency, such as that after multiple debridement operations for septic arthritis of the subtalar joint, or a severely malunited and impacted calcaneal fracture may require supplemental bone graft. Patients with symptomatic anterior ankle impingement due to severe malalignment from a calcaneal fracture may require subtalar distraction arthrodesis to restore the normal talar declination angle.

## PREOPERATIVE PLANNING

Patients with subtalar arthritis typically complain of "pain on the outside of the ankle." Symptoms are mechanical in nature, increased with weight bearing, and relieved with rest. Patients often complain of more difficulty ambulating on uneven terrain, such as the yard, gravel, or side of the road. There is often swelling about the hindfoot and ankle. Patients may notice an uneven wear pattern of the shoes, inability to fit into usual footwear, and improved symptoms with use of boots or high top shoes that limit hindfoot motion.

It is important to distinguish subtalar from ankle disorders. This may be accomplished by physical examination that reveals tenderness localized to the sinus tarsi, absence of tenderness in the joint line of the ankle, and absence of instability during ankle stress testing. There is often painful and restricted hindfoot motion with or without crepitus and painless ankle movement. Passive motion of the hindfoot and deep palpation of the sinus tarsi may reproduce the patient's characteristic symptoms. It is important to distinguish subtalar from transverse tarsal joint disease (e.g., calcaneocuboid, talonavicular). Patients may have an antalgic gait and atrophy of the affected leg musculature. Hindfoot deformity may be quantitated clinically with a standing tibiocalcaneal angle and measured with a goniometer. Neurovascular examination must be documented along with the condition of the soft tissue envelop about the hindfoot.

Radiologic assessment includes standing anteroposterior, lateral, and oblique views of the foot and standing anteroposterior, lateral, and mortise views of the ankle. These may demonstrate findings typical for subtalar arthritis (e.g., osteophytes, joint space narrowing, subchondral cysts, subchondral sclerosis) and are useful for determining the presence of coexisting problems of the ankle, hindfoot, or midfoot. Weight-bearing views are also useful for assessing the alignment of the ankle and hindfoot. Special diagnostic studies, such as tomography of the hindfoot, computed tomography, magnetic resonance imaging, technetium bone scan, and stress views of the ankle or subtalar joint, are occasionally useful.

When there is uncertainty about the extent with which the subtalar joint disorder contributes to the patient's symptoms, a diagnostic injection of a local anesthetic into the subtalar joint may be performed. This test is not always reliable, because it is recognized that the anesthetic agent often migrates into tissues well beyond the subtalar joint. There appears to be a significant difference in postoperative hindfoot and ankle mobility and in the occurrence of complications in patients who have subtalar arthrodesis compared with the more extensive triple arthrodesis. Careful preoperative assessment is warranted.

## SURGERY

Subtalar arthrodesis is usually performed under a spinal or general anesthetic. It is usually performed in an inpatient setting because postoperative care requires neurovascular observation, significant postoperative analgesic medications, and ambulation training and physical therapy.

The patient is placed laterally on the operating table. In some instances, when there is a

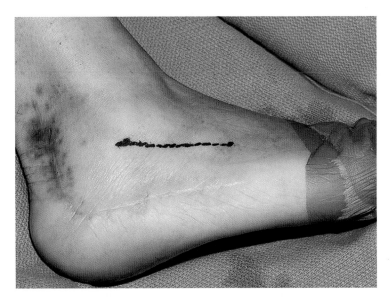

**Figure 28-1.** Oblique hindfoot skin incision. The incision extends from the tip of the lateral malleolus toward the base of the fourth metatarsal.

question of whether the arthrodesis must be extended to the other hindfoot joints, the patient is positioned supine with folded sheets under the buttocks to internally rotate the extremity. A 4-inch elastic wrap is used to exsanguinate the extremity, and a pneumatic thigh tourniquet is used to obtain hemostasis. The leg is prepped in the usual manner, and the leg is draped free at about the knee level.

## Technique

An oblique skin incision is made that is centered over the sinus tarsi (Fig. 28-1). The incision begins at the tip of the lateral malleolus and is extended anteriorly and distally toward the base of the fourth metatarsal. Subcutaneous tissue is incised along the line of the skin incision. Extensor digitorum muscle, peroneal tendon sheath, and fat in the sinus tarsi are exposed (Fig. 28-2).

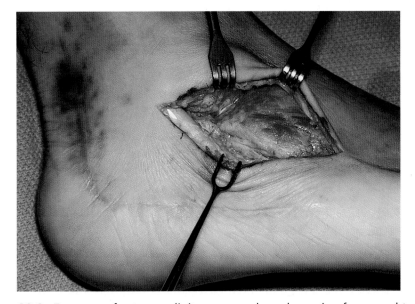

**Figure 28-2.** Exposure of extensor digitorum muscle and margin of peroneal tendon sheath.

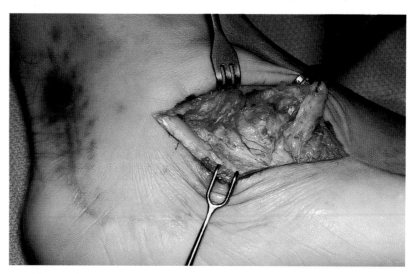

**Figure 28-3.** The extensor digitorum brevis muscle is raised as a distally based flap.

The attachment of the extensor digitorum brevis muscle to the calcaneus is carefully dissected in a distally based flap to allow exposure of the sinus tarsi and anterior process of calcaneus (Fig. 28-3). The fatty tissue from the sinus tarsi is incised longitudinally and preserved. The peroneal tendons and sheath are visualized and protected in the lateral hindfoot (Fig. 28-4). The tendons are retracted posteriorly to allow excellent exposure of the posterior subtalar joint (Fig. 28-4). A lamina spreader is inserted into the sinus tarsi to expose the entire articulation of the subtalar region (Fig. 28-4).

Using a combination of sharp osteotomes, curettes, and rongeurs, the remaining articular cartilage and subchondral bone of the calcaneal and talar joint surfaces are excised (Fig. 28-5). There is particular effort directed toward preserving the contour of the joint surfaces (Fig. 28-6). There is also a specific effort to avoid violating the tibiotalar joint capsule. In selected cases of calcaneal fracture malunion, the displaced, malunited lateral wall of the calcaneus may be resected with a sharp osteotome.

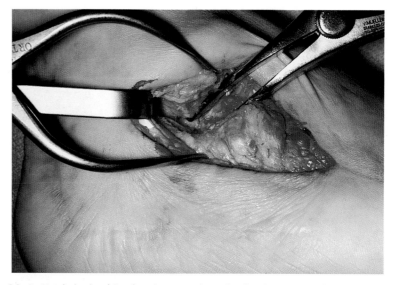

**Figure 28-4.** Fat is incised in the sinus tarsi, and a laminar spreader is inserted to expose arthritis of the subtalar joint.

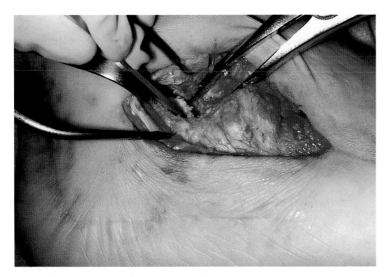

**Figure 28-5.** Peroneal tendons are protected laterally and posteriorly. The remaining articular cartilage and subchondral bone are excised from calcaneal and talar joint surfaces with a sharp osteotome.

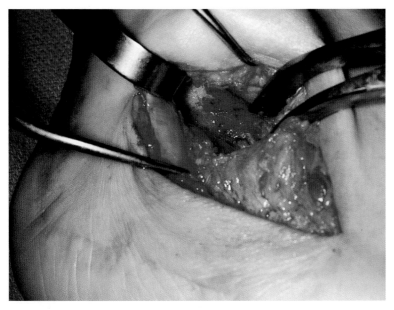

**Figure 28-6.** Calcaneal and talar surfaces. Notice the preservation of the contour of the joint surfaces during the limited resection.

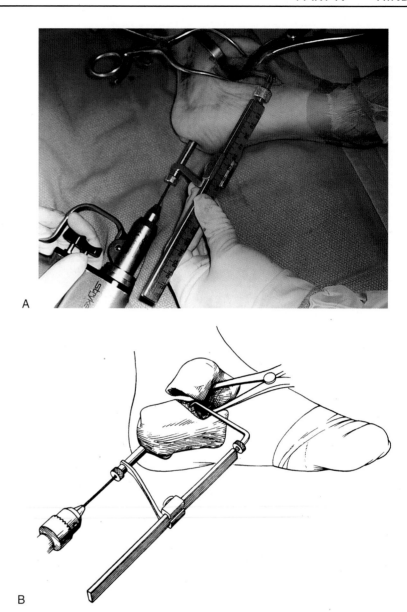

**Figure 28-7. A:** Placement of guide pin through a longitudinal heel incision is facilitated by use of a combined aiming device through a longitudinal heel incision. **B:** Schematic diagram. (**B** from Dahm DL, Kitaoka HB: Subtalar arthrodesis with internal compression for post-traumatic arthritis. *J Bone Joint Surg Br* 80:134–138, 1998, with permission; copyright by the Mayo Clinic and Mayo Foundation, Rochester, Minnesota.)

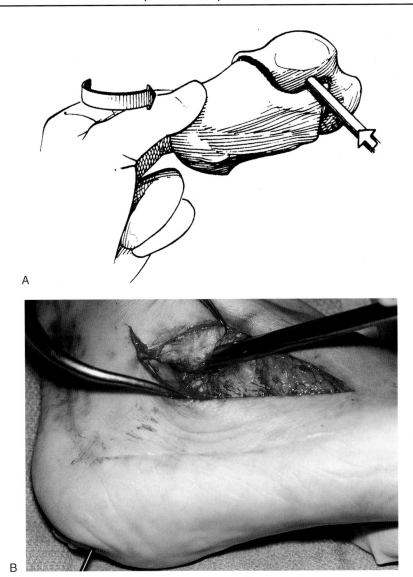

A

B

**Figure 28-8.  A:** The calcaneus is realigned in relation to the talus, usually by internal rotation of the calcaneus. The diagram shows the bone impactor placed against the lateral process of calcaneus to assist in reduction. **B:** Close-up view of the joint reduction. (**A** from Dahm DL, Kitaoka HB: Subtalar arthrodesis with internal compression for posttraumatic arthritis. *J Bone Joint Surg Br* 80: 134–138, 1998, with permission; copyright by the Mayo Clinic and Mayo Foundation, Rochester, Minnesota.)

Using a combined aiming device, a guide wire is passed through a longitudinal incision in the heel through the posterior facet of the calcaneus (Fig. 28-7). The calcaneus is then rotated internally in relation to the talus so that adequate bony apposition is achieved (Fig. 28-8), and the heel is ultimately placed in a position of 5° to 10° of valgus. The guide wire is advanced across the subtalar joint into the body of the talus (Fig. 28-9). A cannulated drill is passed over the guide wire and across the subtalar joint into the talus (Fig. 28-10). A cannulated, 7.0-mm, cancellous screw with a 16-mm thread length is then passed over the guide wire for fixation (Fig. 28-11). The subtalar joint bony apposition and hindfoot position are inspected, and fixation stability is tested with a hindfoot supination-pronation force. If necessary, a second screw may be inserted through the same heel incision. If there is still a question about the adequacy of stability, hardware is removed, and a dorsal-to-plantar oriented screw may be placed through a dorsal incision over the talar neck.

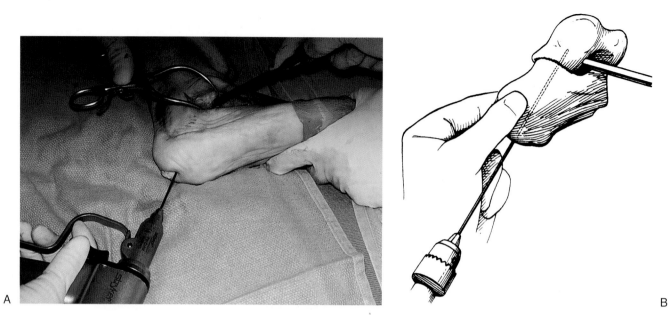

A

B

**Figure 28-9.** **A:** Advancement of the guide pin across the subtalar level in a corrected position. **B:** Schematic diagram. (**B** from Dahm DL, Kitaoka HB: Subtalar arthrodesis with internal compression for post-traumatic arthritis. *J Bone Joint Surg Br* 80:134–138, 1998, with permission; copyright by the Mayo Clinic and Mayo Foundation, Rochester, Minnesota.)

The magnitude of bony deficiency is then assessed. It varies considerably, depending on the underlying pathology. A large deficiency from multiple debridement operations for septic arthritis and osteomyelitis or from a displaced intraarticular calcaneal fracture may necessitate the use of supplement bone graft. The nonarticular portion of the anterior process of the calcaneus is exposed (Fig. 28-12), then morcellated, and placed in the sinus tarsi for bone graft (Fig. 28-13 and 28-14). If additional graft is needed, such as in patients with original central depression–type intraarticular fractures, a proximal tibial graft is used. In a series of patients who underwent isolated subtalar arthrodesis for posttraumatic arthritis, only the anterior process of the calcaneus was used for graft in 15 of 25 feet. The bone graft is morcellated and placed into the deficit. Bony impingement such as that between the calcaneus and the fibular is treated by realignment of the hindfoot or rarely by exostectomy of the lateral wall of the calcaneus.

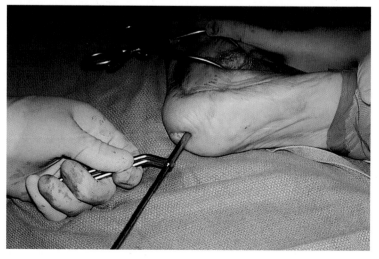

**Figure 28-10.** A cannulated drill is passed over the guide pin.

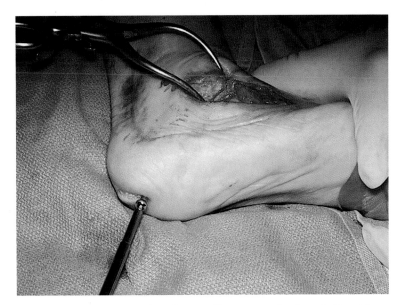

**Figure 28-11.** A 7.0-mm, cannulated, cancellous screw is placed. Good bony apposition is usually achieved.

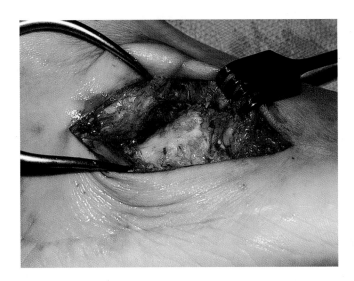

**Figure 28-12.** The anterior process of the calcaneus is exposed.

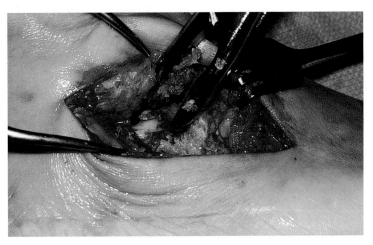

**Figure 28-13.** The nonarticular portion of anterior process of the calcaneus is removed, morcellated with rongeurs, and placed into the sinus tarsi.

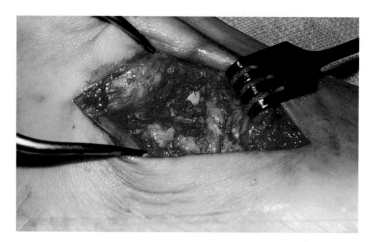

**Figure 28-14.** Morcellated bone graft in the sinus tarsi.

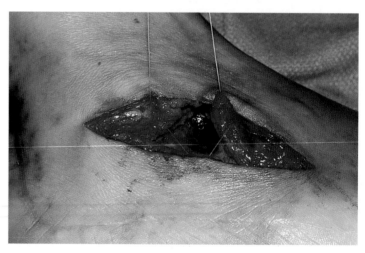

**Figure 28-15.** Soft tissues are reapproximated over the bone graft, including the extensor digitorum brevis muscle and fat over the sinus tarsi.

The proximal tibial graft is obtained through a longitudinal, 2-cm incision anteromedially, distal to the tibial tubercle. A round window is placed in the cortex with a 12-mm Cloward dowel cutter or osteotome. Cancellous bone graft is harvested for transfer to the recipient area of the subtalar joint. This bone graft, including the cortical window, is morcellated with a rongeur. The tibial incision is closed. The arthrodesis site is packed with the autogenous bone graft. Occasionally, Achilles tendon lengthening is necessary, and this may be performed percutaneously with three small incisions posteriorly.

An intraoperative lateral radiograph of the foot is obtained to confirm fixation placement, alignment, and bony apposition. The flap of the extensor digitorum brevis muscle and its aponeurosis are repaired with 2-0 Vicryl sutures (Fig. 28-15). Subcutaneous tissue is reapproximated with interrupted simple 2-0 Vicryl sutures. Skin is closed with interrupted 3-0 nylon sutures or staples.

## POSTOPERATIVE MANAGEMENT

A Robert Jones compression dressing with plaster splints is applied for the first 48 hours after surgery. At that point, the dressing is removed, the incisions are examined, and a well-padded, non–weight-bearing, short-leg cast is applied. The cast is changed, and the sutures are removed at 3 weeks after surgery. A below-knee walking cast is applied at 6 weeks postoperatively and for an additional 4 to 5 weeks until there is radiologic evidence of arthrodesis union.

Patients are encouraged to begin a foot and ankle rehabilitation program after the removal of the final cast, with or without the assistance of a physical therapist. Gentle, progressive range of motion exercises are included in the postoperative regimen. Patients universally experience swelling and aching after cast removal and should be educated about the expected course of recovery.

In a series of patients who underwent this operation for posttraumatic arthritis at this institution, union was achieved in 24 (96%) of 25 feet with this technique (2). In a series of patients who underwent arthrodesis for posterior tibial tendon dysfunction and flatfoot using this method without supplemental iliac crest or tibial graft, union was achieved in all 21 feet (5).

## COMPLICATIONS

As with any operation, failures and complications can occur. The sometimes tedious, meticulous resection of the talar and calcaneal joint surfaces may be accomplished with speed and efficiency using a large osteotome. This may be applicable in patients with severe cavus feet, but in most others, excessive bone removal creates a marked *hindfoot valgus* malposition or larger bony deficiency.

Improper positioning of the hindfoot can lead to later difficulties in ambulation and with footwear restrictions. *Hindfoot varus* can lead to painful callus on the lateral margin of the foot. There is evidence that malposition of the hindfoot after triple arthrodesis is associated with ankle pain, and this may also apply to patients who undergo subtalar arthrodesis. The use of a cannulated screw fixation system allows careful inspection of hindfoot position with a guide wire in place, before definitive screw fixation is applied. Additional visual and radiographic inspection after screw placement can prevent the complication of improper positioning.

As with any arthrodesis procedure, *nonunion* can occur. With this particular technique, nonunion is rare. The careful preparation of joint surfaces allows viable bone surfaces of the talus and calcaneus to be in direct contact, which encourages rapid and successful union. Compression screw fixation is effective and does not require removal. It is not usually necessary to place intercalated nonviable bone between the joint surfaces, but when there is a large deficiency, autogenous bone from the proximal tibia is effective and has low potential morbidity.

The unusual anatomy associated with malunited calcaneal fractures can lead to the inadvertent dissection of the tibiotalar joint instead of the subtalar level. Extensive dissection of soft tissues about the lateral ankle and hindfoot may lead to ankle instability. In patients who have extensive resection of the soft tissues over the sinus tarsi, the skin may adhere to the underlying bone, with long-standing sensitivity to minor trauma.

A major source of dissatisfaction is the presence of associated pathology that is a persistent source of symptoms long after the subtalar joint pain is successfully addressed. The severe force causing the original calcaneal or talar fracture undoubtedly severely traumatizes the soft tissue envelop as well. This may lead to long-standing pain related to smashed heel syndrome in which the heel pad is severely injured. There may be injuries and late arthritis to the adjacent joints, such as the calcaneocuboid joint from extension of the calcaneal fracture into this joint or the lateral joint line of the ankle from calcaneofibular impingement. Patients may have persistent pain from nerve injuries, such as the posterior tibial, sural, or medial calcaneal nerves from the initial trauma. The reconstruction operation may precipitate sympathetically maintained pain. Successful subtalar arthrodesis may theoretically accentuate overloading of joints distal (i.e., talonavicular and calcaneocuboid) and proximal (i.e., ankle), but more often, concomitant pathology in these adjacent areas can be

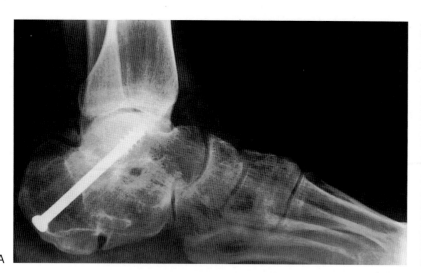
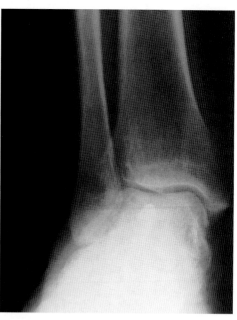

A

B

**Figure 28-16.  A:** Lateral radiograph shows the foot of a 49-year-old man with post-traumatic subtalar arthritis 2 years after an intraarticular calcaneal fracture. There is loss of heel height but no symptoms of anterior ankle impingement. **B:** The antero-posterior view of the ankle shows calcaneofibular impingement from displacement of the lateral wall of the calcaneus laterally. (**A** and **B** copyright by the Mayo Clinic and Mayo Foundation, Rochester, Minnesota.)

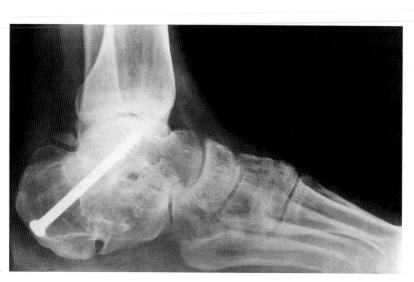
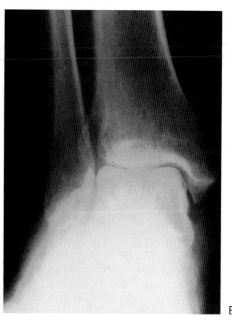

A

B

**Figure 28-17.  A:** Lateral view 3 years after a subtalar arthrodesis without supplemental bone graft shows successful union. The patient had an excellent clinical result. **B:** The anteroposterior radiograph of the ankle 3 years after surgery shows that the calcaneus was realigned in relation to the talus to address the calcaneofibular impingement. (**A** and **B** copyright by the Mayo Clinic and Mayo Foundation, Rochester, Minnesota.)

identified preoperatively and patients properly educated. It is not advisable to consider operative treatment when expectations are unrealistic.

Patients who have severe malalignment and subtalar arthritis may occasionally benefit from more involved reconstruction operations. In the rare instance when there is anterior ankle pain from anterior ankle impingement after a calcaneal fracture with loss of talar declination angle and calcaneal pitch angle, subtalar distraction arthrodesis is indicated. This is a more difficult operation with a much higher published complication rate, and patients must be carefully selected.

## ILLUSTRATIVE CASE

A 49-year-old man sustained a displaced intraarticular calcaneal fracture of the right foot. The fracture was treated nonoperatively, and the patient presented 2 years after injury with lateral hindfoot and ankle pain, swelling, and stiffness. He had difficulty bearing weight, particularly on uneven terrain. He had an obvious limp, calf atrophy, severe restriction of hindfoot motion, painful hindfoot motion, crepitus with hindfoot movement, and tenderness in the sinus tarsi and lateral joint line of the ankle. Weight-bearing radiographs of the lateral foot and anteroposterior ankle views show fracture malunion with subtalar arthritis, loss of heel height, and calcaneofibular impingement (Fig. 28-16). The clinical result was excellent 3 years after internal compression subtalar arthrodesis, and radiographs demonstrate solid union, improved alignment, no calcaneofibular impingement, and satisfactory ankle joint space (Fig. 28-17). The reduction is not absolutely anatomic; this position was acceptable because there were no symptoms or signs of anterior ankle impingement, and a larger reconstruction operation such as subtalar distraction arthrodesis was not indicated.

## ACKNOWLEDGMENT

The author acknowledges the contribution of Gary R. Kitaoka.

## RECOMMENDED READING

1. Chandler JT, Bonar SK, Anderson RB, et al.: Results of in situ subtalar arthrodesis for late sequelae of calcaneus fractures. *Foot Ankle Int* 20:18–24, 1999.
2. Dahm DL, Kitaoka HB: Subtalar arthrodesis with internal compression for post-traumatic arthritis. *J Bone Joint Surg Br* 80:134–138, 1998.
3. Easley ME, Trnka HJ, Schon LC, et al.: Isolated subtalar arthrodesis. *J Bone Joint Surg Am* 82: 613–624, 2000.
4. Flemister AS Jr, Infante AF, Sanders RW, et al.: Subtalar arthrodesis for complications of intra-articular calcaneal fractures. *Foot Ankle Int* 21:392–399, 2000.
5. Kitaoka HB, Patzer GL: Subtalar arthrodesis for posterior tibial tendon dysfunction and pes planus. *Clin Orthop* 345:187–194, 1997.
6. Mangone PG, Fleming LL, Fleming SS, et al.: Treatment of acquired adult planovalgus deformities with subtalar fusion. *Clin Orthop* 341:106–112, 1997.
7. Mann RA, Beaman DN, Horton GA: Isolated subtalar arthrodesis. *Foot Ankle Int* 19:511–519, 1998.
8. Marti RK, de Heus JA, Roolker W, et al.: Subtalar arthrodesis with correction of deformity after fractures of the os calcis. *J Bone Joint Surg Br* 81:611–616, 1999.
9. Russotti GM, Johnson KA, Cass JR: Isolated talocalcaneal arthrodesis, a moldable bone graft technique. *J Bone Joint Surg Am* 70:1472–1478, 1988.

# 29

# Talus-Calcaneus-Cuboid (Triple) Arthrodesis

James Michelson and James A. Amis

## INDICATIONS/CONTRAINDICATIONS

A triple arthrodesis is the fusion of the subtalar, calcaneocuboid, and talonavicular joints. The indications for a triple arthrodesis are correction of a fixed hindfoot deformity, such as that resulting from a posterior tibialis tendon rupture with an acquired flat foot; hindfoot arthritis, such as rheumatoid arthritis, osteoarthritis, posttraumatic arthritis, and adult symptomatic tarsal coalition; control of progressive hindfoot deformities in neuromuscular diseases such as Charcot-Marie-Tooth or cerebrovascular accident; and failed operative procedures such as tarsal coalition resection.

Arthrodesis should be reserved for instances in which all conservative measures have failed. In cases involving hindfoot deformity, consideration should be given to motion-sparing procedures, such as tendon transfers or osteotomies or limited hindfoot arthrodeses, before deciding on a triple arthrodesis. If only one of the three joints is the source of clinical symptoms, that specific joint usually should be fused rather than doing a triple arthrodesis. However, if two of the hindfoot joints are symptomatic, fusing all three joints often is preferable because the functional consequences of fusing two joints is about the same as fusing three, whereas fusing only two carries a higher risk of clinically significant nonunion.

A contraindication is a patient with inadequate vascular supply to the foot; appropriate evaluation and vascular specialist referral may be indicated. Advanced patient age is not a contraindication for surgery, nor is the presence of diabetes mellitus, although it has implications for postoperative regimen.

J. Michelson, M.D.: Orthopaedic Surgery and Clinical Informatics, The George Washington University School of Medicine and Health Sciences, Washington, DC.

J. A. Amis, M.D.: Department of Orthopaedic Surgery, University of Cincinnati; and Department of Orthopaedic Surgery, Good Samaritan Hospital, Cincinnati, Ohio.

## PREOPERATIVE PLANNING

The history and examination are useful in providing clues to the diagnosis and to indicate the specific concerns that need to be treated. A routine foot and ankle physical examination should be undertaken. This encompasses observing the patient in a standing position anteriorly and posteriorly, which frequently demonstrates a deformity, such as hindfoot varus or valgus (Figs. 29-1 and 29-2), which can be estimated with a standing tibiocalcaneal angle measurement with a goniometer. Whether the foot is plantigrade should be determined. A varus hindfoot may have a compensatory forefoot valgus with a plantarflexed first ray. The secondary compensatory changes may require additional corrective surgery to produce a plantigrade foot after the triple arthrodesis. Claw toes may also be present. A cavus foot should raise suspicion about an underlying neuromuscular cause, such as Charcot-Marie-Tooth disease or a spinal lesion.

Similarly, a valgus hindfoot is usually associated with a compensatory varus forefoot deformity (Fig. 29-3) and an abducted forefoot. Generally, these compensatory deformities occur through the Chopart joint and can be corrected with the triple arthrodesis without the need for additional surgery in the anterior foot. There may also be a secondary Achilles tendon contracture due to the valgus, laterally deviated calcaneus with the Achilles tendon in a shortened position. In a rigid valgus hindfoot, this contracture sometimes cannot be definitively determined preoperatively, but restricted dorsiflexion of the ankle should be ascertained intraoperatively. Inadequate dorsiflexion due to tendon contracture may require tendo-Achilles lengthening.

Observing the patient's gait can confirm the functional derangements causing symptoms. The patient should be observed for signs of an antalgic gait. The inability to perform a single-leg heel rise is a reliable test for posterior tibial tendon dysfunction.

The non–weight-bearing examination focuses on the measurement of ankle and hindfoot range of motion and stability. It is useful to determine painful joint motions, numbness, swelling, and the presence of callosities in the medial or lateral forefoot associated with malalignment and deformities such as claw toes. On manual correction of hindfoot varus deformity, a pronated forefoot may indicate the need to correct the deformities with a triple arthrodesis rather than a limited hindfoot arthrodesis (e.g., subtalar). In the cavus foot, a fixed, plantarflexed first metatarsal may indicate the need to correct the deformity with triple arthrodesis rather than a limited hindfoot arthrodesis. Muscle strength testing, sensation assessment, and palpation of pulses should be part of the examination.

All patients should have weight-bearing radiographs of their feet and ankles: anteroposterior foot, lateral foot, and anteroposterior ankle views. Oblique foot and a mortise view

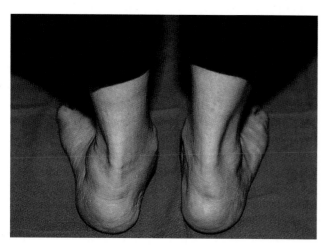

**Figure 29-1.** Severe hindfoot valgus is observed in the left foot. Abduction of the forefoot produces the "too many toes" sign.

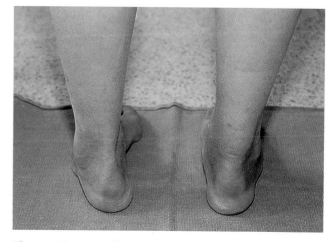

**Figure 29-2.** Hindfoot varus as a component of a cavus-type deformity of the left foot.

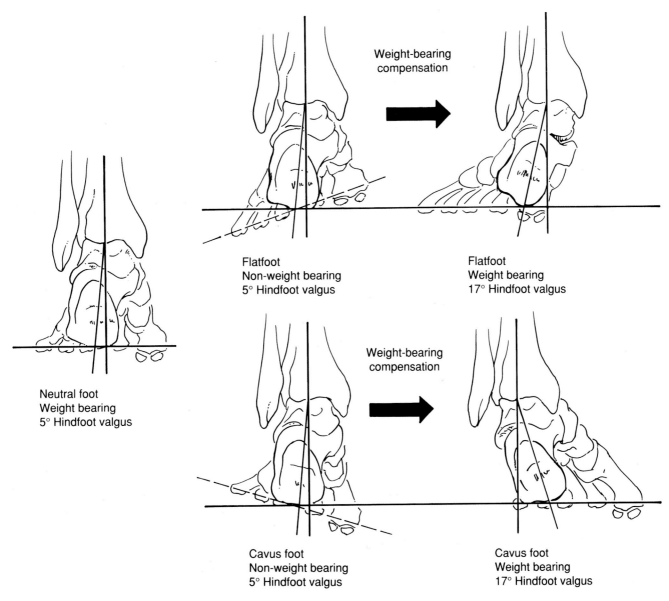

Weight-bearing
compensation

Flatfoot
Non-weight bearing
5° Hindfoot valgus

Flatfoot
Weight bearing
17° Hindfoot valgus

Neutral foot
Weight bearing
5° Hindfoot valgus

Weight-bearing
compensation

Cavus foot
Non-weight bearing
5° Hindfoot valgus

Cavus foot
Weight bearing
17° Hindfoot valgus

**Figure 29-3.** Generally, the hindfoot and forefoot are linked, and one compensates for the other. For example, the "flatfoot" with its hindfoot valgus attains a plantigrade position by a compensatory forefoot varus.

of the ankle are also useful. In the flatfoot, the anteroposterior (Fig. 29-4) and lateral talo-calcaneal angles (Fig. 29-5) diverge, whereas in the cavus foot, these angles tend to be parallel or converge. The ankle radiographs are necessary because some patients with hindfoot deformity (i.e., valgus or varus) have instability or arthritis in the ankle (Fig. 29-6). Failure to appreciate this preoperatively can lead to an unhappy outcome because of persistent ankle complaints. The anteroposterior view of the ankle can also detect calcaneofibular impingement in the flatfoot (Fig. 29-7).

The weight-bearing ankle radiographs provides insight into the overall alignment of the lower extremity. The usual goal for a triple arthrodesis is a plantigrade foot. The optimal position of the foot has to be determined with respect to the entire lower extremity. Whether the proximal surgery (e.g., total knee arthroplasty, tibial osteotomy) precedes or succeeds the triple arthrodesis is determined by the clinical requirements of each case. Failure to appreciate the interaction of proximal alignment on ultimate plantigrade position can lead to a foot that is placed in uncompensatable valgus or varus by the triple arthrodesis (Fig. 29-8).

*(Text continued on page 408.)*

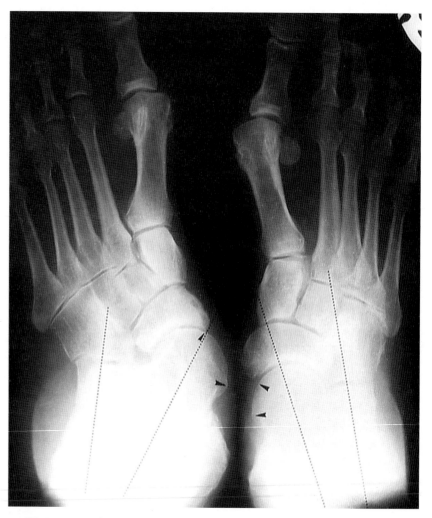

**Figure 29-4.** A standing, anteroposterior radiograph reveals a talocalcaneal divergence *(dotted lines)* in the left foot. Notice the talar head is uncovered *(arrows)*.

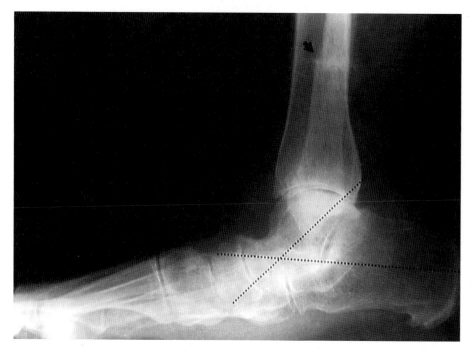

**Figure 29-5.** Standing, lateral radiographs of the feet show divergence of the lateral talocalcaneal angle *(dotted lines)*. Notice the "sag" of the foot at the talonavicular joint. There is also a stress fracture of the fibula *(arrow)* as a result of prolonged lateral impingement.

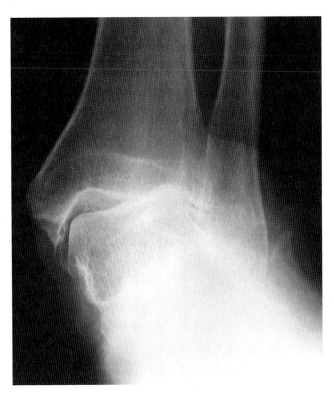

**Figure 29-6.** Ankle valgus may produce all or part of the "flatfoot" deformity observed clinically. Standing, anteroposterior radiographs of the ankle should be part of the routine workup.

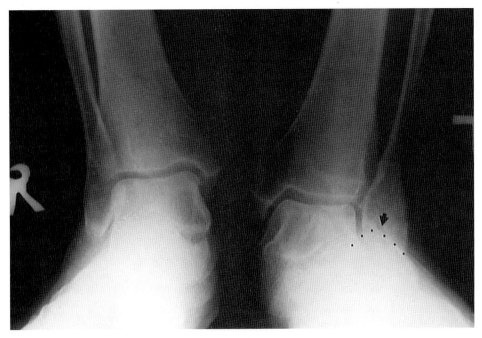

**Figure 29-7.** Standing, bilateral, anteroposterior radiographs of the ankles are an essential part of the workup. The left hindfoot demonstrates calcaneofibular impingement *(black arrow)* compared with the normal right foot. The *black dots* demonstrate the outline of the calcaneal tuberosity.

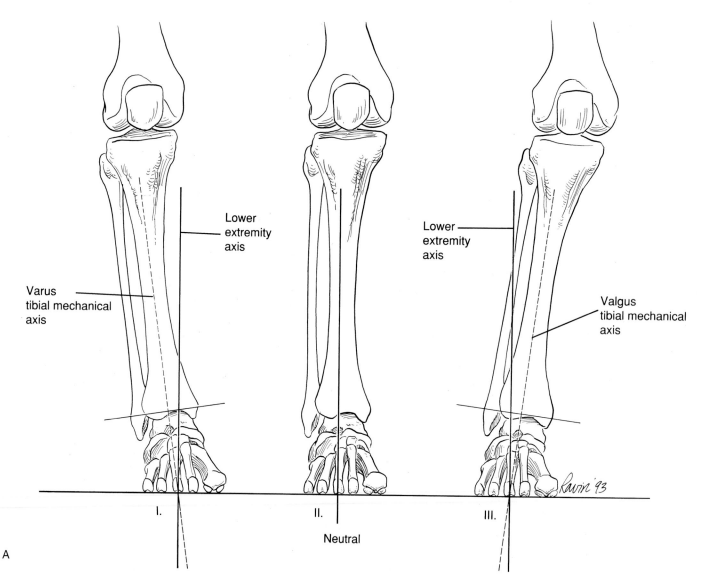

**Figure 29-8.** Tibial mechanical axis in relation to plantigrade positioning of the foot. **A:** The tibial mechanical axis is demonstrated in its three basic forms: I, varus tibial mechanical axis; II, neutral tibial mechanical axis; III, valgus tibial mechanical axis. The position of the forefoot at the time of a triple arthrodesis must take into consideration the angle of the tibial mechanical axis and its relation to the forefoot axis. *(continued)*

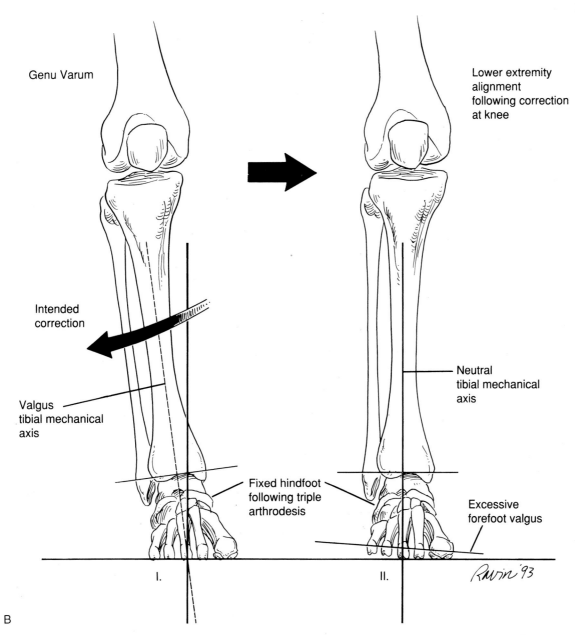

Genu Varum

Lower extremity
alignment
following correction
at knee

Intended
correction

Valgus
tibial mechanical
axis

Neutral
tibial mechanical
axis

Fixed hindfoot
following triple
arthrodesis

Excessive
forefoot valgus

I.

II.

*Ravin '93*

B

**Figure 29-8.** *Continued.* **B:** Preoperative valgus tibial mechanical alignment has an effect on the ultimate position of the foot after triple arthrodesis. Even if the tibial malalignment is not corrected, foot malalignment can be avoided, because the foot has been placed into a plantigrade position with respect to the preexisting proximal lower extremity alignment. *(continued)*

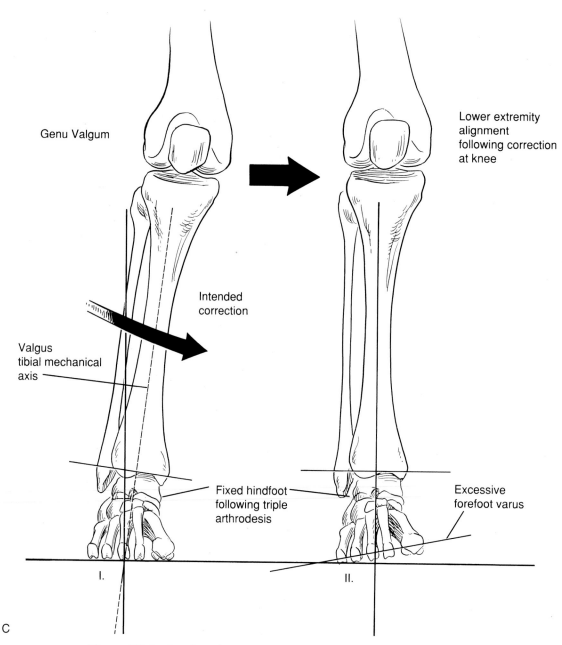

Genu Valgum

Lower extremity
alignment
following correction
at knee

Intended
correction

Valgus
tibial mechanical
axis

Fixed hindfoot
following triple
arthrodesis

Excessive
forefoot varus

I.

II.

C

**Figure 29-8.** *Continued.* **C:** Preoperative varus tibial mechanical alignment has an effect on the ultimate position of the foot after triple arthrodesis. Even if the tibial malalignment is not corrected, foot malalignment can be avoided, because the foot has been placed into a plantigrade position with respect to the preexisting proximal lower extremity alignment.

Computed tomography, radio-isotope bone scanning, and magnetic resonance imaging usually are unnecessary for preoperative assessment. Selective joint injections with a long acting local anesthetic (e.g., mepivacaine [Carbocaine], bupivacaine [Marcaine] ) may useful diagnostically to help determine the most symptomatic joints.

Bone graft is often not required. It can be harvested from the iliac crest, proximal tibia, or demineralized bone graft allograft. The latter option has the advantage of avoidance of an additional, sometimes painful incision with attendant blood loss, and it carries no risk of viral infection transmission. The union rates for grafting technique are equivalent. A tendo-Achilles lengthening may be needed if an Achilles contracture prevents neutral ankle positioning after the hindfoot deformity is corrected intraoperatively. This can be done as an open procedure or percutaneously and should be discussed preoperatively with the patient.

The goals and limitations of surgery should be discussed with the patient. These goals may include correcting a deformity, stabilizing an arthritic joint, and reducing pain. Patients' expectations must be realistic, or they are likely to be unsatisfied with the result.

## SURGERY

Every effort should be made to use sharp dissection and to gently handle the soft tissues. The approach is made with a minimum of blunt dissection and avoidance of raising subcutaneous skin flaps. The closure should be performed carefully. The use of 5-0 chromic sutures for skin closure has been found to yield excellent cosmetic results.

The tourniquet can be placed on the upper calf with adequate soft roll underpadding to protect the common peroneal nerve as it wraps around the proximal fibular head. This allows use of lower cuff pressures, typically 250 mm Hg, and results in less ischemic tissue compared with the use of thigh tourniquets. In addition to the usual surgical skin preparation and draping, it is generally easiest to drape the surgical field using a nonimpermeable stockinette and an extremity drape that is reversed so that the long end of the drape is unfolded cephalad. The stockinette can be opened distally and rolled proximally, and the toes and forefoot can be covered using a surgical glove or iodine adhesive plastic. This reduces the potential for contamination of the surgical field from debris adjacent to the toenails. Preoperative antibiotics are administered.

The procedure requires the following instruments:

Surgairtome (or equivalent) with a 5-mm-long shaft, pineapple-shaped cutting burr
Minidriver (or equivalent) with a quick-release chuck
Large-fragment Synthes AO set with at least one long, 3.2-mm drill bit
15 cc of demineralized bone matrix (250- to 400-$\mu$m particles)
Two 6.5-inch, baby Inge lamina spreaders
Towel roll for the ipsilateral buttock
Hand instrument set, including small Hohman retractors, Littler scissors, Senn retractors, small Key elevator, osteotomes, and a Freer elevator
Tourniquet (18 or 24 inch) for calf

The patient is placed in a semilateral decubitus position by pacing the towel roll under the ipsilateral buttock. This internally rotates the leg to permit easier access to the lateral hindfoot. The tourniquet is placed on the upper calf, with underlying soft roll padding. The leg is exsanguinated using an elastic wrap, and the tourniquet is inflated to 250 mm Hg.

### Technique

The operation is accomplished through two incisions: the dorsal lateral sinus tarsi incision for the subtalar, calcaneocuboid, and lateral talonavicular joints, followed by the dorsomedial approach to the talar neck and medial talonavicular joint.

The calcaneocuboid joint and talonavicular joint are palpated externally and marked (Fig. 29-9). The intermediate branch of the superficial peroneal nerve can frequently be palpated as it runs over the anterior lateral aspect of the ankle and runs inferiorly and laterally over the region of the sinus tarsi. The extensor tendons dorsally and the peroneal tendons posterolaterally should be palpated and marked, as should be the inferior aspect of the lateral malleolus (Fig. 29-9A). The incision runs obliquely along the lines of Langer from the peroneal tendons posterolaterally to the lateral margin of the extensor tendons.

An alternative incision runs from 1 cm distal to the fibula toward the base of the fourth metatarsal (Fig. 29-9B). This approach has the advantage of completely avoiding the intermediate branch of the superficial peroneal nerve, to which it runs parallel. With this inci-

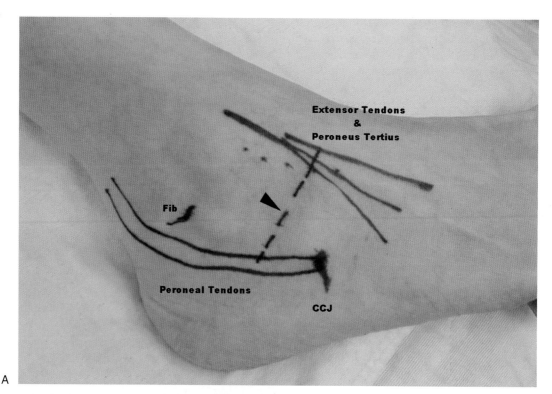

A

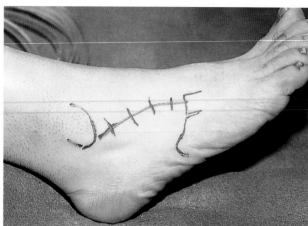

B

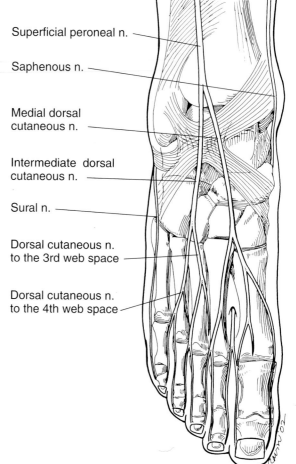

Superficial peroneal n.

Saphenous n.

Medial dorsal
cutaneous n.

Intermediate dorsal
cutaneous n.

Sural n.

Dorsal cutaneous n.
to the 3rd web space

Dorsal cutaneous n.
to the 4th web space

C

**Figure 29-9.** View of the foot preoperatively. **A:** A lateral view shows the boundaries of the incision (arrowhead). The intermediate branch of the superficial peroneal nerve courses along the medial aspect of the incision and can be retracted during the exposure. CCJ, calcaneocuboid joint; Fib, tip of the fibula. **B:** An alternate lateral skin incision extends from the tip of the lateral malleolus to the base of the fourth metatarsal. **C:** Diagram of topographic neural anatomy, indicating the branches of the superficial peroneal nerve and the sural nerve. The sural nerve courses along the inferior aspect of either incision, and care should be taken to prevent its laceration.

sion, the talonavicular joint can be exposed, although not as easily as with the dorsal lateral sinus incision. However, the talonavicular joint can be exposed through a separate dorsal medial incision. Trauma to the intermediate branch of the superficial peroneal nerve using the oblique sinus tarsi incision can occur, and transection of the nerve is not recommended. If there is concern regarding damaging the nerve, the alternative longitudinal incision is a good option.

The incision is made sharply through the skin and subcutaneous tissues with a scalpel and Littler scissors, taking care to isolate and coagulate the traversing veins. The intermediate branch of the superficial peroneal nerve is frequently encountered and can be retracted superiorly through the remainder of the approach. The fascia investing the extensor hallucis brevis (EDB) is sharply incised along the lines of the original skin incision (Fig. 29-10). Care is taken at the upper and lower boundaries of this incision to not incise the peroneus tertius and peroneal tendon sheath, respectively. The EDB muscle attachment to the calcaneus can be sharply dissected and raised as a distally based flap, or alternatively, the EDB muscle can be detached using electrocautery. The preservation of the fascia of the EDB and its muscle belly is useful in preparation for the ultimate wound closure.

The sinus tarsi fat is sharply excised longitudinally to expose the entrance to the tarsal canal, which contains the interosseous ligament running vertically between the calcaneus and talus as well as the artery of the tarsal canal (Fig. 29-11). The posterior facet can be seen in the posterior wound, just lateral to the tarsal canal. The anterior tubercle of the calcaneus is located deep in the anterior aspect of the wound. The bifurcate ligament attaches to this structure, with its two limbs extending to the navicular and cuboid. This is an important landmark for performing a triple arthrodesis, because it locates the entry point to debride the talonavicular joint and naviculocuboid articulation.

Further exposure of the subtalar joint is accomplished by subperiosteal dissection along the lateral border of the posterior facet, typically using a small Key elevator. The lateral soft tissues are then retracted using a small Hohman retractor, which protects the peroneal tendons laterally and the flexor hallucis longus posteriorly. Distraction of the subtalar joint is accomplished by placing a small lamina spreader into the canal of the sinus tarsi or later-

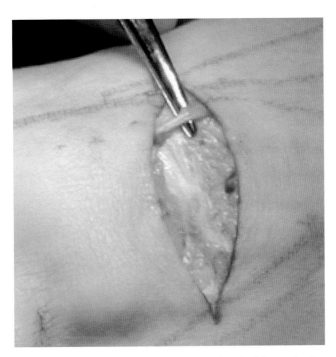

**Figure 29-10.** After performing the skin incisions, the intermediate branch of the superficial peroneal nerve (i.e., over tip of scissors) is exposed and is superficial to the fascia of the extensor hallucis brevis.

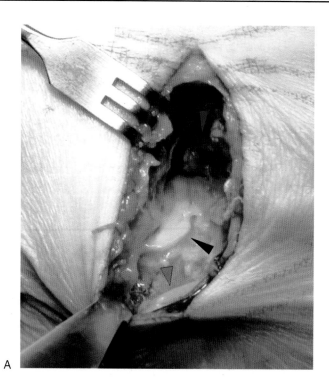

A

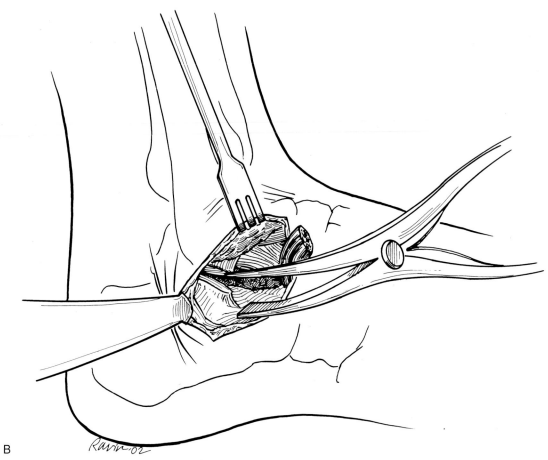

B

**Figure 29-11. A:** Deeper dissection exposes the sinus tarsi and anterior margin of the posterior facet *(black arrowhead)* while the peroneal tendons *(orange arrowhead)* are retracted inferiorly using a small Hohman retractor. The leading edge of the interosseous ligament *(blue arrowhead)* is indicated. **B:** Diagram of the surgical exposure. Figure shows extensor digitorum muscle raised as a distally based flap.

ally into the posterior facet (Fig. 29-12A). This provide wide exposure of the posterior facet, which can be seen to be running in an inferior-to-superior plane as the surgeon progresses posteriorly. The middle facet of the subtalar joint can also be seen in the medial aspect of the wound. This typically merges into the anterior facet of the subtalar joint, which is seen underneath the talar head (Fig. 29-12B). Satisfactory distraction of the subtalar joint may require specific transection of the interosseous ligament within the canal of the sinus tarsi, although this ligament often is already incompetent and need not be directly addressed. Mobilizing the talocalcaneal articulation by soft tissue dissection is critical in reducing a fixed planovalgus deformity, which generally includes a significant lateral calcaneal subluxation that must be corrected.

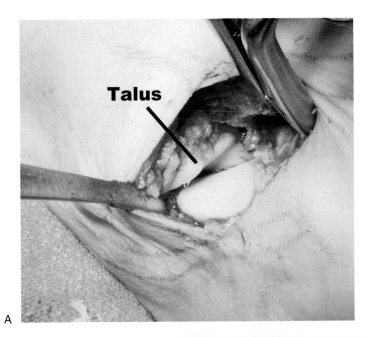

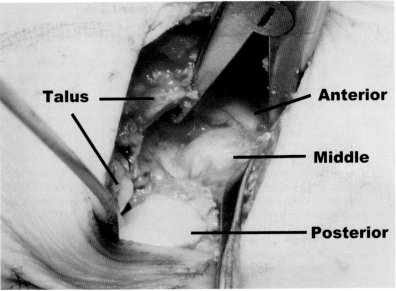

**Figure 29-12.** Subtalar joint (STJ) exposed. **A:** View of the distracted posterior facet of the subtalar joint. The baby lamina spreader is placed in the region of the talocalcaneal interosseous ligament. Notice the curved shape of the posterior facet. The posteromedial corner of the facet must be debrided to permit apposition of the joint surface. **B:** Moving the lamina spreader anteriorly exposes all three facets of the STJ.

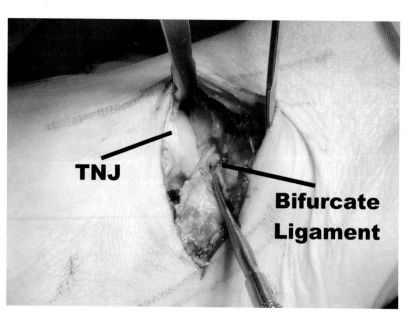

**Figure 29-13.** The calcaneocuboid joint, located at the blade of the Freer elevator, is shown with the bifurcate ligament and lateral talonavicular joint (TNJ). The dorsally placed Hohman retractor is within the capsule of the TNJ to retract and protect the overlying neurovascular bundle.

Subperiosteal dissection is then extended distally over the lateral border of the calcaneus to the level of the calcaneocuboid joint. A small Hohman retractor is placed just distal to this joint to allow visualization of the capsule of the calcaneocuboid joint. The capsule can then be released sharply off its insertion on the calcaneus laterally and dorsally to expose the entire articulation and the bifurcate ligament (Fig. 29-13). Proceeding medially, the bifurcate ligament is again visualized and transected to gain access to the lateral talonavicular joint, as well as the naviculocuboid articulation (Fig. 29-14). Exposure of this region can be improved by using a rongeur to resect the medial projection of the anterior calcaneal tubercle where it abuts the talar head.

The dissection is carried further medially to expose the talonavicular joint. The lateral talonavicular capsule is incised and subperiosteally dissected off its insertion on the talar head dorsally. A small Hohman retractor is placed into the joint dorsally to provide easier dissection of the capsular insertions as well as protect the overlying neurovascular structures. A similar capsular release off of the navicular and placement of a second dorsal Hohman retractor then provides a full exposure of the dorsal and lateral talonavicular joint. The joint can be distracted by placement of a small lamina spreader, permitting debridement of the talonavicular articulation (Fig. 29-15). At least three fourths of the joint can be debrided through this approach.

For most patients, the preoperative deformity can be passively corrected after the soft tissue release has been performed. In those in whom the deformity is passively correctable, debridement of the joints is undertaken so as to minimize the loss of underlying bone. Starting with the talonavicular joint, the joint is distracted using the small lamina spreader, and the pineapple-shaped burr is used to debride the cartilage and subchondral bone down to healthy, bleeding cancellous bone (Fig. 29-15). Care is taken to maintain the normal contours of the articulations, because this makes it easy to position the foot subsequently while maintaining good apposition of the fusion surfaces. On the talonavicular joint, particular attention must be paid to the dorsum of the talar head where an osteophyte is often present, which may block reduction of this articulation if not removed. The osteophyte removal can be accomplished by use of a small osteotome or rongeur.

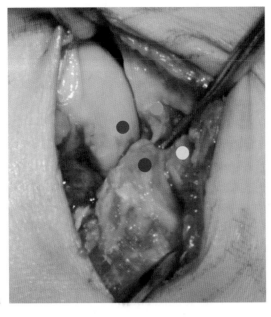

A

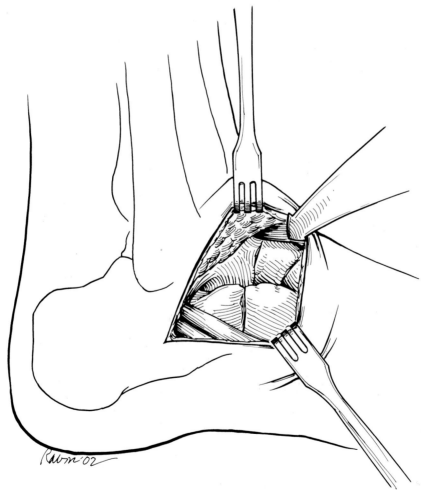

B

**Figure 29-14.** Exposure of the naviculocuboid articulation. **A:** The surgery is a quadruple, rather than triple, arthrodesis. The Freer elevator is placed into the joint between the navicular *(green dot)* and cuboid *(yellow dot)*. The talus *(red dot)* and calcaneus *(blue dot)* are seen. **B:** Diagram of the Chopart joint exposure.

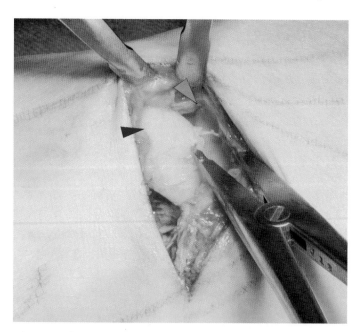

**Figure 29-15.** View of the distracted talonavicular joint through lateral incision using the baby Inge lamina spreader for exposure. The joint surfaces of the navicular *(orange arrowhead)* and talar head *(blue arrowhead)* can be debrided.

Avoidance of thermal necrosis is accomplished by using a light touch with the burr. Some surgeons prefer to use sharp osteotomes, curettes, and rongeurs to debride the joint surfaces.

After talonavicular debridement, attention is turned to the articulation between the cuboid and navicular. This constitutes a true diarthrodial joint and should be included as part of the fusion mass because it completes the circle of stability in the hindfoot (Fig. 29-16). For this reason, some authors have called this procedure a quadruple, rather than triple,

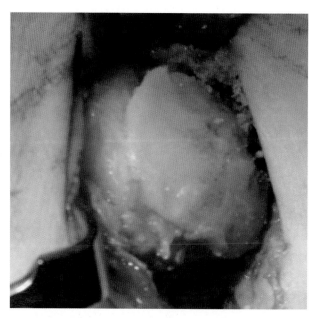

**Figure 29-16.** Most of the talar joint surface can be debrided through the lateral incision. An osteophyte is visible dorsally, and it should be resected to permit adequate positioning of the joint. The most medial portion (20%) of the talar surface can be debrided through the second, dorsomedial incision.

arthrodesis. The naviculocuboid articulation is easily debrided by curettage or rongeur, being careful to limit the amount of bony resection.

At this point, a small Hohman is placed on the lateral border of the cuboid and a small lamina spreader placed within the calcaneocuboid joint. This joint is then debrided using a burr. As shown in Figure 29-17, the calcaneocuboid joint is not a flat joint, and care must be taken to debride the most plantar aspect of the cuboid as it curves underneath the calcaneus. Failure to do so can prevent complete apposition of this fusion site. The lamina spreader must first be placed laterally to debride the medial aspect of the joint and then medially to debride the lateral aspect of the joint. Leaving a small lateral ridge on this joint prevents satisfactory apposition of the bony surfaces. It should be possible to hold the transverse tarsal joints in a reduced position with good apposition of the fusion surfaces.

The small Hohman retractor is then placed around the lateral border of the posterior facet of the subtalar joint and the small lamina spreader placed in the sinus tarsi for exposure of the subtalar joint (Fig. 29-12A). The articular surfaces are debrided using the burr and the curette. The curve and the angle of joint surfaces of the posterior facet lead to the tendency to resect too much calcaneus and too little talus. This can be avoided by providing appropriate joint distraction, which permits direct visualization of the entire joint space. The posteromedial aspect of the posterior facet must be debrided to allow good apposition of the fusion surfaces. It is helpful to place the lamina spreader directly in the posterior lateral corner of the posterior facet to gain better visualization of the middle and anterior facets of the subtalar joint (Fig. 29-12B). These joints are then debrided of cartilage and subchondral bone using the burr. The subtalar joint should be reducible into an anatomic position with good apposition of the posterior facet noted. After adequate reduction can be achieved, the dorsal anterior surface of the calcaneus and inferior lateral surfaces of the talar neck are decorticated using the burr in preparation for later bone grafting. This wound is then copiously irrigated, and attention is turned to the final debridement of the talonavicular joint.

A dorsomedial incision is made centered over the talonavicular joint and extending proximally up the talar neck (Fig. 29-18A). The saphenous vein is almost always directly underneath this incision and must be retracted or cauterized (Fig. 29-18B). The dissection is carried out until the talonavicular joint capsule is identified. This is then incised in longitudinal fashion, and a small Hohman is placed medially and dorsally to expose the medial aspect of this articulation. The small lamina spreader can then be placed in the joint, typically from its superior surface, and the remaining articular surfaces of this joint debrided of

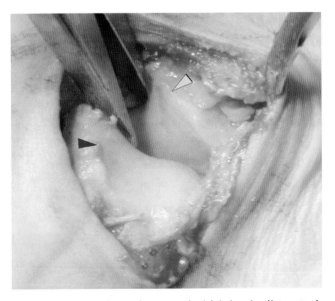

**Figure 29-17.** The calcaneocuboid joint is distracted, demonstrating the saddle-shaped articulation between the calcaneus *(blue arrowhead)* and the cuboid *(yellow arrowhead)*. The joint surfaces are debrided.

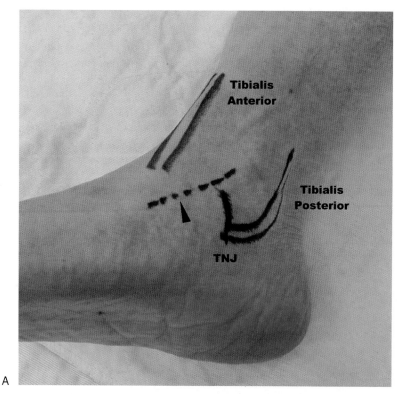

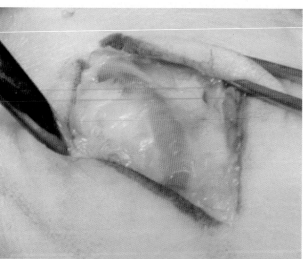

**Figure 29-18.** Dorsomedial incision. **A:** Medial view shows the skin incision *(arrowhead)* centered over the talonavicular joint dorsal to posterior tibial tendon. **B:** After the skin incision, the saphenous vein is identified and retracted.

cartilage and subchondral bone (Fig. 29-19). At this point, it should be possible to hold the foot in a reduced position.

If a tight heel cord prevents neutral positioning of the ankle and foot, an open tendo-Achilles lengthening can be undertaken at this juncture. This is accomplished through a posteromedial incision adjacent to the Achilles tendon, with a Z-lengthening cut performed with minimum of 5 cm overlap in the Z portion. The tendon is not resutured until after the fusion has been stabilized. I prefer to repair the lengthening using no. 2 Ethibond sutures with the knots buried in the overlapped portions.

Through the medial incision, a small Hohman retractor is placed laterally, exposing the dorsum of the talar neck. The subtalar joint is then held in a reduced position (correcting

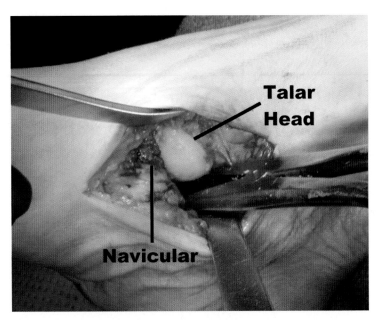

**Figure 29-19.** Medial exposure of the talonavicular joint through a longitudinal capsulotomy, made dorsal to the posterior tibial tendon. This permits debridement of the most medial aspect of the talar head.

the valgus-varus and axial rotation deformities), and a cancellous screw with a 6.5-mm-long thread is placed from the dorsomedial talar neck directed in a posterior and lateral direction to engage the calcaneus. The long, 3.2-mm drill bit is very useful for this step, because the total depth is frequently in excess of 80 mm. The calcaneus is lateral to the talus, and the tendency to drill straight posteriorly into the calcaneus will result in a screw that placed medial to the calcaneus (Fig. 29-20). It is helpful to place a finger on the posterior margin of the calcaneus and aim for it while placing the screw. The hole in the talus should be pretapped, even in osteopenic bone, because the placement of a 6.5-mm screw can cause a talar neck fracture. Care must be taken to avoid placing this screw too posterior in the talar neck because it can easily cause anterior impingement in the ankle.

The subtalar screw can be placed in a dorsal to plantar direction, as described previously, or in a plantar to dorsal direction, as has been described in the literature. The advantage of the antegrade placement is that the surgeon can use a screw with more threads (32 mm), and there is little danger if the screw is a bit too long. The risk of avascular necrosis after placement of such a screw has been reported, but it is a rare event. The disadvantage to the retrograde screw is that the surgeon is limited to using a short (16-mm), threaded screw because of the small size of the talar body, and there is a potential for penetration into the ankle joint by misplacement of the screw.

After the subtalar joint stabilization, attention is turned to the talonavicular joint. It is stabilized with a 4.5-mm cortical screw using lag technique in retrograde direction. The talonavicular joint is held in a reduced position with respect to plantarflexion to restore the longitudinal arch, as well as abduction-adduction and varus-valgus positions. There is a tendency to stabilize this with a forefoot in too much supination, which results in weight bearing on the lateral margin of the foot. The screw must be placed at a shallow angle in the medial-lateral plane (i.e., close to the axis of the talus) and slightly upward to engage the neck of the talus. A cortical screw longer than 40 mm is unnecessary. A misdirected long screw that exits the inferior surface of the talar neck and abuts the calcaneus can cause distraction of the subtalar joint. The entrance hole in the navicular is also countersunk to prevent breaking the long bridge of navicular bone as it is tightened (Fig. 29-21).

The calcaneocuboid is stabilized using an antegradely placed, 4.5-mm cortical screw from the anterior process of the calcaneus into the cuboid. A screw length of more than 40 mm is unnecessary.

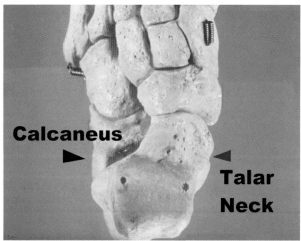

A

**Figure 29-20.** Fixation of the subtalar joint with screw oriented from a medial to lateral direction and from anterior (on the talar neck) to posterior to engage the body of the calcaneus. **A:** Dorsal view of a foot skeleton demonstrates the lateral position of calcaneus *(black arrowhead)* relative to the talus *(blue arrowhead)*. **B:** Exposure of the talar neck through medial incision is achieved with a small Hohman retractor placed on the lateral surface of the talar neck, aiming the subtalar screw laterally and posteriorly. **C:** View of the foot from underneath demonstrates the degree of lateral inclination required to center the screw in the calcaneal body.

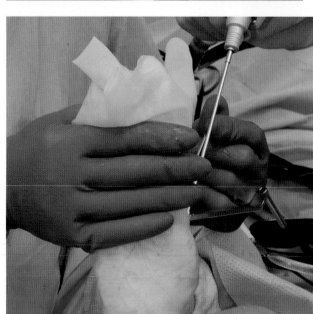

B

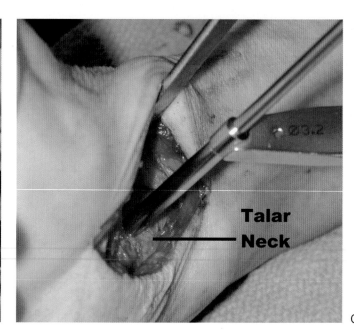

C

The wounds are irrigated and the tourniquet deflated. If a tendo-Achilles lengthening was performed, the ankle is held in a neutral position and the tendon repaired. The bone graft is placed about all the fusion surfaces if desired. Radiographs of the feet are obtained in anteroposterior and lateral planes, as are radiographs in the tangential plane of the calcaneus (Fig. 29-22), to judge fixation placement, bony apposition, and alignment.

The lateral wound is closed using 0 Vicryl in the fascia of the extensor digitorum brevis, 3-0 Monocryl (poliglecaprone 25) in the subcutaneous tissue, and 5-0 chromic in the skin. The dorsal medial incision is closed using 0 Vicryl suture in the capsule and deep fascia, 3-0 Monocryl (poliglecaprone 25) subcutaneous tissue, and 5-0 chromic in the skin. If a tendo-Achilles lengthening was undertaken, the tendon sheath is closed using a running 3-0 Monocryl suture, the subcutaneous tissue with 3-0 Monocryl, and the skin with 5-0 chromic suture. In patients with potentially compromised healing (e.g., diabetes, steroid use), the skin layer is closed using 4-0 nylon sutures rather than the chromic sutures. No drains are used. The leg is then placed into a short-leg, non–weight-bearing cast with the ankle in neutral position. I warn the patients and the nurses that some bleeding into the cast is expected but that it usually does not reflect significant blood loss. Because of the expected swelling, others prefer a compressive dressing with a plaster splint, such as a Robert Jones dressing, and then application of a short-leg, non–weight-bearing cast 2 days later.

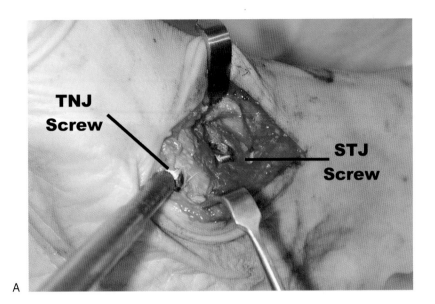

TNJ
Screw

STJ
Screw

A

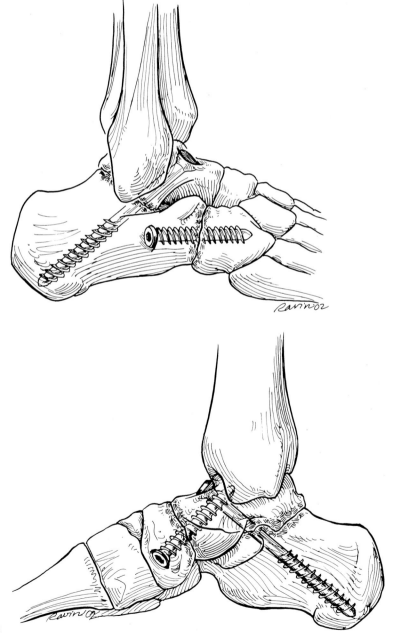

B

**Figure 29-21. A:** The talonavicular joint (TNJ) screw is placed from distal to proximal retrograde into the talar neck starting laterally enough to miss the subtalar joint (STJ) screw. For corrections of pes planus with collapse at the TNJ, the navicular is realigned relative to the talus by adducting plantarflexion and inversion. Consequently, the screw must be directed from inferior to superior to fully engage the talar neck. **B:** Placing the screw in a horizontal direction results in limited purchase of the talar neck, because it traverses inferior to the neck into the subtalar joint.

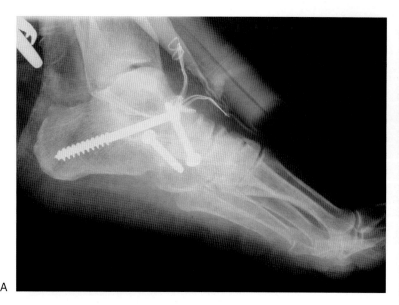

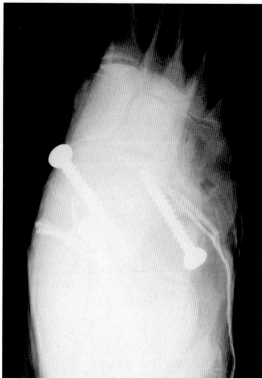

**Figure 29-22.** The calcaneocuboid screw is placed from proximal to distal through a separate 1-cm, longitudinal incision or by extending the lateral incision over the cuboid. Intraoperative lateral **(A)** and anteroposterior **(B)** radiographs show placement of calcaneocuboid subtalar and talonavicular screws.

I attempt to correct the deformities through the fusion sites. For instance, a hindfoot varus deformity is corrected by resecting more of the lateral facet of the subtalar joint so as to place the calcaneus into greater valgus position. The corrective resection can be undertaken with burr or sharp osteotome. In the more severe cases, it may be necessary to use an osteotome to resect the joints in their entirety. Because a considerable amount of bone is lost to this technique (which results in shortening), it should be reserved for only the most severe deformities.

## POSTOPERATIVE MANAGEMENT

A triple arthrodesis is a major surgery, and I routinely admit these patients postoperatively for pain control. They are generally placed on patient-controlled analgesia for the first 24 hours and then progressed as rapidly as possible to oral analgesics. Patients are seen by physical therapy on the first postoperative day for crutch training and are discharged from hospital as soon as they are comfortable and able to ambulate without bearing weight.

Postoperative antibiotics are administered for 24 hours. Routine deep venous thrombosis prophylaxis is not undertaken because the risk is very low.

The patient is maintained in a short-leg cast and not allowed to bear weight for 6 weeks, at which point radiographs are obtained. If the radiographs are satisfactory, the patient is placed into a short-leg walking cast for the next 6 weeks. At that juncture radiographs are taken (Fig. 29-23), and if satisfactory healing is appreciated and no significant tenderness at the fusion sites is elicited, all external support is discontinued. The patient is allowed to wear shoes and gradually increase activities as tolerated.

Physical therapy is used after this procedure only for gait training. Long-term rehabilitation for maximal recovery is not generally necessary. Occasionally, it is useful to refer patients to physical therapy after cast removal to learn foot and ankle rehabilitation exercises.

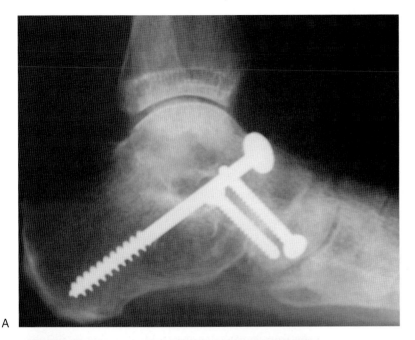

A

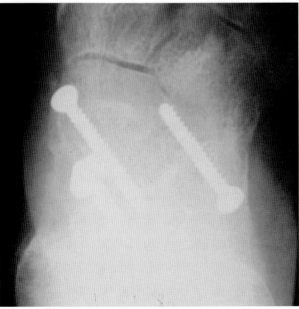

B

**Figure 29-23.** Postoperative radiographs demonstrate good alignment and arthrodesis union. **A:** Lateral view of the foot. **B:** Anteroposterior view of the foot.

## COMPLICATIONS

The triple arthrodesis is an involved procedure with a significant potential for complications related to the soft tissues and the bones. Each of these should be discussed with the patient.

The most common site of *nonunion* in triple arthrodesis is at the talonavicular joint, occurring in 5% to 10% in most of the reported series in the literature. It is likely that the use of adequate bone grafting and the establishment of satisfactory stabilization can minimize this complication intraoperatively. Observing standard surgical technique to obtain healthy cancellous fusion surfaces is essential, because the dense subchondral bone of the articular surfaces is not well vascularized and not conducive to fusion.

If there is doubt about the healing of the fusion at 3 months based on radiographs and persistent tenderness, the patient could be immobilized further into another short-leg walking cast for 4 to 6 weeks. If there is no significant healing by 6 months, revision surgery with debridement, intraoperative cultures, and restabilization may be indicated.

*Malalignment* is a preventable complication, because it is almost always a result of malpositioning at the time of surgery. Patients tolerate some residual valgus in the hindfoot and a somewhat flattened arch medially. I advise them that their foot alignment cannot restore the normal foot appearance. However, the existence of a supinated forefoot, which results in overloading of the lateral foot, persistent hindfoot varus, or a rocker-bottom deformity, are not well tolerated. Initially, attempts may be made to handle these problems by accommodative footwear, but it may be necessary to revise the position of the fusions.

*Nerve damage* and subsequent numbness postoperatively may be caused by injury to the intermediate branch of the superficial peroneal nerve. The nerve should be protected during the procedure to avoid hypesthesia in the dorsal lateral foot or a painful incisional neuroma. Occasionally, the sural nerve has a more superior course than normal and may be seen in the inferior margins of the sinus tarsi incision. Care must be taken in this region to ensure that it is not inadvertently lacerated.

*Wound healing* may be a problem. The incisions used for this procedure are well tolerated by the skin and heal without difficulty. The issues in patients with potentially compromised healing abilities, such as diabetics, are primarily related to the increased time of healing. This is addressed intraoperatively by using nonabsorbable skin sutures rather than the usual chromic sutures. Adequate vascularity must be ensured in all patients. A vascular consultation should be obtained preoperatively if there are any questions in this regard. I also counsel my patients that smoking increases their chances of experiencing problems with healing of the skin and the fusions.

Although there has been some concern about the potential for ankle *arthritis* after triple arthrodesis, the most recent data suggest that this is not a significant problem. In patients who have other reasons for joint degeneration, such as in rheumatoid arthritis, I caution that they may end up with other joints affected; the triple arthrodesis may or may not contribute to this process. It is important to view preoperative radiographs to ensure that ankle or midfoot pathology does not exist before the triple arthrodesis.

## RECOMMENDED READING

1. Figgie MP, O'Malley MJ, Ranawat C, et al.: Triple arthrodesis in rheumatoid arthritis. *Clin Orthop* 292: 250–254, 1993.
2. Frey C, Halikus NM, Vu-Rose T, et al.: A review of ankle arthrodesis: predisposing factors to nonunion. *Foot Ankle Int* 15:581–584, 1994.
3. Jahss MH: Surgical principles and the plantigrade foot. In: Jahss M, ed. *Disorders of the foot and ankle: medical and surgical treatment,* 2nd ed. Philadelphia: WB Saunders, 1990:236–279.
4. Johnson KA: *Surgery of the foot and ankle.* New York: Raven Press, 1989.
5. Jones CK, Nunley JA: Osteonecrosis of the lateral aspect of the talar dome after triple arthrodesis: a report of three cases. *J Bone Joint Surg Am* 81:1165–1169, 1999.
6. Michelson JD, Curl LA: Use of demineralized bone matrix in hindfoot arthrodesis. *Clin Orthop* 325: 203–208, 1996.
7. Saltzman CL, Fehrle MJ, Cooper RR, et al.: Triple arthrodesis: twenty-five and forty-four-year average follow-up of the same patients. *J Bone Joint Surg Am* 81:1391–1402, 1999.
8. Sangeorzan BJ, Smith D, Veith R, et al.: Triple arthrodesis using internal fixation in treatment of adult foot disorders. *Clin Orthop* 294:299–307, 1993.
9. Siffert RS, del Torto U: "Beak" triple arthrodesis for severe cavus deformity. *Clin Orthop* 181:64–67, 1983.
10. Wetmore RS, Drennan JC: Long-term results of triple arthrodesis in Charcot-Marie-Tooth disease. *J Bone Joint Surg Am* 71:417–422, 1989.

# 30

# Open Reduction and Internal Fixation of Calcaneal Fractures

Bruce J. Sangeorzan

## INDICATIONS/CONTRAINDICATIONS

Fractures of the os calcis are common and disabling injuries. They occur most frequently in employed laborers and with increasing frequency in motor vehicle accidents. These fractures account for about 2% of all fractures. Some fracture types, such as extraarticular and stress fractures, have a favorable prognosis. Displaced, intraarticular fractures are most concerning, and there are differing opinions about fracture classification, specific treatment, and indications for operative management.

Fractures of the os calcis are troublesome for several reasons. The soft tissue envelope about the hindfoot is thin, with little muscle and with highly specialized plantar soft tissues (i.e., heel pad). The medial side of the os calcis is covered by a thin layer of skin and intimately associated with artery, nerves, vein, and tendon. The medial side also has a complex surface, with thick, stabilizing ligaments attaching the calcaneus to the talus.

The calcaneus also has complex articular surface anatomy. The articulation with the talus has three facets: the posterior, middle, and anterior facets that require a fixed relationship to function effectively as a joint. A fracture that disrupts the relationship between the three facets is an intraarticular fracture. The middle and anterior facets, although smaller than the posterior facet, function at a much higher joint contact pressure. The relationship of these facets must be restored for full function of the joint. The calcaneus also articulates with the cuboid. Although this calcaneocuboid joint is less complex and more forgiving, a split in this joint widens the heel and limits the function of the transverse tarsal joint.

The mechanism of injury usually involves an axial load where the talus impacts the calcaneus, creating an oblique primary fracture line and often multiple secondary fracture lines (Figs. 30-1 through 30-3).

---

B. J. Sangeorzan, M.D.: Department of Orthopaedics and Sports Medicine, University of Washington; and Harborview Medical Center, Seattle, Washington.

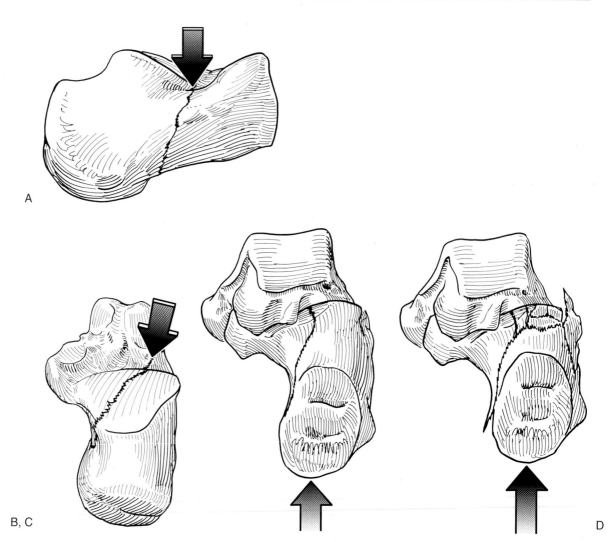

**Figure 30-1.** Drawings of an intraarticular right calcaneus fracture viewed laterally **(A)**, dorsally **(B)**, and posteriorly **(C and D)** show the mechanism of injury and primary fracture line. The *arrows* indicate the point of impact. The primary fracture line, also called the separation fracture, begins at the point of impact from the talus and progresses posteriorly and medially **(A–C)**. With more severe impact, greater displacement and comminution occurs **(D)**, along with a decrease in calcaneal height and increase in width.

Indications for open reduction and internal fixation (ORIF) of calcaneal fracture, although not without controversy, have become more widely accepted. Operative treatment is chosen for injures that would do poorly without open treatment. The characteristics of the calcaneus fracture that suggest a poor outcome include a high-energy mechanism, substantial depression of the tuber or joint angle of Bohler, widening of the heel, horizontally oriented talus, contiguous fractures of multiple bones, severe soft tissue injury, and systemic medical conditions. Contraindications include a severely comminuted fracture, impaired vascularity, infection, severe neuropathy, and a patient who is unable to comply with the limited weight-bearing requirement in the immediate postoperative period.

There are many classification systems for calcaneus fractures, some based on fracture pattern seen on plain film radiographs and others based on the computed tomography (CT) scan. However, no classification system has definitively demonstrated a role in determining which fractures need to be repaired and which can be treated closed.

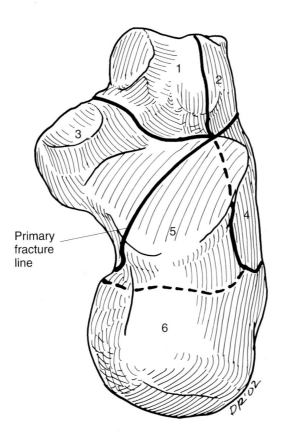

**Figure 30-2.** Dorsal view of the calcaneus shows a primary fracture line *(black)*. The secondary fracture lines progress outward from the point of impact and divide the anterior process (1 and 2) and the middle facet (3) and shear off the lateral wall (4). In central depression fractures, the posterior facet is depressed (5), and the tuberosity fragment is displaced (6).

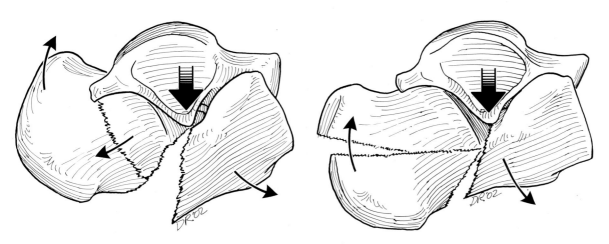

**Figure 30-3.** Lateral view of central depression *(left)* and tongue-type *(right)* fractures.

It is generally agreed that fractures involving the articular surface of the calcaneus with displacement of more of than 3 mm in a young, active person should be treated operatively. The threshold for open treatment increases for patients older than 50 years of age, because the functional expectations recede and the likelihood of soft tissue complications increases. However, age is a minor factor. Gross widening of the heel with dislocation of the tuberosity laterally may be an indication for open treatment even in a relatively sedentary individual. If the tuberosity is allowed to heal in a grossly lateralized position, weight bearing of any kind, even household ambulation, may exceed the functional ability of the hindfoot in this position. Conversely, the calcaneus fracture with multiple lines of comminution but only limited displacement and widening may be amenable to treatment by closed means in a healthy, active individual. In short, ORIF should be chosen as an appropriate treatment technique when there is displacement of the articular surface, widening of the heel, lateral displacement of the tuberosity, flattening of the talar axis, or threatened soft tissue.

## PREOPERATIVE PLANNING

The physical examination of the injured part should include an assessment of the dorsalis pedis and posterior tibial arteries as well as a sensory examination of the plantar surface of the foot. The tibial nerve crosses the medial side of the calcaneus below the sustentaculum tali and may be injured at the time of displacement of the fracture. In our institution, this typically manifests as incomplete loss of sensation on the plantar surface of the foot. Other musculoskeletal injuries commonly occur in patients with calcaneus fractures, particularly those sustained in a fall.

A complete examination should be performed on the rest of the musculoskeletal system, as well as the head, chest, and abdomen. Spine fractures occur in approximately 10% to 15% of patients with calcaneus fractures. Patients involved in motor vehicle accidents with intrusion of the floor pan should be thoroughly evaluated like all other trauma patients for concomitant injuries.

Important aspects of the patient history unique to patients with calcaneus fracture include smoking history; systemic diseases such as diabetes mellitus, vascular disease, and inflammatory diseases; prior history of deep vein thrombosis; and medication history. Although there are no absolute indications or contraindications for open reduction, operative treatment should be approached with great caution in patients with diseases that limit healing of the extremities.

The timing of surgical intervention varies with the fracture pattern and mechanism of injury, as well as more practical matters. Surgery is best performed when the soft tissue swelling has begun to recede. This varies from 3 to 14 days. Patients with fracture blisters may require a longer interval before surgery. Although there is no scientific basis for the approach to patients with fracture blisters, treatment usually is performed when the blisters have dried and the underlying tissue his epithelialized. Fracture patterns that threaten the skin, particularly tongue-type patterns that tent the skin above the Achilles tendon, may be suitable to operative treatment in an urgent fashion.

The treatment of open fractures is performed in staged fashion. Typically, the open wound is debrided and irrigated within 8 hours of the injury. At the time of debridement, the fracture fragments should be repositioned to remove tension from the skin. After skin closure, the patient is treated in the same way as the patient with a closed calcaneus fracture. A well-padded splint is applied with the foot in a neutral position. Alternatively, a commercial brace and Ace elastic bandage may be applied. The patient is instructed in non–weight-bearing ambulation using crutches and asked to maintain elevation of the injured part.

Preoperative planning begins with an understanding of the anatomy of the calcaneus, good-quality imaging, and an understanding the pattern of the fracture. The calcaneus has a long tuberosity that does not have an articular surface but there are important attachments of the Achilles tendon and the plantar fascia. The medial wall of the calcaneus is curved and covered with tendons nerves and ligaments. The lateral wall of the calcaneus is relatively accessible, flat, and relatively well suited to internal fixation. Most often, the fracture pattern is characterized by a primary fracture line that begins in the sinus tarsi and is oriented posteriorly and medially, dividing the lateral half of the posterior facet from the medial part of the posterior facet, the tarsal canal, and the medial and anterior facet. There are many secondary fracture lines that may enter the other facet or enter the calcaneocuboid joint.

Although the anatomy of the calcaneus should be familiar to the surgeon, imaging studies are used to understand the fracture lines. Appropriate plain film evaluation includes views of the foot in anteroposterior, lateral, and axial projections, as well as comparison radiographs of the uninjured heal (Figs. 30-4 and 30-5). The lateral view shows the degree of

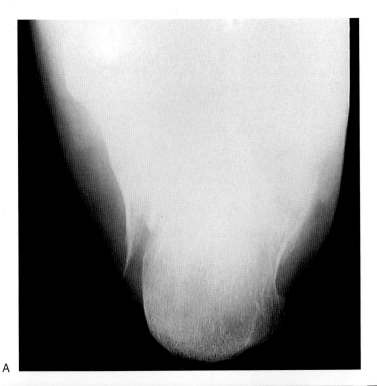

A

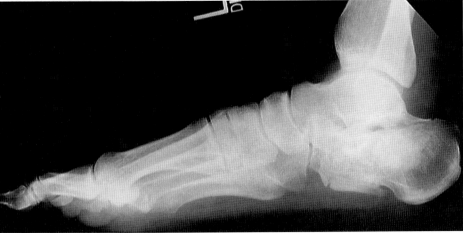

B

**Figure 30-4.** Fractures should be characterized by plain film radiographs obtained with consistent, standard radiologic techniques. **A:** Axial calcaneal view. **B:** Lateral view of the foot. *(continued)*

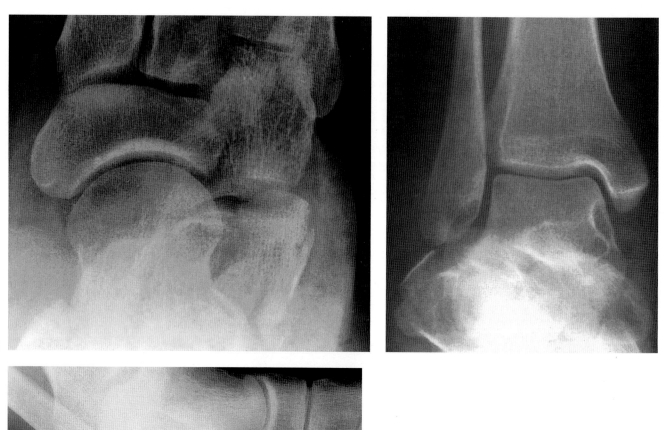

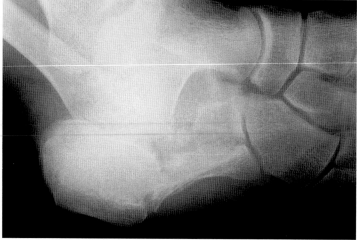

**Figure 30-4.** *Continued.* **C:** Anteroposterior view of the foot. **D:** Oblique view of the foot. **E:** Ankle mortise.

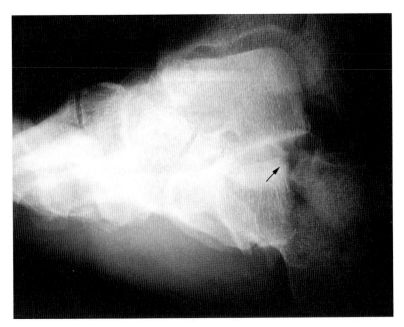

**Figure 30-5.** An oblique radiograph of the calcaneus, such as the Broden's view, can demonstrate fractures of the posterior facet *(arrow)*.

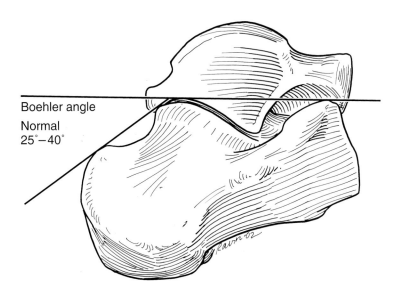

Boehler angle
Normal
25°–40°

**Figure 30-6.** The degree of malalignment can be estimated by the Boehler angle.

displacement as changes in Boehler's angle and the angle of Gissane (Fig. 30-6). The axial view demonstrates the degree of lateral migration of the tuberosity. The CT scan has largely replaced specialized views such as Broden's oblique views of the subtalar joint (Fig. 30-7).

Obtaining CT images in two planes is important: the semicoronal view, which cuts through the posterior and middle facets, and the transverse plane, which shows the position of the tuberosity fragment, the involvement of the anterior process in the fracture, and the size of the sustentacular fragment (Fig. 30-7). Sagittal reconstruction images may be performed along the medial side of the calcaneus, through the posterior facet, and along the

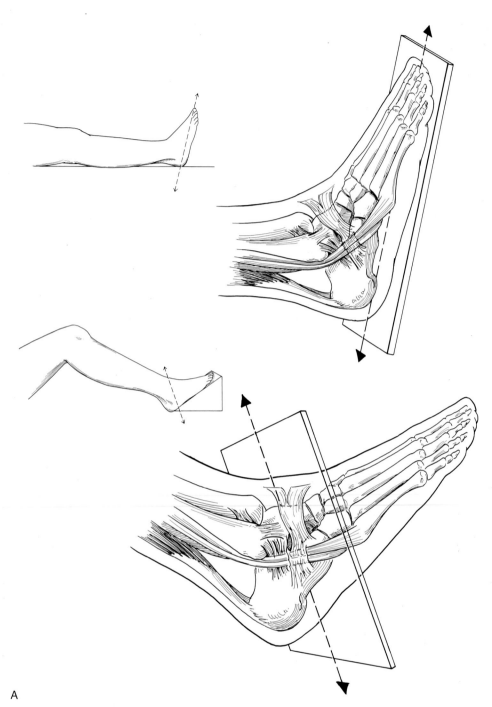

A

**Figure 30-7. A:** Technique of positioning the extremity for CT scans in transverse *(top)* and coronal *(bottom)* plane views. *(continued)*

lateral side of the calcaneus (Fig. 30-7). These reconstructions may be very helpful in complex fractures and in assisting the less-experienced surgeon.

Modern CT software can readily perform three-dimensional reconstructions (Fig. 30-8). These also may be helpful to the surgeon, particularly those with somewhat less experience. The quality of images depends on the original scan parameters, the quality of the scanner, and how the study is performed (Fig. 30-9). If the patient moves during the scanning process, the three-dimensional reconstructions, sagittal reconstructions, and even the coronal or transverse plane images will be of limited value.

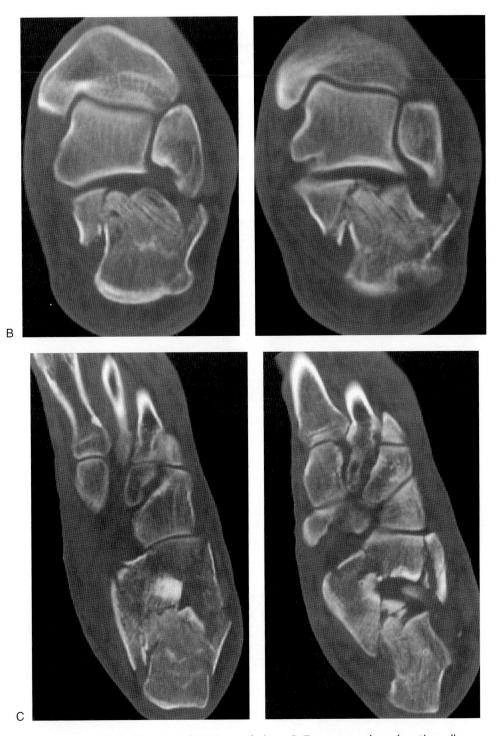

**Figure 30-7.** *Continued.* **B:** Coronal view. **C:** Transverse view. *(continued)*

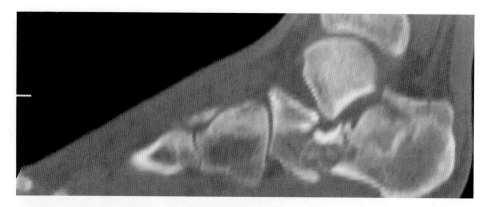

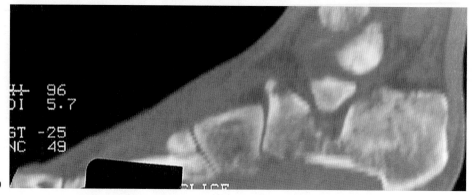

**Figure 30-7.** *Continued.* **D:** Sagittal reconstruction views.

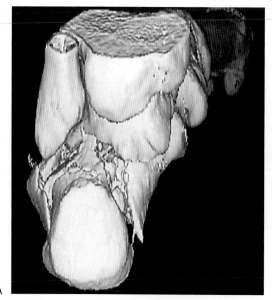

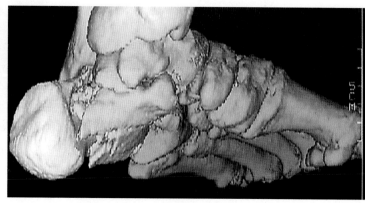

**Figure 30-8.** Axial **(A)**, medial **(B)**, lateral **(C)**, and oblique lateral **(D)** CT views and three-dimensional reconstruction. *(continued)*

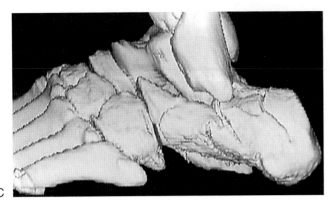
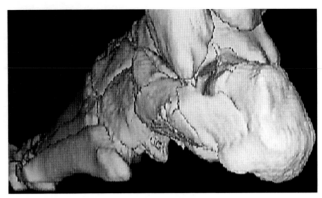

C

D

**Figure 30-8.** *Continued.*

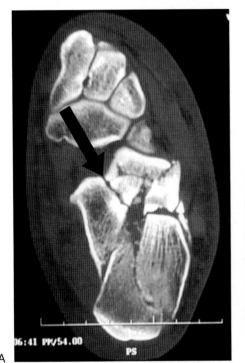
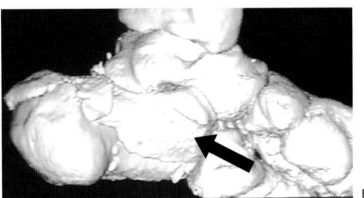

A

B

**Figure 30-9. A:** CT scan in the transverse plane shows the fracture line between anterior calcaneus and sustentaculum, which is not visible. **B:** In the CT scan and three-dimensional reconstruction, the fracture line *(A)* has been erased by the image reconstruction process. This process, by which the CT downgrades low-intensity findings, may in part account for the fact that many do not acknowledge the existence of this fracture line.

## SURGERY

The patient is placed in the lateral decubitus position, with the affected side up (Fig. 30-10). A tourniquet is placed on the thigh. The potential site for the bone graft, such as the iliac crest or proximal tibia, should be selected and prepped. The dependent limb is padded and protected. The operative limb is elevated on blankets or commercial padding such that a platform is created that prevents obstruction by the other limb. A stable platform also allows appropriate positioning for intraoperative radiographs of the foot.

A curved incision is designed with vertical and horizontal limbs (Fig. 30-11). The vertical limb is oriented halfway between the posterior aspect of the peroneal tendons and the

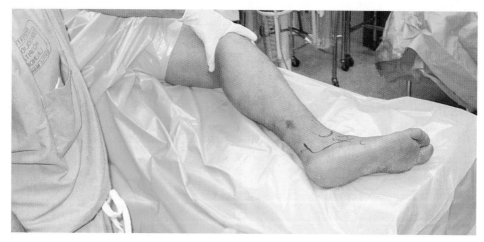

**Figure 30-10.** The patient is positioned on the lateral side with the fractured extremity up. A vacuum bag and an axillary roll are used to protect the shoulder. A tourniquet is applied to the thigh. The operative limb is elevated on a radiolucent pad or folded blankets as shown here. The opposite limb is padded and flexed so that it is not below the operative limb.

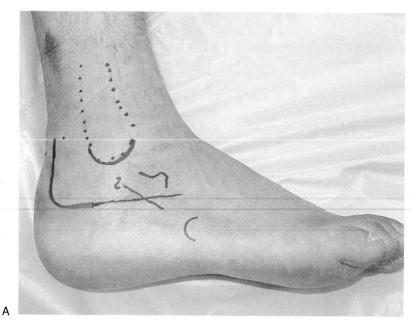

A

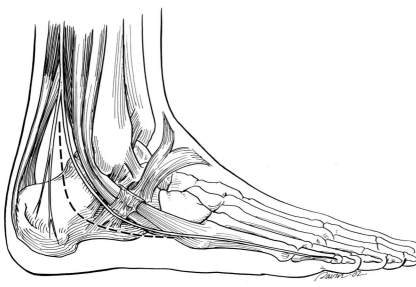

B

**Figure 30-11. A:** The extensile approach allows access to the lateral wall, tuberosity, posterior and middle facets, and the calcaneocuboid joint. The incision is curved, with vertical and horizontal limbs. The vertical limb is halfway between the peroneal tendons and the Achilles tendon. At the superior margin of this incision, the sural nerve courses in the subcutaneous tissue. The horizontal limb parallels the plantar foot, angling slightly dorsally at its anterior aspect. It should be adequately positioned plantarward to allow placement of a plate on the lateral wall but dorsal enough to allow visualization of the subtalar joint. Its distance from the plantar foot varies with the pitch angle and fracture pattern. In this example, it is relatively cephalad. The sural nerve *(s)* crosses at the junction of the middle and distal thirds of the horizontal limb of the incision. If the horizontal limb is more plantar, the sural nerve will cross it more distally or not at all. The fibula is outlined by the *dotted line.* The anterior process is marked by the *irregular line* above the incision. **B:** Extensile approach to the lateral calcaneus, showing the proximity of the sural nerve.

anterior aspect of the Achilles tendon. At the superior margin of this incision, the sural nerve passes in the subcutaneous tissue. The horizontal limb of the incision parallels the plantar surface of the foot and is inclined slightly at the anterior margin. It should be plantar enough to allow application of fixation, such as a plate to the lateral wall after the calcaneus fracture is reduced, but dorsal enough to allow visualization of the subtalar joint. The sural nerve crosses at the junction of the middle and distal thirds of the horizontal limb of the incision. The sural nerve is very closely associated with the subcutaneous tissue above the peroneal tendons.

The incision should be brought sharply to bone on its vertical limb and on the curved portion of the incision and then carried distally to the area of the peroneal tendons. Careful dissection should be performed overlying the peroneal tendons in the area of the sural nerve. The skin is dissected and raised as a full-thickness flap from the periosteum of the calcaneus and should include the calcaneofibular ligament (Fig. 30-12). The subtalar joint can be seen as the flap is raised. Two 0.062-inch Kirschner wires are placed into the talus to maintain retraction of the flap without excessive tension. The first Kirschner wire is inserted from lateral to medial into the lateral process of the talus, advanced into the bone approximately 1.5 cm, and bent proximally. The second Kirschner wire is inserted into the talar body posterior to the fibula and peroneal tendons. These Kirschner wires maintain retraction of the flap without excessive tension that requires only limited supplemental retraction to visualize the reduction.

If the comminution of the fracture extends into the calcaneocuboid joint, the horizontal limb of the incision is carried distally, superficial to the peroneal tendons and then deepened by blunt dissection on the distal dorsal side of the peroneals. The calcaneocuboid joint can be seen through this part of the incision. Visualization is aided by placing a blunt elevator into the joint and levering distally on the cuboid. Typically, the lateral aspect of the calcaneus is displaced in a more lateral and distal position to its native position and tends to block visualization of the joint until the fracture is reduced.

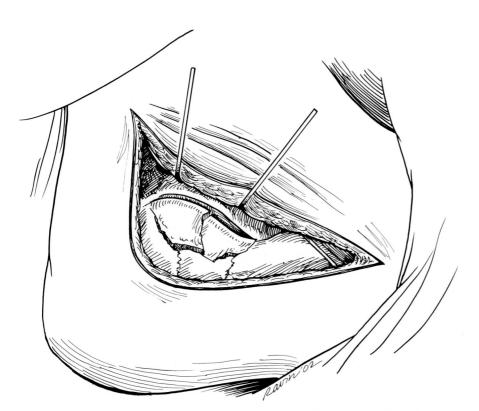

**Figure 30-12.** Lateral calcaneus exposure. The peroneal tendons and sural nerve are retracted anteriorly with a skin flap.

After exposing the subtalar joint, the organizing hematoma and small fracture fragments are removed by suction, irrigation, and use of a pituitary rongeur. The lateral aspect of the posterior facet typically is depressed into the body of the calcaneus. Depression of the posterior facet initially allows improved visualization of the anterior process.

There are multiple steps to reducing and fixing a displaced fracture. First, the surgeon should identify the fracture lines involving the anterior process of the calcaneus that extend medially (Fig. 30-13). These should then be reduced and held with a Kirschner wire. Next, the surgeon identifies the fracture lines that progress toward the calcaneocuboid joint. The lateral wall of the anterior process should be reduced and provisionally fixed with

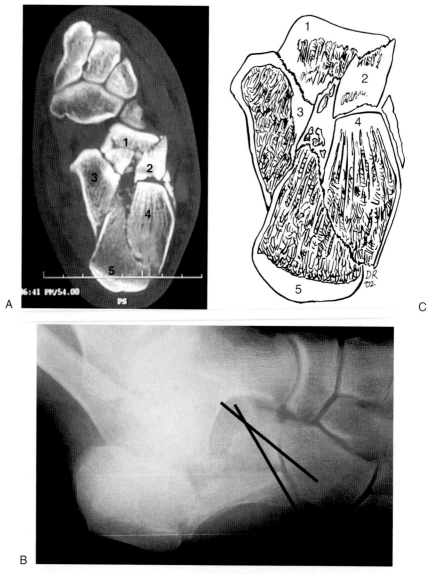

**Figure 30-13. A:** There are three phases to fracture reduction. The first step is to create an intact anterior calcaneus, which includes the anterior and middle facets, calcaneocuboid joint, and sinus tarsi. These are the fracture lines anterior to the point of impact shown in Figure 30-1A. In simple fracture patterns, there are no fracture lines in this area, and this step of the reduction is not necessary. The CT scan in transverse plane **(A)** and drawing **(B)** show an image of a calcaneus similar to that in Figure 30-1A. The fracture line between 1 and 3 should be reduced first to correct the relationship among the anterior, middle, and medial part of the posterior facets. After these parts are reduced, the fracture extending into calcaneocuboid joint (between 1 and 2) is reduced, and Kirschner wires are placed from lateral to medial **(C)** to create a construct to which the tuberosity (fragment 5) and posterior facet (fragment 4) can be reduced.

Kirschner wires (Fig. 30-13). The entire anterior process is typically elevated toward the talus. To reduce the remaining fractures to the anterior process, the anterior process can be retracted plantarward using a Langenbeck retractor or a laminar spreader placed between the lateral aspect of the talar head and the anterior process of the calcaneus. Fracture hematoma is evacuated to improve visualization.

The next step is to identify a fracture line progressing from lateral to medial, separating the medial part of the posterior facet from the middle and anterior facets. The posterior facet is usually plantarflexed relative to the anterior part of the calcaneus. This is reduced by upward pressure on the front of the posterior facet using a periosteal elevator. It is reduced as it is held with Kirschner wire directed from the anterior process laterally toward the posterior facet medially. Next, the lateral part of the posterior facet is retracted away from the fracture or is removed altogether. This allows visualization of the relationship of the medial part of the posterior facet to the medial wall. A 4.0-mm Schantz pin is inserted into the tuberosity fragment and used to reduce the fragment plantarward, medially, and into slight valgus (Fig. 30-14). When the medial wall on the tuberosity fragment lines up with the me-

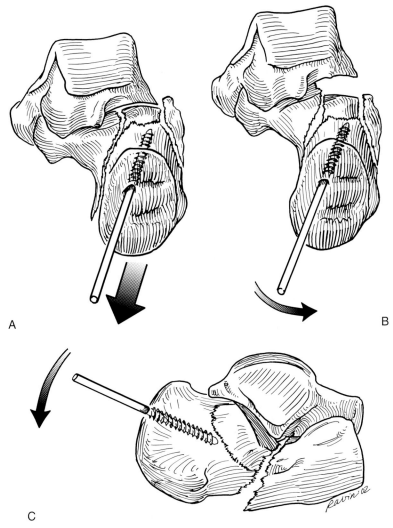

**Figure 30-14.** The second step of fracture reduction is realignment of the tuberosity by placing a Schantz pin in the posterior tuberosity. There is a step-off in the medial wall, with the tuberosity translated laterally, dorsally, and into varus. The tuberosity must be moved in three directions (arrows) for anatomic reduction by applying manual axial traction **(A)**, correcting varus **(B)**, and restoring height **(C)**. The posterior facet cannot be reduced until this is done because the tuberosity occupies the anatomic position of the posterior facet fragment.

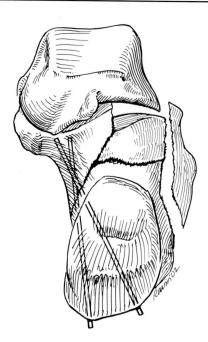

**Figure 30-15.** Reduction is maintained temporarily with 0.062-inch Kirschner wires from tuberosity to sustentaculum.

dial wall on the facet fragment, it is held with two 0.62-inch Kirschner wires (Fig. 30-15). These Kirschner wires enter the posterior aspect of the tuberosity and are directed upward toward the sustentaculum tali.

After the medial wall and the anterior process are reduced, reduction of the posterior facet can be performed (Fig. 30-16). Reduction of the posterior facet is the last step of the fracture reduction sequence. The posterior facet cannot be reduced properly until the front of the medial part of the posterior facet is elevated to its proper relationship with the anterior calcaneus and the tuberosity is reduced medially and plantarward, resulting in unen-

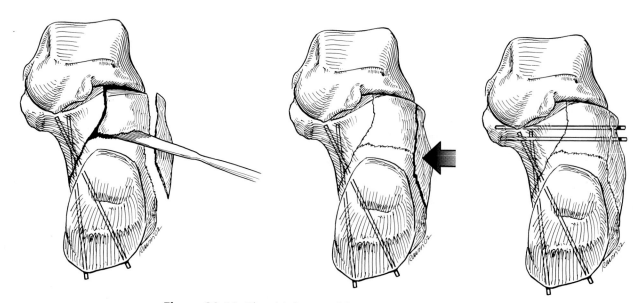

**Figure 30-16.** The third step of fracture reduction is realignment of posterior facet and lateral wall. The posterior facet is raised with an elevator *(left)*, the lateral wall *(arrow)* is replaced *(center)*, and transverse pins are inserted *(right)*.

cumbered space in which to position the posterior facet. If there are more than two pieces of posterior facet, the surgeon attaches the intercalated fracture fragment to the part of the posterior facet that has the best match. If this happens to be the lateral half of the posterior facet, the intercalary segment can be held with a 2.7-mm, cortical lag screw. The lateral fragment of the posterior facet should then be matched with the medial piece (Fig. 30-16). Kirschner wires are inserted in the anterior and posterior margins of the fracture, and intraoperative radiographs are obtained (Fig. 30-16).

Portable intraoperative radiographs are performed in two planes. The lateral view is straightforward, and an effort should be made to obtain a true lateral projection. The axial view is performed by placing the foot on a towel pack. The cassette is placed behind the ankle. The x-ray beam is aimed from plantar-distal to dorsal-posterior at an angle approximately 45° from the cassette, with the beam centered on the anterior part of the heel. This creates the Harris axial view, which used to be performed for evaluation of tarsal coalition, although from a reversed direction. The axial view determines whether the tuberosity has been adequately repositioned medially and shows the surface of the posterior and middle facets (Fig. 30-17). The lateral view allows visualization of the middle facet, posterior facet, and calcaneocuboid joint, as well as the adequacy of reduction of Boehler's angle.

If the fracture reduction is successful, a lag screw is placed across the posterior facet just beneath the subchondral surface. A plate is selected and contoured to fit the lateral wall of the calcaneus. The plate should usually be left straight and not contoured in the coronal plane. Keeping the plate straight reduces varus malposition of the heel. The best bone for fixation is found in three areas: the subchondral bone deep to the calcaneal cuboid joint, the subchondral bone near the Achilles insertion, and the dense bone of the sustentaculum tali. One screw should be directed into each of these areas through the plate and the radiographs repeated in multiple views as before. If the reduction is satisfactory, additional screws are placed in the plate to make the construct sufficiently more rigid to the extent that early mo-

*(Text continued on page 445.)*

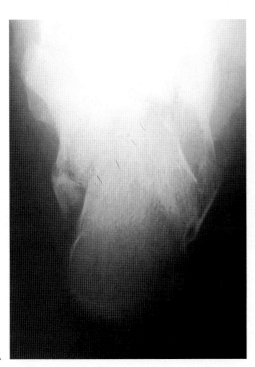
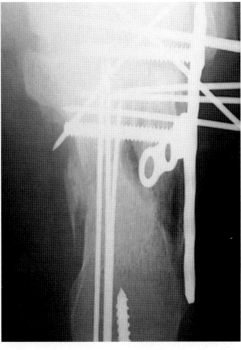

A                                                                                                          B

**Figure 30-17. A:** Intraarticular calcaneal fracture. The axial view shows shortening and varus malalignment before reduction. **B:** The same fracture after the reduction maneuver. Notice the Schantz pin in the tuberosity, multiple Kirschner wires fixing the tuberosity to the sustentaculum, and the posterior facet to the sustentaculum. A Y plate has also been applied.

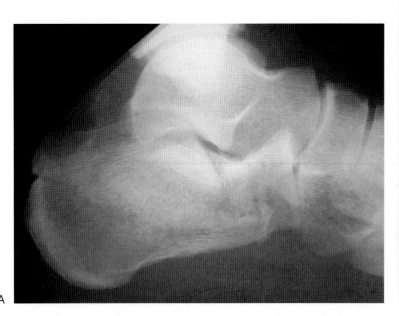

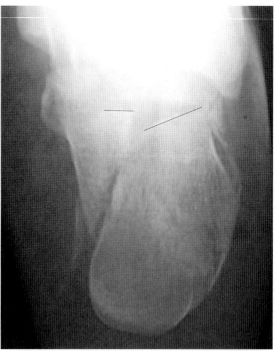

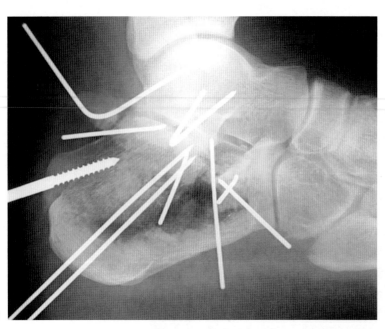

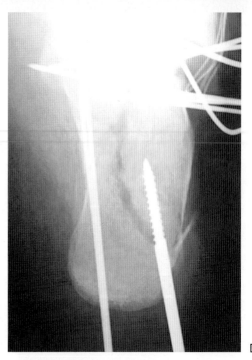

**Figure 30-18. A:** The lateral radiograph shows a displaced intraarticular calcaneal fracture. **B:** The axial view shows shortening and varus malalignment. *Lines* show joint incongruity of the posterior facet. **C:** The lateral view shows reduction and provisional fixation with multiple Kirschner wires through the tuberosity from posterior to anterior and transversely through the posterior facet fragment into the sustentaculum tali. Two Kirschner wires are maintaining the reduction of the anterior calcaneus, and bent Kirschner wires in the talus are used for traction on the skin flap. **D:** The axial view shows the reduced fracture and temporary fixation with Kirschner wires. *(continued)*

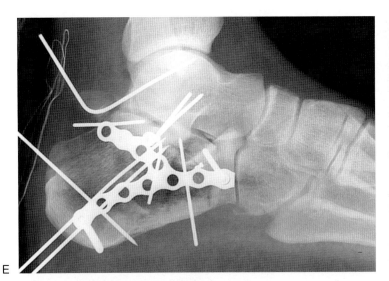

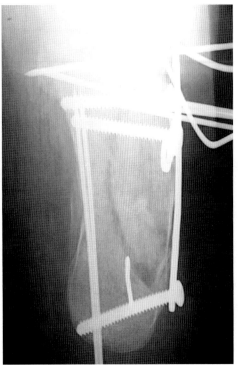

E

F

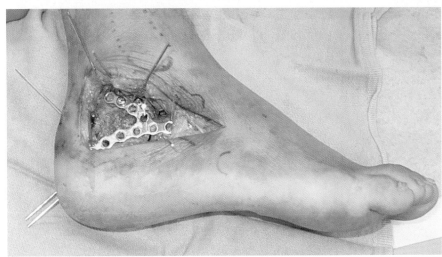

G

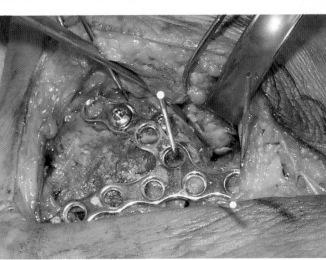

H

**Figure 30-18.** *Continued.* **E:** The lateral radiograph shows placement of the Y-shaped plate and screws. **F:** The axial view shows Y-plate fixation. **G:** Intraoperative photo showing provision reduction and Kirschner wire fixation. Three screws secure the plate to the bone. One is anterior, under the peroneal tendons; a second is posterior in the tuberosity; and a third is in the superior limb of the plate. The two most superior Kirschner wires are in the talus, retracting the skin flap. The two anterior Kirschner wires are maintaining reduction of the anterior process. The two Kirschner wires directed from the plantar tuberosity hold the medial wall reduction. The Kirschner wire from posterior superior maintains the relationship of the medial half of the posterior facet and the sustentacular fragment. **H:** A closer intraoperative photograph shows placement of the Y plate. A no. 2 Penfield elevator is in the posterior facet (from above left), which has the same radius of curvature as the posterior facet and is smooth. With this instrument in the joint, it is possible to look across the posterior facet to directly view the joint surface. A Langenbeck retractor is directly over the lateral process of the talus. The sural nerve is visible on the right in the soft tissue superficial to the peroneal tendons. *(continued)*

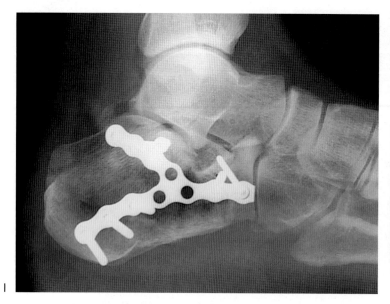

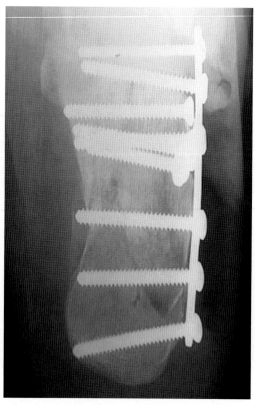

I

J

**Figure 30-18.** *Continued.* **I:** A lateral view shows the final fixation and good reduction. Temporary fixation has been removed. **J:** The axial view shows the final fixation. Notice the calcaneal length has been restored and varus corrected. Multiple screws have been placed transversely into sustentaculum tali.

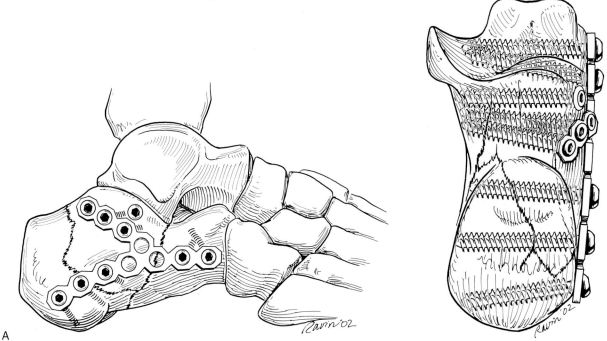

A                                                                                          B

**Figure 30-19.** Lateral **(A)** and posterior **(B)** views of Y-plate fixation.

tion can be performed postoperatively (Fig. 30-18). No construct should be accepted that requires cast treatment postoperatively.

Many different plates can be used for treatment of calcaneus fractures. The preferred plate should have a low profile, particularly in the area of the peroneal tendons. The plate should be stiff enough to correct varus alignment, and it should have a superior limb that prevents depression of the posterior facet. Tongue-type fractures require the plate to prevent rotation of the tongue fragment. This can be accomplished with a traditional Y-shaped plate augmented with a screw from dorsal to plantar or by use of one of the more recently designed plates that allows multiple screws to be placed in tongue fragment anteriorly and posteriorly (Fig. 30-19).

A 0.125-inch, closed suction drain is placed deep in the wound and brought out through the skin overlying the sinus tarsi. The skin flap should be closed in layers. If there is a substantial period of time between injury and treatment, there may be considerable gap in the wound at the completion of the procedure. A towel clip can be placed in the deep tissue of the flap and gently pulled toward the apex of the wound. The deep layer of absorbable suture should be placed beginning at the proximal end of the wound and at approximately 8- to 10-mm intervals. This pattern is then carried distally. The skin should be closed with a nonabsorbable flap stitch such as Donati-type suture. A nonstick dressing should be applied with lateral pressure over the flap to prevent swelling. A plaster splint or commercial boot is then applied for the first 48 hours.

## POSTOPERATIVE MANAGEMENT

At the completion of the operation, the patient is placed into a posterior plaster splint. A femoral sciatic block is helpful to maintain postoperative comfort. The block may last 12 to 20 hours. The acute pain from surgery lasts approximately 30 hours. A femoral sciatic block may allow the patient to have comfort during the first evening and make the first postoperative day much more tolerable. Patient-controlled analgesia (PCA) is used. Typically, there is significant postoperative pain for approximately 30 hours. The block lasts from 12 to 18 hours. The PCA is used until pain control is achieved with oral medications.

The limb is elevated on the day of surgery and until the next day. On the first postoperative day, the patient is allowed out of bed and into a chair with the limb elevated and allowed bathroom privileges. The degree of ambulation depends on the patient's motor control of the limb and degree of comfort. The goals of physical therapy are safe ambulation with no weight bearing on the injured side. Patients with contralateral injuries or upper extremity injuries that do not allow the use of crutches may be instructed in wheelchair ambulation. Alternatively, a commercially available roller device that allows the injured limb to bear weight through the knee may be used.

If a drain has been placed, it is removed on the first or second postoperative day. The drains are removed when there is output of less than 30 mL per shift. The drains are generally not removed on the first postoperative day. The plaster splint is removed on the second postoperative day and replaced by a light compressive dressing with an elastic wrap. Active ankle range of motion exercises are begun at this time. The physical therapist instructs the patient in subtalar range of motion exercises using the uninjured foot. The subtalar range of motion exercises include figure-of-eight motion and drawing the alphabet with the great toe. These exercises are begun in the injured foot when the wound stops draining. No plaster is used at any point in the rehabilitation.

Sutures are removed at 2 to 3 weeks postoperatively. Non–weight-bearing and active range of motion exercises are maintained for 6 weeks after surgery. The fracture pattern and operation determine the period of non–weight-bearing ambulation. A young, healthy person with only moderate comminution and no buttressing or bone graft required may begin weight bearing at 6 weeks postoperatively. If a sufficient defect is present and bone graft is required or a buttressing plate is required, weight bearing is delayed until 12 weeks postoperatively. When weight bearing is begun, only 50% of the body weight is allowed in the first week. If this is reasonably comfortable, the patient progresses to full weight bearing based on his or her level of tolerance.

## COMPLICATIONS

Complications after ORIF of calcaneal fractures are relatively common. These include infection, wound healing problems, pain, swelling, malunion, and nonunion. To some extent, these complications depend on technique. Treatment of these fractures should not be undertaken by surgeons without familiarity with techniques for reconstruction of complex intraarticular fractures or without experience in treating foot and ankle disorders.

*Infection* rate should be between 1% and 2% for ORIF of closed fractures. Infection rates for ORIF of open fractures have been reported to be as high as 45%, but 10% to 15% is probably more reasonable. As with other complex intraarticular fractures, treatment of infection should include antibiotics and debridement, if necessary. The implant should usually not be removed until the fracture is healed. Most infections are superficial and can be treated with antibiotic therapy alone.

*Delayed wound healing* may occur in 5% to 10% of patients after ORIF. This may be related to systemic factors such as shock, polytrauma, blood transfusion, smoking, diabetes mellitus, peripheral vascular disease, or a compromised immune system. It may also be associated with excessive retraction of the skin or poor placement of the incision. The severity of the original injury may also play a role in poor wound healing in this area. Because the calcaneus bone is nearly subcutaneous, it has little in the way of protection and a relatively poor blood supply. Very careful surgical technique is required to limit the negative impact of the original injury and subsequent treatment.

The *sural nerve* crosses the horizontal limb of the incision in the area of the peroneal tendons. Its location is very superficial, and an incision that is misplaced and deep will cut the nerve. Excessive soft tissue retraction may create unpleasant sensations in the course of the nerve but should be transitory. Most cases of sural nerve dysesthesias resolve within 9 weeks.

The *tibial nerve* is closely associated with the primary fracture line as it exits the medial wall of the calcaneus. It is much more likely to be injured by the initial fracture than it is to be injured by treatment. However, the surgeon should take care in drilling through the medial cortex of the calcaneus, particularly in the area that is plantar and posterior to the sustentaculum tali.

The initial trauma and the edema subsequent to the trauma have adverse consequences for the soft tissues of the foot. Direct injury or subclinical compartment syndrome may lead to development of contractures of the lesser toes. These contractures may respond to stretching. If not, it is occasionally necessary to treat the claw toes operatively, such as with a transfer of the flexor digitorum longus tendon into the extensor hood, the Girdlestone-Taylor procedure.

## RECOMMENDED READING

1.  Buckley RE, Meek RN: Comparison of open versus closed reduction of intraarticular calcaneal fractures: a matched cohort in workmen. *J Orthop Trauma* 6:216–222, 1992.
2.  Folk JW, Starr AJ, Early JS: Early wound complications of operative treatment of calcaneus fractures: analysis of 190 fractures. *J Orthop Trauma* 13:369–372, 1999.
3.  Hildebrand KA, Buckley RE, Mohtadi NG, et al.: Functional outcome measures after displaced intra-articular calcaneal fractures. *J Bone Joint Surg Br* 78:119–123, 1996.
4.  Kitaoka HB, Schaap EJ, Chao EY, et al.: Displaced intra-articular fractures of the calcaneus treated non-operatively: clinical results and analysis of motion and ground-reaction and temporal forces. *J Bone Joint Surg Am* 76:1531–1540, 1994.
5.  Levine DS, Malicky ES, Sangeorzan BJ: Intraoperative axial radiograph during fixation of fractures of the calcaneus. *Am J Orthop* 28:429, 1999.
6.  Mittlmeier T, Morlock MM, Hertlein H, et al.: Analysis of morphology and gait function after intraarticular calcaneal fracture. *J Orthop Trauma* 7:303–310, 1993.

7. Sangeorzan BJ, Ananthakrishnan D, Tencer AF: Contact characteristics of the subtalar joint after a simulated calcaneus fracture. *J Orthop Trauma* 9:251–258, 1995.
8. Sangeorzan BJ, Benirschke SK, Carr JB: Surgical management of fractures of the os calcis. *Instr Course Lect* 44:359–370, 1995.
9. Taylor RG: The treatment of claw toes by multiple transfer of flexor into extensor tendons. *J Bone Joint Surg* 33B:539, 1951.
10. Thermann H, Krettek C, Hufner T, et al.: Management of calcaneal fractures in adults: conservative versus operative treatment. *Clin Orthop* 353:107–124, 1998.
11. Thordarson DB, Krieger LE: Operative vs. nonoperative treatment of intra-articular fractures of the calcaneus: a prospective randomized trial. *Foot Ankle Int* 17:2–9, 1996.

# 31

# Calcaneal Realignment and Arthrodesis for Malunited Calcaneal Fracture

Michael M. Romash

## INDICATIONS/CONTRAINDICATIONS

The numerous and often disabling problems caused by malunited calcaneal fractures become clear once the pathomechanics of this fracture are understood. An axial load on the foot causes the shearing fracture of the calcaneus. From the axial view of the calcaneus, this main fracture line often runs from superior-lateral to inferior-medial, and from a dorsal view, it extends in an anterior-lateral to posterior-medial direction through the posterior facet. The sustentaculum tali stays in anatomic relationship to the talus and remainder of the foot. The tuberosity fragment of the calcaneus displaces laterally, upward, anteriorly, and into varus. As this tuberosity displacement occurs, the lateral half of the talus impacts the lateral aspect of the posterior facet, creating secondary fracture lines in the calcaneus. This results in depression and rotation of the posterior facet. Fractures through the anterior aspect of the calcaneus also occur. The resultant displacement and destruction of the posterior facet, if not reduced, interferes with the function of the calcaneus and subtalar joint (Fig. 31-1). A three-dimensional computed tomography (CT) reconstruction of the malunited calcaneus (Fig. 31-2) demonstrates the deformity from all sides.

The calcaneus is a primary point of support for the body weight from initial heel contact to midstance during ambulation. It is a pedestal in that it supports the talus at an appropriate position relative to the midfoot and forefoot. This support of the talus by the calcaneus establishes the alignment of the talus relative to the floor (i.e., talar declination) and presents the appropriate portion of the articular surface of the talus to the tibia. Satisfactory ankle motion in plantarflexion and dorsiflexion is related to some degree to the proper height of the calcaneus. The calcaneus is also important as a center for hindfoot motion. Its joint surfaces articulate with the talus, cuboid, and tarsal navicular. These articulations must be

M. M. Romash, M.D.: Department of Surgery, Uniformed Services University of Health Sciences, Bethesda, Maryland; and Orthopaedic Foot and Ankle Center of Hampton Roads, Chesapeake General Hospital, Chesapeake, Virginia.

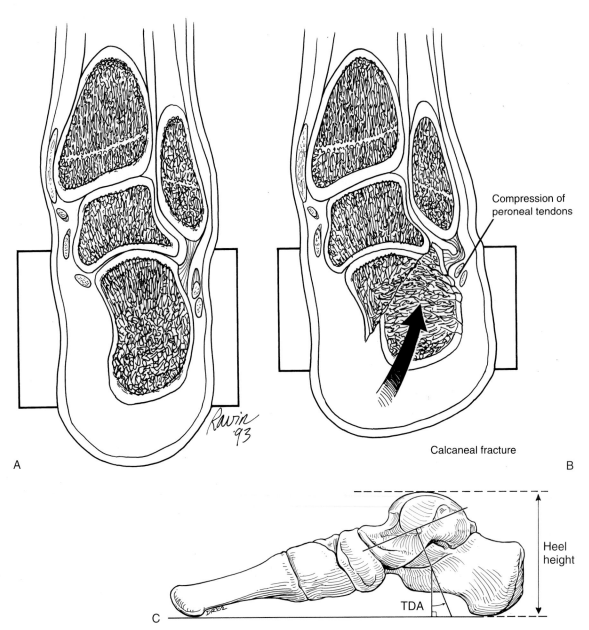

**Figure 31-1.** Schematic drawings of calcaneus in coronal plane. **A:** Normal shape of the calcaneus. **B:** View of displaced fracture, with calcaneofibular impingement and compression of peroneal tendons. **C:** Talar declination is the angle (TDA) formed between a line perpendicular to the talar axis and a line perpendicular to the floor. Heel height measurement is shown.

smooth and correctly arranged in their three-dimensional spatial array to ensure that the coordinated movement about these joints occurs with normal supination and pronation of the foot. The shape of the calcaneus also permits unfettered passage of tendons about its medial and lateral sides and permits standard shoes to be worn. The relationship of the tuberosity to the foot provides the lever arm for the triceps surae and establishes appropriate length relationships for normal gait.

The malunited calcaneal fracture is associated with multiple functional deficits. Shortening of the calcaneus diminishes the lever arm for the triceps surae, making it inefficient in plantarflexion of the foot. With the loss of support for the posterior aspect of the talus, the arch becomes flattened as the pedestal function of the calcaneus is lost. Rather than the normal talar declination, it becomes aligned more horizontally or even inclined and affects

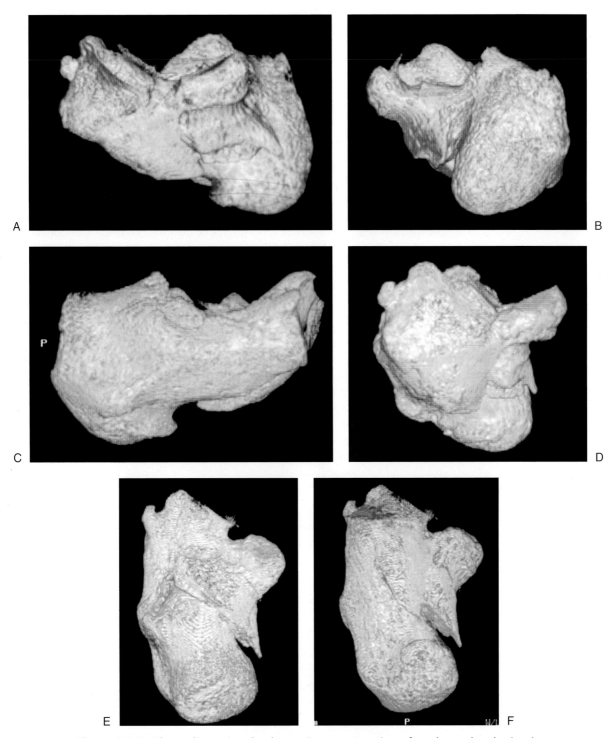

**Figure 31-2.** Three-dimensional volumetric reconstruction of a calcaneal malunion in medial **(A)**, posterior **(B)**, lateral **(C)**, anterior **(D)**, dorsal **(E)**, and plantar **(F)** views. This fracture malunion is amenable to the oblique sliding osteotomy.

the ankle joint function. As a result, there may be impingement anteriorly between the tibia and the neck of the talus and limited ankle dorsiflexion. The talonavicular joint is also adversely affected as the talus is dorsiflexed, while the tarsal navicular remains in its normal position relative to the midfoot. This causes a subluxation at the talonavicular joint. Disruption of the posterior facet of the calcaneus results in posttraumatic arthritis. The lateral, cephalad, and anterior displacement of the tuberosity fragment can cause direct impingement on the fibula (i.e., calcaneofibular impingement) and peroneal tendons (Fig. 31-3). Calcaneal tuberosity displacement also causes widening of the heel and loss of its height. This makes standard shoe fitting difficult because the normal counter of a shoe impinges on the malleoli in the deformed foot, which is flat, short, and wide. Disruption of the three-dimensional spatial arrangement of the subtalar, calcaneocuboid, and talonavicular joints adversely affects coordinated multicentric motion through these joints.

Surgical treatment of the malunited calcaneal fracture should address all the previously described functional losses. Operative correction should ablate the painful, arthritic joint and reestablish the architectural relationships of the hindfoot to the midfoot and ankle. It should reestablish the height of the calcaneus and the normal declination of the talus and its relationship to the navicular, tibia, and fibula. It is important to relieve the fibular impingement and concomitantly narrow the heel.

There are several approaches to addressing the painful, malunited calcaneus. Arthrodesis *in situ* has the advantage of simplicity, does not always require supplemental bone graft, and has high union and relatively low complication rates. It has application for the arthritic subtalar joint with limited displacement. Arthrodeses *in situ*, whether subtalar or triple arthrodeses, are met with limited success for the severely malunited calcaneus because these procedures are not designed to reestablish the height of the calcaneus and its relationship to the other tarsal bones.

A procedure to diminish the width of the heel by removing the lateral wall of the calcaneus impinging on the peroneal tendons and fibula may be useful for carefully selected patients who do not have severe subtalar arthritis or severe malalignment. This operation is also met with limited success for the severely displaced fracture, because the posttraumatic arthritis and architectural derangement of the foot are not corrected (Fig. 31-4).

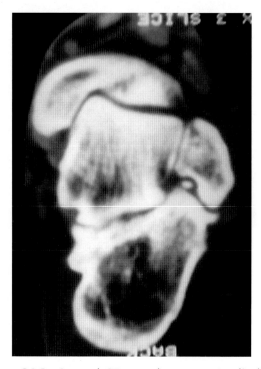

**Figure 31-3.** Coronal CT scan demonstrates displaced subtalar arthritis and calcaneofibular impingement.

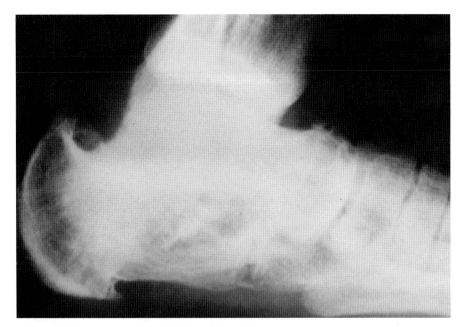

**Figure 31-4.** Lateral radiograph of the foot in a patient who underwent triple arthrodesis with less than optimal alignment. Notice the abnormal architecture and the failure to restore a normal talar declination angle and normal calcaneal pitch angle.

The procedure described here addresses the deformity of the malunited calcaneal fracture by recreating the primary oblique shearing fracture with an osteotomy. The tuberosity fragment is then shifted medially, caudally, and posteriorly under the talus. Subtalar arthrodesis also is done (6). This procedure restores height and length to the heel, decompresses the lateral calcaneus by shifting the tuberosity away from the fibula, and ablates the posttraumatic arthritis by the arthrodesis.

The indication for the osteotomy and arthrodesis is a painful malunion of a calcaneal fracture in which there has been loss of height of the calcaneus and lateral displacement of the tuberosity fragment. Most displacement of the fragment should be along the primary fracture line, the plane of the proposed osteotomy. The tuberosity fragment should be implicated in calcaneofibular impingement. Previous joint depression type fractures may lend themselves better to this treatment than tongue-type fractures in which there is significant cephalad displacement of the tongue fragment.

A contraindication for the procedure is a malunion in which the posterior facet is driven directly downward into the body without an identifiable primary oblique fracture line or lateral shift of the tuberosity. This situation may be better treated by an interpositional distraction bone block arthrodesis, in which corrective medial shift of the tuberosity is not as important. In this case, the focus is on reestablishing calcaneal height and talar declination. Another contraindication is malunion with more than 1.5 cm loss of heel height, because the magnitude of the shift is limited by the geometry of the osteotomy and size of the calcaneus. If greater correction is to be obtained, the surgeon should consider an interposition bone block arthrodesis.

## PREOPERATIVE PLANNING

Preoperative evaluation of patients who may be candidates for this procedure focuses on the patient's symptoms, signs, and radiographic evaluation. The patient's pain should be significant and disabling. Patients usually have difficulty walking on uneven surfaces. Problems such as difficulty with footwear because of impingement on the malleoli should be assessed. Range of motion of the ankle and hindfoot should be measured. Alignment of the calcaneus relative to the tibia, or the tibiocalcaneal angle, should be measured. Stability of the ankle and hindfoot, swelling, muscle atrophy, and heel pad atrophy should be identified. Neurovascular examination is important because it is not unusual for patients to have neuropathy of the posterior tibial or its branches or sural nerve. Localizing the patient's pain and tenderness to the anterior ankle suggests anterior impingement, to the sinus tarsi suggests subtalar arthritis, to the subfibular region indicates impingement, and to the calcaneocuboid joint indicates posttraumatic arthritis.

Radiographic evaluation is much the same as for the acute calcaneal fracture. Weightbearing, anteroposterior and lateral views of the foot along with non–weight-bearing, oblique and Broden's views are obtained. An axial calcaneal view may be obtained. Ankle radiographs are usually obtained in weight-bearing, anteroposterior and non–weight-bearing, mortise views. CT scans in the axial, coronal, and sagittal planes are also helpful. A three-dimensional CT reconstruction is helpful in planning the repositioning of the calcaneus.

Radiographic abnormalities that are typically observed in the malunited calcaneal fracture include the loss of Bohler's angle, dorsiflexion of the talus (identified by loss of the normal talar declination angle), disruption of the alignment of the talonavicular joint on the lateral projection, anterior ankle impingement (may be demonstrated on a lateral radiograph obtained in maximum dorsiflexion), and arthritis of the subtalar (and sometimes calcaneocuboid) joint. A standing, anteroposterior view of the ankle demonstrates the calcaneofibular impingement. Although the focus of attention is on the hindfoot, it is vital to not overlook ankle pathology. CT further demonstrates three-dimensional displacement such as the lateral shift of the tuberosity, as well as calcaneofibular impingement, subtalar arthritis, and calcaneocuboid arthritis.

The calcaneocuboid joint may develop radiologic evidence of arthritis in about 20% of patients, but it does not produce symptoms as often or as severely as arthritis affecting the subtalar joint. If the calcaneocuboid joint has advanced symptomatic arthritis, extension of the operation to include calcaneocuboid arthrodesis could be considered. In equivocal instances, a technetium bone scan or differential joint injection with a local anesthetic may help to determine whether the calcaneocuboid arthrodesis should be added.

## SURGERY

Appropriately small surgical instruments are used: no. 15 scalpel blades, small tenotomy scissors, Freer elevators, small key elevators, and Joker elevators. Joseph skin hooks (10 mm wide), Ragnell retractors, somewhat larger right-angle retractors such as Mason or Army-Navy, and a baby Inge lamina spreader are used. A small drill, such as a 3M-type minidriver, Kirschner wires, and Steinmann pins should be available. A small-fragment screw set is also used. Small, curved osteotomes and motorized burrs to denude the subtalar cortical and articular surfaces are useful. A cannulated, 7-mm, cancellous screw for tuberosity fixation, and cannulated, 4.5- or 4.0-mm screws for osteotomy fixation should be available. An anterior cruciate ligament guide is used to place the guide wire for the 7.0-mm, cannulated screws.

This procedure is done with the patient placed in a lateral decubitus position, with the affected limb toward the surgeon on a bolster. This position allows easier passage of the screw through the tuberosity of the calcaneus into the talus. The lower extremity to the knee and the ipsilateral iliac crest are sterilely prepared and draped with a pneumatic tourniquet about the thigh.

### Technique: Calcaneal Osteotomy with Subtalar Arthrodesis

After exsanguination and tourniquet inflation, an oblique incision is made centered over the sinus tarsi (Fig. 31-5). This allows access to the anterior process, body, and posterior facet of the calcaneus. This may be extended posteriorly for more exposure. The extensor digi-

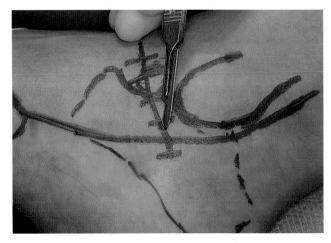

**Figure 31-5.** A lateral view shows an oblique skin incision in the hindfoot.

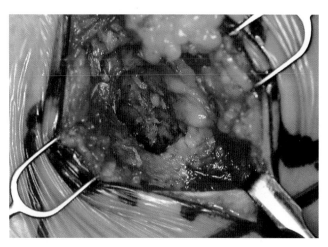

**Figure 31-6.** The sinus tarsi is debrided of adhesions and osteochondral fragments. The anterior margin of the lateral talar process is observed.

torum brevis is reflected, and the fat in the sinus tarsi is excised as necessary. Incision of the soft tissue structures between the talus and calcaneus is done, proceeding from anterior to posterior, deep to the retracted peroneal tendons (Figs. 31-6 and 31-7). A lamina spreader in the sinus tarsi between the talus and calcaneus provides distraction of the joint and exposure to the sustentaculum tali (Fig. 31-8).

At this point, the displaced articular surface of the posterior facet is exposed. The scar tissue within the joint is removed with a pituitary rongeur. After the posterior facet surface has been uncovered, the site of the primary fracture line, which runs obliquely across the calcaneus from dorsolateral to plantar-medial and anterolateral to posteromedial, can be identified. It is not usual for this primary fracture line to be ununited or partially united, to the extent that the line can be followed in its entirety with a small, sharp curette.

The remaining articular cartilage and subchondral bone surfaces of the talus and calcaneus are removed. Special care is taken to denude the sustentaculum tali of the calcaneus and the undersurface of the talar neck. Small, curved osteotomes and a powered burr are particularly helpful in preparing the subtalar joint surfaces (Figs. 31-9 and 31-10).

A Steinmann pin is then placed into the calcaneus in the plane of the primary fracture line (Fig. 31-11). The position of this pin is confirmed by an axial radiograph or fluoroscopy in the operating room (Fig. 31-12). After the pin position is judged to be satisfac-

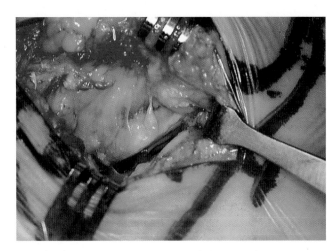

**Figure 31-7.** The lateral aspect of the subtalar joint is exposed.

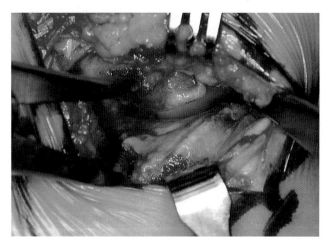

**Figure 31-8.** The arthritic subtalar joint is distracted using a baby Inge lamina spreader.

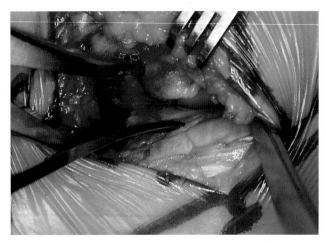

**Figure 31-9.** A curved Lambotte osteotome used to decorticate the calcaneal and talar joint surfaces.

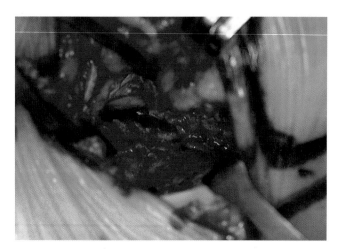

**Figure 31-10.** Joint surfaces after decortication.

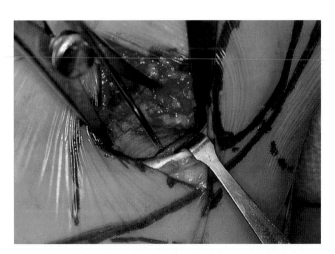

**Figure 31-11.** The primary fracture line is marked with ink on the posterior facet of the calcaneus. A Steinmann pin is placed obliquely in the old primary fracture line.

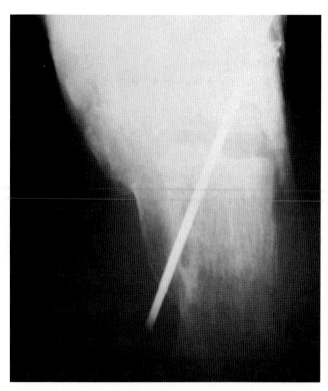

**Figure 31-12.** An intraoperative axial calcaneal radiograph confirms the correct placement of a pin.

tory, an osteotomy of the calcaneus is performed in the plane of the previous primary fracture line, which frees the tuberosity from the sustentaculum (Fig. 31-13). The osteotomy exits the calcaneus anteriorly through the lateral wall. Posteriorly and inferiorly, it exits through the medial wall of the calcaneus beneath and posterior to the neurovascular bundle (Figs. 31-14 and 31-15). The soft tissues about the tuberosity fragment are then released as necessary to permit mobilization and realignment of that fragment. It is not unusual for the primary fracture line to be ununited or partially united, which facilitates identification of the correct plane of dissection.

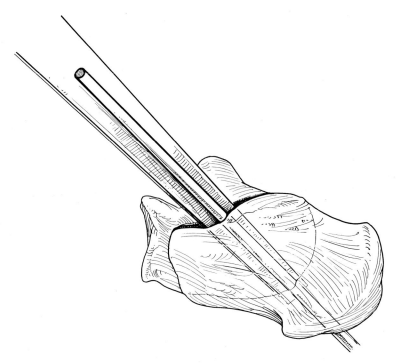

**Figure 31-13.** The osteotomy was performed along a Steinmann pin.

One of the most difficult portions of the operation is shifting or realignment of the tuberosity fragment relative to the sustentacular fragment. It may be helpful to obtain provisional fixation of the sustentacular fragment to the talus with Kirschner wires that are placed through the lateral body of the talus and into the sustentacular fragment. This stabilizes the sustentacular fragment and prevents its motion as the tuberosity is manipulated.

It is often helpful to use osteotomes as levers to distract the tuberosity from the sustentaculum. A lamina spreader is placed in the osteotomy and opened (Fig. 31-16) to distract the fragments relative to each other. This stretching of the soft tissue envelope facilitates the reduction of the tuberosity. A Steinmann pin is often placed through the tuberosity from anterolateral to posteromedial, parallel to the plane of the osteotomy, to gain control of this fragment as the shift or reduction is performed (Fig. 31-17). A lamina spreader between the sustentaculum and the tuberosity fragment helps reposition the tuberosity. Placing a lam-

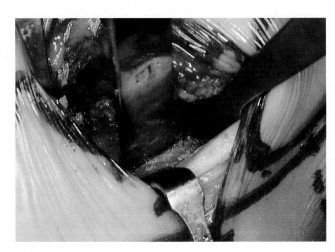

**Figure 31-14.** An osteotome is placed in the osteotomy; the Steinmann pin is not visible.

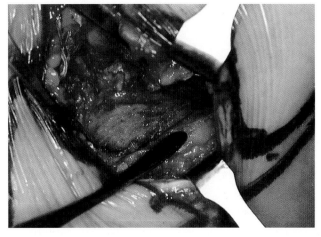

**Figure 31-15.** The osteotomy is complete and reveals the calcaneus before realignment.

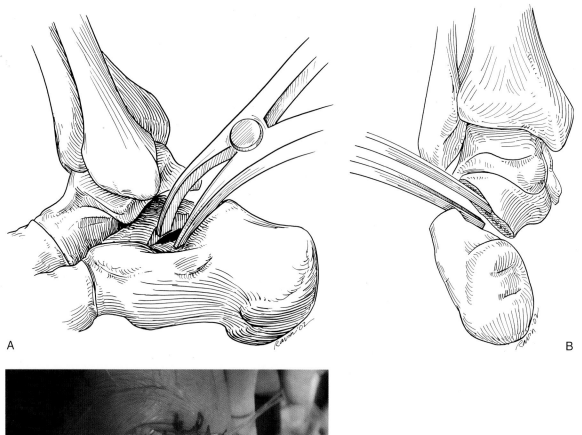

A

B

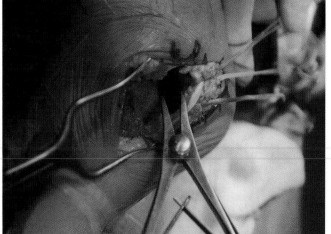

C

**Figure 31-16.** Diagrams of the baby Inge lamina spreader between the osteotomy fragments, creating a gap between the fragments and stretching the soft tissue envelope to facilitate the tuberosity re-alignment. **A:** Lateral view. **B:** Axial calcaneal view. **C:** Photograph shows an example of the lamina spreader placed into the osteotomy to stretch soft tissues adjacent to the osteotomy.

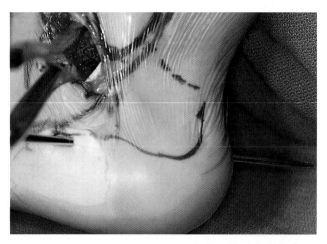

**Figure 31-17.** A Steinmann pin is placed in the tuberosity to assist in mobilizing the tuberosity fragment.

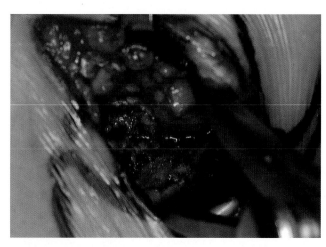

**Figure 31-18.** The osteotomy is shifted with the assistance of a lamina spreader placed between the tip of the fibula and the tuberosity fragment.

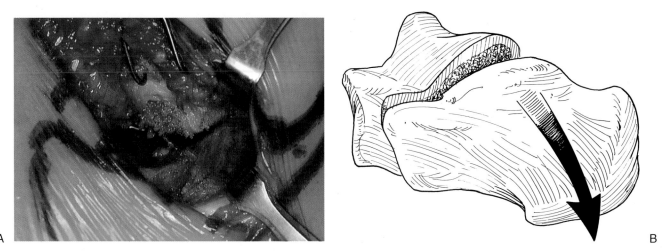

**Figure 31-19. A:** Reduction of the osteotomy is held by Kirschner wires. **B:** The tuberosity is repositioned posteriorly, inferiorly, and medially *(arrow)*.

ina spreader between the tip of the fibula and the tuberosity posteriorly can help effect the shift (Fig. 31-18). If necessary, an external fixation–type distractor can be applied between the tibia and the tuberosity fragment to help in moving the tuberosity fragment into its new position. Plantarflexion of the midfoot and talus helps effect the appropriate translation and rotation of the tuberosity fragment. Because of the obliquity of the osteotomy from dorso-lateral to plantar-medial, the tuberosity fragment moves away from its abnormal location abutting the peroneal tendons and the fibula as it is displaced. A space develops under the lateral aspect of the talus and the lateral aspect of the shifted tuberosity fragment (Fig. 31-19).

After the shift has been achieved, transverse fixation is performed through the lateral wall of the calcaneus into the sustentaculum tali with small-fragment screws or cannulated, 4.0- or 4.5-mm screws (Fig. 31-20). Next, a large, cannulated, 7-mm screw is placed through the tuberosity, through the sustentacular fragment, and into the body of the talus. This screw placement can be done under direct visualization or with image intensification (Figs. 31-21 through 31-24). An anterior cruciate ligament drill guide helps to position this guide wire. After satisfactory position has been obtained, morcellated cancellous bone graft is placed in the decorticated subtalar level, sinus tarsi, and the space created under the lat-

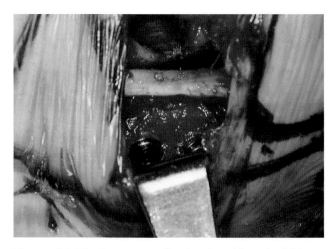

**Figure 31-20.** Osteotomy fixation is achieved with two screws oriented transversely into the sustentacular fragment.

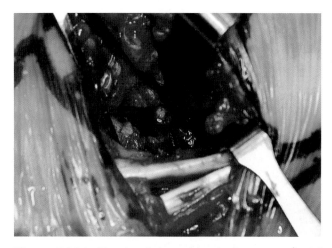

**Figure 31-21.** The tip of the guide pin for a cannulated screw is passed through the tuberosity and into the sustentacular fragment. The pin is advanced into the talus.

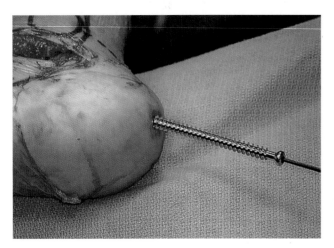

**Figure 31-22.** A cannulated drill is used, and then a fully threaded, cannulated screw is inserted over the guide pin.

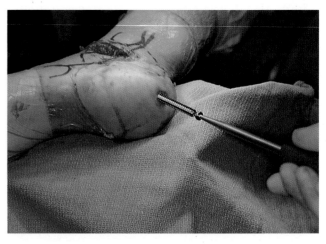

**Figure 31-23.** A screw is placed into the heel and across the subtalar joint.

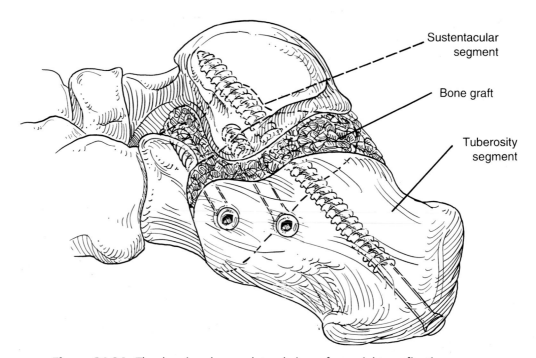

Sustentacular segment

Bone graft

Tuberosity segment

**Figure 31-24.** The drawing shows a lateral view of an axial transfixation screw.

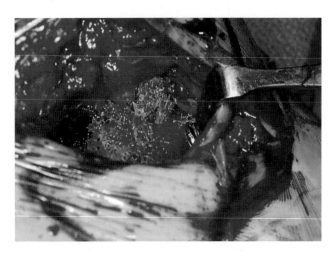

**Figure 31-25.** The cancellous bone graft is placed in a space created by the repositioned tuberosity fragment.

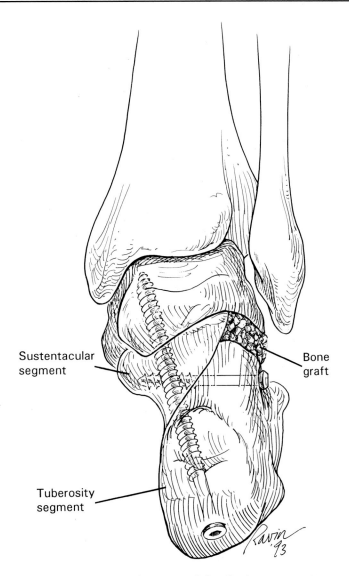

**Figure 31-26.** Posterior view of the final construct. Notice the position of the transfixion screws across osteotomy and subtalar level and into the body of the talus. The preferred position of the transversely oriented screws is also seen. Notice also the morcellated bone graft placement.

eral aspect of the talus and the lateral aspect of the shifted tuberosity fragment (Fig. 31-25). The bone graft is obtained from the ipsilateral iliac crest. The repositioned tuberosity does not depend on the bone graft for structural support to maintain its position (Fig. 31-26). The wound is closed using absorbable suture in the subcutaneous tissue and nylon mattress sutures for the skin.

## POSTOPERATIVE MANAGEMENT

Postoperative management is similar to that used for the surgically treated acute calcaneal fracture. The patient is initially placed in a compressive dressing with plaster splints or in a short-leg cast with a foot pump such as the Arterial-Venous Impulse System Foot Pump Inflation Pad (Kendall Co., Mansfield, MA). After about 3 days, the cast is changed, and the foot is not allowed to bear weight for 8 to 12 weeks. When casting is discontinued, graduated weight-bearing and range of motion exercises are begun.

With this realignment and arthrodesis of the calcaneus, the result depends to a large degree on obtaining a solid subtalar arthrodesis with the calcaneus narrowed and the tuberosity in an improved position (Fig. 31-27). As with a subtalar arthrodesis alone, the subtalar motion is lost, and compensation of the hindfoot to uneven ground surfaces is difficult. However, most of these patients have severe restriction of subtalar motion before reconstruction. Pain relief is emphasized as the primary goal of treatment. Restoration of heel height and improvement in footwear are secondary goals.

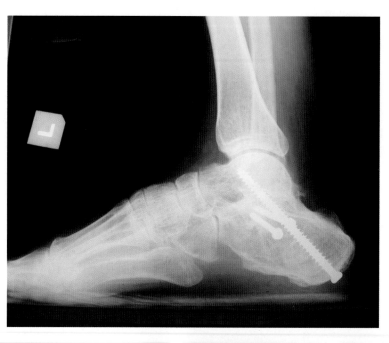

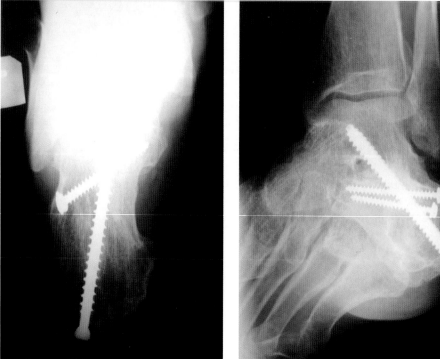

**Figure 31-27.** Radiographs after an oblique sliding calcaneal osteotomy show lateral **(A)**, axial calcaneal **(B)**, and Broden's **(C)** views. The patient had a good result.

Another approach to the malunited calcaneal fracture that could be considered in carefully selected patients is the subtalar distraction arthrodesis (SDA) (Fig. 31-28). A procedure was described by Carr et al. in 1988 (5) and has been used by others subsequently. It is a modification of the Gallie technique of subtalar arthrodesis (7), which involves arthrodesis with a structural bone graft inserted into the subtalar joint designed to realign the heel. It is indicated in patients with pain and impairment due to a severely malaligned calcaneus in which there is loss of the talar declination angle, loss of heel height, and symptomatic anterior ankle impingement with subtalar arthritis. There may also be calcaneofibular impingement.

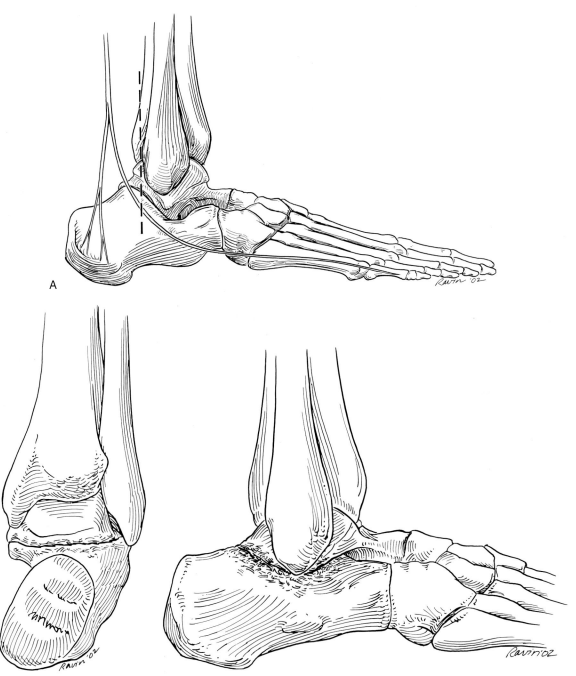

**Figure 31-28.** Drawings show a subtalar distraction arthrodesis operation. **A:** The posterolateral, longitudinal incision *(dotted line)* is near the sural nerve. **B:** Posterior *(left)* and lateral *(right)* views show fracture malunion with calcaneofibular impingement, heel varus, loss of talar declination, and loss of calcaneal inclination (i.e., pitch angle). *(continued)*

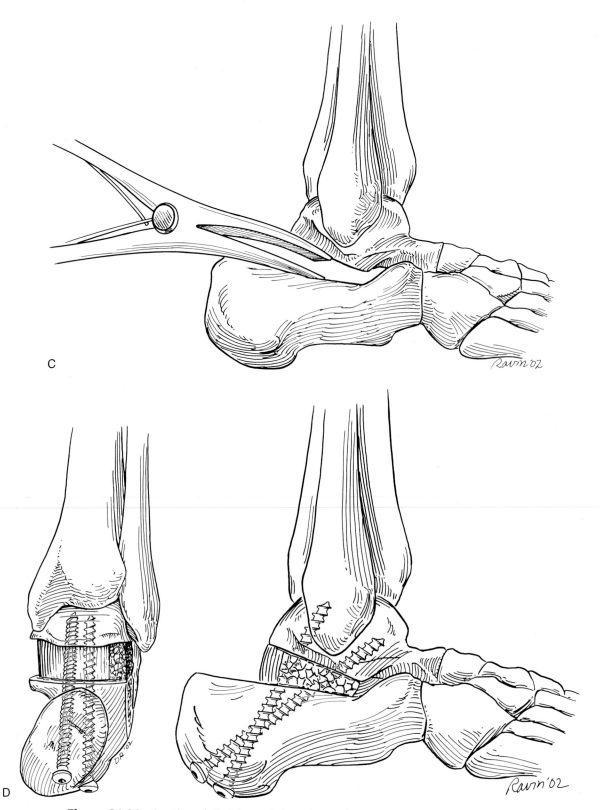

**Figure 31-28.** *Continued.* **C:** A lateral view shows distraction of the posterior margin of the subtalar joint with a lamina spreader. **D:** Posterior *(left)* and lateral *(right)* views demonstrate realignment, insertion of a bone block in the posterior subtalar joint, and fixation with two fully threaded, 6.5-mm, cancellous screws passed through a heel incision. Additional morcellated bone graft is packed around the structural graft.

Patients report difficulty walking on uneven terrain, a widened heel, difficulty with footwear, stiffness, and swelling. On examination, there is reduced hindfoot and ankle motion, painful motion of these joints, and tenderness in several areas: sinus tarsi, lateral ankle, and anterior ankle. It is often possible to reproduce the anterior ankle pain with passive dorsiflexion. An abrupt block with dorsiflexion can be observed.

Contraindications include patients with infections, skin ulceration, dysvascular extremity, neuropathy, and widespread arthritis of the hindfoot and ankle joints. Another contraindication is a patient who has fracture malunion with subtalar arthritis but does not have pain attributable to impingement in the anterior ankle. In these patients, a more conventional arthrodesis with intercalated bone graft is preferable (see Chapter 28). Patients who have fracture malunion with dislocation or severe displacement of the tuberosity fragment laterally with impingement against the fibula would benefit from the oblique sliding calcaneal osteotomy rather than the SDA procedure. Compared with the *in situ* arthrodesis, the SDA is a more complex operation with higher reported complication rates, and it should therefore be considered only in carefully selected patients.

Preoperatively, the degree of deformity should be quantitated by measuring a standing tibiocalcaneal angle with a goniometer. Anteroposterior and lateral, weight-bearing radiographs of the foot should be examined to determine the degree of malposition, including the talar declination angle and heel height, which is the distance between the dorsal margin of the talar dome and plantar margin of calcaneal tuberosity (Fig. 31-1C). There may be loss of the heel height to the extent that the axis of the talus is oriented horizontally or even in dorsiflexion on the lateral-view, weight-bearing radiograph of the foot. Axial calcaneal and oblique foot radiographs; an anteroposterior, weight-bearing ankle view; and a CT scan of the hindfoot in coronal and axial planes are helpful.

A posterolateral approach to the subtalar joint is made through a vertical incision. The joint surfaces of the talus and calcaneus are denuded of remaining articular cartilage and subchondral bone. This exposure permits distraction of the calcaneus from the talus posteriorly, creating a gap between the calcaneus and talus equal to the height lost from compression of the fracture (Fig. 31-29). The distraction may be accomplished with a lamina

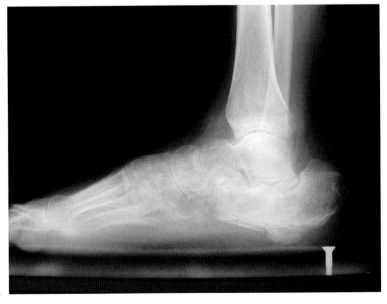

A

**Figure 31-29.** The patient had a painful lateral hindfoot. **A:** The lateral radiograph shows a malaligned calcaneus and subtalar arthritis. The talar axis is inclined dorsally rather than the usual talar declination angle. *(continued)*

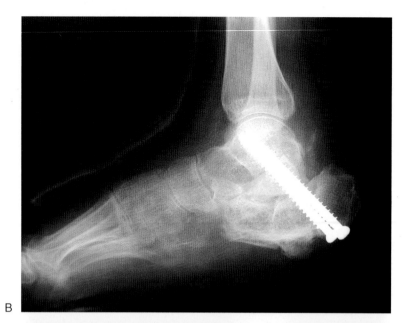

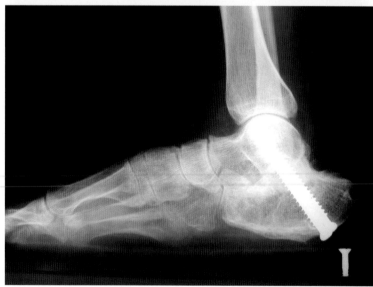

**Figure 31-29.** *Continued.* **B:** A lateral view immediately after subtalar distraction arthrodesis shows a large block of tricortical iliac crest bone graft fixed with two fully threaded, cancellous screws. **C:** Weight-bearing lateral view 1 year postoperatively shows normal talar declination has been restored. The patient had a good result, with no hindfoot pain or symptoms of anterior ankle impingement.

spreader or an invasive bone distractor such as a femoral distractor. An intraoperative lateral radiograph is obtained to assess the realignment, such as restored talar declination angle (Figs. 31-28 and 31-29). If good connection is achieved, the gap is then filled with a block or wedge of tricortical bone graft harvested from the iliac crest as a structural graft to maintain the position (Figs. 31-28 and 31-29). The graft may be fashioned in a trapezoidal shape, with more distraction medially to avoid varus malalignment. Fixation is accomplished by two fully threaded, 6.5- or 7.0-mm screws through the tuberosity into the body of the talus. Supplemental morcellated bone graft is placed around the bone block. If there is lateral impingement and widening of the heel from the displaced lateral wall of the calcaneus, this bone may be removed. It is important to gauge the size of the wedges to ensure that the heel is not placed into varus or valgus. It may be necessary to lengthen the Achilles tendon.

Patients are immobilized in a Robert Jones compressive dressing for 2 days, followed by a non–weight-bearing, short-leg cast for 6 weeks. If radiographs are suboptimal at 6 weeks postoperatively, a short-leg walking cast is applied for another 6 weeks.

The results have been favorable in terms of pain relief, improved alignment, and successful union (Fig. 31-29). However, there is a much higher complication rate than with *in situ* subtalar arthrodesis, with problems such as wound dehiscence, sural neuropathy, varus malunion, loss of correction postoperatively, infection, and nonunion. It is unusual for the final alignment to be anatomic. The operation is technically demanding and should be considered in carefully selected patients who have severe malalignment, anterior ankle impingement, and subtalar arthritis.

## COMPLICATIONS

Complications of realignment with arthrodesis such as infection, wound dehiscence, loss of correction, incomplete correction, and nonunion may occur. The potential for *infection* can be reduced by use of prophylactic antibiotics during the operative procedure and 24 hours afterward. Careful operative technique to prevent tissue damage and ischemia and the use of a compression dressing with an Arterial-Venous Impulse Pump have helped to decrease the incidence of infection and wound healing problems.

*Pseudarthrosis* has not been a major problem, probably because of the large surface area of exposed bone at the subtalar joint and the use of bone graft and stable fixation.

*Inadequate realignment* is probably the most common postoperative problem. A thorough understanding of the fracture position by preoperative radiographs and CT scan allows proper planning of the repositioning. Where secondary fracture lines are present, realignment is not ideal but should be improved.

*Breakage of fixation devices* sometimes occurs with a bone block procedure and early weight bearing. This has not been observed with the oblique sliding osteotomy and arthrodesis. Perhaps this is because the final construct is not as dependent on a structural bone graft for stability or correction.

*Neurologic injury* has not been a problem with the oblique sliding osteotomy and arthrodesis, but it occurred in the early experience of subtalar distraction arthrodesis.

## RECOMMENDED READING

1. Amendola A, Lammens P: Subtalar arthrodesis using interposition iliac crest bone graft after calcaneal fracture. *Foot Ankle Int* 17:608–614, 1996.
2. Bednarz PA, Beals TC, Manoli A: Subtalar distraction bone block fusion: an assessment of outcome. *Foot Ankle Int* 18:785–791, 1997.
3. Bradley SA, Davies AM: Computerized tomographic assessment of old calcaneal fractures. *Br J Radiol* 63:926–933, 1990.
4. Burton DC, Olney BW, Horton GA: Late results of subtalar distraction fusion. *Foot Ankle Int* 19:197–202, 1998.
5. Carr JB, Hansen ST, Benirshke SK: Subtalar distraction bone block fusion for late complications of the os calcis fractures. *Foot Ankle* 9:81–86, 1988.
6. Chan SC, Alexander IJ: Subtalar arthrodesis with interposition tricortical iliac crest graft for late pain and deformity after calcaneus fracture. *Foot Ankle Int* 18:613–615, 1997.
7. Gallie WE: Subtalar arthrodesis in fractures of the os calcis. *J Bone Joint Surg* 25:731–736, 1943.
8. Hansen ST Jr: Calcaneal osteotomy in multiple planes for correction of major postraumatic deformity. In: Hansen ST Jr. *Functional reconstruction of the foot and ankle.* Philadelphia: Lippincott, Williams & Wilkins, 2000, 380–383.
9. Leung K, Chan W, Shen W, et al.: Operative treatment of intra articular fractures of the os calcis. The role of rigid internal fixation and primary bone grafting: preliminary results. *J Trauma* 3:232–240, 1989.
10. Romash MM: Calcaneal fractures: three-dimensional treatment. *Foot Ankle* 8:180–197, 1988.
11. Romash MM: Reconstructive osteotomy of the calcaneus with subtalar arthrodesis for malunited calcaneal fractures. *Clin Orthop* 228:157–167, 1993.

# 32

# Talus Fracture: Open Reduction and Internal Fixation

David B. Thordarson

## INDICATIONS/CONTRAINDICATIONS

Fractures of the talus are relatively uncommon fractures of the foot, but they have potentially serious complications. Any displaced fracture of the neck or body of the talus requires open reduction and internal fixation. A common treatment goal is urgent anatomic reduction to restore congruity to the ankle and subtalar joints and to reduce risk of avascular necrosis by preserving the remaining blood supply. Although these fractures occur relatively infrequently, the consequences may be disastrous, it is important for surgeons who manage patients with acute trauma to be knowledgeable of treatment. This chapter focuses on talar neck fractures, which are among the most challenging to treat.

Fractures of the neck of the talus account for approximately 50% of significant injuries to the talus. They are commonly caused by high-energy trauma such as motor vehicle or motorcycle accidents or falls from a height. Although it has been theorized that hyperdorsiflexion of the ankle with abutment of the neck of the talus against the anterior lip of the tibia causes this fracture, it has been found in the laboratory to be caused by axial loading of the ankle in the neutral position while compressing the calcaneus against the overlying talus and tibia.

Because of the severe disability after nonoperative treatment of a displaced fracture, there are few contraindications for operative treatment of this fracture. Because the fracture is associated with high-energy trauma, a patient occasionally is too unstable to undergo any operative treatment on presentation to the hospital. After the patient's condition has stabilized, he or she should be treated in an urgent fashion to minimize the risk of complications, including especially skin necrosis and avascular necrosis.

D. B. Thordarson, M.D.: Foot and Ankle Trauma and Reconstructive Surgery, Department of Orthopaedic Surgery, Keck School of Medicine, University of Southern California, Los Angeles, California.

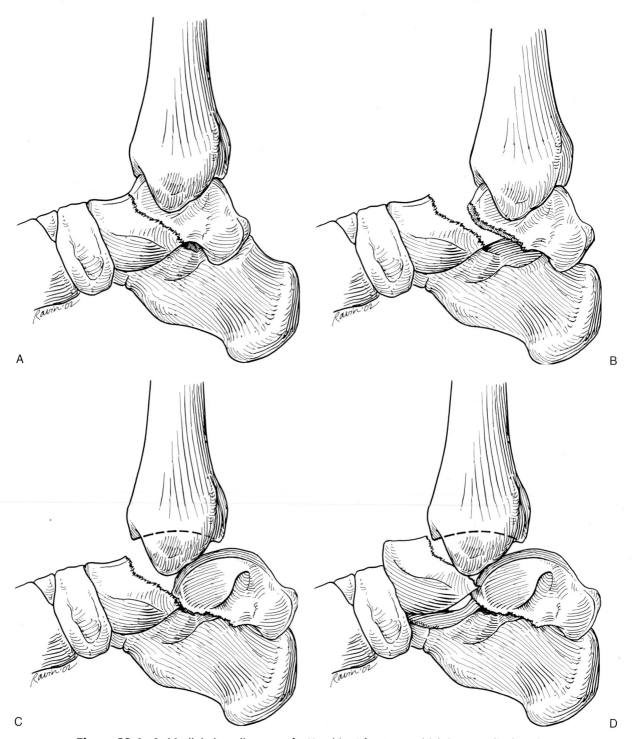

**Figure 32-1.** **A:** Medial-view diagram of a Hawkins I fracture, which is a nondisplaced fracture of the neck of talus that has a congruent ankle and subtalar joint. **B:** Medial view of a Hawkins II fracture demonstrates displacement of the fracture at the neck of the talus and subluxation of the subtalar joint. Notice that the ankle joint is congruent. **C:** Medial view of a Hawkins III fracture demonstrates complete dislocation of the body of the talus posteromedially with disruption of the ankle and subtalar joints. **D:** Medial view of the foot shows a Hawkins IV fracture with dislocation of the ankle, subtalar, and talonavicular joints.

## PREOPERATIVE PLANNING

Talar neck fractures usually result from high-energy trauma and occur more frequently in young adults. They occur more often in men than women (3:1) and most frequently in the third decade of life. Many have associated injuries of the musculoskeletal system. Approximately 20% to 30% of patients have associated medial malleolar fractures, especially in Hawkins type III fractures. It is not unusual for patients with severe lower extremity injuries to have an overlooked talus fracture.

Physical examination frequently reveals severe swelling of the foot. Fracture displacement can be masked by this swelling, making palpation of fracture dislocations difficult or impossible. The neurovascular structures are generally spared from serious injury. Soft tissue damage can be extensive with a significant incidence of open fractures. Compartment syndrome of the foot sometimes occurs.

Radiographic evaluation includes anteroposterior, lateral, and oblique radiographs of the foot and an anteroposterior view of the ankle. These views allow the fracture to be characterized, such as type, displacement, comminution, and incongruity of the subtalar, ankle, and/or talonavicular joints (Fig. 32-1). Varus or valgus displacement of the talar neck can be difficult to demonstrate on a routine anteroposterior radiograph. Canale described a modified anteroposterior radiograph (Fig. 32-2) that can be particularly beneficial in the intraoperative assessment of reduction.

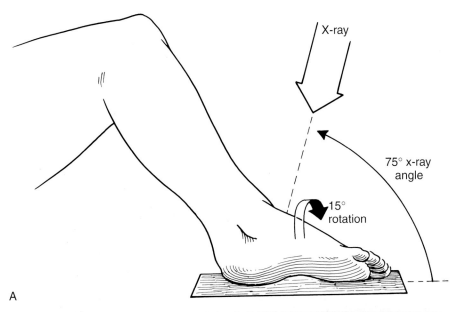

A

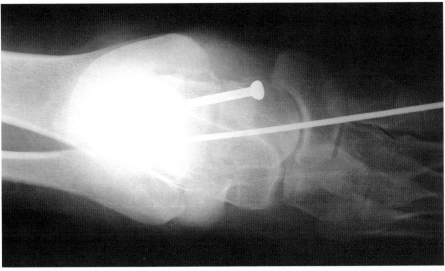

B

**Figure 32-2. A:** With a cassette placed beneath the foot, the ankle is place in maximum plantarflexion; the foot is pronated 15°, and the radiograph beam is angled cephalad in a 75° angle relative to the cassette to obtain the modified Canale anteroposterior radiograph of the neck of talus. **B:** Canale view of the talus was obtained intraoperatively. This view can be useful in demonstrating the adequacy of fracture reduction and fixation placement.

Treatment of fractures of the neck of the talus are predicated on their classification. Hawkins described a classification system based on displacement of the fracture and the congruency of the subtalar and ankle joints (Fig.32-1). Higher grades are associated with more severe trauma, greater displacement, and a worse long-term prognosis.

A Hawkins type I fracture is a vertical fracture at the neck of the talus that is nondisplaced with the ankle in neutral position (Fig. 32-1). In theory, this fracture disrupts only the blood vessels entering the dorsal and lateral aspects of the neck of the talus and has the lowest rate of avascular necrosis and best overall prognosis. These fractures can be treated nonoperatively.

In a Hawkins type II fracture, the talar body fragment is displaced with subtalar joint subluxation or frank dislocation (Fig. 32-1). This fracture disrupts the blood supply from the dorsal and lateral aspects of the talar neck and from the vascular sling in the sinus tarsi and tarsal canal. They therefore have a worse prognosis, with avascular necrosis rates of 20% to 50%.

In Hawkins type III fractures, the talar body fragment is displaced with subtalar and ankle joint dislocation or subluxation. Usually, the body of the talus is dislocated and is found posteromedially between the posterior aspect of tibia and the Achilles tendon (Fig.32-1). These are frequently open injuries and often have an associated fracture of the medial malleolus. The blood supply of the talus is completely disrupted, with the possible exception of branches that enter through the deltoid ligament. These deltoid branches may be affected by fracture displacement, and urgent reduction may restore some degree of the blood supply to the body of the talus. Avascular necrosis rates of 80% to 100% have been reported for this type of fracture.

A Hawkins type IV fracture includes subtalar, ankle, and talonavicular subluxation or dislocation. In addition to all of the possible problems related to a Hawkins III fracture, type IV fractures carry the risk of damage to the blood supply to the head of the talus.

In patients with fractures of the body of the talus, a preoperative computed tomograph (CT) scan in the transverse and coronal planes can be helpful in defining the fracture anatomy and the degree of comminution. In patients with clearly defined fractures of the talar neck or body based on plain film radiography, the CT scan is generally unnecessary and may delay urgent operative treatment of these fractures.

## SURGERY

The common treatment goal of all fractures of the neck and body of the talus is urgent anatomic reduction with rigid internal fixation. In patients with a Hawkins type II fracture with a subluxated or dislocated subtalar joint, an attempt at closed reduction in the emergency room with distraction and plantarflexion is warranted. If anatomic or near-anatomic reduction of the fracture is achieved, the patient can then be taken to surgery in a semi-elective fashion, because theoretically, little remaining tension on the blood supply of the talar body will persist. Open reduction should be performed even if an anatomic closed reduction of a Hawkins II fracture has been achieved, because it avoids the inevitable equinus contracture that develops after a prolonged period of casting in plantarflexion. In Hawkins type III fractures with a dislocated body of the talus, closed reduction is often unsuccessful and may even further traumatize articular cartilage and soft tissue. These cases are surgical emergencies, as the dislocated body of the talus can lead to skin necrosis and any potential remaining blood supply to the body of the talus through the deltoid branches remains embarrassed until it is reduced.

### Technique: Fracture without Dislocation of the Talar Body

The patient is placed in a supine position, with a bump under the ipsilateral hip to orient the foot perpendicular to the floor. A thigh tourniquet is applied, and the leg is prepped and draped above the level of the knee. Intraoperative fluoroscopy should be available and can be a full-sized C-arm or a mini-image, depending on the surgeon's preference. Figure 32-3 shows the high quality of images that are typically obtained with contemporary fluoroscopy units. A combined anteromedial and anterolateral approach to the neck of the talus should be used. The anteromedial approach is made from the anterior aspect of the medial malleolus to the dorsal aspect of the navicular tuberosity (Fig. 32-4). The dissection is car-

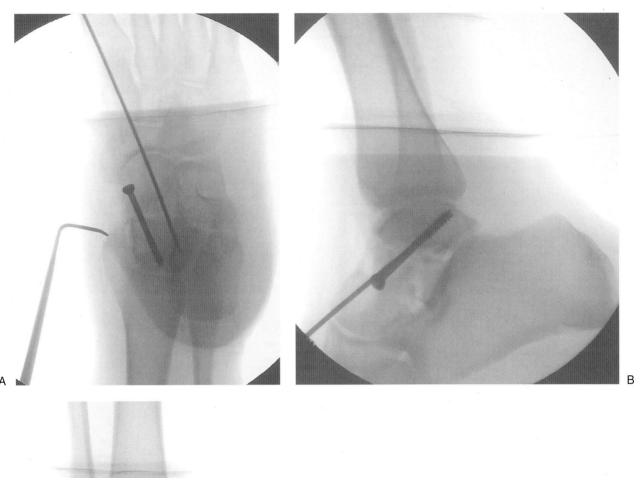

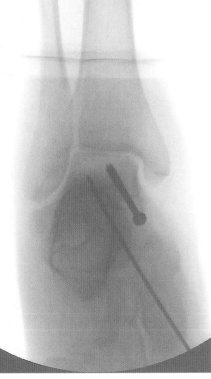

**Figure 32-3.** Intraoperative fluoroscopic views of the foot and ankle in patient with a displaced type II fracture during fixation. **A:** Anteroposterior view of the foot. **B:** Lateral view of the foot. **C:** Anteroposterior view of the ankle.

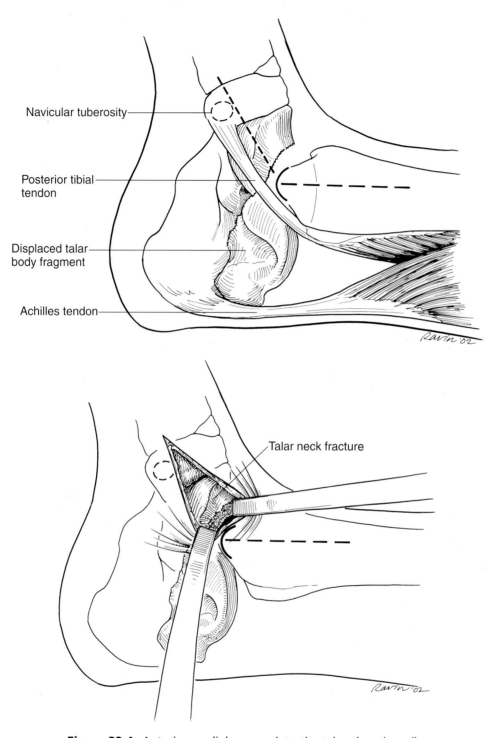

Navicular tuberosity

Posterior tibial
tendon

Displaced talar
body fragment

Achilles tendon

Talar neck fracture

**Figure 32-4.** Anterior-medial approach to the talus. *(continued)*

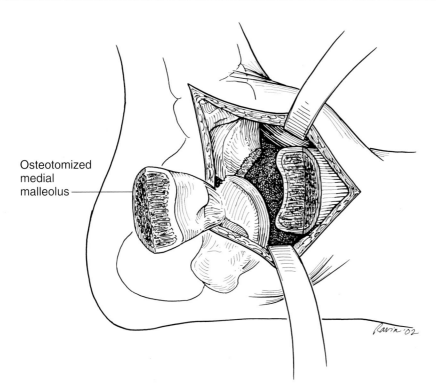

Osteotomized
medial
malleolus

**Figure 32-4.** *Continued.*

ried down to the bone, just dorsal to the posterior tibial tendon (Fig. 32-4). Disruption of the deltoid ligament should not be performed, because it will violate some of the remaining blood supply to the body of the talus. The fracture can be visualized and subsequently mobilized through this incision to allow removal of fracture hematoma and to begin mobilizing the fracture. Dissection of soft tissues at the talar neck dorsally or plantarly should not be performed to avoid disrupting the blood supply any further.

An anterolateral hindfoot incision is made (Fig. 32-5) that allows for confirmation of the accuracy of the reduction of the fracture by visualizing the fracture reduction opposite the medial incision. Because of limited exposure medially, the fracture often is initially malreduced. This second incision also permits removal of any osteochondral fragment debris from the subtalar joint. Fracture comminution is frequently present on the medial neck of the talus, and visualizing the lateral aspect of the neck can provide a more accurate gauge of the adequacy of reduction because there is rarely comminution laterally.

The anterolateral hindfoot incision is made starting from the anterior margin of the lateral malleolus toward the base of the third or fourth metatarsal. The inferior extensor retinaculum is incised. The extensor digitorum longus tendon and peroneus tertius tendon are retracted (Fig. 32-5). The extensor digitorum brevis muscle is retracted dorsally and distally. An angled retractor (Army-Navy) can be placed deep in this incision to facilitate exposure of the neck. If osseous fragments are evident in the subtalar joint preoperatively, they should be located and removed, perhaps with the aid of a lamina spreader in the sinus tarsi. The subtalar joint is routinely probed blindly with a blunt instrument such as a hemostat and irrigated to remove any articular debris that may be present.

The fracture is reduced under direct visualization through the medial and lateral incisions (Figs. 32-6 through 32-8). The surgeon must beware comminution of the medial neck of the talus, because it can lead to a varus malreduction of the neck of the talus that subsequently leads to a rigid, supinated foot. The fracture site often has a diastasis or gap if the fracture is malpositioned in varus. Once provisional reduction is performed, it should be stabilized with 0.062-inch Kirschner wires. After provisional pin stabilization, the clinical alignment of the foot should be assessed to make certain there is no tendency toward varus

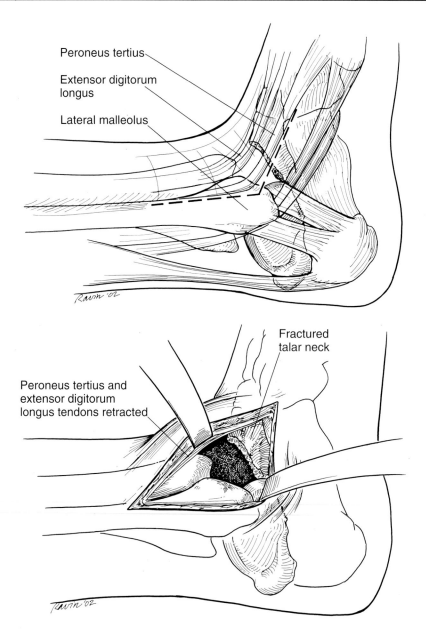

Peroneus tertius

Extensor digitorum
longus

Lateral malleolus

Fractured
talar neck

Peroneus tertius and
extensor digitorum
longus tendons retracted

**Figure 32-5.** Anterior-lateral approach to the talus.

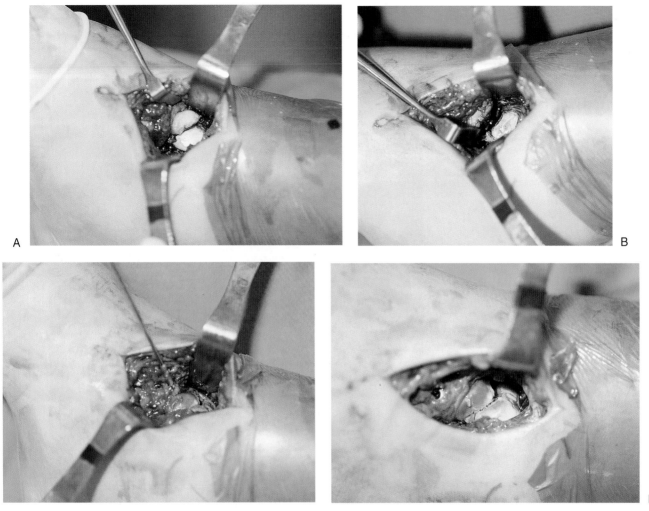

**Figure 32-6. A:** Intraoperative photograph demonstrates the appearance of a displaced talar neck and body fracture through the medial approach. Notice the dissection spares the region of the deltoid ligament, which carries some of the remaining blood supply to the body of the talus. **B:** Intraoperative photograph demonstrates the appearance of the fracture after it has been distracted, allowing for debridement of the hematoma and osseous debris. **C:** Medial intraoperative photograph demonstrates a Kirschner wire and screw across the reduced talar neck. **D:** Medial photograph after placement of a cortical screw through the distal medial aspect of the talar neck.

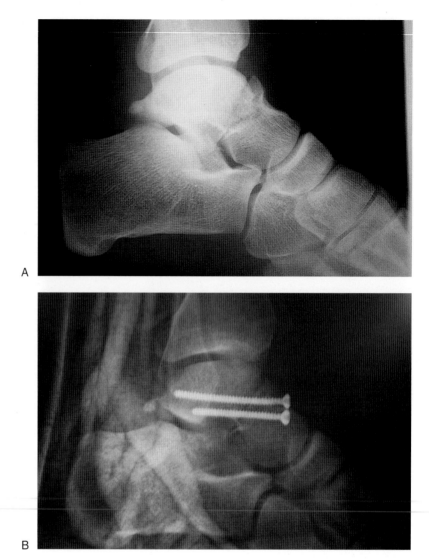

**Figure 32-7. A:** Lateral preoperative radiograph of a patient with a Hawkins II fracture demonstrates subluxation of the talar dome fragment. **B:** Postoperative radiograph of the same patient after open reduction and internal fixation with two fully threaded cortical screws inserted from anterior to posterior.

or supination. Subsequently, intraoperative lateral foot, anteroposterior foot, and Canale fluoroscopic views should be obtained to assess the quality of reduction (Fig. 32-2). If it is adequate, fully threaded titanium screws may be placed for definitive fixation (Figs. 32-9 and 32-10). Because medial comminution is frequently present, lag screw fixation typically is not used, because it may displace the fracture into varus. A minimum of two screws should be placed across the fracture site. A hard, cortical ridge of bone may be present along the dorsal aspect of the sinus tarsi that allows for excellent fixation with one or two screws inserted from the lateral neck of the talus across the fracture site. Titanium screws allow for postoperative magnetic resonance imaging (MRI) of the talus to assess for presence of avascular necrosis. Stainless steel screws may also be used, but with MR scanning, signal abnormalities adjacent to the screws is expected and precludes visualization of part of the talus.

If the fracture is located in the distal neck of the talus, the head of the screw should be countersunk into the head of the talus. As an alternative, a different method of fixation such as a polylactic acid (PLA) bioabsorbable screw (Bionix Implants, Inc., Blue Bell, PA), Herbert screw (Zimmer Corp., Warsaw, IN), or Acutrak screw (Acumed, Beaverton, OR), can be used in an antegrade direction. Although placement of the screws from the posterolateral approach from the posterior tuberosity of the talus into the head has been shown to provide good mechanical stability, it is a more difficult approach, and fracture reduction may be more challenging.

### Technique: Fracture with Dislocated Talar Body

In Hawkins type III fractures, in which the body of the talus is dislocated posteromedially, the medial approach must be extended over the medial malleolus and the distal aspect of the tibia (Fig. 32-4). The body of the talus is identified in the subcutaneous tissue between the posterior aspect of the tibia and the Achilles tendon. If the medial malleolus is fractured, it is retracted distally to facilitate reduction of the body of the talus back into the mortise (Fig. 32-8). Despite the excellent exposure of the talar body with this approach, reduction is frequently very difficult. A large, smooth Steinmann pin can be placed transversely in the posterior-inferior aspect of the calcaneus to act as an intraoperative traction device. A femoral distractor may be used, with pins in the calcaneus and tibia (Fig. 32-11). With vigorous traction applied and direct manual pressure over the body of the talus, reduction of the body back into the mortise can be achieved with some difficulty. If a patient has an intact medial malleolus, the traction pin is still placed in an attempt at reducing the body of the talus through the tear of the joint capsule. If it is still not possible to reduce the body of the talus, a medial malleolar osteotomy should be performed.

Although an oblique malleolar osteotomy can be performed quickly, a step-cut osteotomy allows for a larger cancellous bone surface that can be easily reduced with good initial stability (Fig. 32-12). This osteotomy is performed by first identifying the level of the ankle joint anteriorly and posteriorly. Before making the osteotomy, two retrograde parallel drill holes are made with a 2.5-mm drill bit in the tip of the medial malleolus to allow for osteotomy reduction and fixation at the conclusion of the procedure. The anterior ankle capsule from the axilla to the anterior aspect of the deltoid ligament is released, as well as a portion of the posterior tibial tendon sheath posteriorly. A blunt retractor is placed anterior to the posterior tibial tendon to prevent inadvertent damage. The periosteum is incised approximately 5 to 10 mm superior to the ankle joint, and a narrow, oscillating saw blade is used to cut transversely through the tibia to the level of the ankle joint. The vertical portion of the osteotomy is then made from anterior to posterior with a narrow, straight osteotome. The medial malleolus is reflected distally, taking care not to damage the ligament. To properly mobilize the medial malleolar fragment, the anterior joint capsule and the posterior tibial tendon sheath must be released as described previously.

After the body of the talus is manually placed back into the ankle mortise, the anterolateral incision is made to facilitate exposure of the fracture, if necessary. A medial malleolar osteotomy allows visualization of the dorsal aspect of the fracture. When the extended medial incision is made, it may not be necessary to add the lateral incision unless osseous debris is expected in the subtalar joint. After reducing and fixing the fracture of the neck of the talus, the medial malleolar fracture or osteotomy is fixed with two partially threaded, 4.0-mm, cancellous, titanium screws (Fig. 32-13). The skin incisions are closed with multiple, interrupted, nonabsorbable mattress sutures.

## POSTOPERATIVE MANAGEMENT

A posterior splint with ankle in neutral position is applied. A cast may be applied in 1 to 2 days. After the incisions have healed, approximately 2 to 3 weeks after surgery, the sutures are removed, and a splint or boot is applied. At this time, the patient begins ankle and subtalar range of motion exercises, provided that rigid internal fixation is achieved at the time of surgery. Range of motion exercises are not advised until wound healing has occurred. Patients should be kept on a non–weight-bearing program for approximately 8 to 12 weeks

*(Text continued on page 484.)*

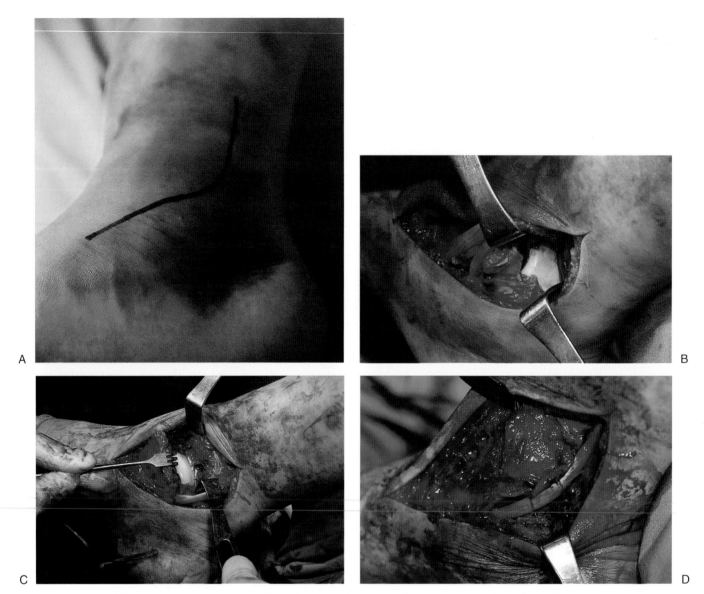

**Figure 32-8. A:** Preoperative photograph demonstrates ecchymosis and swelling overlying the dislocated body of the talus medially in the right foot. The patient also had a medial malleolar fracture. Notice the extension of the medial incision more proximally. **B:** Intraoperative photograph through a medial incision after dissecting through the subcutaneous tissues. The severely displaced dorsal articular surface of the talus is visible through the subcutaneous tissues. The posterior tibial and flexor digitorum longus tendons are retracted anteriorly. Notice the proximal extension of the incision over the distal medial aspect of the tibia to facilitate exposure of the dislocated body of the talus. **C:** Intraoperative photograph through a medial incision after the medial malleolar fracture is retracted distally and the body of the talus is reduced into the mortise. Notice the large, smooth traction pin in the posterior aspect of the calcaneus that facilitates reduction of the talar body. **D:** Intraoperative photograph after open reduction and internal fixation of the medial malleolar fracture with two partially threaded cancellous screws. The posterior tibial tendon can be seen in its proper location just before repair of its sheath, which was disrupted at the time of injury.

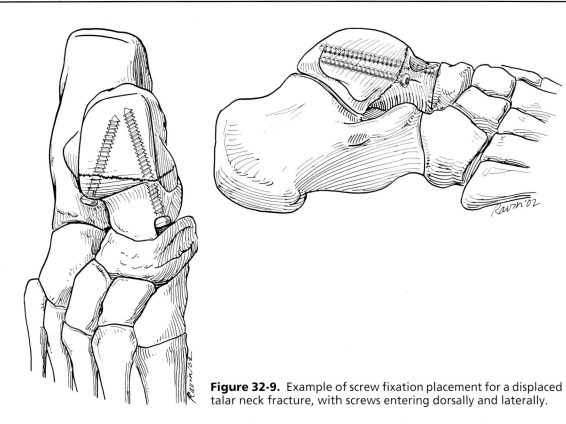

**Figure 32-9.** Example of screw fixation placement for a displaced talar neck fracture, with screws entering dorsally and laterally.

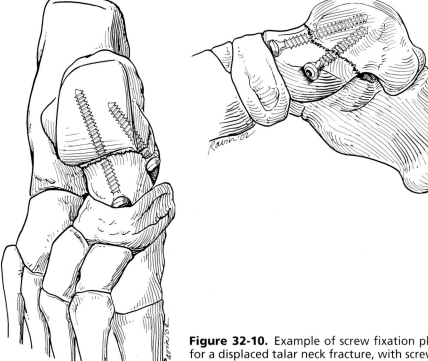

**Figure 32-10.** Example of screw fixation placement for a displaced talar neck fracture, with screws entering dorsally and dorsomedially.

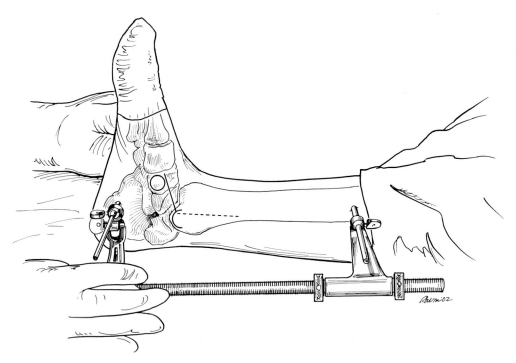

**Figure 32-11.** The femoral distractor is applied for traction to facilitate difficult fracture reduction with a pin in calcaneus and in tibia.

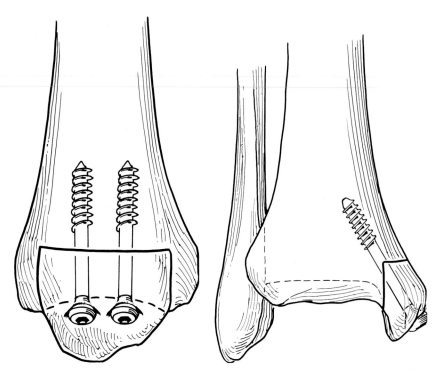

**Figure 32-12.** For the step-cut osteotomy, the transverse portion is made 5 to 10 mm proximal to the joint line to the level of the axilla with a narrow oscillating saw. The vertical portion is made with an osteotome. The anterior joint capsule and posterior tibial tendon sheath are released to mobilize the fragment.

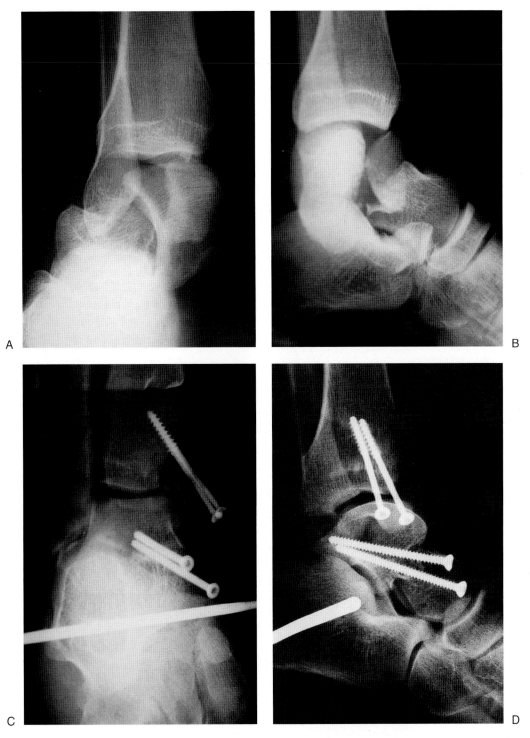

**Figure 32-13. A:** Preoperative anteroposterior radiograph of the ankle after a Hawkins III fracture. Notice the body of the talus is dislocated medially and rotated approximately 90° on its deltoid ligament attached to the fractured medial malleolus. **B:** Preoperative lateral radiograph demonstrates posteromedial dislocation of the body of the talus. The medial malleolar fragment is visible as a crescent-shaped density anterior to the ankle joint. Notice the congruent talonavicular joint. **C:** Intraoperative anteroposterior radiograph after open reduction and internal fixation of the talar neck and medial malleolar fractures shows the large, smooth Steinmann pin that was placed for traction. **D:** Intraoperative lateral radiograph demonstrates congruent reduction of the ankle and subtalar joint with a large, smooth Steinmann traction pin still in place. Notice the fully threaded cortical screws used for neutralization fixation of the talar neck fracture and partially threaded cancellous screws for fixation of the medial malleolar fracture.

after surgery, until there is radiographic evidence of union such as trabeculae crossing of the fractures.

Ideally, the patient should be able to perform activities of daily living without significant pain. Because of the severe soft tissue injury, most patients have some subtalar and ankle stiffness and are limited in performing high-impact activities to some degree in the long term. Because of the severe nature of the injury, patients should be counseled that it is unlikely the foot condition will be restored to normal.

## COMPLICATIONS

Complications after fractures of the neck and body of the talus include avascular necrosis, subtalar and ankle joint arthritis and arthrofibrosis, skin necrosis, osteomyelitis, nonunion, and malunion. *Avascular necrosis* of the body of the talus after a fracture of the neck can occur in patients after Hawkins II, III, and IV fractures. The diagnosis has classically been made on plain radiographic evaluation. The Hawkins sign, a subchondral radiolucency, is an active process and therefore rules out the presence of avascular necrosis (Fig. 32-14). It should be evaluated on an anteroposterior radiograph of the ankle without a cast 6 to 8 weeks after injury. Absence of the Hawkins sign, however, does not always indicate avascular necrosis (Fig. 32-15). Magnetic resonance (MR) scans performed can reliably demonstrate avascular necrosis. MR scans can also detect partial avascular necrosis of the talar body. Although it may be impossible to prevent the occurrence of avascular necrosis, the revascularization process can be enhanced by an accurate, stable reduction of the fracture.

Long-term prognosis of patients with avascular necrosis is uncertain. Some authors state it takes 2 years for the talus to revascularize completely. Others state that the development of avascular necrosis does not guarantee a poor result. However, collapse of the dome of the talus generally leads to a poor result. Because of the risk of collapse, some surgeons have recommended prolonged periods without weight bearing after these injuries. One report described a patient who experienced segmental collapse 2.5 years after injury on commencing weight bearing. The current protocol for weight bearing after operative treatment of talar neck fractures without avascular necrosis includes weight bearing as tolerated after

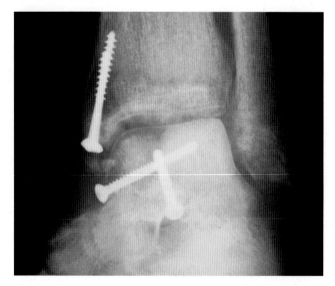

**Figure 32-14.** Anteroposterior radiograph of a patient demonstrating avascular necrosis of the lateral half of the body of the talus. Notice the subchondral radiolucency (i.e., Hawkins sign) in the medial half of the body of the talus. The sclerotic lateral portion of the body of the talus has evidence of avascular necrosis.

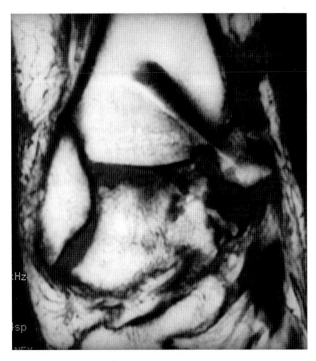

**Figure 32-15.** Coronal MR scan of a patient with avascular necrosis of the body of the talus. Notice the minimal scattering about the titanium screws, evident in the distal medial aspect of the tibia, that had been placed across the medial malleolar fracture. Notice the decreased signal in the avascular portion of the dorsal body of the talus.

fracture consolidation. Patients with avascular necrosis involving more than one third of the talar body are advised of the risk of late segmental collapse after weight bearing and are offered a patellar tendon bearing brace to be used during the period of revascularization. Most patients, however, choose to begin bearing weight after the fracture has healed.

All patients who sustain a fracture of the neck of the talus are at risk for developing *arthrofibrosis* of the subtalar and ankle joints. More than one half of all patients in some series have developed subtalar degenerative changes. Severely decreased range of motion of the ankle and/or subtalar joints is associated with a poor result. Although some degree of stiffness of these joints can be expected, early and aggressive range of motion exercises after wound healing has occurred can limit stiffness. Because of chondral injury at the time of fracture, arthritis of the ankle and subtalar joints can occur in the absence of avascular necrosis of the talus or joint incongruity.

*Malunion* of a talar neck fracture is a preventable complication with proper operative technique. It results in incongruity and degenerative arthritis of the ankle and subtalar joints. Varus malalignment is most common because of the medial talar neck fracture comminution that has not been properly aligned. More severe deformity is associated with more severe stiffness and is difficult to treat even with a salvage operation such as an arthrodesis.

*Nonunion* may occur after talar neck fractures. Patients with avascular necrosis of the body of the talus may have fracture union between the viable neck and avascular body. *Delayed union* is more common than nonunion, occurring in approximately 10% of patients.

*Skin necrosis* can occur after delayed treatment of a Hawkins III fracture with a dislocated body of the talus (Fig. 32-16). When present, these wounds require aggressive debridement and early soft tissue coverage. Delayed treatment of these wounds can lead to deep infection that is difficult to eradicate and generally requires additional operations and protracted recovery.

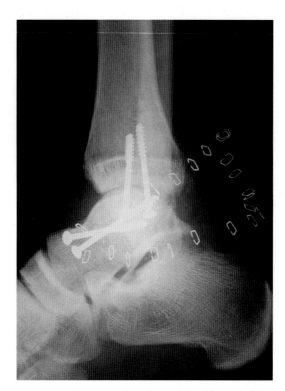

**Figure 32-16.** Postoperative lateral radiograph of a patient after a split-thickness skin graft for full-thickness skin slough after delayed treatment of a Hawkins III fracture. The skin necrosis occurred directly above the dislocated body of the talus. Staples outline the margin of the skin graft.

## RECOMMENDED READING

1. Alexander IJ, Watson JT: Step-cut osteotomy of the medial malleolus for exposure of the medial ankle joint space. *Foot Ankle* 11:242–243, 1991.
2. Canale ST, Kelley FB: Fractures of the neck of the talus. *J Bone Joint Surg Am* 68:143–156, 1978.
3. Hawkins LG: Fractures of the neck of the talus. *J Bone Joint Surg Am* 52:991–1002, 1970.
4. Penny JN, Davis LA: Fractures and fracture dislocations of the neck of the talus. *J Trauma* 20:1020–1037, 1980.
5. Peterson L, Goldie I, Lindell D: The arterial supply of the talus. *Acta Orthop Scand* 45:260–270, 1974.
6. Thordarson DB, Triffon M, Terk M: Magnetic resonance imaging to detect avascular necrosis after open reduction and internal fixation of talar neck fractures. *Foot Ankle Int* 17:742–747, 1996.

# PART V

## Ankle

# 33

# Ankle Instability Repair: The Bröstrom-Gould Procedure

## William G. Hamilton

## INDICATIONS/CONTRAINDICATIONS

In 1964 to 1966, Lennart Bröstrom wrote a series of six articles on ankle sprains in the *Acta Chirurgica Scandinavica* (1–6). In the last of these, he reported successful results for 58 of 60 patients with the use of a new operation for the correction of "chronic" ankle instability. In one of the earlier articles, he discussed the use of a similar operation for the acute ankle sprain (2).

His procedure involved isometrically tightening the stretched-out lateral ankle ligaments to restore their normal anatomy without the use of supplemental tissues or "weaving" procedures. It was based on the fact that the anterior talofibular ligament lies within the anterolateral ankle capsule (similar to the anterior glenohumeral ligaments of the shoulder), and when the anterior talofibular ligament is torn, it heals within the capsule in an elongated form. The operation shortened the stretched-out anterior talofibular and calcaneofibular ligaments to their normal lengths and sutured them to their anatomic locations, thereby restoring the normal anatomy and maintaining full range of motion without sacrificing the peroneus brevis tendon.

In 1980, Nathaniel Gould reported his modification of the Bröstrom repair (7). It consisted of Bröstrom's operation followed by mobilizing the lateral portion of the extensor retinaculum and suturing it to the distal fibula over the ligament repair. This approach reinforces the repair; limits inversion, which is the position of reinjury; and helps correct the subtalar component of the instability. The latter factor is important, because the calcaneofibular ligament is one of the main stabilizers of the subtalar joint (9). When it is torn, as in third-degree lateral sprains, a combined instability is usually present in the tibiotalar and subtalar joints. The retinacular reinforcement helps correct this combined instability because it runs parallel to the calcaneofibular ligament and inserts in the lateral calcaneus.

W. G. Hamilton, M.D.: Department of Orthopaedic Surgery, Columbia University College of Physicians and Surgeons; St. Luke's-Roosevelt Hospital Center; and Orthopedic Associates of New York, New York, New York.

There are several advantages to the modified Bröstrom procedure. It is a relatively easy procedure; it uses a small cosmetic incision; the sural nerve should not be in any danger of injury; it does not require the sacrifice of a peroneal tendon; it is anatomic and maintains a full range of motion in the ankle and subtalar joints; and contrary to the various weaving procedures, it is difficult to make the repair so tight that the subtalar joint is locked in eversion.

Because of these factors, it is an ideal procedure for the athlete who needs ankle stability with a full range of motion and no loss of peroneal function, such as the ballet dancer, gymnast, or ice skater. We now use it routinely on all our patients. It has recently been modified in patients who weigh over 200 pounds by adding the split Evans repair over the Bröstrom repair. Bröstrom and Gould described the use of their procedures for acute third-degree sprains in selected cases as well.

The indications for this procedure include chronic symptomatic lateral ankle instability that has not responded to physical therapy and rehabilitation (especially proprioceptive training and peroneal strengthening) and selected cases of acute third-degree ankle sprains (usually professional-level athletes).

This procedure is not recommended for the patient with a fixed heel varus without correction of this deformity. In this instance, a valgus osteotomy (Dwyer procedure) of the os calcis should be performed along with the repair. The procedure is also not recommended for patients of increased body weight, such as athletes who weigh more than 200 to 250 pounds. For these individuals, I recommend doing the modified Bröstrom and then adding an Evans type repair using one half of the peroneus brevis tendon. Peroneal weakness due to peroneal nerve palsy and neurologic dysfunction such as Charcot-Marie-Tooth disease are relative contraindications.

## PREOPERATIVE PLANNING

The patient who is being considered for this surgical procedure has a history of multiple sprains involving the lateral aspect of the ankle, which limits the functional ability to a significant degree. This type of surgical repair is particularly appropriate for the athlete because it does not restrict subtalar motion to the degree that some of the procedures involving tendon weaving on the lateral aspect of the ankle can do. During the physical examination, it is particularly important to be aware that a fixed heel varus can contribute to recurrent instability and, if present, should be corrected with a Dwyer lateral closing wedge osteotomy at the same time as the ligament reconstruction, placing the tuberosity of the calcaneus in a normal slight valgus position. During physical examination, the strength of the peroneal mechanism should be assessed. Weakness in peroneal strength should be corrected before contemplation of any surgical procedure. Sometimes, peroneal strengthening can control the instability and obviate the need for surgical treatment.

Instability of the hindfoot can be evaluated by an inversion stress test to determine the degree of talar tilt versus the contralateral (normal) ankle. The anterior drawer sign is an accurate way to determine the amount of laxity in the lateral ligaments. This sign is elicited by stabilizing the tibia and fibula with one hand while pulling the talus forward on the tibia with the ankle held in about 20° of plantarflexion. In my experience, this is the best predictor of instability of the ankle and can be compared with the joint laxity present in the opposite, undamaged ankle. It is also important to assess subtalar motion, which should be normal. If it is decreased, other diagnoses such as a tarsal coalition should be suspected. Chronic ankle instability is often associated with an unrecognized tarsal coalition.

Routine radiographs are taken to be certain osteochondral fractures, anterior process fractures of the calcaneus, or other associated injuries that may need to be corrected are not present. Inversion stress views of the ankle are frequently done to look for abnormal talar tilt. Because this test primarily stresses the calcaneofibular ligament, the talar tilt may not be increased and ankle instability can still be present because of the subtalar component of the instability. For this reason, stress views of the ankle are usually evaluated in association with a history and physical findings supporting a diagnosis of instability and are not an absolute contraindication to surgical treatment if they do not show an increased talar tilt. Stress Broden's views of the subtalar joint can show the subtalar component of the instability problem.

## SURGERY

The operation is usually performed as an outpatient procedure. The patient is placed supine, with a sandbag under the hip if the patient has increased external rotation of the hip, so that the foot is in a vertical or slightly internally rotated position (Fig. 33-1). A thigh tourniquet is used over cast padding, and general, spinal, or epidural anesthesia is needed.

### Technique

After exsanguination of the leg, a curvilinear incision is made along the anterior border of the distal fibula, stopping at the peroneal tendons (Figs. 33-2 and 33-3). The sural nerve is just below the distal margin of the incision, lying adjacent to the peroneal tendons and

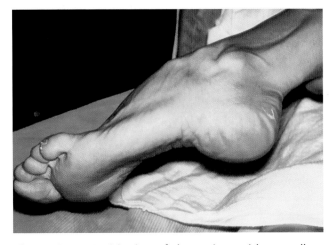

**Figure 33-1.** Positioning of the patient with a sandbag under the affected hip allows access to the anterolateral aspect of the ankle.

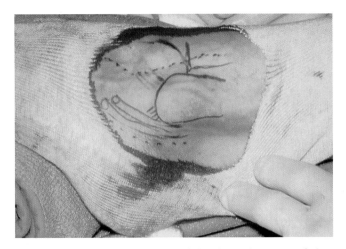

**Figure 33-2.** The structures of the lateral aspect of the ankle are drawn with the skin-marking pen. Starting inferiorly, the *dotted line* shows the usual location of the sural nerve. Next, the peroneal tendons and the calcaneofibular ligament attached to the tip of the fibula are marked. More anteriorly, the dome of the talus along with the lateral branch of the superficial peroneal nerve *(dotted line)* is shown.

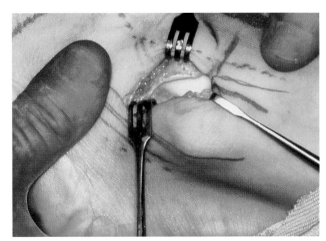

**Figure 33-3.** An oblique skin incision is made down through the capsule anterior to the fibula.

should be avoided (Fig. 33-4). The lesser saphenous vein usually crosses the distal fibula at this level and must be ligated. In several cases I have observed, the sural nerve crossed in the middle of this incision, so the surgeon should always be prepared for anatomic variations. The sural nerve may not always course where it is supposed to be.

If it is necessary to perform the split Evans procedure, an alternate incision is necessary that can allow access to the peroneal tendons (Fig. 33-5, incision B). It extends longitudinally from the posterior margin of the fibula distally toward the base of the fourth metatarsal. Incision A is the standard Bröstrom incision, and incision C is the incision used for the Dwyer operation.

The dissection is carried down to the joint capsule along the anterior border of the lateral malleolus. Laxity of the anterior talofibular and frequently the calcaneofibular ligaments are found (Fig. 33-6). The capsule is divided along the anterior border of the fibula down to the peroneal tendons, leaving a 2- to 3-mm cuff of tissue. The anterior talofibular ligament lies within this capsule, similar to the anterior glenohumeral ligaments of the shoulder. It usually is seen as a thickening in the capsule. It is best to leave a small cuff of tissue on the fibula rather than take the capsule off the bone by sharp dissection so that an isometric repair can be performed that does not limit motion.

The calcaneofibular ligament must now be identified (Fig. 33-7). It lies deep to the peroneal tendons, running obliquely downward and posteriorly to its insertion in the calcaneus (Fig. 33-8). It will often be stretched out and attenuated, or it may be dislodged so that it lies outside the peroneals. On rare occasions it can be found avulsed from its calcaneal origin with a bone fragment. If it is in continuity, it is divided, leaving a cuff at its insertion on the fibula. By leaving a cuff of tissue at the insertion of the ligaments, the surgeon will

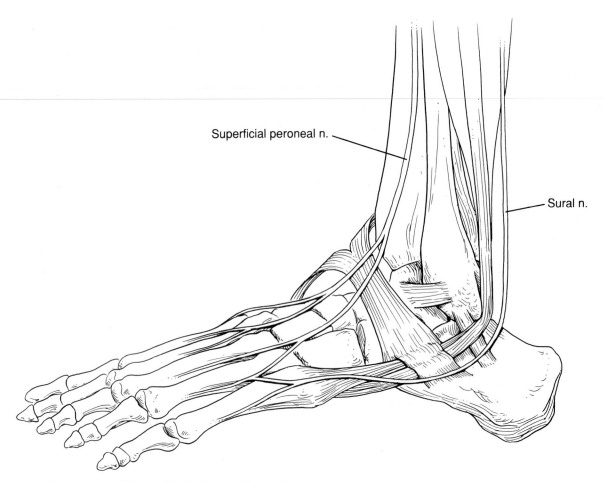

Superficial peroneal n.

Sural n.

**Figure 33-4.** The relative positions of the sural nerve, the lateral branch of the superficial peroneal nerve, and the inferior extensor retinaculum are shown.

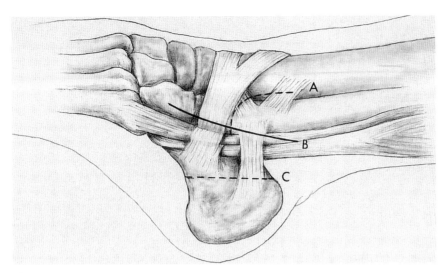

**Figure 33-5.** The typical and two alternate incisions are shown for the standard Bröstrom procedure *(A)*, if an Evans procedure reinforcement is needed *(B)*, and for the Dwyer operation *(C)*.

be able to repair the ligaments in their exact anatomic locations, preserving isometry and an unrestricted range of motion, analogous to an anterior cruciate ligament reconstruction in the knee.

The ligaments must now be shortened and repaired. The ankle should be placed in the fully reduced position in neutral dorsiflexion and slight eversion. The stumps of the ligaments are pulled up and the redundancy is trimmed. The ligaments are then sutured to their

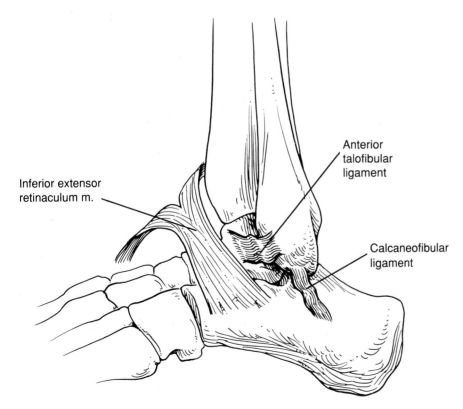

Inferior extensor
retinaculum m.

Anterior
talofibular
ligament

Calcaneofibular
ligament

**Figure 33-6.** The diagram shows the position of the elongated anterior talofibular ligament and calcaneal fibular ligament.

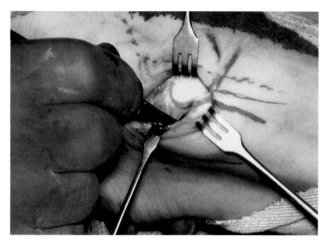

**Figure 33-7.** Deep to the tip of the fibula in the plane of the joint capsule, the tear of the calcaneofibular ligament is identified.

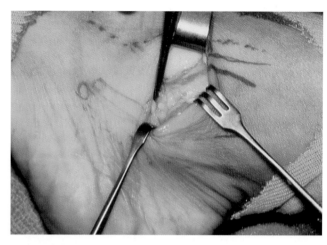

**Figure 33-8.** The torn distal portion of the calcaneofibular ligament is brought up in the wound, and the ends are "freshened" by removing the scar tissue.

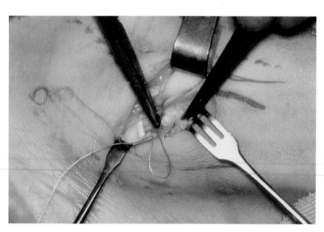

**Figure 33-9.** The two ends of the calcaneofibular ligament are sutured, reestablishing its continuity.

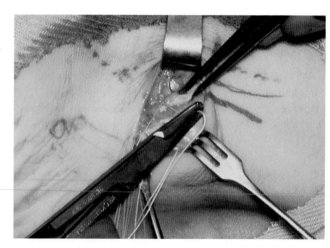

**Figure 33-10.** The anterior talofibular ligament, represented as a thickening of the anterior joint capsule, is also sutured to reestablish its proper length.

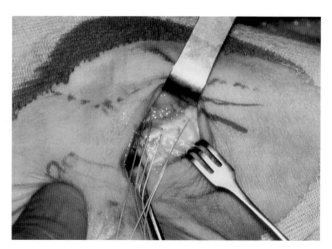

**Figure 33-11.** Multiple sutures are used to reattach the anterior talofibular ligament and anterior lateral joint capsule.

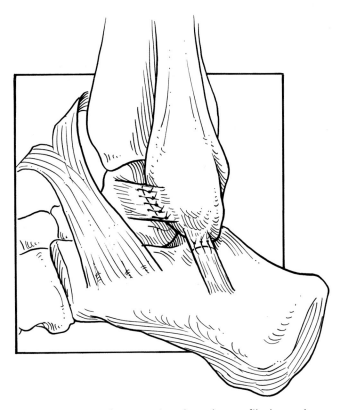

**Figure 33-12.** After suturing the calcaneofibular and anterior talofibular ligaments, the ankle is ready for inferior extensor retinaculum translocation.

anatomic locations with 2-0 nonabsorbable sutures, starting with the calcaneofibular ligament (Fig. 33-9), because it is the most difficult to visualize, and then proceeding to the anterior talofibular ligament within the capsule (Figs. 33-10 and 33-11). This repair can be done by end-to-end suture, "pants over vest," or into drill holes (Figs. 33-12 and 33-13). Occasionally, the capsular insertion on the fibula is completely torn away or missing, and it is impossible to leave a cuff for repair. In this instance, the capsule and anterior talofibular ligament needs to be attached where the soft tissue cuff should be present. It is necessary to make a small trough in the fibula with drill holes so that the capsule can be pulled into the trough and reattached or else secured with the use of suture anchors. I like to use a

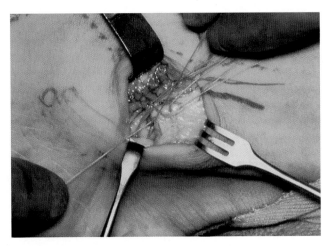

**Figure 33-13.** The inferior extensor retinaculum is seen just beneath the wide, more distal retractor.

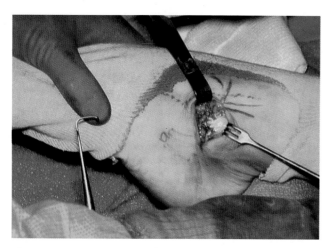

**Figure 33-14.** This view shows the exposure of the inferior extensor retinaculum superficial to the anterolateral joint capsule.

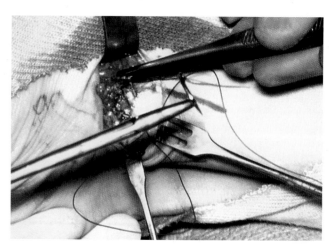

**Figure 33-15.** The retinaculum is mobilized and sutured to the anterior aspect of the fibula.

small bolster behind the distal tibia when performing this procedure. The bolster lifts the heel off the table so that the talus is not displaced forward in the anterior drawer position when the ligaments are repaired.

At this point, the ankle should be examined for stability and a full range of dorsiflexion and plantarflexion. The lateral portion of the extensor retinaculum is then identified. It is dissected off the capsule and mobilized so that it can cover the repair at the end of the procedure (Figs. 33-14 and 33-15). Care should be taken when operating anterior to the malle-

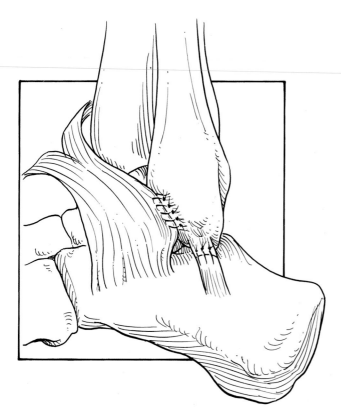

**Figure 33-16.** Suturing of the inferior extensor retinaculum to the anterior aspect of the fibula.

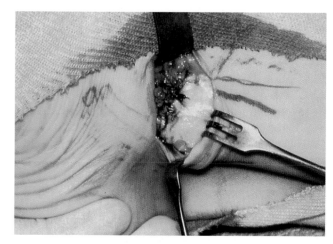

**Figure 33-17.** With completion of the procedure, the lateral ligaments and inferior extensor retinaculum are in the appropriate positions, which will allow full motion of the ankle.

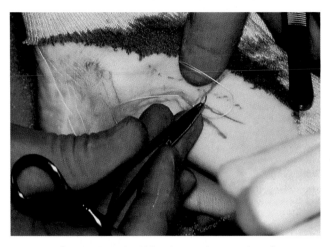

**Figure 33-18.** Skin closure is completed.

olus because of the proximity to the lateral branch of the superficial peroneal nerve in the subcutaneous tissues, which can be damaged by dissection or a sharp retractor. Sometimes, the extensor retinaculum can be somewhat difficult to identify. Its fibers run at right angles to the fibers of the anterior talofibular ligament and joint capsule. If it cannot be identified, extending the incision can help. The mobilization of the extensor retinaculum can be performed before or after the capsular incision.

The previously identified extensor retinaculum mechanism is then pulled over the repair and sutured to the tip of the fibula with 2-0 chromic catgut (Figs. 33-16 and 33-17). This accomplishes three things: it reinforces the repair, it limits inversion (the position of injury), and it helps correct the subtalar component of the instability. (If the calcaneofibular ligament is attenuated, there will be some degree of subtalar instability.) The ankle is again checked for stability and moved through a full range of motion.

A layered closure is then performed with an absorbable subcutaneous suture and Steri-Strips (Fig. 33-18). The patient is placed in anterior-posterior plaster splints and discharged with crutches to maintain a non–weight-bearing program.

## POSTOPERATIVE MANAGEMENT

When the swelling has subsided in 3 to 5 days, a short-leg walking cast or a removable short-leg walker (in reliable patients) is applied for 3 to 4 weeks. The cast is removed 1 month postoperatively, and the ankle is protected with an air stirrup-type of splint for another month. Swimming, range of motion, and isometric peroneal exercises are begun. Unrestricted activities are allowed at 8 to 12 weeks if full peroneal strength is present.

We started using this procedure in ballet dancers in 1980, and because of good results, we began to use it on all of our ligament repairs. As of 1992, we had more than 40 cases, 55% of which were high-level professional ballet dancers. The rest were recreational athletes and nonathletic patients. Average follow-up was 7 years. Of the 28 operations reviewed and reported (8), there were 26 excellent, 1 good, and 1 fair result. All of the professional dancers obtained excellent results and returned to their careers. My colleagues and I have performed more than 70 procedures, and there have been only 3 failures (due to significant reinjury) that were revised, but no serious complications occurred. Two patients have loosened the repair with time, but they are not symptomatic and have not required revision. They both have generalized ligamentous laxity, and for this type of patient, I now recommend adding the split Evans procedure to act as a "check-rein."

This operation is felt to be an excellent choice for the dancer, athlete, and nonathlete who needs a stable ankle with a full range of motion and normal peroneal function. Other investigators report success with the technique. Hennrikus et al. (10), in a randomized prospective study of 40 patients, found that the operation provided stability to chronically unstable ankles and had better clinical results with fewer complications than those treated with the Chrisman-Snook operation. Karlsson et al. (11) reported that most patients with chronic ankle instability can be successfully treated with anatomic reconstruction of the lateral ankle ligaments with retraction of mechanical stability. Girard et al. (7) reported good results of the operation augmented with a portion of the peroneus brevis tendon to provide greater stability to inversion stress in patients who are overweight, hyperflexible, or involved in strenuous work or athletic activities.

## COMPLICATIONS

Complications as a result of this procedure have been minimal. It is possible to overtighten the capsule when doing the repair of the capsule and anterior talofibular ligament structures. If this is done, *plantarflexion of the ankle may be limited.* To avoid this complication, the ankle should be tested at the time of surgery to be certain it can move into full plantarflexion while the hindfoot is in a neutral position. It is felt that the essence of this procedure is not only the static support to the ankle, but also the replacement of proprioception to the soft tissues about the ankle and subtalar joint.

The other complication that may occur involves *injury to the superficial sensory nerves* about the lateral aspect of the ankle. If the incision is extended too far dorsally on the top of the foot, injury to the lateral branch of the superficial peroneal nerve can occur. Being aware of this risk and protecting the nerve from excessive stretching at the time of surgery is important. The sural nerve must also be protected. Limiting the distal portion of the incision to the level of the peroneal tendons, but not below that level, decreases the possibility of sural nerve damage. Identifying the nerve at the inferior aspect of the wound should avoid transection of the nerve and resulting hypesthesia in the lateral aspect of the foot distally.

## RECOMMENDED READING

1.  Bröstrom L: Sprained ankles. I. Anatomic lesions in recent sprains. *Acta Chir Scand* 128:483–495, 1964.
2.  Bröstrom L: Sprained ankles. III. Clinical observations in recent ligament ruptures. *Acta Chir Scand* 130: 560–569, 1965.
3.  Bröstrom L: Sprained ankles. V. Treatment and prognosis in recent ligament ruptures. *Acta Chir Scand* 132: 537–550, 1966.
4.  Bröstrom L: Sprained ankles. VI. Surgical treatment of "chronic" ligament ruptures. *Acta Chir Scand* 132: 551–565, 1966.
5.  Bröstrom L, Liljedahl S, Lindvall N: Sprained ankles. II. Arthrographic diagnosis of recent ligament ruptures. *Acta Chir Scand* 129:485–499, 1965.
6.  Bröstrom L, Sundelin P: Sprained ankles. IV. Histological changes in recent and "chronic" ligament ruptures. *Acta Chir Scand* 131:483–490, 1966.
7.  Girard P, Anderson RB, Daris WH, et al.: Clinical evaluation of the modified Bröstrom-Evans procedure to restore ankle stability. *Foot Ankle Int* 20:246–252, 1999.
8.  Gould N, Seligson D, Gassman J: Early and late repair of lateral ligament of the ankle. *Foot Ankle* 1:84–89, 1980.
9.  Hamilton W, Thompson FM, Snow SW: The modified Bröstrom procedure for lateral ankle instability. *Foot Ankle* 14:1–7, 1993.
10. Hennrikus WL, Mapes RC, Lyons PM, et al.: Outcomes of the Chrisman-Snook and modified Bröstrom procedures for chronic lateral ankle instability: a prospective, randomized comparison. *Am J Sports Med* 24: 400–404, 1996.
11. Karlsson J, Eriksson BI, Bergsten T, et al.: Comparison of two anatomic reconstructives for chronic lateral instability of the ankle joint. *Am J Sports Med* 25:48–53, 1997.
12. Kleiger B: Mechanisms of ankle injury. *Orthop Clin North Am* 5:127–146, 1974.

# 34

# Fibular Derotational and Lengthening Osteotomy

Lex A. Simpson, Timothy J. Bray, and Bernhardt Weber

## INDICATIONS/CONTRAINDICATIONS

Concepts of posttraumatic ankle malalignment have changed dramatically in the last 20 years, with the anatomic repositioning of the fibula assuming a vital role. Comminuted Weber type B and C fibular fractures challenge fixation methods, especially with involvement of the interosseous membrane. Late complications of fibular shortening and malrotation can be avoided by anatomic reduction and rigid fixation of the comminuted fractures in the initial surgical intervention (Figs. 34-1 and 34-2). Surgical techniques to regain anatomic length in the initial surgical fixation are well described. These techniques involve preservation of the soft tissue envelope and distraction methods of regaining fibular length.

Traumatic displacement of the talus is associated with displacement of the lateral malleolus, and malalignment of the ankle mortise is therefore characterized by distal fibular shortening, lateral shift, or malrotation. This is clinically relevant in that malalignment as contact pressures of the tibiotalar joint increase with lateral shift of the fibula. Models simulating fibular shortening, malrotation, and lateral shift with physiologic loads applied to the ankle show significant increases in contact pressure in the mid-lateral and posterolateral quadrants of the talar dome. Left untreated, the risk of pain and degenerative changes due to abnormal talar dome loading is significant. The goal of surgical correction of fibular malalignment is to restore this sensitive weight-bearing area to normal anatomic relationships.

Abnormalities of talar position within the ankle mortise are typically visible on plain film radiographs. Using the involved ankle radiographs, the surgeon can measure widening of

L. A. Simpson, M.D.: Department of Orthopaedic Surgery, Cleveland Clinic Florida, Weston, Florida.

T. J. Bray, M.D.: University of California-Davis Medical Center, Sacramento, California; and Reno Orthopaedic Clinic, Reno, Nevada.

B. Weber, M.D.: Department of Orthopaedic Surgery, University of Bern, Bern; and Department of Orthopedic Surgery, Orthopedics at Rosenberg, St. Gallen, Switzerland.

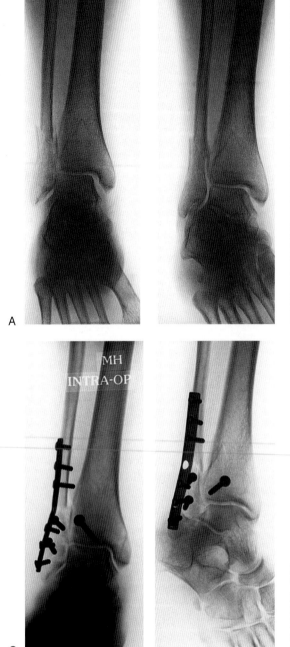

**Figure 34-1** Comminuted and shortened acute Weber type B fibular fracture in anteroposterior and mortise views **(A)** and lateral view **(B)**. Fibular length and rotation are regained with lag screws and a lateral plate. Postsurgical radiographs confirm the anatomic joint mortise **(C)**.

the medial joint space, talar tilt, and fibular shortening compared with the opposite, normal ankle radiographs. Because rotational malalignment of the distal fibula is more difficult to visualize, rotation can be assessed with computed tomography (CT) scanning with three-dimensional reconstruction. With an absence of metal implants at the joint, magnetic resonance imaging (MRI) offers the added advantage of joint cartilage assessment. This may be helpful when discussing surgical outcomes during preoperative planning.

Assuming that ankle malalignment has been well-defined and that pain and disability are present or anticipated, the next major issue is the degree of degenerative joint disease. If only mild to moderate, the physician can proceed with realignment based on the experience that symptoms will often improve and the progression of posttraumatic arthritis can be

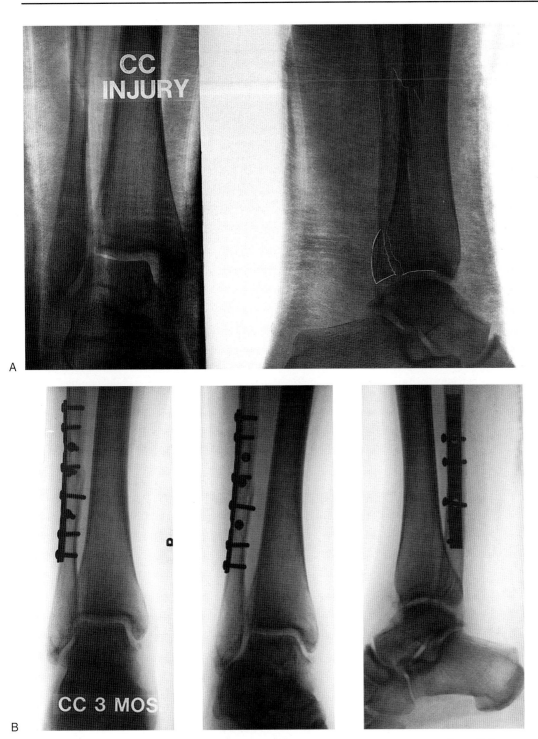

**Figure 34-2. A:** Comminuted Weber C fibular fracture with shortening and medial mortise widening. **B:** After open reduction and internal fixation, fibula length is regained, and the syndesmosis integrity is confirmed in anteroposterior, mortise, and lateral views. Notice that the fibula healed with anatomic length and rotation.

slowed or stopped. In the absence of advanced arthritis, experience indicates that the interval from the original injury to the date of realignment is not a significant factor in the eventual outcome. If, however, degenerative change is advanced, the surgeon should plan and surgically execute a well-aligned ankle arthrodesis.

The involved extremity is assessed for acceptable vascularity and soft tissue viability. Infection is always possible and must be excluded with appropriate testing. Neuropathic joints caused by diabetes mellitus or other neurologic disorders are contraindications to this technique. The physician must ensure that the patient is of appropriate age, in reasonably good health, and understands that complete relief of symptoms may not ensue. The surgeon should explain the possible need for subsequent procedures, such as ankle arthrodesis, to treat symptoms not resolved by the initial operation.

## PREOPERATIVE PLANNING

Preoperative planning begins with the history and physical examination, attempting to confirm the ankle as the source of symptoms and eliminating other causes of lower extremity pain. Pain and tenderness should be localized to a specific area and correlated, if possible, to documented areas of malalignment. The examiner records the pain level, gait, activity restrictions, and range of motion of the ankle and subtalar joints. The same evaluation technique is used in the late follow-up period to assess the overall results and presence or absence of late degenerative change. Several foot and ankle functional scoring systems are available for quantitating the results.

The surgeon scrutinizes plain film radiographs, including anteroposterior, lateral, and mortise (internally rotated 20°) views of involved and uninvolved ankles. The mortise view demonstrates at least four characteristics to compare between the normal and involved ankle. The first characteristic is an equidistant and parallel joint space with no medial widening. Lateral displacement of the talus within the mortise due to fibular shortening or medial tissue interposition is noted. Any increase in medial widening, even subtle, compared with the joint space laterally is considered abnormal (Fig. 34-3). The second characteristic demonstrates a *Shenton's line of the ankle*. The dense subchondral supporting bone of the tibia creates a radiographic line that can be followed over the syndesmotic space to the fibula, where a small spike points to the tibial subchondral bone (Fig. 34-4). The third char-

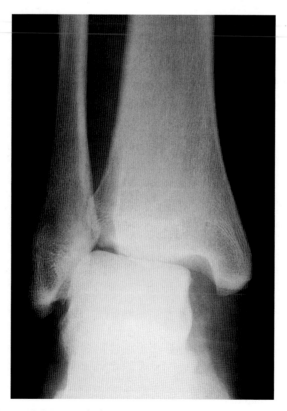

**Figure 34-3.** Medial joint space widening is associated with lateral shift of the talus.

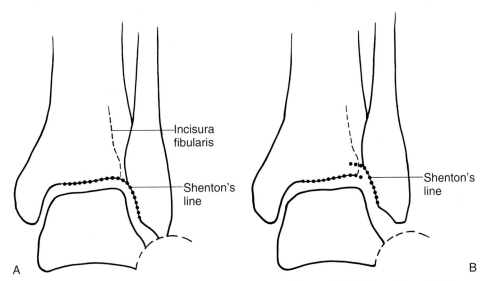

**Figure 34-4.** **A:** In a mortise view, Shenton's line of the ankle is the subchondral bone contour of the tibial plafond and fibula, which should be a curved, unbroken line *(dotted line)* in the intact ankle. **B:** The fibula is shortened, with a broken Shenton's line and broken curve representing the lateral process of the talus and distal fibular recess.

acteristic is an unbroken curve between the lateral part of the articular surface of the talus and the distal fibular recess (Fig. 34-4). The fourth characteristic is talar tilt. This is measured by lines drawn along the dome surface of the talus and the tibial plafond. In neutral stress with the ankle at 90°, these lines should be parallel or within 3° of parallel (Fig. 34-5).

The surgeon should look for evidence of abnormal seating of the fibula in the incisura fibularis of the tibia representing the tibiofibular or syndesmotic interval (Fig. 34-4). Two parameters involving this tibiofibular interval are diminished overlap of the distal fibula and anterior tibial tubercle and an increase in the tibiofibular clear space. Of these, the latter appears to be more reliable, with the normal width being less than 6 mm as measured 1 cm above the plafond (Fig. 34-6). Because the clear space represents the posterior aspect of the tibiofibular interval, its width can also vary with rotational deformity of the fibula. Internal fibular rotation, for instance, may contribute to an increase in this distance, and ex-

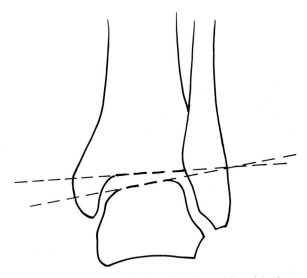

**Figure 34-5.** Abnormal talar tilt *(dotted lines)* is shown. Lines should be parallel or within 3° of parallel.

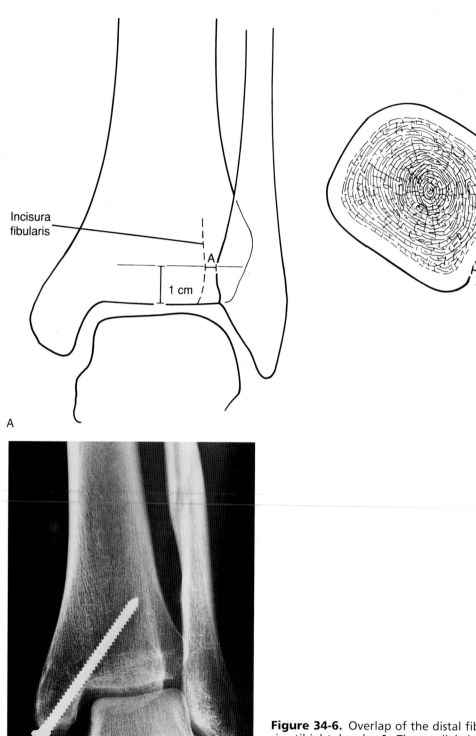

A

B

**Figure 34-6.** Overlap of the distal fibula and anterior tibial tubercle. **A:** The medial clear space measured 1 cm above the plafond is the distance between the medial margin of the distal fibula and incisura fibularis (A, A$_1$). **B:** Radiograph shows the widened medial clear space.

ternal fibular rotation is possible in association with this interval appearing normal or diminished.

Although plain film radiographs usually provide useful information about the nature of the malunion, the definitive study is the CT scan or MRI, or both. Axial cuts across the tibiofibular interval and ankle mortise with comparison views of the normal ankle can accurately determine the amount of talar shift as well as the position of the fibula relative to

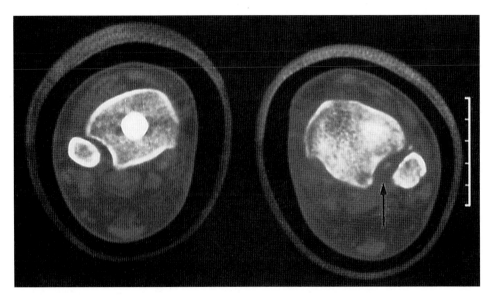

**Figure 34-7.** CT scan of the lower legs of an individual after open reduction and internal fixation of a pronation–external rotation ankle fracture on the left. Axial cuts across the distal tibiofibular interval reveal residual lateral translation and internal rotation of the distal fibula, which is indicated by more widening of the tibiofibular interval posteriorly *(arrow)* than anteriorly.

the tibia. Malrotation of the fibula with internal and external rotation being encountered can be assessed by noting the width of the tibiofibular interval at the anterior and posterior aspects of the syndesmosis. External rotation of the relatively oval fibula manifests as asymmetric widening anteriorly and as versus internal rotation, which appears as asymmetric widening posteriorly (Fig. 34-7). Sagittal or coronal cuts can help to determine the size and position of posterior malleolar fragments. Three-dimensional reconstructions help to visualize the correct surgical plan preoperatively.

## SURGERY

The patient is positioned supine, with support beneath the buttock or in a half-lateral position if a posterolateral dissection is anticipated to correct a posterior malleolar malunion (Fig. 34-8). The ipsilateral anterior iliac crest is also prepped and draped. Under tourniquet control, the distal fibula is exposed subperiosteally through a lateral longitudinal approach (Fig. 34-9).

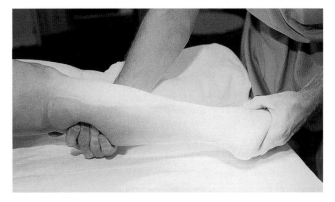

**Figure 34-8.** Patient positioning for the lateral approach.

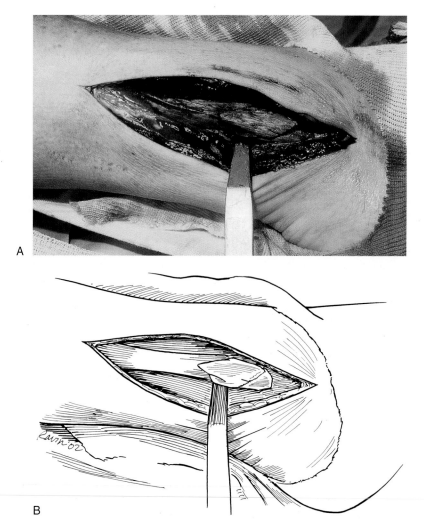

**Figure 34-9. A:** Operative approach to the lateral ankle with dissection through an incision long enough distally to expose ankle joint and of sufficient length proximally for distractor positioning. Notice the displaced fracture. **B:** Diagram of the lateral approach.

## Technique

The incision can be shifted anteriorly or posteriorly to expose pertinent abnormalities, such as fractures of the anterior tibial tubercle or posterior malleolus. Usually, the fibula is malpositioned in the incisura fibularis of the tibia with some degree of widening of the syndesmosis. It is imperative to remove all interposed scar in this area to obtain and maintain a good reduction. When there has been a proximal fibula fracture with little displacement, such as a Maisonneuve injury, or a diastasis without fracture, the surgeon may expose the syndesmosis anteriorly, progressively removing scar from anterior to posterior throughout the length of the syndesmotic interval.

In cases of distal fibula fracture with displacement and shortening, a fibular osteotomy is necessary. This may be done in an oblique fashion through the fracture site, but this approach will only gain 3 to 5 mm of lengthening. This technique is reserved for the most minor deformities.

Transverse osteotomy in the distal one third of the fibula supplemented with iliac bone graft is able to restore the original fibular length in virtually all cases. Before lengthening of the distal fibula, the surgeon removes any obstruction medially between the talus and the tibia so that the talus may be restored to its original position. Resection of scar tissue, osteotomy, or osteosynthesis of the malleolus may be required (Fig. 34-10). An anteromedial

arthrotomy is used to completely debride scar, including a portion of the deep deltoid ligament if necessary. If a malunion or nonunion of the medial malleolus exists, it is taken down
and correctly positioned and stabilized with cancellous screws or Kirschner wires with tension band fixation. A small, cancellous bone graft is used if indicated for any significant osseous defect. Stabilizing the medial fragment before reduction and stabilization of the fibula
may be advantageous in terms of defining a buttress against which the talus may be reduced.
If malalignment of the medial malleolar fragment is not obvious, it may be better to initially
reduce and stabilize the fibula, realizing that the common error is to not adequately seat the
fibula in the incisura fibularis and not adequately reduce the talus from a position of lateral
shift and tilt. If the incisura fibularis has been well debrided and correct fibula position and
length have been regained, the talus should be correctly positioned beneath the plafond and
can then be used as a buttress against which to reduce the medial malleolar fragment.

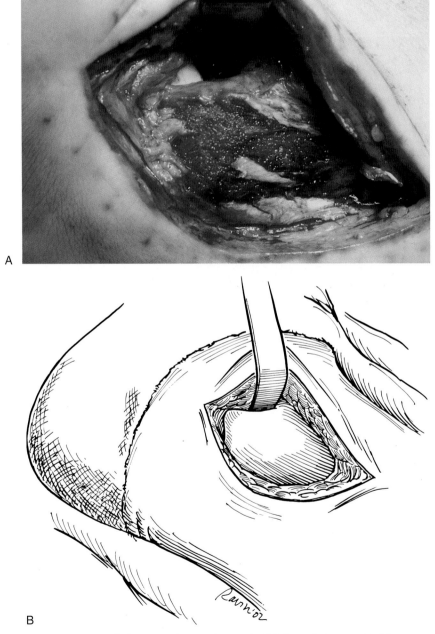

A

B

**Figure 34-10.  A:** Medial approach to a clear talotibial medial space. **B:** Diagram of the
medial approach to the ankle.

The distal fibula is exposed with an incision long enough to accommodate the ankle orthosis (AO) tensioning device. Keep in mind that osteotomy or exposure of the middle and distal one third of the fibula must avoid the peroneal artery and the superficial peroneal nerve. The superficial peroneal nerve remains anterior to the lateral fibula, and it then moves anterolaterally into the dorsum of the foot. The peroneal artery is adjacent to the medial border of the fibula until it courses anteriorly, away from the danger zone.

As a first step with the fibula, any interposed scar tissue in the area of the incisura fibularis is cleared. The syndesmosis is exposed anteriorly, and scar is progressively removed until the distal fibula is mobile around the joint area (Fig. 34-11). The goals in correction of fibular malunions are adequate seating of the fibula in the incisura fibularis, restoration of fibular length, and correction of fibular malrotation. These depend on adequate debridement of the syndesmosis, adequate mobilization of the distal fibula, and an appropriate preoperative analysis of the rotational status of the fibula. After the debridement and osteotomy have been accomplished, some method for applying forceful traction to the distal fibula with distraction at the osteotomy site is needed. With only mild shortening, manual traction through a bone clamp may be satisfactory. When greater length needs to be regained, a distraction

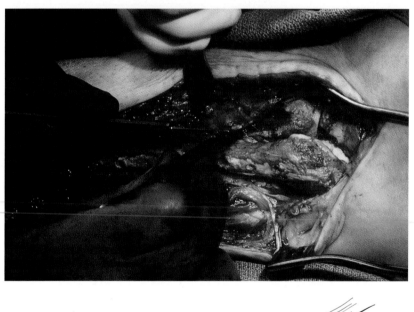

A

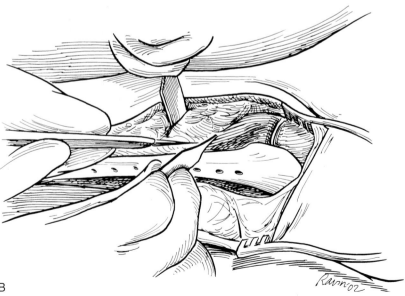

B

**Figure 34-11.** **A:** Surgical approach to a lateral syndesmosis and removal of scar tissue after fibular mobilization. **B:** Diagram of the lateral approach, allowing reduction of the talus within the medial mortise.

device is very helpful. The AO articulating tension device attached to bone at the end of a plate and reversed to a distraction mode has been the procedure of choice. Defining normal length intraoperatively may be difficult, and intraoperative radiographs with the distractor in place compared with preoperative planning is helpful. The more common error is to underestimate rather than overestimate the amount of lengthening necessary.

Rotational assessment of the distal fibula is done preoperatively with plain radiographs and CT. These images help to define rotational malalignment of the distal fibula. Most common is an external rotational malalignment of the distal fragment.

Assess the need for a bone graft in the fibular defect created in the preoperative plans. Small gaps (i.e., several millimeters) can be grafted with cancellous bone, whereas larger defects require a structural corticocancellous strut graft. Although small grafts may be harvested from the distal tibia, larger grafts are best obtained from the iliac crest. A narrow, 3.5-mm, five- or six-hole AO dynamic compression or 3.5-mm reconstruction plate is used. Before applying the plate to the fibula, the oscillating saw is used to create a small step-cut in the distal fibular lateral surface to allow the distal end of the plate to be more recessed into the bone and the length of the plate to lie smoothly against the fibular shaft. If the reconstruction plate is used, the step-cut is less. If the distal fragment is to be derotated from an externally rotated position, the plate is applied slightly posterior on the distal fragment to provide 10° to 15° of internal rotation of this fragment. Internal rotation of the distal fragment (rare) requires the plate to be applied distally slightly anterior. The plate is secured to the distal fibula with at least two screws through the last two holes of the plate (Fig. 34-12).

The AO articulating distraction-compression device is then applied proximally, with the hook engaged on the end of the plate and the device collapsed to its smallest size (Fig. 34-13). The osteotomy site is planned for the middle of the plate once distracted. The surgeon performs the osteotomy with an oscillating saw, using cooling irrigation to prevent thermal necrosis (Fig. 34-14). The articulating tool is lengthened until the distal fibula fits at the joint line. Plain radiographs or fluoroscopic images are checked to confirm the correct length and complete restoration of joint space (Fig. 34-15). Corticocancellous graft is excised from the iliac crest and shaped until it is 1 mm longer than the measured gap of the

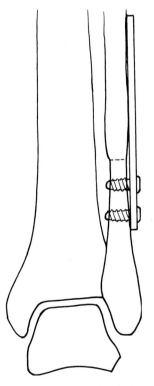

**Figure 34-12.** The plate is applied distally before osteotomy.

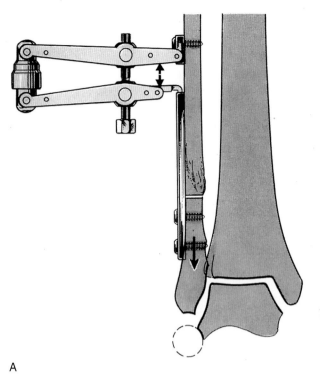

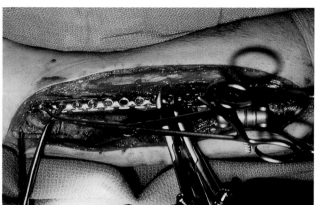

**Figure 34-13. A:** A distraction hook is in place for lengthening. **B:** The intraoperative photograph shows distraction.

A

B

**Figure 34-14.** Interval space after lengthening.

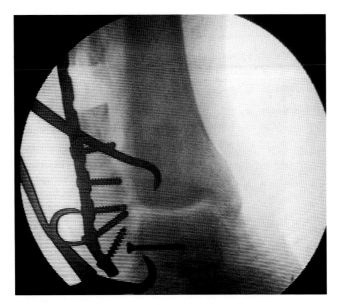

**Figure 34-15.** An intraoperative image is obtained to confirm reduction.

lengthened fibula. The gap is distracted another 1 to 2 mm, until the graft interposes easily (Fig. 34-16), and the distractor is reversed to a compression mode to apply compression to the end of the green scale (Fig. 34-16). The remaining screws are inserted to complete the fixation, allowing distractor-compressor removal.

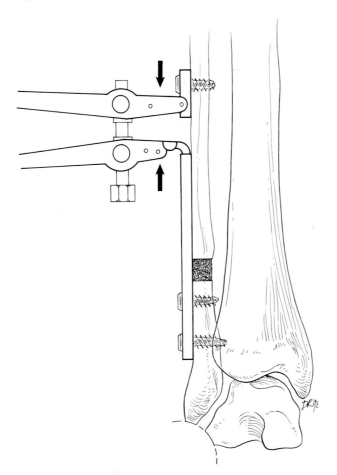

**Figure 34-16.** The iliac graft is placed, the distractor hook is switched, and compression is applied.

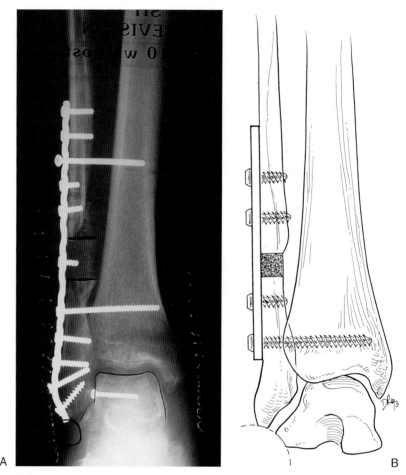

**Figure 34-17. A:** Syndesmosis is stabilized with screws. **B:** The diagram shows completed fixation.

When a significant portion of the syndesmotic ligament has been disrupted and this interval debrided of scar, a transsyndesmotic screw is indicated, placed through or adjacent to the plate (Fig. 34-17). One or two, 3.5-mm cortical screws are used through or proximal to the plate. By penetrating the medial tibial cortex, the screws have stronger fixation, and if breakage occurs, medial retrieval is simplified. Ideally, this should be a position screw placed in a nonlagged fashion. Occasionally, a lag effect with overdrilling of the fibula is necessary to make the fibula seat well in the incisura fibularis and reposition the talus well beneath the tibial plafond. If compression is used across the syndesmosis, the ankle should be held in neutral flexion while the screw is tightened to avoid excessive narrowing and loss of ankle motion. No repair of the syndesmotic or deltoid ligaments is necessary, because both heal well with correct repositioning of the talus and stabilization of the syndesmosis. In cases of severe instability of the interosseous membrane, 4.5-mm cortical screws may be used proximal to the plate.

The subcutaneous tissue and skin are closed with interrupted sutures. Use of a small suction drain is advisable if there is excessive bleeding at the time of surgery. A compressive dressing with plaster splint immobilization is advisable, with the ankle maintained at a neutral 90° position.

## POSTOPERATIVE MANAGEMENT

Postoperative therapy consists of 7 to 10 days in the 90° plaster splint, followed by suture removal. Further postoperative care is somewhat discretionary and depends on the reliability of the patient and the stability of the fixation. Early motion is generally advantageous, using a removable boot and crutch-assisted partial weight bearing for 8 weeks. Patients should expect to be using crutches at least 2 months and to have significant bone graft donor pain for 2 weeks. If patient reliability is a concern, splint initially with therapy supervised range of motion followed by partial weight bearing casting for 6 to 8 weeks. A removable fracture brace may be helpful thereafter, especially if significant bone grafting has been

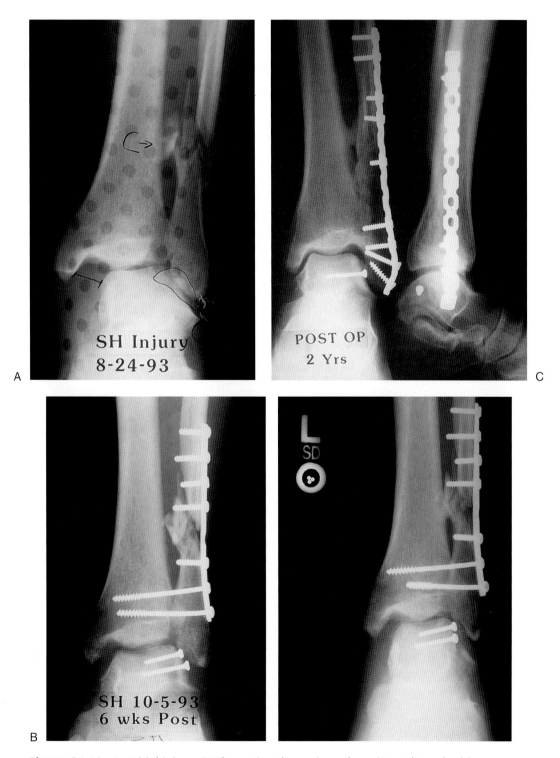

**Figure 34-18.  A:** Initial injury. **B:** The patient has pain and persistent lateral subluxation with shortening. **C:** Fibular lengthening with restoration of the joint 2 years after revision surgery.

necessary. Early, partial weight bearing is encouraged to help prevent bone loss. Transsyndesmotic four cortical screws are left in place for at least 10 to 12 weeks. Screw removal can then be accomplished at any time. Rehabilitation involves a standard physical therapy regimen for ankle and hindfoot motion plus lower extremity strengthening.

A review of published results indicates that approximately 75% of patients undergoing realignment of an ankle malunion will obtain a good or satisfactory result. This appears to be valid despite the length of time from injury to realignment or the age of the patient, assuming that advanced posttraumatic arthritis is not present (Fig. 34-18). There is evidence that the progression of mild to moderate arthritis may be slowed or stopped and ankle function often improved. Patients with severe arthritis and loss of motion should be counseled about the advisability of an ankle arthrodesis.

## COMPLICATIONS

Complications of this procedure include *nonunion* of the osteotomy site in the fibula. This can be prevented by using bone graft from the iliac crest and having the surfaces of the bone graft tightly opposed to the patient's own well-vascularized fibula. *Loss of initial bone position* may occur as a result of inadequate fixation of the syndesmosis. Placement of the screws through the fibula as described should prevent this complication. *Failure of anatomic reduction* of the talus under the tibial plafond may be the result of an inadequate debridement of the medial joint space or the syndesmosis. Inadequate lengthening of the fibula allows persistent lateral displacement of the talus on the tibial plafond.

## RECOMMENDED READING

1. Bray TJ, ed: *Techniques in fracture fixation*, 1st ed. New York: Gower Medical Publishing, 1993.
2. Brunner CF, Weber BG: *Special techniques in internal fixation*. Berlin: Springer-Verlag, 1982.
3. Marti RK, Raaymakers EL, Nolte PA: Malunited ankle fractures: the late results of reconstruction. *J Bone Joint Surg Br* 72:709–713, 1990.
4. Mast J, Jakob R, Ganz R: *Planning and reduction techniques in fracture surgery*. Berlin: Springer-Verlag, 1989.
5. Offierski CM, Graham JD, Hall JH, et al.: Late revision of fibular malunion in ankle fractures. *Clin Orthop* 171:145–149, 1982.
6. Rupp RE, Podeszwa D, Ebraheim NA: Danger zones associated with fibular osteotomy. *J Orthop Trauma* 8:54–58, 1994.
7. Thordarson DB, Motamed S, Hedman T, et al.: The effect of fibular malreduction on contact pressures in an ankle fracture malunion model. *J Bone Joint Surg Am* 79:1809–1815, 1997.
8. Ward AJ, Ackroyd CE, Baker AS: Late lengthening of the fibula for malaligned ankle fractures. *J Bone Joint Surg Br* 72:714–717, 1990.
9. Weber BG, Simpson LA: Corrective lengthening osteotomy of the fibula. *Clin Orthop* 199:61–67, 1985.
10. Yablon IG, Leach RE: Reconstruction of malunited fractures of the lateral malleolus. *J Bone Joint Surg Am* 71:521–527, 1989.

# 35

# Arthroscopic Treatment of Osteophytes and Osteochondral Lesions of the Talus

James W. Stone

## ARTHROSCOPIC TREATMENT OF ANKLE OSTEOPHYTES

### INDICATIONS/CONTRAINDICATIONS

Osteophytes occur most commonly at the anterior margin of the tibia and form as a result of degenerative arthritis in the ankle or after trauma. They appear on plain radiographs as a beaklike prominence on the anterior tibia and may be accompanied by an adjacent talar neck lesion, known as a kissing lesion, which may physically impinge on the anterior tibial osteophyte in ankle dorsiflexion. Less commonly, osteophytes may form at the medial malleolus or lateral malleolus. Posterior tibial osteophytes are least common and tend to cause greatest symptoms in the plantarflexed ankle.

The main indication for osteophyte excision is pain attributable to the presence of this lesion, in the absence of other causes of ankle pain such as severe degenerative arthritis. Patients may complain of limitation of range of motion of the ankle joint, which is particularly noticeable during stair climbing or squatting, and surgical excision of the osteophyte may allow improved ankle dorsiflexion. However, recovery of motion is not as predictable as diminution of pain after osteophyte excision. A contraindication is significant ankle degenerative arthritis affecting most or all of the joint. In this case, osteophyte excision will predictably fail.

### PREOPERATIVE PLANNING

A comprehensive history and physical examination must be performed for any patient with ankle pain and the presence of an osteophyte to determine whether the osteophyte itself is

J. W. Stone, M.D.: Department of Orthopaedic Surgery, Medical College of Wisconsin, Milwaukee, Wisconsin.

responsible for the symptoms or if other abnormalities of the joint must be addressed. Careful evaluation must be performed to differentiate anterior ankle pain arising from a primary ankle joint problem or from a subtalar joint condition.

Patients complain of pain localized over the osteophyte that usually worsens during activities such as stair or hill climbing, squatting, or running. Occasionally, patients complain of instability or giving way of the joint but do not have objective evidence of ligament laxity.

Physical examination must include evaluation of range of motion, stability, localized swelling, and tenderness over the area of the osteophyte. Passive forced dorsiflexion usually causes increased discomfort in patients with symptomatic anterior tibial osteophytes. Patients may have limited ankle dorsiflexion compared with the normal contralateral ankle. There should be no clinical evidence of joint laxity.

Radiographic evaluation should include routine anteroposterior, lateral, and mortise views. Van Dijk (5) observed that most anterior tibial osteophytes occur asymmetrically on the anterior aspect of the tibia, more on the medial compared with the lateral side. He found that routine lateral radiographs tend to underestimate the size of the osteophyte and suggested a modified radiographic technique to better visualize these lesions (Fig. 35-1). Lateral dorsiflexion stress radiographs may demonstrate impingement of the anterior tibial and talar neck osteophytes.

Scranton and McDermott (4) developed a classification of anterior tibiotalar spurs based on the size of the tibial spur, the presence or absence of a talar spur, and the presence of generalized degenerative changes within the ankle joint. In type 1, there is synovial impingement, the tibial spur measures less than 3 mm, and there is no talar spur. In type 2, there are osteochondral reaction exostoses, a tibial spur larger that 3 mm, and no associated talar spur. In type 3, there is significant exostosis with tibial and talar spurs. In type 4, there is pantalocrural impingement, and degenerative changes in the ankle joint are present.

The lateral radiograph may be used as a guide to the amount of osteophyte that should be resected surgically (Fig. 35-2). The lateral radiograph is taken with the ankle in neutral position and the angle between the anterior edge of the tibia and the talar neck is determined. This angle should be at least 60° in the normal ankle. The angle decreases to less than 60° with anterior tibial and talar neck osteophytes. Any bony osteophyte projecting anterior to a 60° angle on the lateral radiograph should be resected surgically.

A bone scan may be helpful in excluding other potential causes of ankle pain, such as an osteochondral lesion of the talus or tibia, and usually shows increased uptake over the area of a symptomatic osteophyte. A computed tomography (CT) scan is usually unnecessary to

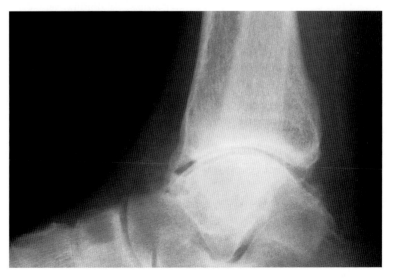

**Figure 35-1.** Lateral radiograph shows a large, anterior tibial osteophyte with a smaller, adjacent talar neck osteophyte (i.e., kissing lesion).

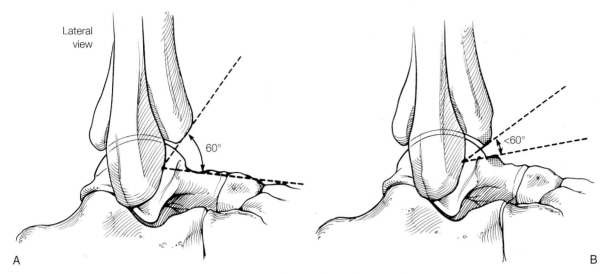

**Figure 35-2.** Artist's depiction of a lateral view of the ankle, showing the normal angle between distal tibia and talar neck as 60° or greater (**A**). The presence of an anterior osteophyte restricts access to the ankle joint with an arthroscope, because the angle is less than 60° (**B**). An intraoperative lateral radiograph can assist the surgeon in determining whether sufficient osteophyte has been removed in restoring this angle to normal. (From Stone JW, Guhl JF, Ferkel RD: Osteophytes, loose bodies, and chondral lesions of the ankle. In: Ferkel RD, ed. *Arthroscopic surgery: the foot and ankle.* Philadelphia: Lippincott-Raven, 1996:175.)

evaluate these lesions but can be useful for precise localization of a spur if required preoperatively or if there is a concern about other pathology. If used, the CT scan should include primary axial and coronal views, along with sagittal reconstruction views. Magnetic resonance imaging (MRI) is not used for preoperative evaluation unless it is for investigating associated chondral or soft tissue pathology.

## SURGERY

Although anterior tibial osteophytes may be removed using open techniques, arthroscopic surgery has largely supplanted open surgery because it may be performed on an outpatient basis with minimal morbidity, while affording a more complete view of the joint than with open surgery. General anesthesia, spinal anesthesia, or a local block may be used. The patient is positioned supine on the operating table, with the ipsilateral hip and knee flexed and supported by a well-padded leg holder beneath the knee. This position allows the leg to hang free with the foot and ankle in a plantigrade position, allowing access to the anterior and posterior ankle for portal placement (Fig. 35-3).

After skin preparation, sterile drapes are applied. A noninvasive ankle distractor strap is applied to the foot and connected to a sterile bar attached to the operating table using a Velcro strap. Appropriate tension is "dialed in" with the Velcro strap that is then fixed to itself. The distraction technique allows better visualization of the ankle joint than that obtained without distraction, and the ankle may be manipulated into any position of dorsiflexion or plantarflexion intraoperatively. Invasive joint distraction using pins placed into the tibia and the talus or calcaneus was used in the past. However, it does not achieve a greater degree of distraction than that obtained with noninvasive devices, is associated with significant potential morbidity, and is no longer recommended.

Anatomic landmarks are marked using a sterile marking pen. The medial malleolus, anterior tibial margin, fibula, tibialis anterior tendon, peroneus brevis tendon, and Achilles tendon are outlined. The course of the superficial peroneal nerve can frequently be identified in its subcutaneous position with plantarflexion and inversion of the ankle. Its position should be marked with a pen to avoid injury to this sensory nerve.

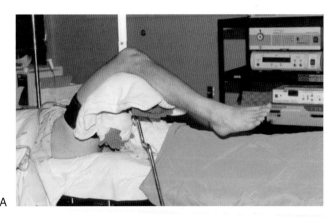

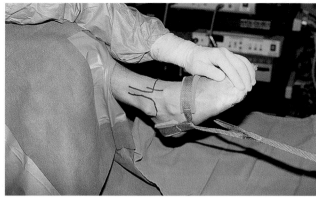

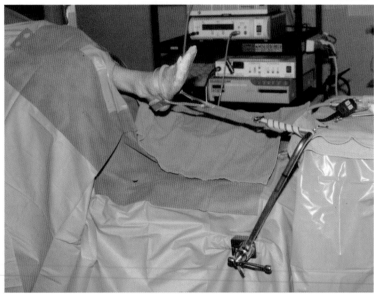

**Figure 35-3.** Noninvasive distraction technique. **A:** View of the lower extremity before prepping and draping. **B:** View after the extremity is draped. **C:** Intraoperative photograph of a patient who is prepped and draped and has the noninvasive strap distractor applied.

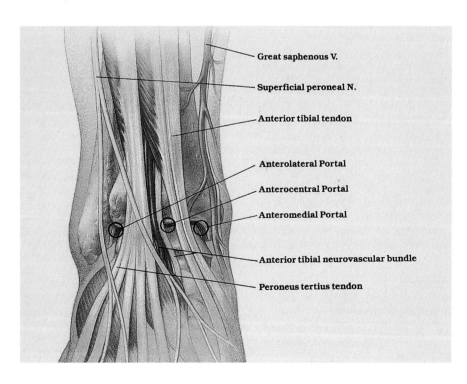

Great saphenous V.

Superficial peroneal N.

Anterior tibial tendon

Anterolateral Portal

Anterocentral Portal

Anteromedial Portal

Anterior tibial neurovascular bundle

Peroneus tertius tendon

**Figure 35-4.** Anatomic drawing shows the locations for the antero-medial and anterolateral arthroscopic portals. (From Ferkel R, Poehling G, Andrews J: *An illustrated guide to small joint arthroplasty.* Andover, MA: Smith & Nephew, Inc., 1997:3.)

The anteromedial portal is created first (Fig. 35-4). It is located adjacent to the medial margin of the tibialis anterior tendon. An appropriate position for the portal is ensured by using an 18-guage needle for localization. The best position allows easy needle passage across the joint without impingement on the tibia or talus. A position too proximal results in instrument impingement on the talus, and a position too distal causes instrument impingement on the tibia. All portals are created in such a manner as to minimize risk of injury to superficial nerves. The skin alone is incised without advancing the scalpel blade into the subcutaneous tissues. The subcutaneous tissues are then bluntly dissected with a small hemostat down to the level of the joint capsule. A cannula with a blunt obturator is then used to penetrate the capsule. The ankle joint capsule is quite thin so a sharp obturator is not required. This technique minimizes the risk of iatrogenic articular cartilage injury during creation of portal.

The arthroscope is introduced into the anteromedial portal, and the anterolateral portal is created under direct visualization, again using an 18-gauge needle first to optimize portal location. The anterolateral portal is placed adjacent to the lateral border of the peroneus tertius tendon. Careful attention to portal creation technique can avoid injury to branches of the superficial peroneal nerve.

The posterolateral portal is then placed under direct visualization (Fig. 35-5). An 18-gauge needle is placed at the lateral margin of the Achilles tendon approximately 1 to 2 cm distal to the level of the anterior portals. This more distal position accommodates the convexity of the talar articular surface. While viewing arthroscopically, the needle is observed to enter the joint just beneath the posterior syndesmotic ligament. The cannula is used for dedicated inflow.

Some surgeons recommend use of the anterior portals without the posterolateral portal. However, more efficient inflow can be obtained using a dedicated posterior portal. All surgeons performing arthroscopic ankle surgery should be comfortable using a posterolateral portal, because this approach is advantageous in approaching other posterior pathology, including osteochondral talar dome lesions, posterior osteophytes, or removal of posterior loose bodies.

A comprehensive joint examination is then performed first from the anteromedial approach and then from the anterolateral approach to rule out other intraarticular pathology. Initial visualization may be difficult secondary to the presence of anterior joint synovitis.

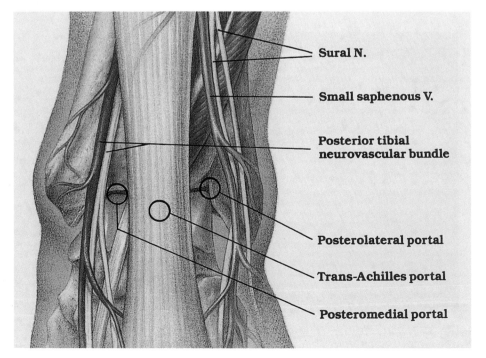

- Sural N.

- Small saphenous V.

Posterior tibial
neurovascular bundle

Posterolateral portal

Trans-Achilles portal

Posteromedial portal

**Figure 35-5.** Anatomic drawing depicts the location of the posterolateral portal. (From Ferkel R, Poehling G, Andrews J: *An illustrated guide to small joint arthroplasty.* Andover, MA: Smith & Nephew, Inc., 1997:3.)

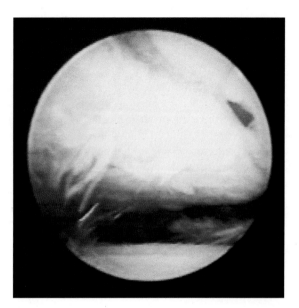

**Figure 35-6.** Arthroscopic view of an anterior tibial osteophyte.

The inflamed synovium is removed using a 2.9- or 3.5-mm shaver. Care must be exercised to avoid directing the shaver anteriorly, causing injury to the anterior neurovascular structures. Anterior joint visualization may be improved by dorsiflexing the ankle, a maneuver that causes the anterior capsule to relax and fill with irrigant fluid.

The extent of the osteophyte is then determined (Fig. 35-6). The anterior capsule is invariably adherent to the superior surface of the osteophyte and must be dissected free. This maneuver is most easily performed using the shaver with the blade directed against the osteophyte, lifting the adherent capsule off the osteophyte proximally.

The osteophyte may be resected using an osteotome or rongeur. An easier technique is to use a 4-mm round burr introduced from the anterolateral portal to remove the lateral portion of the osteophyte while viewing with the arthroscope in the anteromedial portal (Fig. 35-7). The portals are then switched to remove the medial half of the osteophyte. The preoperative radiographs should be studied to determine the extent of the proposed excision.

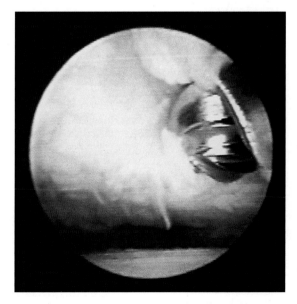

**Figure 35-7.** Intraoperative photograph of a round burr used to remove an anterior tibial osteophyte.

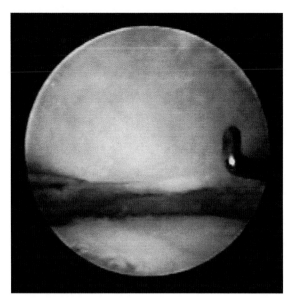

**Figure 35-8.** Intraoperative photograph of a fully resected anterior tibial osteophyte.

With experience, the surgeon is able to identify where abnormal bone constituting the osteophyte ends and the normal contour of the tibia begins (Fig. 35-8). An intraoperative lateral radiograph may assist the surgeon to determine that an adequate amount of osteophyte has been removed.

Care should be taken to examine the medial extent of any anterior tibial osteophyte. Osteophytes often extend onto the anterior surface of the medial malleolus and may cause symptomatic bony impingement with ankle dorsiflexion. After excision of the anterior osteophyte, the arthroscope is inserted into the anterolateral portal, and the anterior aspect of the medial malleolus is visualized. Resection of bone to the normal contour of the medial malleolus must be performed.

Occasionally, an osteophyte of the tip of the medial malleolus may be observed (Fig. 35-9). Such a spur can be removed by viewing with the arthroscope in the anteromedial portal

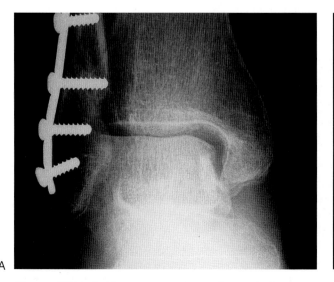
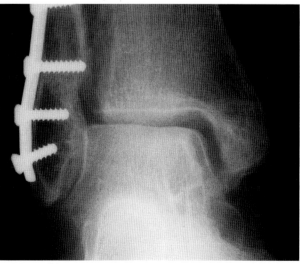

A                                                                                                          B

**Figure 35-9.  A:** The preoperative radiograph shows a posttraumatic medial malleolar osteophyte. **B:** The postoperative radiograph shows resection of the medial osteophyte.

and the instruments placed into an accessory anteromedial portal. The location for the accessory portal is determined by placing an 18-gauge needle approximately 1 to 2 cm medial and slightly distal to the standard portal and directing the needle into the medial gutter. Wound healing problems can be avoided by ensuring that the accessory portal is located at least 1 cm from the standard portal.

The less common posterior tibial osteophyte can be approached with the arthroscope in one of the routine anterior portals and the working instruments inserted into the posterolateral portal. A 70° viewing arthroscope may be helpful in visualizing this area.

## POSTOPERATIVE MANAGEMENT

After irrigating the joint thoroughly, the wounds are closed loosely using nylon suture, and a bulky compressive dressing and posterior plaster splint are applied with the ankle in neutral position. Five to 7 days postoperatively, the dressing is changed, and the sutures are removed. Weight bearing and range of motion exercises are encouraged. Exercises to increase strength and motion may be performed by the patient or with the assistance of a therapist.

Based on published reports and personal observation, most patients can expect to achieve an increase in ankle dorsiflexion of 5° to 10° after excision of a significant anterior tibial osteophyte. Pain relief is a predictable result in patients who do not have any significant co-existing degenerative arthritis in the ankle joint.

# ARTHROSCOPIC TREATMENT OF OSTEOCHONDRAL TALAR DOME LESIONS

## INDICATIONS/CONTRAINDICATIONS

Osteochondral lesions of the talar dome (e.g., osteochondritis dissecans, flake fracture of the talar dome) include abnormalities of articular cartilage and underlying subchondral bone that may cause fragment separation and loose body formation. The cause of the disorder is not fully understood, although trauma has been implicated in most clinical studies. The natural history of untreated osteochondral lesions of the talar dome is not well-defined, and therefore the indications for surgery are controversial.

In their seminal 1959 publication, Berndt and Harty (9) suggested that most osteochondral lesions of the talar dome are best treated surgically. Canale and Belding (10) refined the indications for surgery, suggesting that stage 1 and 2 lesions were best treated nonoperatively and that lateral stage 3 and all stage 4 lesions responded better to surgical treatment. Flick and Gould (11) found that symptomatic patients with radiographs suggesting partially or completely detached lesions did poorly with nonoperative treatment. They agreed with Alexander and Lichtman (6) that a delay in operative treatment resulting from a trial of nonoperative therapy does not adversely affect the result of later surgical treatment. Pettine and Morrey (12) agree that the surgeon should initially attempt to treat lesions of the talar dome with a period of immobilization and suggest that even nondisplaced medial stage 3 lesions have a significant chance of healing.

Indications for surgical intervention for osteochondral lesions of the talar dome include failure of nonoperative treatment for any stage lesion. Nonoperative treatment may include a period of immobilization and weight relief. Lesions that are asymptomatic or that become asymptomatic after nonoperative treatment, do not necessarily require surgical intervention even if radiographic studies fail to document complete healing.

Patients who present with loose fragments, as demonstrated on plain film radiographs, CT, or MRI, are candidates for surgical intervention. Acute talar dome fractures are most commonly seen on the anterolateral surface. If displaced, these lesions are most amenable to surgical treatment with reduction and fixation.

## PREOPERATIVE PLANNING

A patient with an osteochondral lesion of the talar dome may present for evaluation after an acute injury, but more commonly, the presentation is one of gradual onset of symptoms such as pain, catching, or giving way after one or more inversion ankle sprains. Although instability may be a prominent feature, objective evidence of ligament laxity on stress radiography is usually absent. Tenderness over the anterolateral joint line may be noted on physical examination for lateral lesions. Medial lesions may show less tenderness as they are blocked to direct palpation by the medial malleolus. Swelling may be present, along with limitation of range of motion when compared with the opposite ankle.

The evaluation of a patient with acute or chronic ankle pain begins with plain film radiographs. Anteroposterior, lateral, and mortise radiographs should be obtained (Fig. 35-10). Medial dome lesions may be more clearly seen on anteroposterior radiographs obtained with the ankle plantarflexed because of the more posterior location of the typical lesion. Lateral lesions may be more clearly defined on anteroposterior radiographs taken with the ankle in slight dorsiflexion.

Clinical studies have shown that the appearance of an osteochondral lesion of the talar dome on plain film radiographs correlates poorly with the actual appearance of the articular cartilage seen at arthroscopy. Attempts to classify these lesions using CT scan or MRI have been made to predict more accurately the condition of the articular cartilage and underlying bone so as to refine treatment guidelines.

Ferkel and Sgaglione developed a CT classification that reportedly correlates better with the arthroscopic appearance of these lesions than plain film radiographs (Fig. 35-11). Stage I lesions are cystic with an intact roof on all views. Stage IIA lesions show communication of the cystic lesion with the roof. Stage IIB lesions demonstrate an open articular surface lesion with an overlying nondisplaced fragment (Fig. 35-12). Stage III lesions are undisplaced with lucency beneath the entire fragment. Stage IV lesions are displaced fragments.

CT clearly defines the bony anatomy of the osteochondral lesion but does not evaluate the overlying articular cartilage. MRI possesses the advantages of multiplanar imaging without use of ionizing radiation and is able to visualize articular cartilage and the presence of fluid beneath the lesion (Fig. 35-13). However, it is inferior to CT in evaluating the bone. Anderson et al. (7) proposed a staging system using MRI, and they found that MRI was more sensitive in diagnosing the presence of a subtle talar dome lesion.

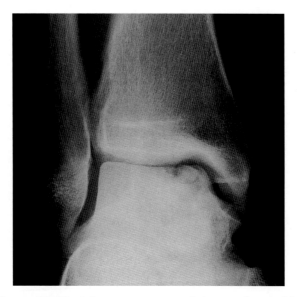

**Figure 35-10.** A large, posteromedial osteochondral lesion of the talar dome is seen on the radiograph.

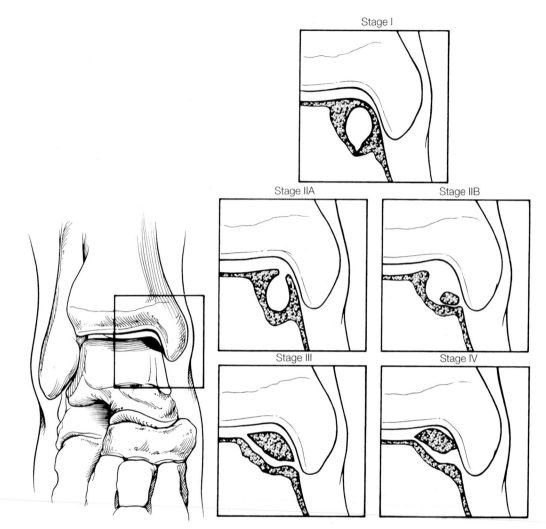

Stage I

Stage IIA          Stage IIB

Stage III          Stage IV

**Figure 35-11.** CT classification of osteochondral lesions of the talar dome. (From Ferkel RD: Osteochondral lesions of the talus. In: Ferkel RD, ed. *Arthroscopic surgery: the foot and ankle*. Philadelphia: Lippincott-Raven, 1996:151.)

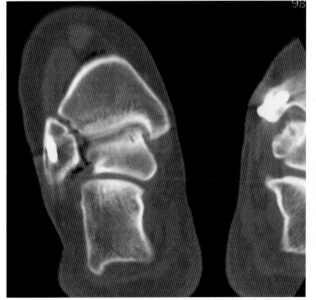

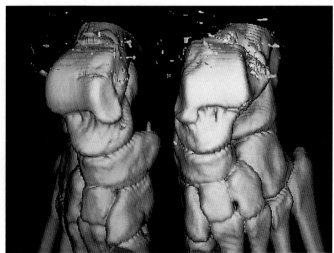

A                                                                                    B

**Figure 35-12.  A:** The CT scan shows a posteromedial talar dome lesion. **B:** The three-dimensional CT reconstruction shows bilateral posteromedial talar dome lesions.

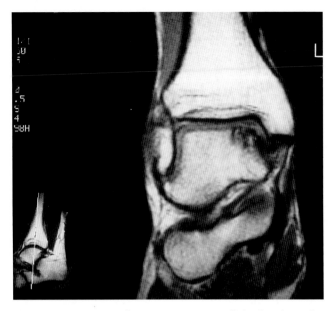

**Figure 35-13.** MRI shows a posteromedial talar dome lesion.

## SURGERY

Arthroscopic surgery for osteochondral lesions of the talar dome is performed under general or spinal anesthesia. The positioning is the same as that described for osteophyte excision, with noninvasive distraction and creation of the standard three portals.

A 2.7-mm-diameter, wide-angle arthroscope is used to examine the joint. Both 30°- and 70°-angle scopes should be available. A complete examination of the joint is performed from the medial and lateral portals, carefully observing and palpating the articular surface of the talus with a small probe. The osteochondral lesion is evaluated regarding the intactness of the articular surface, whether there is a loose bone fragment beneath the articular surface, and for the extent of the lesion over the talar dome (Fig. 35-14).

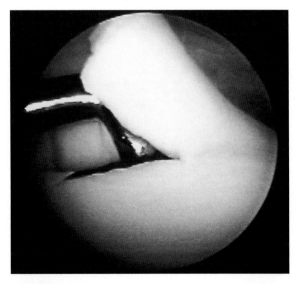

**Figure 35-14.** The intraoperative photograph shows examination of a talar dome lesion with a probe. In this case, the lesion is entirely cartilage, representing a delamination of the cartilage alone from the subchondral bone.

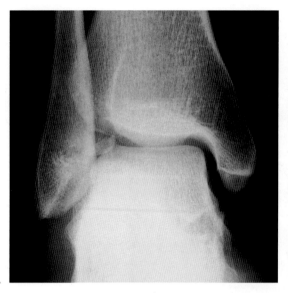
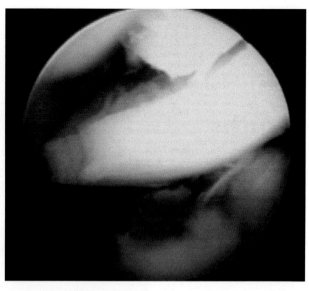

A                                                                                        B

**Figure 35-15. A:** The anteroposterior radiograph shows an acute osteochondral lesion of the anterolateral talar dome. Careful examination reveals that the fragment is flipped 180°, with the articular surface oriented downward toward the base of the lesion. **B:** An intraoperative photograph of same patient shows the inverted osteochondral lesion.

The choice of the surgical procedure for a given type of osteochondral defect is influenced by the chronicity of the lesion, the age of the patient, the quality of the articular cartilage, and the quality of the subchondral bone fragment. An acute lesion is most likely to be anterolateral in location, have a more substantial bone base, and is therefore more amenable to internal fixation (Fig. 35-15). In contrast, a chronic posteromedial lesion is more likely to have a fragmented, necrotic bone base with poor quality articular cartilage (Fig. 35-16). These lesions usually must be removed. Patients who have not reached skeletal maturity may present with intact appearing articular surface, and simple drilling of these

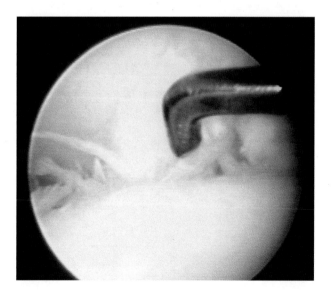

**Figure 35-16.** The intraoperative photograph shows a posteromedial talar osteochondral dome lesion with the overlying articular cartilage of poor quality and a necrotic bone fragment.

lesions to encourage healing may be attempted. There are no good quality clinical studies to document the chances of successful healing after simple drilling of intact lesions.

### Technique: Drilling of Intact Lesions

Intact lesions that show smooth articular cartilage and no loose bone fragment are rare but may be seen, especially in patients before skeletal maturity. Simple drilling of these lesions may be attempted to encourage healing. Anterolateral lesions are usually easily accessible from the anterolateral portal while viewing from the anteromedial portal. A smooth, 0.062-inch Kirschner wire is used to drill multiple holes into the talus to a depth of 1 to 1.5 cm. It is advantageous to place the pin in a guide cannula that minimizes risk of pin breakage and also sets the depth of penetration.

Posteromedial lesions are more difficult to reach. Rarely, the anteromedial portal can be used with the ankle in maximum plantarflexion to reach these lesions. Most, however, require another approach. Drilling across the medial malleolus into the lesion (i.e., transmalleolar approach) has been recommended in the past (Fig. 35-17). It provides an easy method to drill these lesions, especially when using a commercially available drill guide. However, use of this approach is not optimal because it compromises the integrity of the articular cartilage of the medial malleolus. An alternative approach is to drill the lesions from distal to proximal across the talus (i.e., the transtalar approach) (Fig. 35-18). A commercially available guide facilitates aiming a smooth wire that is introduced from the sinus tarsi into the talus while viewing the lesion arthroscopically. Multiple drill holes can be made using the guide system. The pin is advanced until the point where the articular cartilage is noted to vibrate, signaling impending penetration of the cartilage layer.

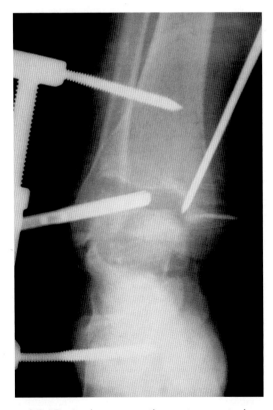

**Figure 35-17.** An intraoperative anteroposterior radiograph of the ankle shows invasive pin distraction applied to the ankle and transmalleolar drilling of a posteromedial lesion of the talar dome. This technique of invasive ankle distraction and transmalleolar drilling is no longer recommended.

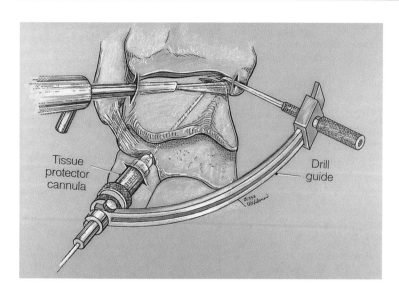

Tissue
protector
cannula

Drill
guide

**Figure 35-18.** Distal-to-proximal transtalar drilling technique. (From Stone JW, Gould JS: Chronic lateral ankle pain. In: Pfeffer GB, Frey CC, eds. *Current practice in foot and ankle surgery.* New York: McGraw-Hill Companies, 1993:1–29, reproduced with the permission of the McGraw-Hill Companies.)

### Technique: Debridement, Abrasion, and Drilling

Most osteochondral lesions of the talar dome are chronic at the time of presentation and on arthroscopic inspection are observed to have poor quality articular cartilage that is soft or flaking and an underlying bone fragment that is loose, fragmented, and necrotic. These lesions cannot be salvaged and must be removed.

The arthroscopic approach is the same as previously described, with routine use of anteromedial, anterolateral, and posterolateral portals. The 70° arthroscope is often useful for viewing posteromedial lesions, or the arthroscope may be inserted through the posterolateral portal while instruments are passed from anterior. A probe is usually sufficient to elevate the articular cartilage and underlying bone fragments, which can then be removed using a loose body forceps. A selection of angled cervical curettes must be available to completely debride the lesion to healthy bone that demonstrates bleeding when the inflow pressure is decreased. (Fig. 35-19) Care must be taken to remove all loose bone fragments. Failure to do so will result in persistent symptoms. Posteromedial lesions usually extend onto the vertical surface of the talus in the medial gutter and are not simple lesions on the weight-bearing surface of the dome. Adequate viewing and palpation of this surface of the talus must be performed to ensure complete removal.

If good bleeding of the cancellous bone bed is demonstrated after removal of the lesion and abrasion of the base using a curette or a round burr, further treatment of the bone base is unnecessary. If good bleeding is not demonstrated from the base, drilling multiple holes is performed using techniques as described earlier.

### Technique: Retrograde Bone Grafting

Some investigators have suggested bone grafting intact osteochondral lesions of the talar dome. To be considered for bone grafting, the lesion should demonstrate intact articular cartilage and be associated with a viable bone fragment or demonstrate only edema of the underlying cancellous bone rather than a distinct bone fragment. Unfortunately, this set of circumstances rarely exists, as most patients present with lesions that show degeneration of the surface cartilage and/or a discrete necrotic fragment of subchondral bone.

Bone grafting may be performed using a retrograde transtalar approach (Fig. 35-20). As in the approach for transtalar drilling, a guide pin is advanced from distal to proximal, starting in the sinus tarsi, and is directed to the posteromedial talar dome lesion. The pin is then overdrilled using a cannulated drill bit or trephine reamer to remove a core of bone. Bone graft is then advanced to a position beneath the lesion and tamped into position.

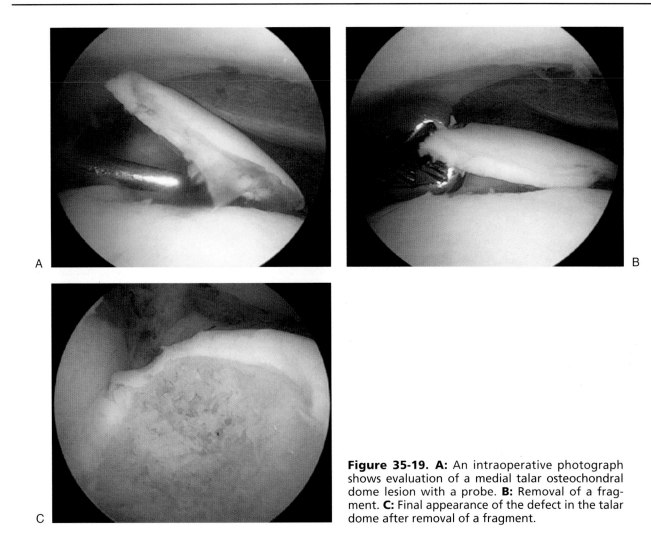

**Figure 35-19. A:** An intraoperative photograph shows evaluation of a medial talar osteochondral dome lesion with a probe. **B:** Removal of a fragment. **C:** Final appearance of the defect in the talar dome after removal of a fragment.

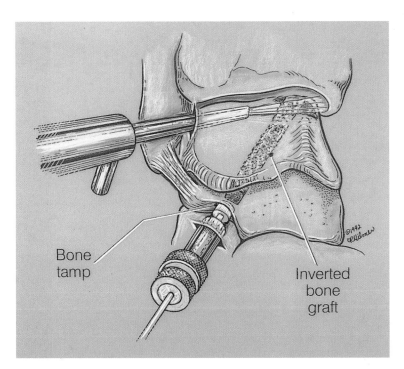

**Figure 35-20.** Artist's depiction of a retrograde bone grafting technique for a posteromedial talar dome lesion. (From Stone JW, Gould JS: Chronic lateral ankle pain. In: Pfeffer GB, Frey CC, eds. *Current practice in foot and ankle surgery.* New York: McGraw-Hill Companies, 1993:1–29, reproduced with the permission of the McGraw-Hill Companies.)

Postoperatively, the patient is not allowed to bear weight for 6 weeks, and then weight bearing is advanced as tolerated with routine postoperative physical therapy for range of motion and strengthening exercises.

### Technique: Osteochondral Grafting with Mosaicplasty and OATS Procedures

The newest method for reconstruction of osteochondral lesions of the talus involves transplantation of autogenous bone and articular cartilage into the defect (see Chapter 43). For

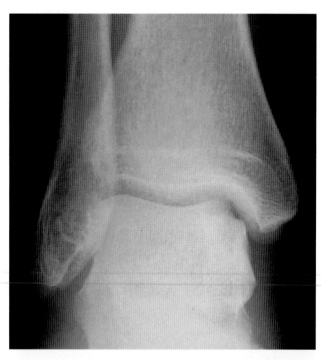

A

**Figure 35-21.** Osteoarticular transplantation for talar osteochondral lesion (i.e., OATS procedure) . **A:** The preoperative radiograph of the ankle shows a medial talar dome lesion. **B:** A longitudinal skin incision is marked for access to the dome of the talus through a medial malleolar osteotomy. **C:** The medial malleolus is exposed. Notice the placement of small Hohman retractors anteriorly and posteriorly, as well as a loose saw blade in the osteotomy. *(continued)*

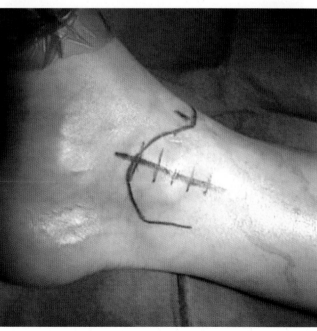

B

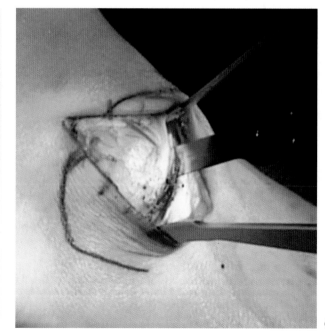

C

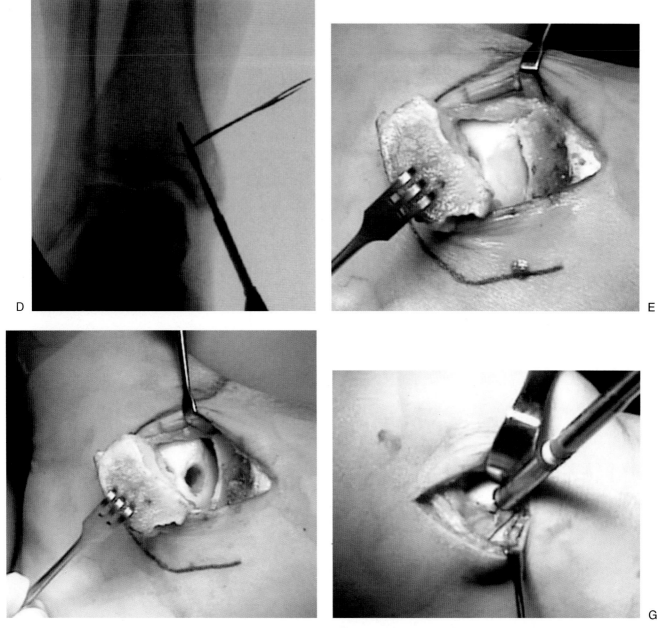

**Figure 35-21.** *Continued.* **D:** Intraoperative fluoroscopy shows a loose microsagittal saw blade marking the position and the angle of the malleolar osteotomy. Notice the drill bit indicating the location of one of the two drill holes placed for later fixation of the osteotomy. **E:** The initial view after medial malleolar osteotomy shows the talar dome lesion. **F:** The photograph shows the posteromedial talar recipient site after removal of diseased bone and cartilage. **G:** Harvesting graft from the ipsilateral knee. *(continued)*

the usual posteromedial lesion, the procedure must be performed using an open approach including osteotomy of the medial malleolus. The lesion is debrided to viable subchondral bone. A single plug of bone and articular cartilage is obtained from a donor site in the knee joint for the OATS procedure (Fig. 35-21), or multiple small plugs are harvested for a "mosaicplasty" reconstruction (Fig. 35-22). Specific instrumentation is commercially available for these procedures. The plug or plugs are placed, carefully reconstructing the normal con-

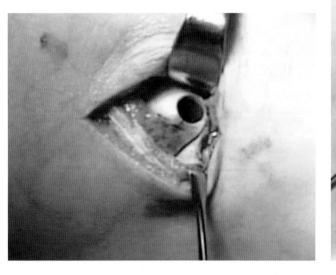

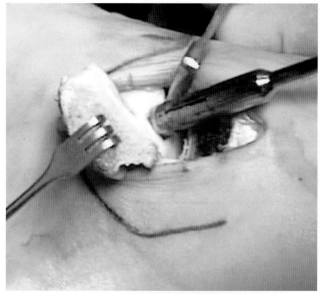

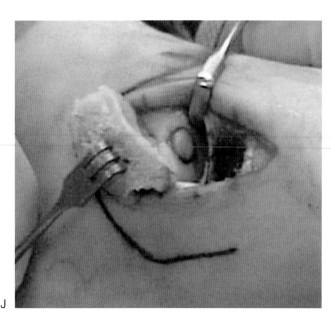

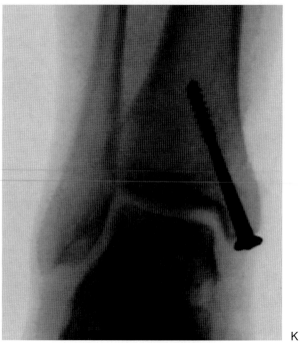

**Figure 35-21.** *Continued.* **H:** Knee donor site after removal of graft. **I:** Insertion of a single graft into the talar defect. **J:** The graft is in place, with the articular surface level compared with the adjacent, intact joint surface. The malleolar osteotomy is fixed with two compression screws, and the incision is closed. **K:** Postoperative anteroposterior ankle radiograph showing screw fixation of malleolar osteotomy.

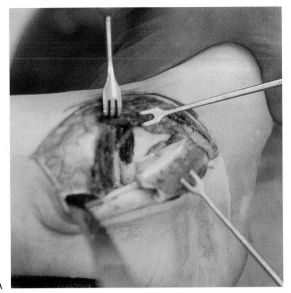
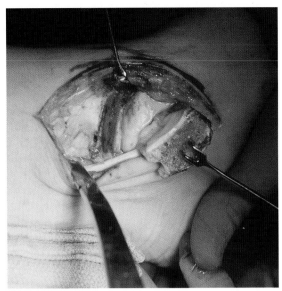

A

B

**Figure 35-22.** Osteoarticular transplantation for talar osteochondral lesion with multiple grafts (mosaicplasty). **A:** An intraoperative photograph shows a posteromedial talar dome lesion that is effectively exposed by medial malleolar osteotomy. **B:** An intraoperative photograph shows a reconstructed talar dome using multiple osteochondral plugs from the ipsilateral knee.

tour of the talar dome, and the malleolar osteotomy is fixed with screws. The patient does not bear weight for up to 12 weeks, although range of motion exercises may be initiated at 6 to 8 weeks postoperatively.

Some investigators consider the results of routine debridement procedures for posteromedial talar dome lesions to be so poor that they recommend this procedure for any sizable (1 to 1.5 cm diameter) lesion. However, the lack of studies with long-term follow-up dictates that this procedure be considered investigational in nature.

## POSTOPERATIVE MANAGEMENT

Patients who undergo drilling for intact lesions are not allowed to bear weight for 6 weeks, but range of motion exercises are begun at approximately 3 weeks postoperatively. Afterward, weight bearing is advanced as tolerated, and a progressive physical therapy program is initiated.

After debridement of an osteochondral lesion, no weight bearing is suggested for 3 to 6 weeks, depending on the size of the lesion, and weight bearing is then advanced as tolerated. After weight bearing has been initiated, passive and active range of motion exercises are instituted, followed by a proprioceptive and agility exercise program. Modalities such as ultrasound, iontophoresis, and phonophoresis may be used to diminish pain and swelling postoperatively.

## COMPLICATIONS

The incidence of complications from arthroscopic ankle surgery has diminished significantly because noninvasive means of joint distraction have replaced invasive distraction techniques in which pins were placed into the tibia and calcaneus and an outrigger device applied the distraction force. This technique was associated with a significant incidence of complications, such as pin tract infection, fracture at the pin site, and nerve injury. We have had no complications directly related to the use of noninvasive strap distraction.

Superficial *nerve injury* is the most common complication of arthroscopic ankle surgery. This complication can be avoided by meticulous operative technique in which the portals are created by first incising the skin only, gently spreading the subcutaneous tissues, and then creating the portals with a blunt trocar. The portals should be large enough to easily pass the instruments into the joint without traumatizing the soft tissues excessively. Soft tissue trauma at the portals may increase the risk of infection and sinus tract formation. We have had no sinus tract complications, no infections, no superficial nerve injuries, and no deep vein thromboses in our series of patients since initiating the noninvasive joint distraction technique.

The most common "complication" of arthroscopic surgery for osteochondral lesions of the talar dome is failure to diminish *pain* to a level that allows the patient to function in his or her chosen occupation or sport. If the patient fails to improve after drilling of an intact lesion or bone grafting in an attempt to save a lesion, the next step is to perform a debridement with abrasion of the base and/or drilling. If this procedure fails to achieve a satisfactory functional state, an osteochondral autografting procedure may be attempted. Ankle fusion can be performed as a salvage procedure.

## RECOMMENDED READING

### Osteophytes

1. Ferkel RD, Karzel RP, Del Pisso W, et al.: Arthroscopic treatment of anterolateral impingement of the ankle. *Am J Sports Med* 19:440–446, 1991.
2. Martin DF, Baker CL, Curl WW, et al.: Operative ankle arthroscopy: long-term follow-up. *Am J Sports Med* 17:16–23, 1989.
3. Ogilvie-Harris DJ, Gilbart MK, Chorney K: Chronic pain following ankle sprains in athletes: the role of arthroscopic surgery. *Arthroscopy* 13:564–574, 1997.
4. Scranton PE, McDermott JE: Anterior tibiotalar spurs: a comparison of open versus arthroscopic debridement. *Foot Ankle* 13:125–129, 1992.
5. van Dijk CN, Tol JL, Verheyen C: A prospective study of prognostic factors concerning the outcome of arthroscopic surgery for anterior ankle impingement. *Am J Sports Med* 25:737–745, 1997.

### Osteochondral Talar Dome Lesions

6. Alexander AH, Lichtman DM: Surgical treatment of transchondral talar dome fractures (osteochondritis dissecans). *J Bone Joint Surg Am* 62:646–652, 1980.
7. Anderson IF, Crichton KJ, Grattan-Smith T, et al.: Osteochondral fractures of the dome of the talus. *J Bone Joint Surg Am* 71:1143–1152, 1989.
8. Baker CL, Morales RW: Arthroscopic treatment of transchondral talar dome fractures: a long-term follow-up study. *Arthroscopy* 15:197–202, 1999.
9. Berndt AL, Harty M: Transchondral fractures (osteochondritis dissecans) of the talus. *J Bone Joint Surg Am* 41:988–1020, 1959.
10. Canale ST, Belding RH: Osteochondral lesions of the talus. *J Bone Joint Surg Am* 62:97–102, 1980.
11. Flick AB, Gould N: Osteochondritis dissecans of the talus (transchondral fractures of the talus): review of the literature and new surgical approach for medial dome lesions. *Foot Ankle* 5:165–185, 1985.
12. Pettine KA, Morrey BF: Osteochondral fractures of the talus: a long-term follow-up. *J Bone Joint Surg Br* 69:89–92, 1987.

# 36

# Ankle Arthrodesis

Ronald W. Smith

## INDICATIONS/CONTRAINDICATIONS

The primary indication for ankle arthrodesis is pain from severe ankle arthritis that limits activities of daily living. The arthrodesis surgical technique described in this chapter is applicable in patients in whom there is significant deformity or subluxation at the tibiotalar joint. In some cases, there is anterior subluxation of the talus relative to the distal tibia due to previous trauma. There may be bony deficiency from previous trauma or surgery. This technique may be used when there is a moderate to severe equinus contracture with associated arthritis. This technique is useful when ankle positioning with posterior subluxation of the talus on the tibia is desired, such as in rheumatoid arthritis patients with ankyloses of the midfoot or younger patients.

Severe arthritis of the ankle may be caused by ankle fractures, tibial plafond fractures, or in rare instances, chronic ankle instability. Rheumatoid arthritis is a less common indication for ankle arthrodesis than the degenerative type, and a patient's complaint of arthritis in the ankle often results from subtalar arthritis.

Deformity is a relative indication for arthrodesis. Occasionally, an equinus, varus, or valgus deformity may interfere with functional activities as much as or more than pain. The deformity may result from trauma or neuromuscular disorders. Arthrodesis and realignment in such cases may lead to significant improvement in walking.

Failure of nonoperative care for the arthritic or paralyzed ankle is usually a prerequisite for recommending arthrodesis. The nonoperative regimen may include antiinflammatory medications, soft-laced ankle gauntlet, or a motion-limiting brace such as a polypropylene ankle-foot orthosis.

The ankle arthrodesis technique described here involves a transverse resection of the distal articular surface of the tibia and is particularly useful in patients with deformity, such as varus-valgus, equinus, or rotational malalignment. The bimalleolar approach presented facilitates full correction of even severe deformities, and it allows posterior displacement of

R. W. Smith, M.D.: Department of Orthopaedic Surgery, University of California at Los Angeles, Los Angeles; Foot and Ankle Service, Department of Orthopaedic Surgery, Harbor-UCLA Medical Center, Torrance, California.

the talus to improve gait. An attribute of this fusion technique described is the orientation of the screws, which allows relatively easy placement of three screws (instead of the commonly used two screws) without impingement between the screws. The use of screws as an alternative to external fixation obviates the occurrence of superficial pin track infections, which may occur with external fixator devices.

There are numerous variations in the internal compression arthrodesis technique with screw fixation. A somewhat simpler method of arthrodesis than the one described previously may be appropriate in patients with severe arthritis without significant deformity or bone loss. An arthrodesis *in situ* can be performed by removing the joint surfaces without complete joint resection of the distal tibia and dome of the talus. In these cases, double screw fixation may be sufficient. Arthroscopic ankle arthrodesis is also applicable when there is no significant deformity or bone loss.

Avascular necrosis involving a significant portion of the talar body may be better treated with an alternative method than the technique described in this chapter. In the Blair technique, the avascular body of the talus is removed, and the tibia is fused to the talar neck with a sliding tibial graft. The term *significant portion* is not well-defined in the literature, but if more than one half of the talar body radiographically appears to be avascular, the Blair technique could be applied. Other techniques have been successful featuring bone graft spanning the affected joint.

Peripheral neuropathy, such as that associated with diabetes mellitus, may be a relative contraindication to arthrodesis because of an increased likelihood of nonunion and complications compared with arthrodesis in patients with normal sensory function. Patients with sensory neuropathies should be treated to the extent possible in immobilizing braces designed for sensory impaired patients. However, a severe deformity may be refractory to brace treatment because of skin breakdown. Ankle arthrodesis in such patients is a reasonable alternative to amputation.

Severe osteoporosis is a relative contraindication to ankle arthrodesis with screw fixation. An external compression fixator is reasonable if the screw fixation is not optimal.

A failed total ankle arthroplasty may be a relative contraindication to screw fixation when there is insufficient talus remaining to effectively engage the threads of the screws. An external fixator may be a better fixation device under those conditions.

Ankle arthritis associated with sepsis is another relative contraindication to screw fixation. An external fixator should be considered.

## PREOPERATIVE PLANNING

Radiographic analysis is performed with weight-bearing anteroposterior and lateral views and with a mortise view. Weight-bearing views allow more critical evaluation of malalignment and loss of cartilage space in the ankle and hindfoot. Typical findings of ankle arthritis are loss of joint space, subchondral sclerosis, subchondral cysts, osteophytes, loose bodies, malposition, or osteopenia. At least a portion of the joint may have complete loss of the cartilage space. Surprisingly, there is an occasional patient with radiographic findings of severe arthritis who does not have enough pain to significantly limit daily activities, and postponement of arthrodesis is recommended.

The patient with ankle arthritis should be evaluated preoperatively for associated pathology such as subtalar arthritis. Sinus tarsi tenderness and "ankle pain" with forced passive hindfoot motion are indicators of subtalar irritability. Plain film radiography is usually adequate, but computed tomography (CT) studies with coronal sections of the hindfoot may be helpful in more critically assessing the subtalar joint condition. If there is evidence of early subtalar arthritis, alert the patient to the possibility of persistent pain that may occasionally progress and require further surgery. When significant radiographic changes are present in the subtalar joint, it is necessary to extend the arthrodesis across both ankle and subtalar levels, with or without supplemental bone graft.

It is useful to test the stability of screw fixation intraoperatively and to have a contingency plan if the fixation is not rigid. An external fixator such as the Calandruccio triangular compression device or uniaxial fixator should be available in the event that screw fixation is not satisfactory. Threaded, 0.1875-inch-diameter, Steinmann pins placed longitudinally have occasionally been used as a last resort in rheumatoid arthritis patients with ankle and subtalar disease if the bone is too osteopenic for conventional fixation.

In patients with a valgus or varus deformity, the alignment is often corrected by adjusting the bone resection of the tibia or talus, or both. The severity of the malalignment influences the amount of bone to be resected to achieve correction. The amount of bone removed influences the degree of limb shortening that will occur.

In postfracture cases, bone grafting of the distal tibia may be necessary if there is significant bone loss. The resected malleoli usually provide enough bone in such circumstances. In contrast, arthrodesis of a failed total ankle arthroplasty usually requires a much larger amount of bone graft such as iliac crest graft.

Scars or areas where previous soft tissue coverage operations were performed may require modifications from the recommended incisions. The surgeon should avoid making parallel incisions close to a surgical or other incision when possible. When necessary to incise across a linear scar, it is important to advise the patient preoperatively of the possibility of delayed wound healing.

The timing of arthrodesis after ankle trauma varies with the fracture severity and degree of patient impairment. In patients with ankle arthritis from severe pilon fractures, delaying operative treatment may allow revascularization of the bone fragments, fracture union, and a greater likelihood of successful arthrodesis. However, severe pain may prompt an earlier arthrodesis operation.

Significant sclerosis, often seen on the tibial side of the ankle joint after severe pilon fractures, may require adjusting the arthrodesis technique, such as intramedullary drilling and more prolonged immobilization. Thermal necrosis may occur during resection of the tibial joint surface or the saw blade may inadvertently deviate when attempting to cut the dense bone.

Preoperative counseling prepares the patient for realistic expectations. Items of information include incidence of infection, nonunion, and neurovascular complications. Patients should be advised about the possibility of needing supplemental bone grafts, alternative fixation technique, prolonged cast immobilization, noticeable shortening, and altered footwear postoperatively.

## SURGERY

The patient is operated with a spinal or general anesthetic and positioned in a semilateral decubitus position with the operative side up (Fig. 36-1). The desired position is such that at rest the lateral side of the ankle is almost parallel to the floor, but with gentle external rotation the toes can be directed toward the ceiling, and the medial ankle is accessible. A beanbag is used to hold the position. A radiograph table facilitates the use of an image intensification device. A pneumatic tourniquet is used on the proximal thigh. Before the surgical scrub and draping, the surgeon repeats the evaluation of rotational alignment of the operative and nonoperative lower extremities by flexing the knee 90° and extending the ankle to neutral or as close to neutral as possible. The rotational position is noted, aligning the tibial tubercle with a landmark of the forefoot such as the web space between the first and second toes. Surgical drapes are applied, leaving the foot, leg, and the knee exposed in the surgical field (Fig. 36-2). This allows flexion of the knee to 90° and comparison of the rotational alignment of the foot to the knee during surgery (Fig. 36-3). If the patient has a previously fused ankle on the other extremity, occasionally it is helpful to scrub and drape the other leg in the surgical field to provide close symmetry in ankle position, if the other ankle is satisfactorily aligned.

### Technique

The lateral incision begins over the distal fibula about 10 cm above the tip of the lateral malleolus (Fig. 36-4). The skin incision extends distally to the tip of the lateral malleolus

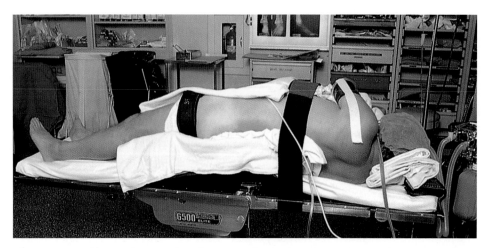

**Figure 36-1.** The patient is placed in a semilateral position. External rotation of the hip allows the toes to be directed toward the ceiling and allows access to the medial side of the ankle. Internal rotation allows easy access to the lateral side of the ankle.

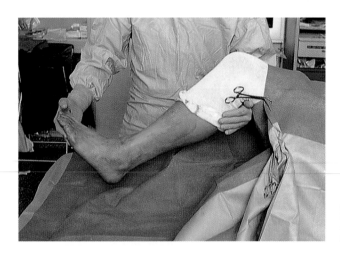

**Figure 36-2.** The lower extremity is draped to expose the knee to allow 90° of knee flexion for rotational alignment assessment.

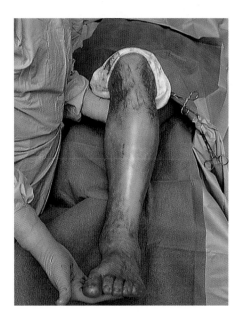

**Figure 36-3.** The frontal view allows assessment of rotational alignment. A mental note is made of how the foot aligns with the tibial tubercle. A similar assessment is made of the other leg and foot before surgery.

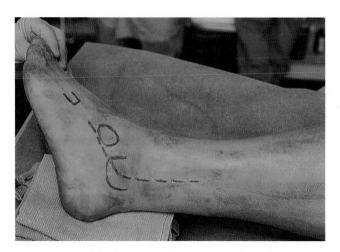

**Figure 36-4.** The lateral landmarks and planned incisions are drawn on the skin. The circle depicts the sinus tarsi, and the partial rectangle marks the base of the fourth metatarsal.

and angles across the sinus tarsi toward the base of the fourth metatarsal, terminating near the dorsum of the cuboid. The soft tissue in the sinus tarsi is not excised, but the incision extends distally to allow easy exposure of the anterolateral surface of the talar body.

The lateral malleolus is osteotomized with an oscillating saw, using a blade that is 0.5 to 1.0 cm wide (Fig. 36-5). The osteotomy begins about 4 cm proximal to the joint line and is directed distally and medially to make a beveled cut. The distal fragment is grasped with a Lewin bone clamp (i.e., a tenaculum similar to a heavy towel clamp) and the soft tissue detached with scalpel, 1.2-cm Key elevator, and rongeurs. Bone spurs and dense soft tissue at the tibiofibular syndesmosis are resected. Visualizing the peroneal tendons limits the possibility of injury to them when dissecting around and excising the lateral malleolus.

Alignment reference guide pins are placed in the tibia before making the medial exposure (Fig. 36-6). Two 0.062-inch, smooth wires are placed in the tibia about 12 cm proximal to the ankle joint. One pin is placed in the anterior cortex in an anterior to posterior direction. It is placed perpendicular to the tibia as the surgeon looks at the lateral surface of the leg. This pin serves to orient for the calcaneus-equinus position as the distal tibial cut is made. The second pin is placed in the lateral cortex in a lateral to medial direction, placing the pin perpendicular to the axis of the anterior surface of the tibia. This pin serves to orient for the varus-valgus position as the distal tibial osteotomy is made.

The leg is externally rotated to access the medial ankle, and an incision is made beginning on the bone about 8 cm above the tip of the malleolus (Fig. 36-7). The incision is extended distally and at the tip of the malleolus it is angled anteriorly along a line parallel to the axis of the talar neck. The skin incision is continued to the level of the navicular to allow easy visualization of the ankle and medial talar neck.

With sharp dissection, free the tibialis posterior and flexor hallucis tendons from the posterior margin of the distal tibia. They may be adherent to the bone and can be injured as the articular surface of the tibia is osteotomized (Fig. 36-8).

Osteotomize the medial malleolus at a 45° angle toward the level of the plafond (Fig. 36-9). The osteotomy facilitates visualization of the vulnerable medial tendons. No further resection of the medial flare of the tibia should be needed at the end of the procedure. The small residual medial flare serves as a solid buttress for the medial screw (Fig. 36-10). Before osteotomizing the tibial articular surface, the ankle joint capsule is dissected anteriorly and posteriorly so that adequate visualization is achieved.

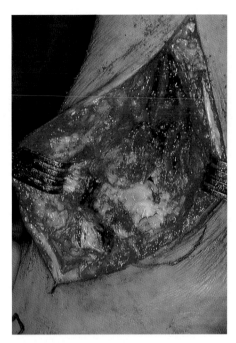

**Figure 36-5.** The lateral malleolus has been resected, exposing the lateral talus. The central white area is the lateral surface of the talus.

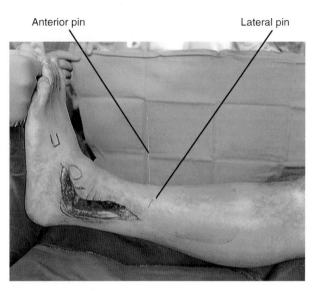

**Figure 36-6.** Guide pins are placed in orthogonal planes.

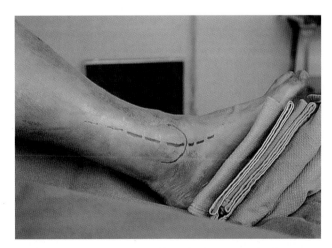

**Figure 36-7.** The planned medial incision is drawn. A smaller incision may be sufficient in cases not requiring extensive hardware removal.

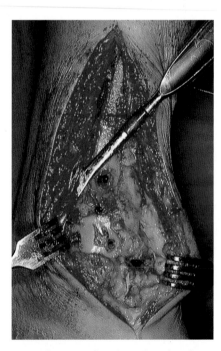

**Figure 36-8.** A fracture fixation plate has been removed from the medial tibia. A periosteal elevator is used to free the tibialis posterior tendon, which is scarred down on the posterior tibia.

Posterior
tibial
tendon

Medial
malleolus
resection

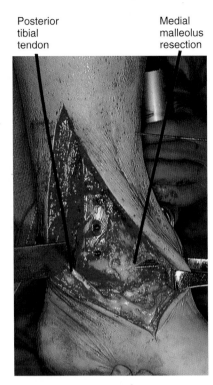

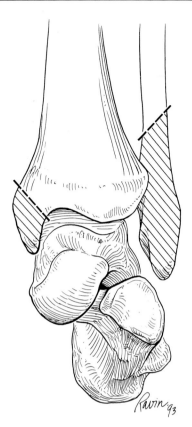

**Figure 36-9.** The medial malleolus has been resected at about a 45° angle.

**Figure 36-10.** The anterior-view drawing shows resection of the malleoli.

Excision of the tibial articular surface is made from lateral to medial using a large oscillating saw with a blade about 3 cm wide (Fig. 36-11). Visualization and protection of soft tissue is accomplished by placing bladelike retractors such as Chandler or Giannestras retractors posteriorly, both medially and laterally, interposed between bone and tendons. Army-Navy retractors are placed in the medial and lateral incisions and traction applied toward the ceiling with one hand of the assistant. The assistant surgeon and scrub assistant are involved in retraction at this point.

The surgeon resects the tibial articular surface, removing only about 3 to 4 mm of bone (Figs. 36-12 and 36-13). Using the guide pins for orientation, the articular surface is cut perpendicular to the axis of the leg. The talar bone cut orientation is critical as it is undesirable to reuse the cut multiple times, reducing the height of the talus. Regardless of the deformity, the distal articular surface of the tibia is usually osteotomized perpendicular to the long axis of the leg. The resected fragment of bone may be wedge shaped, for example, and thicker on the medial side if there was a preoperative valgus deformity. In the past, it was common to place the ankle arthrodesis in slight equinus position in female patients who desired to wear an elevated heel postoperatively or if the leg length was short preoperatively. Many feel that the most consistent satisfaction in walking with a fused ankle is with a neutral flexion-extension position.

After removal of the articular surface of the tibia, the foot is positioned in neutral flexion-extension. The assistant surgeon holds the alignment, the scrub assistant retracts the anterior skin with the medial and lateral retractors while the surgeon resects the dome of the talus, removing about 3 mm of dorsal surface (Fig. 36-14). A 2- to 2.5-cm blade width is used for the talar dome resection. The ankle position should be about 5° of valgus, 5° to 10° of external rotation, neutral to slight posterior displacement of the talus relative to tibia, neutral medial-lateral displacement, and neutral flexion-extension (1).

Temporary fixation is attained with an axial, tibiotalocalcaneal, 0.125-inch, smooth Steinmann pin supplemented with a 0.062-inch, smooth Kirchner wire placed obliquely across the

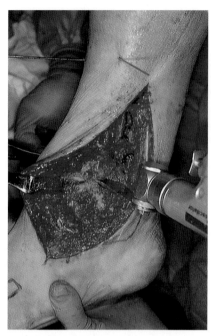

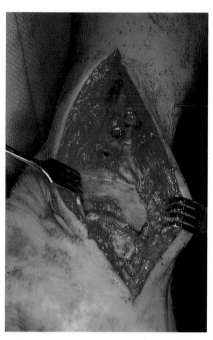

**Figure 36-11.** Resection of the distal tibia from lateral to medial aspects is done with an oscillating saw. Army-Navy retractors are used in the medial and lateral incisions to retract the anterior skin.

**Figure 36-12.** The cut surface of the distal tibial is seen in a medial view, and a central bone defect is visible.

fusion site starting from the lateral talus toward the medial tibia. The Steinmann pin placement is readily accomplished first by directing it antegrade starting in the dorsal surface of the talus and directed plantarward (Fig. 36-15). The lateral location for the axial pin avoids interference with placement of the first two screws; these screws will be directed anterolaterally to posteromedially. If the Steinmann pin is placed too far posterior in the talus, it will cut out of the tibia posteriorly when the pin is advanced proximally after posteriorly displacing the talus on the tibia. The subtalar joint should be aligned in neutral as the pin crosses the subtalar joint. There is a tendency to leave the subtalar joint slightly inverted as the pin is advanced plantarly and this may lead to malpositioning of the ankle arthrodesis (Fig. 36-16). The Steinmann pin is withdrawn plantarward and the talus is displaced posteriorly. With posterior displacement

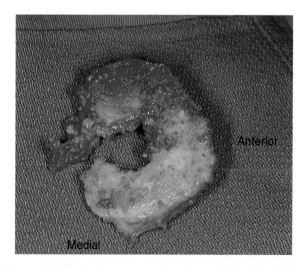

**Figure 36-13.** In the resected surface of the distal tibia, the medial side is thicker to compensate for a valgus deformity.

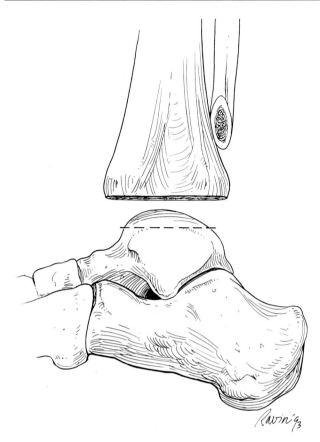

**Figure 36-14.** Lateral-view drawing shows the ankle under traction after resection of the tibial articular surface. The foot is aligned in preparation for resection of the talus.

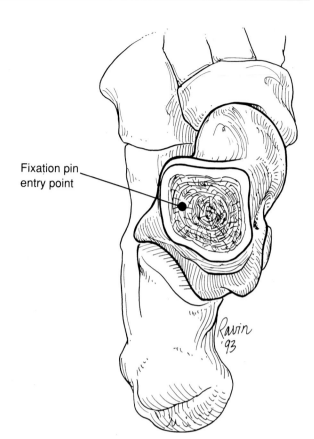

Fixation pin entry point

**Figure 36-15.** A drawing of the superior surface of the talus after resection of the dome shows the location of the temporary fixation pin that will be directed plantarward through the talus.

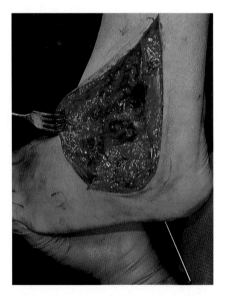

**Figure 36-16.** A 0.125-inch, smooth Steinmann pin is driven plantarward to exit the plantar surface of the calcaneus. In the process, the ankle is adducted and the foot displaced laterally to expose the dorsal surface of the talus. Care is taken to position the hindfoot in neutral and avoid an inversion position when the pin crosses the subtalar joint.

of the talus, the anterior flare of the distal tibia usually lines up near the junction of the head and neck of the talus. The posterior displacement of the talus reduces the length of the anterior lever arm of the foot, which is desirable as it allows a more normal pattern of gait.

The tibiotalar joint surfaces are well apposed, and the Steinmann pin is advanced retrograde into the tibia. Next, rotational alignment is rechecked, and the Kirschner wire is inserted to control the rotational alignment. This Kirschner wire is inserted just lateral to the base of the talar neck on the anterior margin of the talar body and directed into the medial tibia (Figs. 36-17 and 36-18). If the Kirschner wire is started too laterally in the talus, it will interfere with placement of the first screw, which enters in the center of the anterior surface of the lateral talar body. The surgeon can use 7.0-mm, cannulated, stainless steel screws or 6.5-mm, cannulated, titanium screws. A guide pin with a larger diameter is easier to direct because it does not inadvertently deflect or deviate in hard cortical bone, but it seems to penetrate the cortex better than smaller diameter guide pins.

The first cannulated screw is started on the anterior surface of the lateral talar body and is directed toward the posteromedial tibia. In some cases, properly directing the screw from the anterior aspect of the talus to the posteromedial aspect of the distal tibia is difficult because the large head of the screw may abut on the anterior calcaneal process as it is being inserted. In these cases, the guide pin is driven to extend beyond the posteromedial cortex and the screw is inserted in the opposite direction, starting from the posteromedial tibia, toward the anterolateral talar body.

At this point, the image intensifier is useful to evaluate the position of the arthrodesis and the location of the initial guide pin (Figs. 36-19 and 36-20). The standard technique of drilling, tapping, and inserting appropriate-length cannulated screws is used. The opposite cortex is engaged if feasible. The first screw is not tightened until the second screw is inserted and the temporary fixation pins are removed.

The guide pin for the second screw is inserted on the anterolateral surface of the tibia about 2 to 2.5 cm proximal to the arthrodesis site. The pin and subsequent screw are directed into the posteromedial talus with the aid of the image intensifier (Fig. 36-21). After the second screw is placed, the temporary fixation pins are removed, and both lateral screws are tightened.

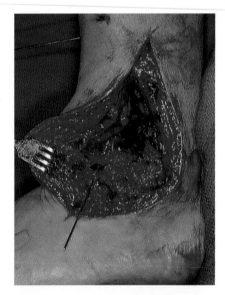

**Figure 36-17.** In a lateral view, the joint surfaces are reduced, with the talus displaced posteriorly 5 to 8 mm, and the tibiocalcaneal pin is advanced into the tibia while applying axial compression. A 0.062-inch Kirschner wire is added across the talotibial interval as temporary fixation to control rotation. The pin enters the talar body adjacent to the talar neck, sufficiently medial to allow entry of the first screw at the lateral surface of the talar body.

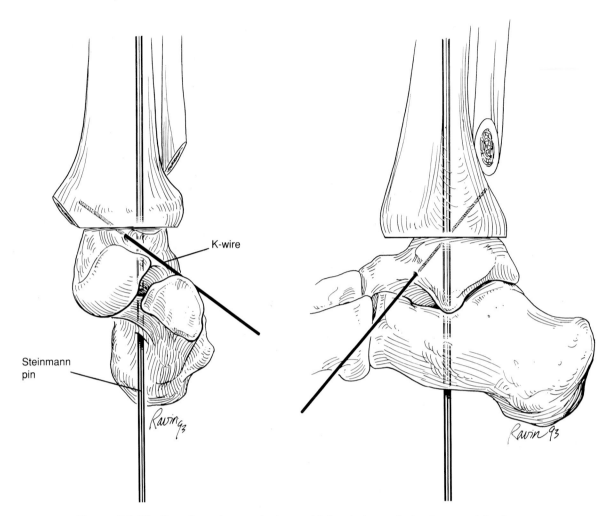

K-wire

Steinmann
pin

**Figure 36-18.** Drawings show anterior and lateral views of pin placement for temporary fixation.

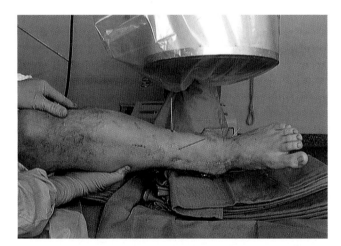

**Figure 36-19.** The leg is internally rotated to place the axis of the foot parallel for a lateral view using the image intensifier. The angle of the image intensifier is adjusted to accomplish a true lateral view.

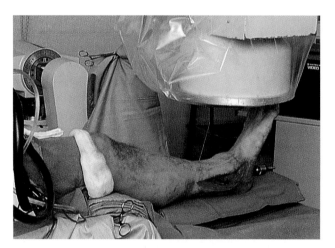

**Figure 36-20.** The leg is externally rotated and positioned for the anteroposterior view.

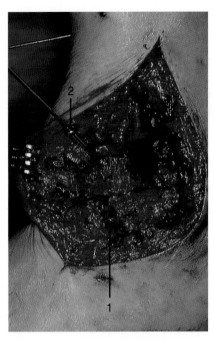

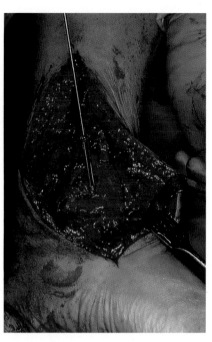

**Figure 36-21.** In this lateral view, the second cannulated screw enters the anterolateral surface of the distal tibia and is directed into the posteromedial talus. The first screw has already been placed, and the screw head is seated on the anterior surface of the talar body and is directed into the posteromedial tibia.

**Figure 36-22.** The third cannulated screw enters the medial tibia and is directed toward the anterolateral body or neck of the talus.

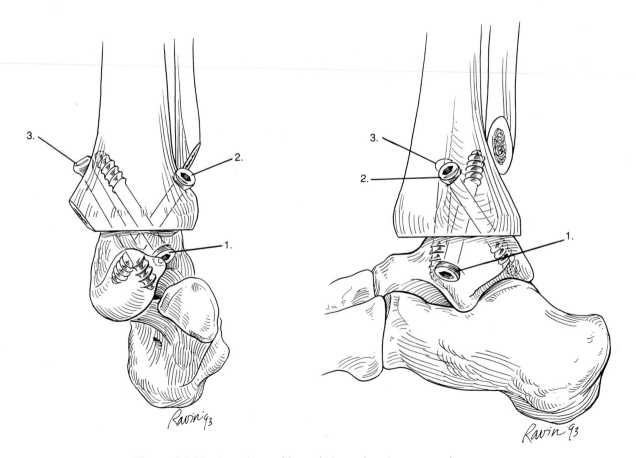

**Figure 36-23.** Anterior and lateral views showing screw placement.

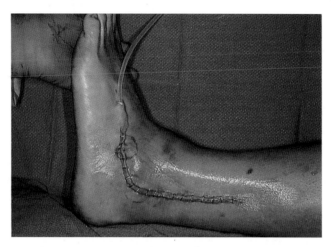

**Figure 36-24.** Lateral view after wound closure.

The pin for the third screw is started in the medial surface of the tibia at about the midline (Fig. 36-22). The pin is directed anteriorly toward the lateral talar neck. The screw may be quite oblique to the tibial cortical surface and may require countersinking for the head of the screw. Countersinking is done with a 4-mm power burr on the proximal side of the drill hole after temporarily removing the guide pin. The use of a burr rather than a countersinking device appears to maintain a better cortical "shoulder" distal to the drill hole. Inserting and tightening the third screw adds stability to the fusion site (Fig. 36-23).

At any of the screw sites, a washer may be necessary if the cortex is soft and allows unacceptable penetration of the head of the screw. The utmost care is taken to avoid penetrating the subtalar joint with the second and third screws (i.e., proximal-to-distal screws). Radiographic imaging and checking subtalar motion help identify inadvertent screw extension into the subtalar joint.

A soft suction drain tube is brought out from the lateral ankle at the dorsum of the foot, just proximal to the base of the fourth metatarsal. The wound is closed with absorbable subcutaneous sutures and nylon sutures or stainless steel staples on the skin (Figs. 36-24 and 36-25).

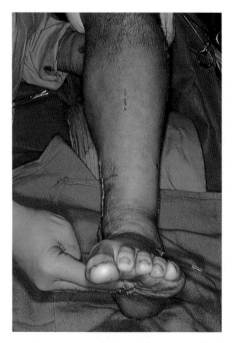

**Figure 36-25.** Frontal view after wound closure.

## POSTOPERATIVE MANAGEMENT

A well-padded, short-leg cast is applied with two rolls of 6-inch plaster and no splints. This lightweight cast is easily univalved and spread open if required because of pain after surgery. As an alternative, a compressive Robert Jones dressing with plaster splints may be used that accommodates some swelling. The drain is usually removed on the first postoperative day. The cast is closed and reinforced with a layer of fiberglass casting material on the second day. The patient usually starts non–weight-bearing ambulation on the second day and is dismissed from the hospital on the second or third postoperative day. Bed rest with elevation of the ankle at a level of at least 12 inches above the heart is emphasized initially. With time, the patient progresses to sitting, using another chair for elevation.

The cast is changed about 2 weeks after surgery, sutures or staples are removed, and a short-leg fiberglass cast is reapplied. Patients are advised to continue non–weight-bearing ambulation for 2 months, and calf isometric exercises are instructed. In our early experience with this procedure, no weight bearing was advised for 3 months, but we may allow earlier weight bearing if the patient's pain and swelling are resolving. Cast changes are made at 4- to 6-week intervals, and weight bearing is usually initiated at 2 months postoperatively. The patient is advised to gradually progress the amount of weight bearing as long as there is no pain.

Three months postoperatively, the patient is expected to be ambulating with full weight bearing in a short-leg cast without pain. The cast is converted to a bivalve cast with anterior and posterior shells of fiberglass that can be used as removable support. This device allows a gradual weaning from immobilization. In the security of the home, the patient can walk cast-free initially for an hour three times the first day and then progress to walking without a cast for a longer time on subsequent days as long as there is no pain. An elastic stocking is worn with and without the bivalve cast for approximately 3 months to minimize swelling.

Physical therapy is started when the bivalve program (i.e., weaning from the cast) is started. Subtalar range of motion exercises and foot and ankle strengthening exercises are emphasized. The surgeon or physical therapist may suggest footwear modifications such as a rocker-bottom sole and SACH heel to assist in resuming a normal gait. In this surgeon's experience, ankle fusion patients improve in walking pattern over a period of 9 to 12 months after surgery. Patients usually walk better with shoes than barefooted.

Conservative guidelines for patient expectations include playing golf at 9 to 12 months and doubles tennis at 1 to 2 years. Stationary bicycle riding or swimming or other low-impact activities are encouraged as a form of aerobic exercise but usually not jogging, even after the arthrodesis is well-healed. The repetitive impact loading of jogging could irritate other joints in the foot or knee, particularly in patients who already have degenerative changes in these joints.

It is reasonable to expect a 10% nonunion rate, and this may be higher in extenuating circumstances, as discussed later. Malalignment complaints may occur in about 15% of patients.

## COMPLICATIONS

*Pseudarthrosis* occurs in about 10% of cases (range, 0% to 30%) of reported ankle fusions. An increased rate of pseudarthrosis is associated with factors such as the severity of the initial trauma, presence of neuropathy, infection, and tobacco use. Several factors may help limit the occurrence of pseudarthrosis. An adequate area of cancellous bone apposition promotes arthrodesis. Removal of only 1 or 2 mm off the dome of the talus to minimize shorting may not provide a large enough surface area of cancellous bone to assure arthrodesis as the cross-sectional area of the talus is larger 3 to 4 mm below the dorsal surface.

If the distal tibia is sclerotic, as may be seen with arthritis after pilon fractures, multiple intramedullary drill holes could be made in the tibial surface. Bone defects can be addressed with morcellated bone from the malleoli in most cases.

Additional protection with a long-leg cast with the knee in flexion may be necessary in patients who are prone to pseudarthrosis. Such patients include those who had a previous failed arthrodesis attempt and difficulties with compliance with non–weight-bearing instructions in the initial postoperative period.

The physician should be suspicious of a delay in union if a patient has significant pain, swelling, or warmth at the ankle 3 months after surgery. A long-leg cast and an electrical stimulator or prolonging short-leg cast immobilization may be occasionally considered if there is a concern about delayed union.

Revision ankle arthrodesis with bone grafting is a consideration for painful nonunion at least 6 months after the primary procedure. Occasionally, a patient with a painless or minimally painful nonunion can be observed rather than revised.

The most common *malalignment* problems associated with ankle arthrodesis are equinus, varus, and internal rotation. Equinus deformity can cause knee hyperextension, laxity of the medial collateral ligament of the knee, midfoot degenerative arthritis, and difficulty in walking barefoot. It can be avoided by carefully aligning the lateral border of the plantar surface of the foot perpendicular to the axis of the leg at the time temporary fixation is accomplished. Resecting the distal articular surface of the tibia perpendicular to the long axis of the tibia is imperative.

A postoperative varus deformity causes the patient to walk on the lateral border of the foot and may contribute to subtalar joint degeneration. This deformity can be avoided by resecting the distal articular surface of the tibia with a minimal valgus angle and double-checking the position intraoperatively visually and radiologically.

Rotational deformity can be lessened by the use of temporary fixation and careful inspections as well as the technique of flexing the knee to 90° while judging the rotation of the foot.

The occurrence of malalignment is treated with footwear modifications if the deformity is mild. An osteotomy just proximal to or at the fusion site may be necessary in more severe circumstances. Occasionally, a slowly developing internal rotation-varus deformity may result from a progressive hindfoot disorder such as subtalar arthritis or neurologic problem.

*Persistent postoperative pain despite a solid fusion* may result from subtalar arthritis. It is not unusual for patients to have a stiff, mildly arthritic subtalar joint before the arthrodesis operation. Occasionally, subtalar irritability can be caused by penetration of the screws into the talocalcaneal joint. Use of the image intensifier while placing the guide pins and screws, as well as checking the subtalar motion after removing the temporary fixation, helps to avoid this problem.

*Tendon lacerations* may occur. The tibialis posterior and flexor hallucis longus tendons are vulnerable to injury during resection of the distal tibial articular surfaces. Carefully resecting of a portion of the medial malleolus clearly exposes the tendons that can then be protected.

## ILLUSTRATIVE CASE

The case of a 51-year-old machine operator is used to illustrate this technique of ankle arthrodesis. The patient sustained an intraarticular fracture of the ankle 3 years before his arthrodesis while cross-county skiing. The fracture was treated surgically, but progressive pain and valgus deformity developed (Fig. 36-26).

The preoperative examination revealed a moderate limp and moderate heel valgus. There was mild lateral translation of the foot relative to the longitudinal axis of the leg. Examination showed a mild loss of ankle dorsiflexion and moderate loss of plantarflexion. Subtalar motion was negligible. Well-healed surgical scars were present over the anteromedial distal tibia and distal aspect of the fibula. There was significant loss of active flexion of the great toe.

At surgery, sclerotic bone and a bone defect were encountered in the distal tibia. The flexor hallucis longus was incarcerated in adhesions at the posterior surface of the distal

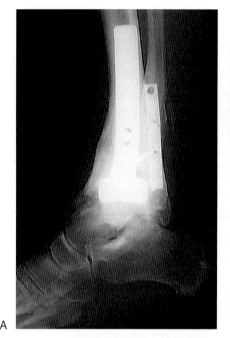
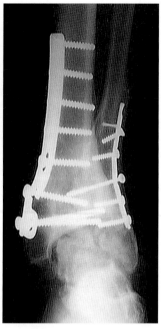

**Figure 36-26. A, B:** Preoperative radiographs.

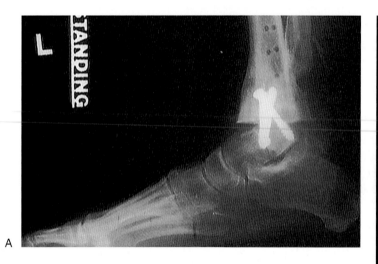
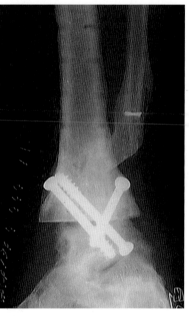

**Figure 36-27. A, B:** Radiographs 2 weeks postoperatively.

tibia, and tenolysis was performed. At the completion of the operation, ankle position was approximately neutral with regard to dorsiflexion-plantarflexion and valgus-varus. The foot was externally rotated about 15° (Fig. 36-27).

The patient was discharged from the hospital on the third postoperative day. He had a good clinical result.

## RECOMMENDED READING

1. Buck P, Morrey BF, Chao EY: The optimum position of arthrodesis of the ankle: a gait study of the knee and ankle. *J Bone Joint Surg Am* 69:1052–1062, 1987.

2. Dennis DA, Clayton ML, Wong DA, et al.: Internal fixation compression arthrodesis of the ankle. *Clin Orthop* 253:212–220, 1990.
3. Holt ES, Hansen ST, Mayo KA, et al.: Ankle arthrodesis using internal screw fixation. *Clin Orthop* 268:21–28, 1991.
4. Kenzora JE, Simmons SC, Burgess AR, et al.: External fixation arthrodesis of the ankle following trauma. *Foot Ankle* 7:49–61, 1986.
5. Kitaoka HB: Arthrodesis of the ankle: technique, complications, and salvage treatment. *Instr Course Lect* 48: 255–261, 1999.
6. Kitaoka HB, Patzer GL: Arthrodesis for the treatment of arthrosis of the ankle and osteonecrosis of the talus. *J Bone Joint Surg Am* 80:370–379, 1998.
7. Mann RA, Rongstad KM: Arthrodesis of the ankle: a critical analysis. *Foot Ankle Int* 19:3–9, 1998.
8. Monroe MT, Beals TC, Manoli A: Clinical outcome of arthrodesis of the ankle using rigid internal fixation with cancellous screws. *Foot Ankle Int* 20:227–231, 1999.
9. Perlman MH, Thordrson DB: Ankle fusion in a high risk population: an assessment of nonunion risk factors. *Foot Ankle Int* 20:491–496, 1999.

# 37

# Tibiotalocalcaneal Arthrodesis

Todd A. Kile

## INDICATIONS/CONTRAINDICATIONS

Simultaneous degeneration or deformity of the ankle and subtalar joints is a debilitating condition, presenting the surgeon with a challenging salvage situation. The appropriate treatment may be an arthrodesis from the tibia to the calcaneus. Tibiotalocalcaneal arthrodesis has proven to be an effective salvage procedure for a variety of disabling conditions involving the hindfoot; including posttraumatic arthrosis, failed total ankle replacement with subtalar intrusion, severe acquired flatfoot deformities associated with posterior tibialis tendon dysfunction, avascular necrosis of the talus after trauma, failed ankle arthrodesis, rheumatoid arthritis, Charcot neuroarthropathy with collapse, and deformity secondary to talipes equinovarus or neuromuscular diseases.

Various fixation methods have been described for this procedure, including external fixators, Steinmann pins, multiple screws, plates and screws, blade plates, and intramedullary devices. The most common approaches used are the combined lateral and medial in the supine position and the posterior approach with the prone position. Frequently, prior surgical procedures or trauma necessitate an alternate approach through previously uninjured tissue with healthy skin. Regardless of the approach or method of fixation, a tibiotalocalcaneal arthrodesis is a versatile procedure that can provide the patient with a large correction of deformity and accurate repositioning of the foot to a plantigrade position.

Contraindications are few, because many of these patients are considering or have received recommendations for a below-knee amputation as their best reconstructive option. Impaired circulation may require revascularization before reconstruction. A current infection, in the joint or the fracture site, or history of previous pin tract infection may best be treated with debridement and external fixation.

T. A. Kile, M.D.: Department of Orthopaedic Surgery, Mayo Graduate School of Medicine, Mayo Clinic, Rochester, Minnesota; and Foot and Ankle Surgery, Department of Orthopaedic Surgery, Mayo Clinic Scottsdale and Hospital, Scottsdale, Arizona.

## PREOPERATIVE PLANNING

Patients who present with ankle pain or deformity are evaluated with a systematic physical examination, paying particular attention to the ankle joint and the subtalar joint. The calcaneocuboid and talonavicular joints are also evaluated and are included in the arthrodesis procedure when needed. Weight-bearing radiographs of the foot and ankle are usually sufficient to evaluate the extent of hindfoot involvement. However, selective diagnostic injections under fluoroscopic guidance can be quite valuable in making this determination.

The examiner makes note of the skin condition preoperatively and considers the placement of previous incisions as they may determine the proper surgical approach. Conditions such as rheumatoid arthritis or diabetes can delay postoperative wound healing, and in these patients, the posterior approach may be inadvisable.

The vascularity of the entire limb is assessed, and a vascular surgery consultation is obtained when indicated before embarking on a complex reconstruction. A below-knee amputation may be preferable to multiple surgical procedures in a patient with severe peripheral vascular disease or diabetes. When avascular necrosis of the talus is suspected, particularly after trauma, a magnetic resonance imaging study is useful in determining the extent of dysvascular bone within the talar body.

A fixed deformity is usually evident on physical examination and plain radiographs. However, a weight-bearing hindfoot alignment view is occasionally helpful in determining the level and extent of the deformity in relation to the mechanical axis of the lower extremity. In those patients with a large hindfoot varus or valgus deformity, osteotomies of the malleoli may be necessary to regain a plantigrade position of the foot. Frequently, arthrosis resulting from trauma causes an equinus deformity, which requires lengthening or release of the Achilles tendon to achieve neutral position. The posterior approach can provide for significant realignment in otherwise healthy patients with severe deformity and intact skin.

Realistic expectations are key to obtaining a successful result, and preoperative counseling may prepare the patients for wound healing difficulties, nonunions, neurovascular damage, and infection.

## SURGERY

Before or immediately after induction of general anesthesia, a knee block (i.e., popliteal block) is performed as described by McLeod et al. (7). This is administered through a lateral, transbiceps approach with the patient in the supine position and an anteromedial field block of the saphenous nerve (Fig. 37-1). The patient is placed supine, with a sandbag beneath the ipsilateral buttock. The biceps femoris tendon is identified on the lateral aspect of the thigh at level approximately one fingerbreadth (2 cm) above the superior pole of the patella. The knee is flexed slightly on a blanket or small sandbag to facilitate identification of the biceps tendon, particularly in heavier patients. A 21-gauge, 4-inch (100-mm), insulated Stimuplex needle (B. Braun Medical, Inc., Bethlehem, PA) is inserted through the tendon in a horizontal plane with a 45° cephalad angulation (Fig. 37-1B). A low-output peripheral nerve stimulator is used to produce biceps femoris contraction, and as the needle is slowly advanced, it produces peroneal nerve branch stimulation with eversion of the foot. The needle is carefully advanced until the tibial nerve branch is stimulated, as evidenced by plantarflexion of the toes (Fig. 37-1C). If the biceps twitch appears and then disappears with needle advancement, the peroneal and tibial nerve twitch will not be present. In those instances, the surgeon withdraws the needle and readvances it in a slightly more anterior or posterior alignment relative to the floor, maintaining a 45° cephalad angulation. With proper stimulation of the tibial nerve branch, a total of 20 mL of 0.5% bupivacaine are injected with epinephrine, and the surgeon observes for abolition of the foot twitching as the initial 1 or 2 mL is placed. The saphenous nerve is blocked with an additional 10 mL of 0.5% bupivacaine with epinephrine using a below-knee subcutaneous field block by infiltrating the region between the tibial tuberosity and medial head of gastrocnemius muscle

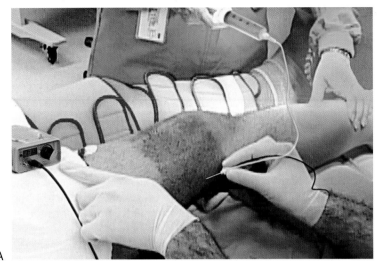

**Figure 37-1. A:** Knee block as described by McLeod et al. to provide postoperative pain relief. This can be administered before or immediately after induction of general anesthesia. **B:** Schematic of lateral popliteal block using transbiceps femoris approach. **C:** Cross-sectional diagram demonstrates proximity of the common peroneal and tibial nerves to the biceps femoris. **D:** Schematic drawing of anteromedial needle placement for a saphenous nerve block.

A

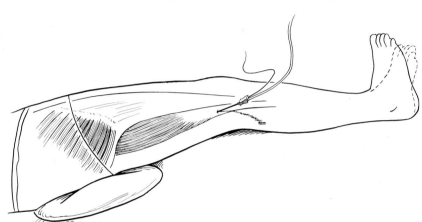

B

C

Vastus medialis

Popliteal artery

Popliteal vein

Semimembranosus muscle

Semitendinosus muscle

Vastus lateralis

Iliotibial tract

Biceps femoris (short head)

Internal intermuscular septum

Tibial nerve

Common peroneal nerve

Needle

Biceps femoris (long head)

Femur

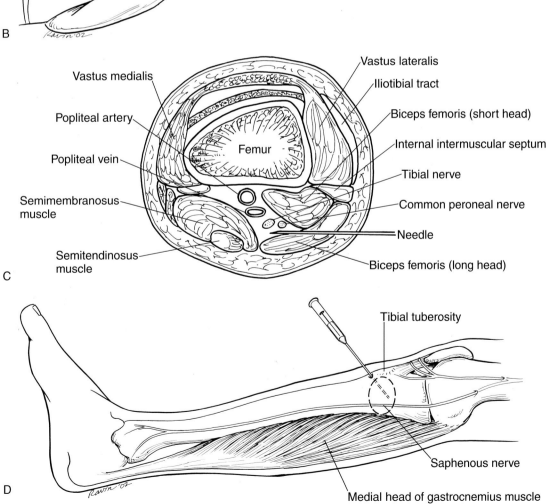

Tibial tuberosity

Saphenous nerve

Medial head of gastrocnemius muscle

D

(Fig. 37-1D). When administered before making the incision, the knee block allows patients to require less perioperative narcotics and, on average, can obtain 15 to 18 hours of postoperative pain relief. Although paresthesias may occur as the block wears off, no patients were found to have any permanent neurologic sequelae in a recent follow-up study of nearly 500 consecutive patients. The knee block provides a significant reduction in the use of postoperative narcotics and a very high patient satisfaction rate.

After successful induction of anesthesia, a tourniquet is placed over cast padding about the proximal thigh, and the patient is placed in the semilateral supine position, with a 10-lb sand bag placed beneath the ipsilateral buttock. This ensures equal access to the medial and lateral aspects of the ankle and allows satisfactory exposure of the iliac crest. Before surgical scrub and draping, the surgeon inspects both lower extremities for alignment in all planes and mentally notes the rotation of the contralateral foot relative to the tibial tubercle. After sterile preparation and draping of the affected limb, an adhesive drape is placed about the forefoot to seal the toes from the surgical wound. The surgeon sterilely prepares and drapes the iliac crest for autologous bone marrow aspiration or for possible open bone graft harvest. We use a radiolucent table and a sterilely draped minifluoroscopy unit for intraoperative radiographic visualization.

## Technique

The lateral incision begins over the fibula, approximately 5 to 10 cm proximal to the tip of the lateral malleolus (Fig. 37-2). The surgeon continues the distal extent of the incision longitudinally, coursing over the lateral malleolus and curving anteriorly toward the base of the fourth metatarsal. He or she must pay attention to creating full-thickness flaps and minimize handling of the skin with forceps. The distal aspect of the fibula is exposed, and in patients with significant deformity, an oblique osteotomy is performed from proximal-lateral to distal-medial, minimizing the lateral prominence (Fig. 37-3). The fibular fragment is grasped and detached with a sharp, square periosteal elevator and scalpel. The fragment is cleaned of soft tissues and saved for later use as bone graft. In patients with minimal deformity, the ankle and subtalar joints are exposed without removing the malleolus, and the remaining articular cartilage and dense subchondral bone is debrided from all joint surfaces using small sagittal saws, osteotomes, rongeurs, and curettes (Figs. 37-4 and 37-5). However, in patients with a more significant deformity, the surgeon aggressively mobilizes the talus and calcaneus to reduce the foot and restore longitudinal alignment. A medial longitudinal incision is made over the medial malleolus to facilitate joint debridement and re-

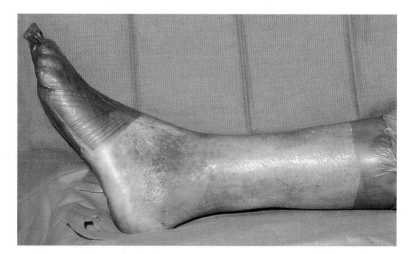

**Figure 37-2.** This patient is placed supine on the operating room table, and the procedure is done under thigh tourniquet hemostasis. The lateral incision is made over the fibula, 10 cm proximal to the tip of the lateral malleolus and distally toward the base of the fourth metatarsal, and allows access to ankle and subtalar joints.

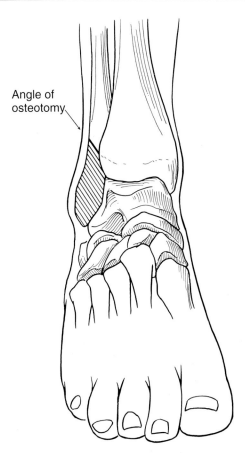

**Figure 37-3.** Fibular osteotomy is performed obliquely, if desired.

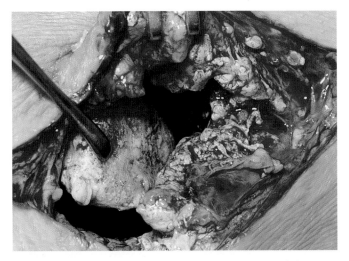

**Figure 37-4.** The lateral view shows exposure of the ankle *(right)* and subtalar *(left)* joints with advanced degenerative arthrosis seen without performing a fibular osteotomy. Elevator is on talus.

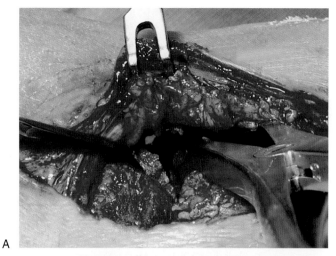

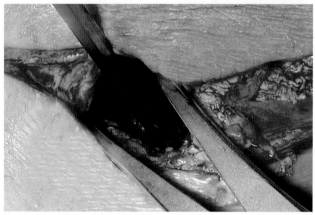

**Figure 37-5. A, B:** A lamina spreader aids visualization during debridement of the tibiotalar and subtalar joints through the lateral incision.

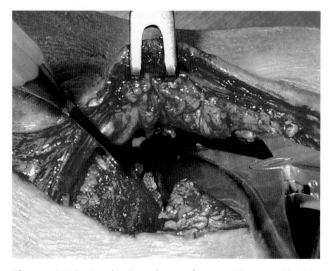

**Figure 37-6.** Feathering the surfaces with a small, thin osteotome facilitates bony union.

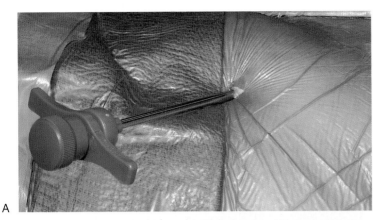

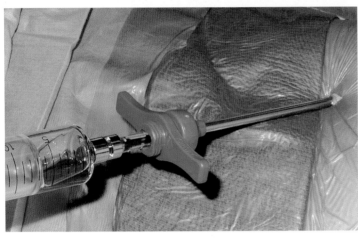

**Figure 37-7. A:** Approach to left anterior iliac crest for bone marrow aspiration. **B:** Bone graft composite is prepared by aspirating 15 mL of autologous bone marrow with an 11-gauge bone marrow aspiration needle and a heparin-soaked syringe from the iliac crest in 5-mL aliquots.

duction, and if needed, the malleolus is resected in patients with severe deformity. Lamina spreaders can aid visualization during debridement of the tibiotalar and subtalar joints (Fig. 37-5). After thorough irrigation, the surgeon should spend additional time feathering the surfaces with a small, thin osteotome to facilitate bony union (Fig. 37-6) and to minimize the chance of nonunion. In patients with avascular necrosis, a trough is created through the body of the talus, debriding all dead bone and replacing it with fresh autologous bone graft. The morcellated graft material (fibula versus iliac crest) is packed throughout the fusion sites to create intraarticular and extraarticular arthrodeses.

The bone graft composite is prepared by aspirating 15 mL of autologous bone marrow with an 11-gauge bone marrow aspiration needle and a heparin-soaked syringe from the iliac crest in 5-mL aliquots (Fig. 37-7). The bone marrow is mixed with rehydrated demineralized bone matrix powder or reconstituted Allomatrix graft, placed into a syringe, and injected into prepared subtalar and ankle joints (Fig. 37-8). In patients with a significant bone defect (i.e., failed total ankle arthroplasty), harvesting structural tricortical or cancellous bone graft in an open fashion from the iliac crest may be required. Soft tissue is removed from the graft with a large rongeur and, after final fitting, placed into the arthrodesis site. A bone mill is helpful for creating small cortical and cancellous bone graft particles. Any additional graft material is placed about the fusion site as needed.

When using a locked intramedullary device for fixation, the surgeon begins by making a plantar incision at the junction of the middle and distal thirds of the heel fat pad, in line with the malleoli (Fig. 37-9). The foot is carefully maintained in the desired position, and a threaded-tipped guide pin is advanced through the calcaneus and talus and up into the center of the tibia (Figs. 37-9 and 37-10). The position is verified with image intensification (Fig. 37-11). Clinical alignment is checked in all planes, and the guide pin and foot are adjusted until satisfactory position is achieved. Residual plantarflexion or equinus results in a back-kneed gait and should be avoided, as should excessive dorsiflexion. After reaming has started, it is not possible to change the alignment of the foot, so the surgeon must plan to spend additional time at this stage to ensure a proper final result.

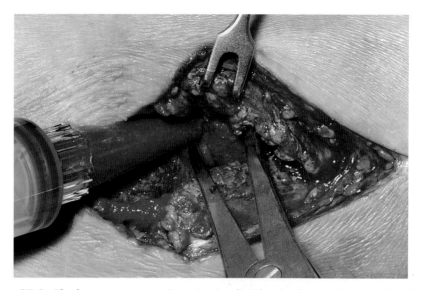

**Figure 37-8.** The bone marrow aspirate is mixed with rehydrated, demineralized bone matrix (Allomatrix) composite graft (i.e., demineralized bone matrix and autologous bone marrow), placed in syringe, and then inserted into the ankle joint. Notice that the composite graft has already been placed in the subtalar joint.

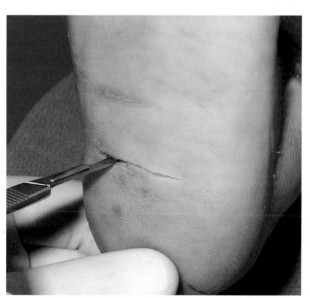

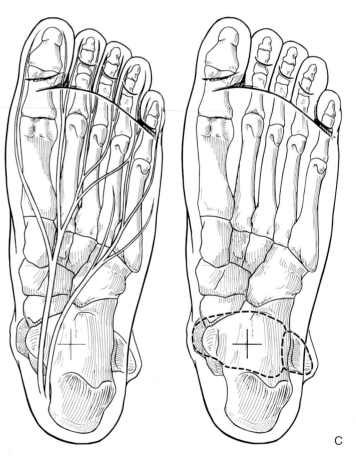

A, B                                                                                                             C

**Figure 37-9. A:** Plantar incision at the junction of the middle and anterior thirds of the heel fat pad, in line with the transmalleolar axis. **B:** The drawing shows the proximity of the lateral plantar nerve to the plantar calcaneal entry site. **C:** The drawing shows the location of the tibia and fibula *(dotted lines)* relative to the entry site.

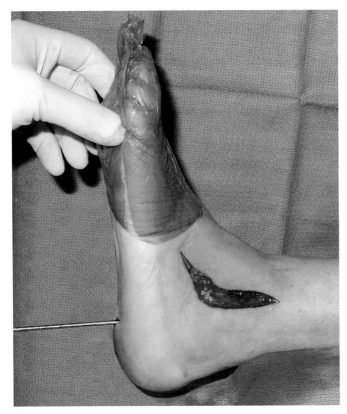

**Figure 37-10.** The guide pin is advanced through the calcaneus and talus and into the tibia with the foot maintained in a neutral position.

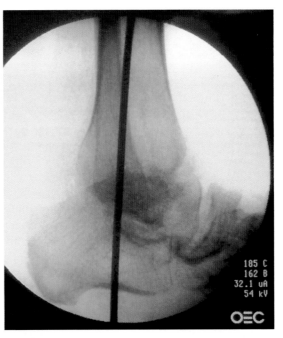

**Figure 37-11.** The surgeon verifies the proper position of the guide pin and foot with image intensification.

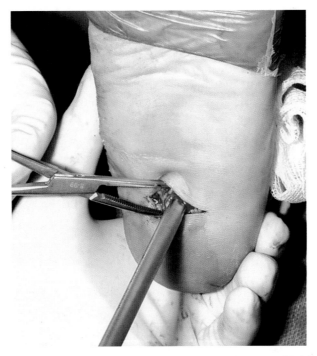

**Figure 37-12.** An end-cutting, cannulated reamer (rigid) is advanced through the calcaneus and talus and into the tibia.

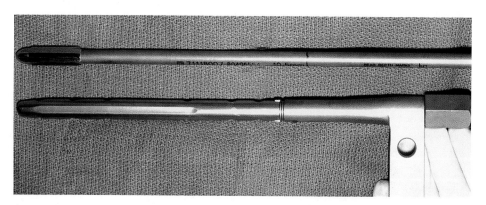

**Figure 37-13.** By measuring the length of the nail and marking the depth of insertion on the reamers, the surgeon ensures that the nail can easily advance to its proper depth.

The surgeon begins reaming with a small, end-cutting cannulated reamer, slowly advancing across the calcaneus and talus and up into the tibia (Figs. 37-12). The threaded guide pin is exchanged for a longer, nonbeaded guide pin, and then the surgeon reams to 0.5 mm less than the selected nail diameter. The length of the nail is carefully measured, and the depth of insertion is marked on the reamers (Fig. 37-13). This ensures that the nail will easily advance to its proper depth without needing to overream the tibia. For an 11-mm-diameter nail, we only ream to 10.5 mm, ensuring a snug fit within the calcaneus and generating compression as the nail is gently tapped into place, before locking screw insertion (Fig. 37-14). By underreaming in this fashion, the press fit of the nail within the calcaneus adds rigidity to the construct. We routinely use an 11-mm-diameter, 15-cm-long ReVision Nail (Smith & Nephew, Memphis, TN) in most patients, although nine sizes are available. During insertion of the nail, the construct is slightly rotated anteriorly such that the external drill guide is positioned just anterior to the fibula, which greatly aids insertion of the proximal locking screws (Fig. 37-15). Proper depth of insertion is confirmed with image intensification, and the surgeon ensures that the distal locking holes are properly aligned within the calcaneus or talus (Fig. 37-16). He or she avoids leaving the nail proud at the plantar aspect of the calcaneus but also takes time to prevent the nail from being driven too far into the calcaneus, which causes the interlocking holes to be within the subtalar or ankle joints. Proper depth of insertion and underreaming are important to obtaining satisfactory distal fixation.

The locking screws are inserted percutaneously with the attached drill guide, after removing the intramedullary guide wire (Fig. 37-17). The operator should avoid placing the

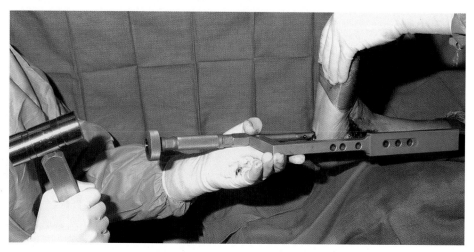

**Figure 37-14.** Advancing the intramedullary nail through the calcaneus after underreaming by 0.5 mm provides satisfactory compression across the construct.

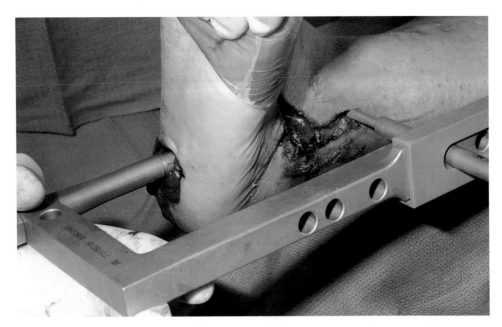

**Figure 37-15.** The construct is rotated just anterior to the fibula for ease of placement of the transverse locking screws. An oblique angle through the calcaneus can improve purchase.

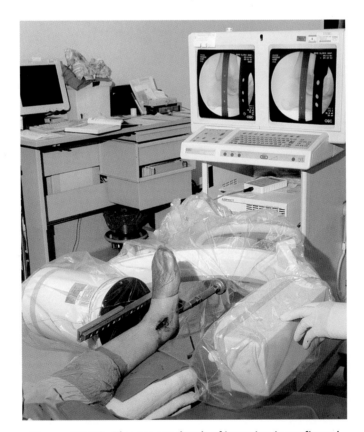

**Figure 37-16.** The proper depth of insertion is confirmed with image intensification. C-arm images demonstrate insufficient depth of insertion on the right screen and proper alignment of the locking screw holes on the left. Notice the medial ankle incision.

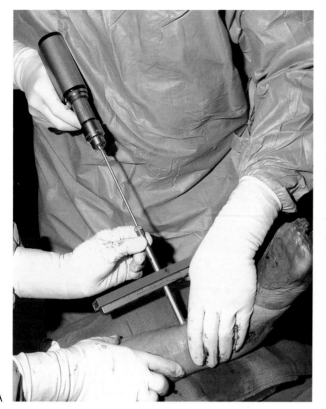

A

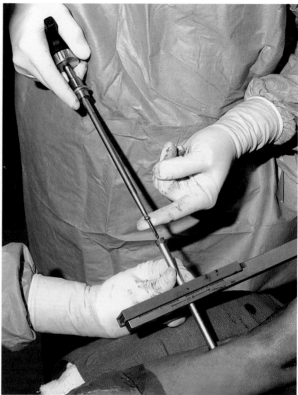

B

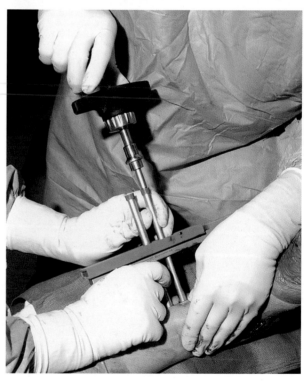

C

**Figure 37-17. A:** The surgeon ensures that the drill sleeves are inserted down to the tibia by gently tapping with a small mallet. Drilling is done for proximal locking screws. Measuring with depth gauge requires that the outer drill sleeve remain tightly against the bone. **B:** Locking screws are inserted through the outer drill sleeve with T-handled wrench. **C:** Adjacent drill sleeves are placed through separate percutaneous incisions. *(continued)*

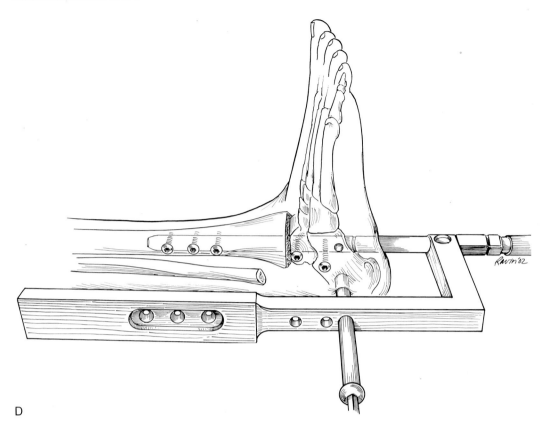

D

**Figure 37-17.** *Continued.* **D:** The drawing shows placement of a distal locking screw with the T-handled wrench. Three proximal locking screws have already been placed.

transverse locking screws through the fibula, because this provides less secure fixation. Attempts to pass the drill bit through the nail without first removing the guide wire will result in frustration and increased tourniquet time. The proximal locking screws are inserted through the tibia, and then the distal two screws are inserted through the calcaneus, with an optional screw through the talus (this hole is rarely used). It is preferable to have good purchase with both of the distal (calcaneal) locking screws. Some surgeons recommend placing the calcaneal screws from posterior to anterior in the sagittal plane to gain additional fixation.

The surgeon checks the final clinical alignment and confirms the final construct under image intensification in all planes (Fig. 37-18). If the position or fixation is unsatisfactory, the operator proceeds with revision and additional fixation as needed. External fixation is always available for patients who may require an intraoperative salvage option. Any remaining bone graft material is placed about the fusion site, and the incision is closed in layers.

Before deflating the tourniquet, the limb is placed in a short-leg Robert Jones compression dressing with stirrup splints maintaining the foot in neutral position (Fig. 37-19). With proper use of the Robert Jones dressing to control swelling and hematoma formation, a drain has not been routinely used.

As a result of using the posterior approach in our initial experience and then later the lateral approach, some aspects of this procedure have become evident. First, the ability to realign severe deformity is present through either approach, with a minimum of periosteal stripping. Osteotomies of the fibula combined with resection of the distal tibial plafond and talar dome and occasional resection of the medial malleolus afford realignment of a significant deformity into a plantigrade position. Second, in patients with avascular necrosis, it is important that the necrotic or dysvascular talar body be adequately debrided or a trough created through the body of the talus from the tibia down to the calcaneus. Filling the re-

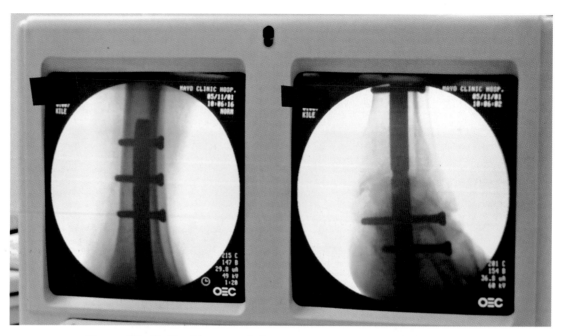

**Figure 37-18.** Final images of the construct are seen with the mini-fluoroscopy unit and demonstrate satisfactory alignment and hardware placement.

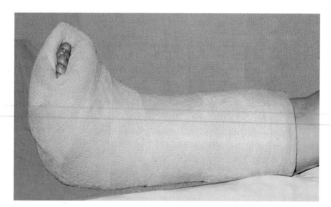

**Figure 37-19.** Modified Robert Jones compression dressing minimizes swelling and hematoma formation, with a stirrup splint maintaining a satisfactory foot position.

sultant defect with fresh autologous bone graft minimizes the chances of delayed or nonunion.

The desire to gain compression across the ankle to stimulate an arthrodesis has been carried over from our experience with external fixation. However, it is not as important as minimizing periosteal stripping, a thorough debridement of the complex joint surfaces, satisfactory bone graft material, and rigid internal fixation. These latter concepts have provided improved results over our earlier experience.

## POSTOPERATIVE MANAGEMENT

The Robert Jones dressing and splint are changed 3 to 5 days postoperatively, and a non–weight-bearing, short-leg cast is placed if swelling allows. Sutures are removed at the next cast change, usually in 2 to 3 weeks. The patient continues non–weight-bearing ambulation for 6 weeks and then begins progressive weight bearing as tolerated in a well-molded, fiberglass walking cast for an additional 4 to 6 weeks. A minimum of 10 weeks is spent in fiberglass cast immobilization. Radiographs obtained at 2, 6, and 12 weeks usually demonstrate early satisfactory bony consolidation. Additional return visits occur at 6-week intervals. An example of a patient who underwent tibiotalocalcaneal arthrodesis is described in Figure 37-20.

A recent review of 61 consecutive patients who underwent tibiotalocalcaneal arthrodesis, at an average follow-up of 6.7 years (range, 4 to 11 years), revealed 78% were satisfied

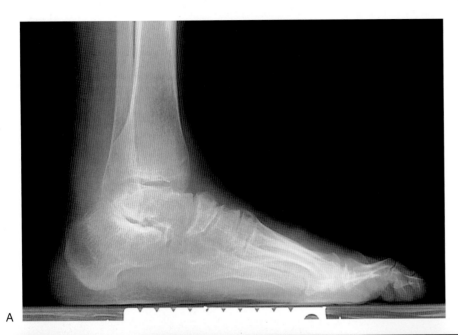

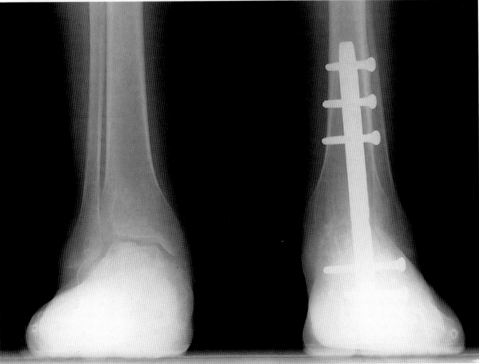

**Figure 37-20. A:** Lateral-view, weight-bearing radiographs show the ankle of a 41-year-old woman with a history of bilateral congenital clubfeet treated with surgical releases when she was a child. She subsequently developed painful, disabling arthritis of the ankle and subtalar joints and failed treatment with an ankle-foot orthosis. **B, C:** Radiographs obtained 2 years after tibiotalocalcaneal arthrodesis with an intramedullary nail show satisfactory union and good alignment. *(continued)*

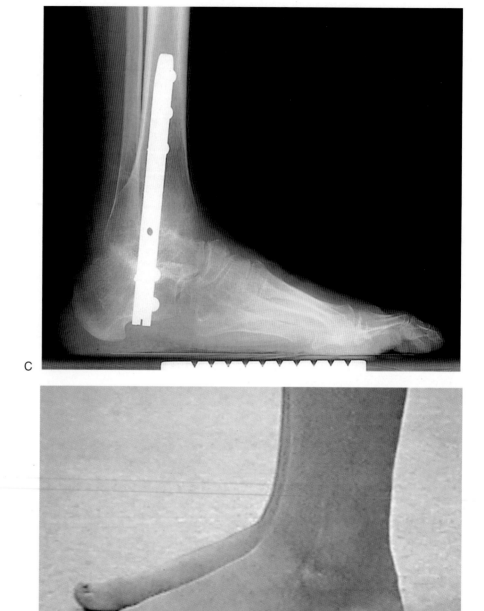

**Figure 37-20.** *Continued.* **D, E:** Clinical photographs were taken with the patient standing and rising up on her toes. The patient had relief of pain and was able to ambulate without a noticeable limp. *(continued)*

or very satisfied, without diminution of results over time. Two of these patients have returned and undergone the same procedure on the contralateral side. The average AOFAS hindfoot score was 54 of a possible 78 (allowing for lack of flexion, extension, supination, and pronation). After a tibiotalocalcaneal arthrodesis, the patients may notice a slight limp with a shorter stride length. However, pain relief is very good, and formal physical therapy is rarely necessary. An extra-depth shoe with a rocker bottom and cushioned heel can com-

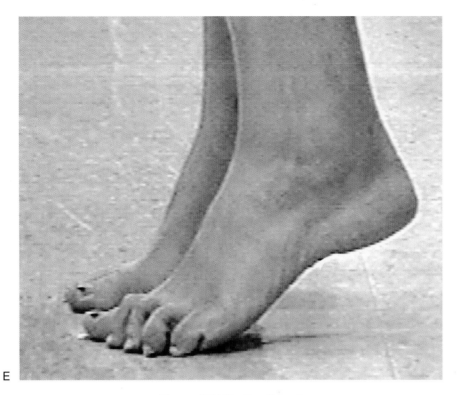

E

**Figure 37-20.** *Continued.*

pensate for any shortening and facilitate gait, but most patients usually opt for a soft lace-up shoe such as an athletic or casual shoe.

The most challenging aspect of the recovery process, particularly for elderly patients, is the initial 6 weeks or longer of a strict non–weight-bearing program and cast immobilization. The physician must resist the temptation to shorten the patient's time spent in a fiberglass cast in favor of early bony union. Intensive physical therapy and occupational therapy during the initial hospitalization, as well as possible transfer to an inpatient rehabilitation facility, may be necessary to ensure compliance and safety for the patient. As weight bearing is advanced, most patients are able to mobilize independently and do not require any further therapeutic intervention.

## COMPLICATIONS

Complications in this relatively high-risk patient population do occur and are discussed with the patients during the preoperative consultation. Wound healing difficulties with eventual deep sepsis, delayed unions, nonunions, malunions, stress fractures, or hardware failure comprise most postoperative complications seen in this group. In a series of 91 procedures, 92% achieved satisfactory clinical and radiographic union, but 35% developed a wound complication, 22% sustained some form of hardware failure, and 9% healed in excessive varus or valgus. Thirty-seven cases of cortical hypertrophy occurred, and 3 of these patients sustained stress fractures. Three patients developed infected nonunions, requiring debridement, revision, or below-knee amputation.

*Nonunions* are infrequent but can develop, particularly in those patients with inadequate bone preparation, graft, or fixation. Infatuation with the intramedullary fixation device can lead to inattention during the preparation of the surfaces for arthrodesis. Early or unprotected weight bearing can also lead to a loss of fixation and eventual nonunion. If a nonunion is evident at 6 months, continued non–weight-bearing cast immobilization and electrical stimulation may be all that is necessary. However, repeat bone grafting and additional internal fixation may be required.

*Malunion* can develop intraoperatively or postoperatively, particularly if the method of fixation allows the ankle to plantarflex during the procedure or during the initial healing period. A mild to moderate equinus deformity can be treated with a simple heel lift or shoewear modifications. The more severe deformities may require corrective osteotomy through the distal tibial metaphysis and repeat fixation.

*Stress fractures*, or more commonly cortical hypertrophic areas, are seen near the proximal aspect of the intramedullary device. They are treated with simple cast immobilization, and weight bearing is allowed to progress based on symptoms. Hardware failure can occur, usually in the form of transverse locking screw breakage. This often allows the fusion site to settle and eventually unite. However, should the nail or screws become proud, hardware removal may be indicated.

*Dehiscence or necrosis* of the incision may occur. The posterior approach seems to be more susceptible to this complication than the lateral approach described previously, particularly in patients with rheumatoid arthritis or diabetes. The surgeon should maintain full-thickness skin flaps, avoid forceps trauma to the skin, and pay attention to the closure, and a few days of compression dressing immobilization can minimize wound problems. When the incision does breakdown, use local wound care with dressing changes and antibiotics to prevent secondary infection. Rarely, split-thickness skin grafting or free-tissue transfer is needed to provide adequate skin coverage.

In the absence of a draining wound, deep *infection* of the hardware can be difficult to diagnose. The physician should maintain a high index of suspicion for patients who present with pain, fracture of the intramedullary nail, backing-out of the hardware or nonunion with radiolucency about the hardware. Aggressive debridement with hardware removal and prolonged, culture-directed antibiotic therapy, combined with rigid external fixation, may provide satisfactory resolution. However, some patients eventually require below-knee amputation as their final salvage procedure.

Dynamization is rarely necessary with this device, because compression is generated during insertion, and a press fit is obtained as the intramedullary nail is passed through the calcaneus. Occasionally, if the locking screws fail distally, the construct self-dynamizes and allows some settling. If the distal end of the intramedullary nail become prominent, hardware removal may become necessary.

## RECOMMENDED READING

1. Acosta R, Ushiba J, Cracchiolo A: The results of a primary and staged pantalar arthrodesis and tibiotalocalcaneal arthrodesis in adult patients. *Foot Ankle Int* 21:182–194, 2000.
2. Blair HZ: Comminuted fractures and fracture dislocations of the body of the talus: operative treatment. *Am J Surg* 59:37–43, 1943.
3. Chou LB, Mann RA, Yaszay B, et al.: Tibiotalocalcaneal arthrodesis. *Foot Ankle Int* 21:804–808, 2000.
4. Johnson KA: Tibiocalcaneal arthrodesis. In: Thompson RC Jr, ed. *Master techniques in orthopaedic surgery – the foot and ankle*, 1st ed. New York: Raven Press, 1994:483–496.
5. Kile TA, Donnelly RE, Gehrke JC, et al.: Tibiotalocalcaneal arthrodesis with an intramedullary device. *Foot Ankle Int* 15:669–673, 1994.
6. Lidor C, Ferris LR, Hall R, et al.: Stress fracture of the tibia after arthrodesis of the ankle or hindfoot. *J Bone Joint Surg Am* 79:558–564, 1997.
7. McLeod DH, Wong DH, Vaghadia H, et al.: Lateral popliteal sciatic nerve block compared with ankle block for analgesia following foot surgery. *Can J Anaesth* 42:765–769, 1995.
8. Otterberg ET, McMullen ST, Fitzgibbons TC: Arthrodesis in the foot using demineralized bone matrix and bone marrow aspirate as an alternative to iliac crest bone grafting. *Orthop Trans* 22:1111, 1999.
9. Papa JA, Myerson MS: Pantalar and tibiotalocalcaneal arthrodesis for post-traumatic osteoarthrosis of the ankle and hindfoot. *J Bone Joint Surg Am* 74:1042–1049, 1992.
10. Russotti GM, Johnson KA, Cass JR: Tibiocalcaneal arthrodesis for arthritis and deformity of the hind part of the foot. *J Bone Joint Surg Am* 70:1304–1307, 1988.
11. Thordarson DB, Chang D: Stress fracture and tibial cortical hypertrophy after tibiotalocalcaneal arthrodesis with an intramedullary nail. *Foot Ankle Int* 20:497–500, 1999.

# 38

# Arthroscopic Ankle Arthrodesis

## James W. Stone

## INDICATIONS/CONTRAINDICATIONS

The most common indication for ankle arthrodesis is persistent ankle pain and disability from severe ankle arthritis unresponsive to nonoperative treatment, including the use of nonsteroidal antiinflammatory medications, orthotics, braces, and corticosteroid injections. Radiographs may reveal loss of joint space, osteophyte formation, loose body formation, and joint malalignment (Fig. 38-1). The most common etiologies of joint degeneration are osteoarthritis, posttraumatic degenerative arthritis, and rheumatoid arthritis. Less common etiologies include hemophilic arthritis, congenital deformity, crystalline arthritis (gout and pseudogout), and osteochondral lesions of the talus. Contraindications to arthroscopic ankle fusion include patients with severe arthritic changes who also have significant ankle malalignment in valgus or varus. Arthroscopic ankle fusion cannot be used to correct deformity greater than approximately 5° to 10°. In particular, preoperative planning must be performed to ensure that the ankle can be placed into a neutral or slight valgus position. Varus position of the ankle fusion is poorly tolerated and results in a painful callus on the lateral aspect of the foot.

Patients with avascular necrosis of the talus have a lower rate of fusion with arthroscopic or open approaches and represent a contraindication to arthroscopic ankle arthrodesis. The procedure is also contraindicated for patients with concomitant hindfoot arthritis leading to infection, neuropathy, or peripheral vascular disease.

## SURGERY

The patient is placed supine on the operating table, with the flexed hip and knee supported by a padded leg holder, as described in Chapter 35 (Fig. 38-2). The noninvasive ankle distractor is applied and routine anteromedial, anterolateral, posterolateral portals are created

J. W. Stone, M.D.: Department of Orthopaedic Surgery, Medical College of Wisconsin, Milwaukee, Wisconsin.

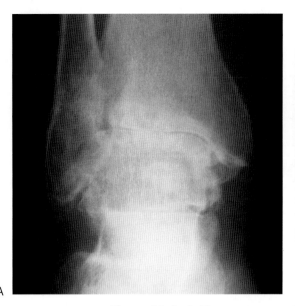
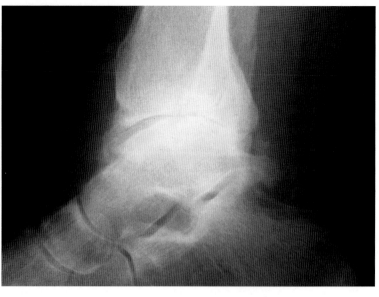

A                                                                                            B

**Figure 38-1.  A:** The anteroposterior radiograph of a patient's ankle with severe post-traumatic degenerative arthritis shows satisfactory alignment. **B:** The lateral view shows anterior osteophytes, which are commonly seen in patients with severe osteoarthritic ankles undergoing arthrodesis.

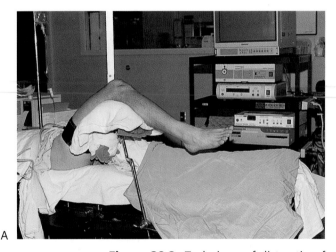
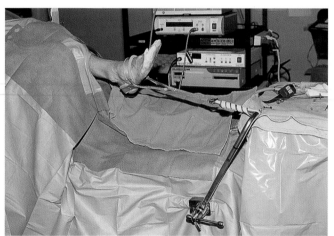

A                                                                                            B

**Figure 38-2.** Technique of distraction for arthroscopic ankle arthrodesis. **A:** The patient is positioned supine on the operating table, with the ipsilateral hip and knee supported by a well-padded leg holder. **B:** After sterile prepping and draping of the lower extremity. *(continued)*

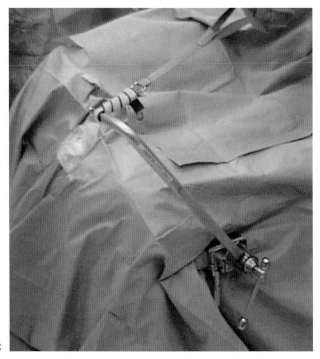

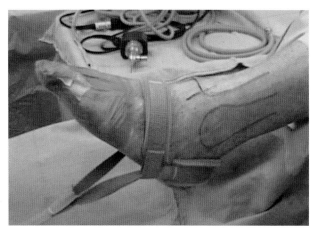

C

D

**Figure 38-2.** *Continued.* **C:** Close-up view of the ankle distractor fixed to the operating table using a sterile clamp. The commercially available strap is placed around the heel and midfoot, and traction is applied using a Velcro strap. **D:** Close-up view of the Velcro strap applied to the foot. The outlines of the tibia and fibula are marked on skin, as well as a line marking the medial-lateral position of the anterolateral portal.

(Fig. 38-2). The arthroscopic view shows large areas of cartilage loss (Fig. 38-3). If a large anterior osteophyte is present, it should be debrided as described in Chapter 35 to allow better joint visualization and better coaptation of the joint surfaces at the conclusion of the case. Initial visualization may also be impaired by anterior joint synovitis. This material should be debrided with a shaver, exercising care to avoid injury to soft tissues anterior to the joint capsule such as neurovascular structures. Scar tissue within the medial or lateral gutter may also impair reduction of the joint surfaces, therefore both gutters should be aggressively debrided using a curette and/or a shaver (Fig. 38-4).

The initial debridement of the joint involves removal of any remaining articular cartilage. This procedure is most efficiently performed using a simple motorized synovial re-

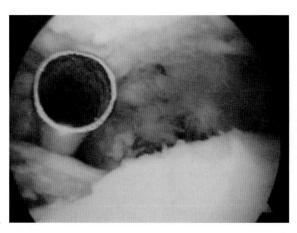

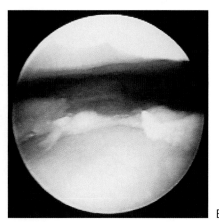

A

B

**Figure 38-3. A:** In the initial arthroscopic view of a severely arthritic ankle joint, the inflow cannula is seen. **B:** Large areas of complete articular cartilage loss are seen over the talar dome.

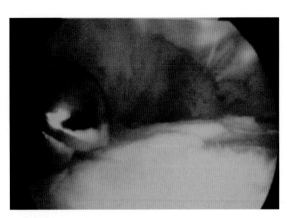

**Figure 38-4.** Various instruments, such as curettes and a shaver, are used to debride ligament, scar tissue, and articular cartilage from the medial and lateral gutters.

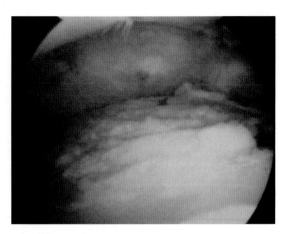

**Figure 38-5.** Tibiotalar joint appearance after initial debridement using a shaver and curettes before debridement with a motorized burr.

sector. The procedure is tedious, and it is important not to get bogged down trying to debride one specific area. Instead, the surgeon should keep the instruments moving, and switch from medial to lateral portals to approach debridement of the talar dome and tibial plafond in a systematic manner. The posterolateral portal can be very useful for debridement of the posterior talar dome and tibial plafond if these areas cannot be reached with instruments through the standard operating portals. Occasionally, an accessory anteromedial or anterolateral portal may be useful for medial or lateral gutter debridement. A combination of straight and angled curettes are used to debride any remaining articular cartilage that was not removed with the shaver (Fig. 38-5).

After complete debridement of all surfaces, the bone must be abraded to bleeding, viable subchondral bone. This procedure is best performed using a round burr (Fig. 38-6). In general, the largest burr that can fit within the joint is the best one to use, because the larger radius of curvature of the burr gives the flattest surface with the least grooving of the surface. Only approximately 1 to 2 mm of bone needs to be removed to achieve a viable bone bed. It is not necessary to expose cancellous bone. The viability of the exposed bony surfaces and the completeness of the debridement can be evaluated by decreasing the inflow pressure and observing the surfaces for bleeding (Fig. 38-7). This procedure allows the surgeon to direct attention to areas not demonstrating adequate bleeding so that further burring can be performed.

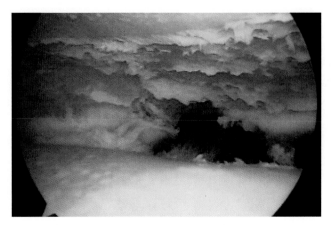

**Figure 38-6.** Arthroscopic appearance of the joint surfaces after abrasion, showing viable, bleeding subchondral bone.

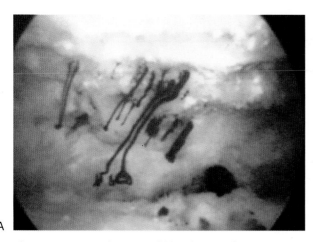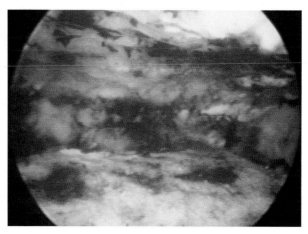

A                                                                                          B

**Figure 38-7.** Evaluation of bleeding surfaces by decreasing inflow pressure. **A:** Bleeding from bony surfaces shortly after inflow pressure was released. Areas that fail to demonstrate adequate bleeding should have additional debridement with the burr. **B:** Bony surfaces after adequate debridement with the burr.

Fixation is accomplished with multiple screws. There are variations in screw types, sizes, orientation, and number. Cannulated screws of 6.5 mm or larger are typically used for fixation of the arthrodesis. I prefer a self-drilling, self-tapping, 6.5-mm cancellous screw with a large guide pin. The large-diameter guide pin allows easy repositioning if necessary and is unlikely to bend or break.

Several screw configurations have been described and advocated in the literature. A crossed two-screw technique involves directing one of the screws across the medial malleolus into the talar body and a second screw across the lateral malleolus into the talar neck. A second technique uses two screws placed from the medial side into the talar neck and body in a parallel fashion. A third technique uses the crossed transmalleolar screw construct, with a third screw placed from posterior to anterior, entering adjacent to the lateral border of the Achilles tendon or through the Achilles tendon. Although this third screw has been shown to impart a greater degree of rigidity to the fixation construct, surgeons have found that the two-screw technique is adequate and has a high union rate.

Accurate guide pin placement can be facilitated by visualizing placement of the pins with the arthroscope as they enter the joint (Fig. 38-8). The entry point medially should be at the angle of curvature where the tibial plafond and medial malleolus meet. The entry point lat-

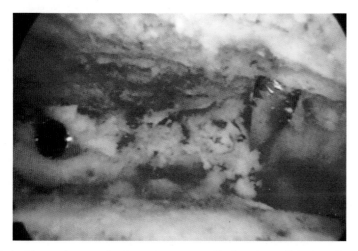

**Figure 38-8.** The arthroscopic view shows a well-placed medial pin. The pin ideally should enter the joint at the angle of curvature of the medial malleolus and should engage the talus well as it is advanced. After ensuring a good position, the pin is backed out to beneath the surface of the tibia.

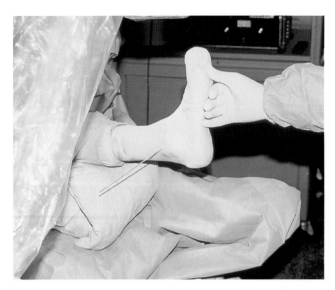

**Figure 38-9.** After guide pin placement, the distraction device is removed, the leg is removed from the leg holder, and the fluoroscope is used to monitor pin advancement.

erally should be at the level of the tibial-fibular articulation. The pins are inserted at an angle of approximately 45° in the coronal plane and 45° in the sagittal plane. They are visualized arthroscopically to confirm that the entry point in the joint will allow passage into the talus at the appropriate location and angle. After ascertaining that the pins are in appropriate position, they are withdrawn to a position just beneath the bone surface.

At this point, the noninvasive distraction device is removed, and the leg is taken out of the leg holder. Intraoperative radiographs are obtained using a fluoroscope (Fig. 38-9). The surgeon stabilizes the ankle in the appropriate position for fusion: neutral dorsiflexion-plantarflexion and slight valgus. Varus positioning is assiduously avoided. As longitudinal

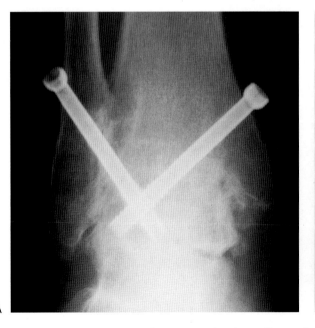
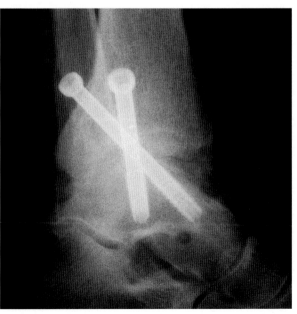

A                                                                                                    B

**Figure 38-10.** The radiographs show transmalleolar screw placement. **A:** Anteroposterior view. **B:** Lateral view.

compression is applied across the joint, the medial pin is advanced into appropriate position, engaging the maximum amount of talar bone while carefully avoiding penetration of the subtalar joint. The screw is then advanced over the guide pin and tightened. Anteroposterior, lateral, and oblique radiographic views are obtained to ensure good screw position without subtalar joint penetration. The second medial screw (or the lateral screw if bimalleolar fixation is chosen) is advanced in a similar fashion and radiographs obtained (Figs. 38-10 and 38-11). As an alternative, two screws may be inserted posteromedial to anterolateral, parallel to each other (Fig. 38-12).

Incisions are closed with nylon suture. A bulky compressive dressing with a posterior plaster splint is applied.

*(Text continued on page 579.)*

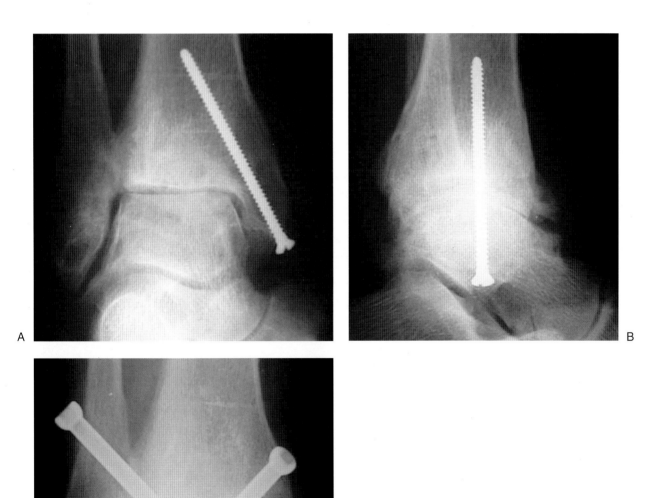

**Figure 38-11.** Transmalleolar screw placement. **A:** In the anteroposterior ankle radiograph obtained preoperatively, severe ankle arthritis is seen. **B:** Lateral view obtained preoperatively. **C:** Anteroposterior view shows crossed screws, good alignment, and good bony apposition. *(continued)*

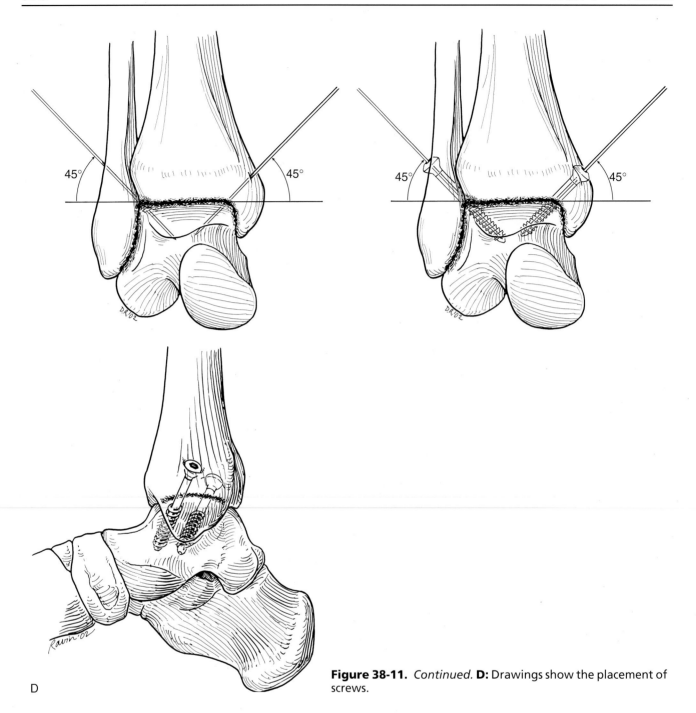

D

**Figure 38-11.** *Continued.* **D:** Drawings show the placement of screws.

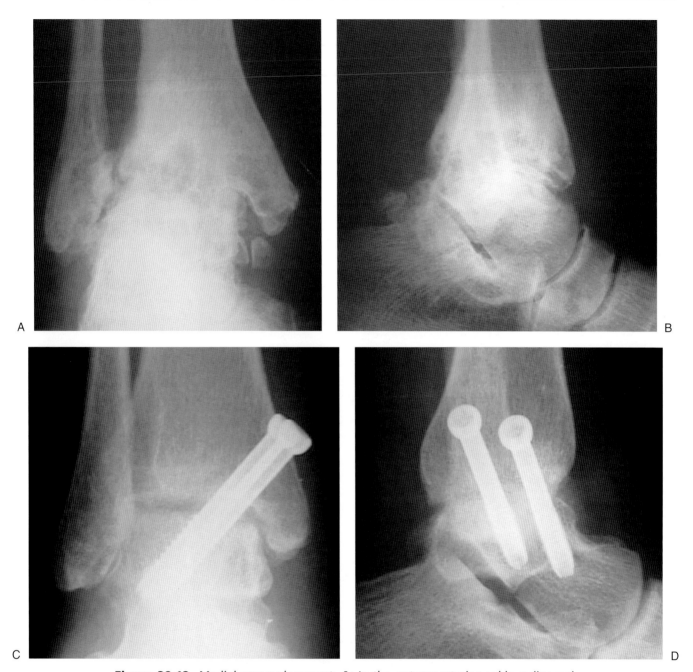

**Figure 38-12.** Medial screw placement. **A:** In the anteroposterior ankle radiograph obtained preoperatively, severe arthritis affects the ankle. **B:** Lateral view obtained preoperatively. **C:** Anteroposterior view in the early postoperative period shows progressive union of arthrodesis, parallel screws, good alignment, and good bony apposition. **D:** Lateral view in early postoperative period. *(continued)*

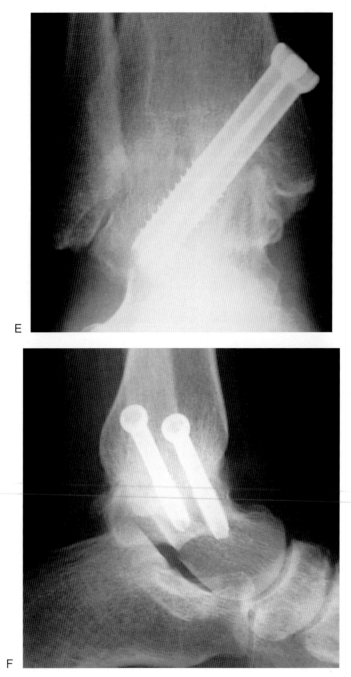

**Figure 38-12.** *Continued.* **E:** An anteroposterior radiograph at final follow-up shows a solid union. **F:** Lateral radiograph at final follow-up. *(continued)*

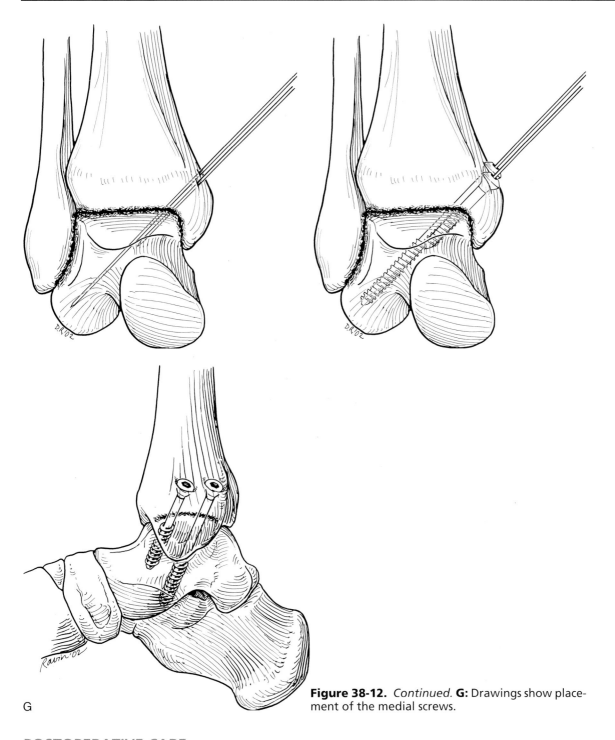

G

**Figure 38-12.** *Continued.* **G:** Drawings show placement of the medial screws.

## POSTOPERATIVE CARE

The postoperative dressing is removed in 5 to 7 days, when the sutures are removed. A removable, short-leg walking boot is applied. Non–weight-bearing ambulation using crutches or a walker is suggested for the first 4 weeks postoperatively, and weight bearing is then increased as tolerated. Radiographs are obtained at monthly intervals to monitor healing. The walking boot is used until radiographic union is achieved, usually 8 to 12 weeks postoperatively. Afterward, a regular shoe is used or a shoe with a rocker-bottom sole.

Several published studies have documented the utility of arthroscopic ankle arthrodesis, with high rate of fusion of more than 90% and a low incidence of complications. These operations were generally performed in patients who had one joint affected, little or no deformity, and few other complicating factors. Studies that compared open with arthroscopic techniques found a more rapid rate of fusion with the arthroscopic method. It is difficult to draw firm conclusions from these comparative reports that were nonrandomized, retrospective studies. Although unproved, the rapid rate of fusion has been attributed to the minimal soft tissue dissection compared with open techniques, the large surface area of joint coaptation obtained by the *in situ* method, and the rigid fixation achieved using the compression screw technique.

We compared a group of 19 arthroscopic ankle fusions with a group of 17 fusions performed through standard arthrotomy and resecting the joint surfaces with flat cuts. All of the patients in the open group would otherwise have qualified for the arthroscopic procedure based on the limited degree of preoperative deformity and the ability to achieve a neutral position preoperatively. There were no significant differences in distribution by age, gender, weight, deformity, smoking history, or diagnosis between the two groups. We found significant differences in intraoperative blood loss, tourniquet time, and hospitalization. Most of the arthroscopic fusions were performed as outpatient procedures or as 24-hour admissions in the hospital. There were three nonunions in the open group and one nonunion in the arthroscopic group. The one nonunion in the arthroscopic group occurred in a patient with avascular necrosis of the talus. Analysis of ankle position on postoperative radiographs suggested the position of the ankle fusion in the arthroscopic was more consistent compared with the open fusion group.

## COMPLICATIONS

Complication rates as high as 55% have been reported with this operation, although most are considered minor and manageable. In a report of 42 procedures, there were nonunions (3), fractures (2), pin site infections (4), deep infection (1), hardware problems (4), and painful subtalar joints (4). The common complication after arthroscopic ankle surgery is superficial nerve injury at the portal site. This complication can be avoided by careful attention to the technique of portal creation. The portal must be created by incising the skin only, spreading the subcutaneous tissues with a hemostat and then penetrating the capsule with a blunt trocar. The portal should be large enough to easily pass the instruments. Inserting a large shaver or burr through a small portal causes soft tissue trauma, increasing the likelihood of skin problems, nerve injury, and sinus tract formation.

There were no infections or deep vein thrombosis in our series. One patient with *avascular necrosis* of the talus went on to *nonunion* of the fusion, and an open procedure was performed to achieve successful fusion. *Delayed union* may occur, and externally applied electrical stimulation may enhance healing potential in some patients.

## RECOMMENDED READING

1. Crosby LA, Yee TC, Formanek TC, et al.: Complications following arthroscopic ankle arthrodesis. *Foot Ankle Int* 17:340–342, 1996.
2. Ewing JW, Tasto JA, Tippett JW: Arthroscopic surgery of the ankle. *Instr Course Lect* 44:325–340, 1995.
3. Fitzgibbons TC: Arthroscopic ankle debridement and fusion: indications, techniques, and results. *Instr Course Lect* 48:243–248, 1999.
4. Glick JM, Ferkel RD: Arthroscopic ankle arthrodesis. In: Ferkel RD, ed. *Arthroscopic surgery: the foot and ankle.* Philadelphia: Lippincott-Raven, 1996:215.
5. Glick JM, Morgan CD, Myerson MS, et al.: Ankle arthrodesis using and arthroscopic method: long-term and follow-up of 34 cases. *Arthroscopy* 12:428–434, 1996.
6. Morgan CD, Henke JA, Bailey RW, et al.: Long-term results of tibiotalar arthrodesis. *J Bone Joint Surg Am* 67:546–550, 1985.
7. Myerson MS, Quill G: Ankle arthrodesis—a comparison of an arthroscopic and an open method of treatment. *Clin Orthop* 268:84–95, 1991.
8. O'Brian TS, Hart TS, Shereff MJ, et al.: Open versus arthroscopic ankle arthrodesis: a comparative study. *Foot Ankle Int* 20:368–374, 1999.
9. Ogilvie-Harris DJ, Lieberman I, Fitsialos D: Arthroscopically assisted arthrodesis for osteoarthrotic ankles. *J Bone Joint Surg Am* 75:1167–1174, 1993.

# 39

# Total Ankle Replacement

Carl T. Hasselman, Yue Shuen Wong, and Stephen F. Conti

## INDICATIONS/CONTRAINDICATIONS

First-generation total ankle arthroplasty produced a rather disappointing long-term survival despite various designs. Earlier designs, including cemented, uncemented, constrained, and nonconstrained types, had high failure rates compared with hip and knee replacements. However, newer prostheses that have shown lower failure rates at almost 5-year follow-up have given hope for longer survival rates (6).

Total ankle arthroplasty is indicated for patients with severe ankle arthritis whose pain limits their activities of daily living despite attempts at nonoperative treatment. This may include weight loss, activity modification, nonsteroidal antiinflammatory pain medication regimens, corticosteroid injections, modalities such as ice or heat, bracing, orthoses, and footwear modification. Ankle arthritis may be primary osteoarthritis, posttraumatic, inflammatory, or result from hemophilia or avascular necrosis of the talar dome. Varus or valgus deformity must be less than 20° for successful correction using an ankle prosthesis. Although some physicians have successfully performed ankle arthroplasty after previous ankle arthrodesis, we have little experience with this (3). The ideal candidate for ankle arthroplasty is older than 50 years of age, has a smaller build or is of average size, weighs less than 250 pounds, has no expectations of return to impact sports or manual labor, and whose only other option is ankle arthrodesis.

Absolute contraindications to total ankle arthroplasty are lower extremity neuropathy, avascular necrosis involving a significant portion of the body of the talus, active or chronic infection involving the ankle joint, absent or inadequate leg muscle function, previous ankle fusion with removal of the malleoli, and severe ankle deformity with varus or valgus tilt of more than 20° (5). The operation is relatively contraindicated for younger patients, heavier patients, preoperative total ankle range of motion less than 20°, a history of a pre-

C. T. Hasselman, M.D.: Department of Orthopaedic Surgery, University of Pittsburgh; and Three Rivers Orthopaedic Associates, Pittsburgh, Pennsylvania.

Y. S. Wong, M.B., B.S., F.R.C.S. (Edin): Department of Orthopaedic Surgery, Alexandra Hospital, Singapore.

S. F. Conti, M.D.: Department of Orthopedic Surgery, University of Pittsburgh School of Medicine; and Division of Foot and Ankle Surgery, University of Pittsburgh Physicians, Pittsburgh, Pennsylvania.

vious ankle infection, severe osteoporosis, inadequate soft tissues around the ankle joint, poor vascular supply to the leg, segmental bone loss of the talus or distal tibia, and those expecting to return to heavy manual labor or aggressive weight-bearing activity.

## PREOPERATIVE PLANNING

Planning for ankle arthroplasty is similar to that involved in other joint arthroplasties, with some significant differences. The main difference is that rather than a two-bone system like that found in the hip and knee, the ankle has a complex arrangement of 26 bones and 35 joints below it, which contributes significantly to the loading characteristics of the prosthesis. Another consideration, which usually does not apply to hip and knee arthroplasty, is that the most common form of ankle arthritis is posttraumatic rather than osteoarthritis. This is important because the soft tissue envelope that exists around the ankle is naturally thin and often damaged from trauma before ankle arthroplasty. Ligament balancing and range of motion are often compromised and must be accurately assessed before surgery.

The first step in preoperative planning for ankle arthroplasty should be to evaluate the entire lower extremity for any deformities. Previous tibial shaft fractures may also have resulted in the tibial plafond not being parallel to the ground. Angulation of the plafond in any direction in relationship to the axis of the tibia greater than 10° may require a correctional osteotomy before ankle arthroplasty. The distal tibia may be deformed from a tibial pilon fracture. If there is any question about the integrity of the bone in the distal tibial metaphysis, computed tomography (CT) of the distal tibia should be done. The CT scan can be useful in planning surgery for orientation of bone cuts and likelihood of requiring bone graft. Subtalar varus from a cavus foot or subtalar valgus from a severe flatfoot may also cause abnormal loading of the prosthesis and early failure. If the deformity is small and passively correctable, often correction is achieved by simply completing the arthroplasty. If the deformity is large, corrective osteotomies are needed to obtain a plantigrade foot (2).

Generally, if the hip or knee is arthritic and significantly symptomatic, the joint should undergo replacement before ankle arthroplasty. If the ankle is replaced first, correction of any valgus or varus of the knee at the time of subsequent knee arthroplasty will effect the alignment of the ankle replacement with respect to the ground. If one suspects that other joints such as subtalar or talonavicular are a source of significant symptoms, further investigation is warranted such as plain radiography of the foot and ankle and sometimes special studies such as CT, magnetic resonance imaging (MRI), or radionuclide imaging. Selective lidocaine injections into suspect joints may also assist in localizing the source of the pain. If the subtalar and talonavicular joints are significantly affected by arthritis, fusion of these joints should be considered before, during, or after ankle replacement. The decision is based on whether the ankle arthritis has caused symmetric or asymmetric collapse of the tibiotalar joint and the surgeon's ability to perform arthroplasty and arthrodesis. If the arthritis has caused symmetric narrowing and the alignment is close to normal, performing these other fusions can be done before or during the arthroplasty procedure. If the arthritis has caused asymmetric narrowing with malalignment, the fusions are best performed during or after the ankle arthroplasty procedure to ensure that a plantigrade foot is obtained (4).

The ligaments and tendons around the ankle must be evaluated before arthroplasty. If the ankle cannot be restored to at least neutral position during active-assisted dorsiflexion, an Achilles tendon contracture, posterior capsular contracture, or anterior ankle osteophytes must be considered as possible causes. Lengthening of the Achilles tendon may be performed proximally or distally if the contracture is considered a significant part of the deformity. Lateral ligamentous laxity may be a cause for ankle arthritis. If the lateral ligament complex is felt to be incompetent by anterior drawer and talar tilt testing, or in cases of severe varus and ankle arthritis, reconstruction using a peroneus brevis tenodesis procedure or ligament repair such as the modified Bröstrom repair must be planned as a part of the arthroplasty surgery.

Scars from previous surgical procedures must also be taken into consideration. The stan-

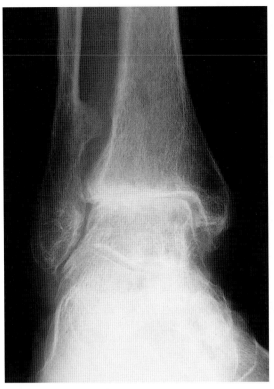
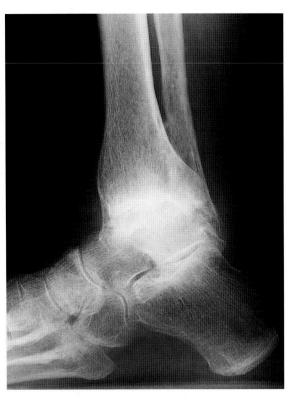

A                                                                                    B

**Figure 39-1.** **A:** Mortise view of the ankle shows severe loss of the normal joint space and partial erosion of the lateral tibia. **B:** Lateral view reveals tibial erosion with mild joint space loss in the subtalar region and significant osteophyte formation in the anterior ankle.

dard incision for ankle arthroplasty is the anterior approach; however, modifications of the standard incision may be needed to avoid creating parallel incisions around the ankle that are within 5 cm of each other. If it is necessary to cross a previous incision, crossing at a 90° angle may lessen the potential for creating devascularized skin flaps.

The Agility Ankle replacement (DePuy, Warsaw, IN) has six possible implant sizes to accommodate most ankle sizes and shapes. Before surgery, standard weight-bearing, anteroposterior, mortise, and lateral ankle radiographs should be obtained (Fig. 39-1). Full-length lower extremity radiographs should be obtained when significant alignment difficulties are expected. Standard radiographic templates are available from the manufacturer that can be used to estimate the size of the implant needed (1).

We use the Agility Ankle replacement. If a different prosthesis is used, the surgeon should review the surgical technique of the specific prosthesis before its use.

## SURGERY

Patient positioning involves placing the patient supine on a radiolucent table, with a soft bolster placed under the ipsilateral hip. A thigh tourniquet is placed on the leg, and the anterior and lateral ankle is shaved. The skin is prepped with alcohol and a povidone-iodine solution, and sterile plastic adhesive is used to cover the toes and knee where the sterile drapes meet the skin.

An ankle distraction device such as the EBI external fixator is used to distract and stabilize the ankle during surgery. The first pin is placed medially through the talar neck and in line with the deformity so that, if a varus angle needs to be corrected, it can be angled inferiorly and laterally parallel with the talar dome (Fig. 39-2). By attaching the first pin to the external fixator, the proper position of the second pin into the posterior calcaneus is al-

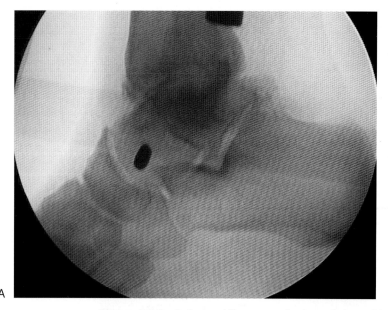
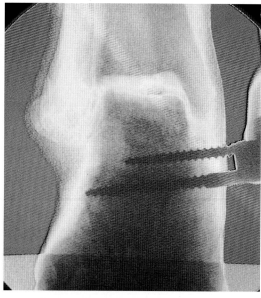

**Figure 39-2.  A:** Lateral fluoroscopic view of the ankle shows placement of the first external fixation half pin into the talar head-neck junction. **B:** Anteroposterior view of the fixation pins in the talus and calcaneus with attempted manual correction of the joint space before completing the fixation device.

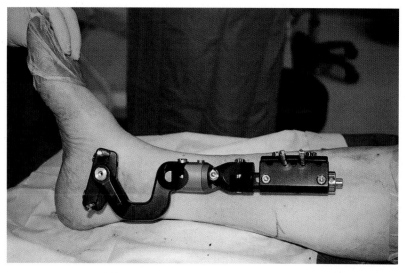
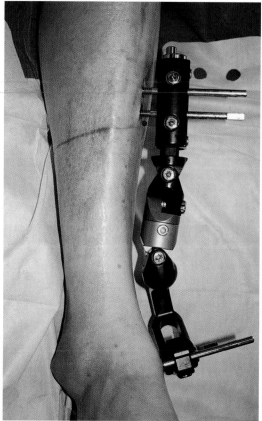

**Figure 39-3.  A:** Lateral view of the leg shows proper placement of the external fixator. Notice the direct medial placement of the tibial pins so they do not interfere with the cutting alignment jig. **B:** An anterior view of the leg and fixator shows partial distraction of the device to restore ankle joint space and alignment.

ready determined by the hole in the fixator for the second pin. The external fixator is then attached to both distal pins, and the proximal distraction-compression device is placed in the middle of compression and distraction mode (2.5 cm long, with a possible range of 0 to 5 cm). Two pins are placed in the tibia from medial to lateral using the guide holes in the fixator. The external fixator is then removed from the pins, the leg is exsanguinated, and the thigh tourniquet cuff is inflated. The external fixator is then reattached to all four pins and securely tightened. The foot is placed in neutral with any angular deformity of the ankle corrected (Fig. 39-3). At this point, the mobile joints of the external fixator are tightened to hold the foot in this position. The ankle is now distracted sufficiently to recreate the normal ankle joint space as determined by an anteroposterior radiograph using C-arm fluoroscopy.

Exposure of the ankle is achieved through a 15-cm anterior incision centered over the ankle joint and lying between the tibialis anterior and extensor hallucis longus tendons (Fig. 39-4). The superficial peroneal nerve lies within the subcutaneous fat and must be protected during dissection (Fig. 39-5). The extensor retinaculum is longitudinally incised within the tendon sheath of the extensor hallucis longus in an attempt to keep the tibialis anterior within its own tendon sheath (Fig. 39-6). The anterior tibial artery and deep peroneal nerve are located deep to the extensor hallucis longus tendon. These structures are identified and retracted laterally during the operation. The joint capsule is divided longitudinally and subperiosteal dissection is used to expose the distal tibia, fibula, and talus to the talar head and from the medial malleolus to the syndesmosis (Fig. 39-7). All osteophytes are removed from the tibia and talus so the joint is clearly visualized.

A second incision is made longitudinally over the distal fibula, maintaining at least a 5-cm skin bridge with the anterior incision (Fig. 39-8). The incision is carried directly down

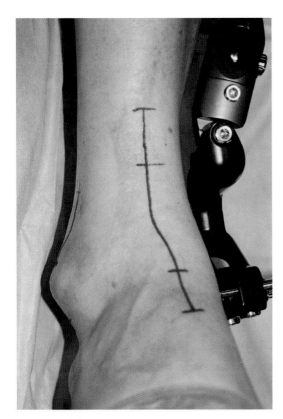

**Figure 39-4.** The skin incision for anterior exposure of the ankle is centered over the extensor hallucis longus tendon and is about 15 cm long.

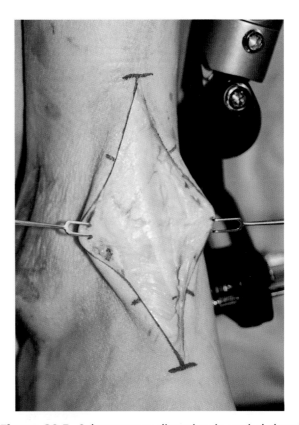

**Figure 39-5.** Subcutaneous dissection is carried sharply to the extensor retinaculum. The superficial peroneal nerve (lateral edge of the wound) is identified and retracted laterally in this dissection.

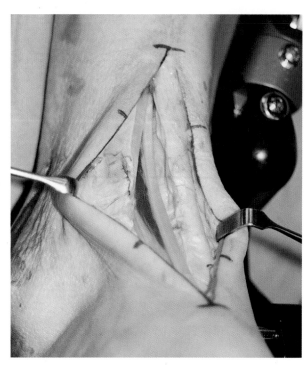

**Figure 39-6.** The sheath of the extensor hallucis longus tendon is opened to gain access to the ankle joint.

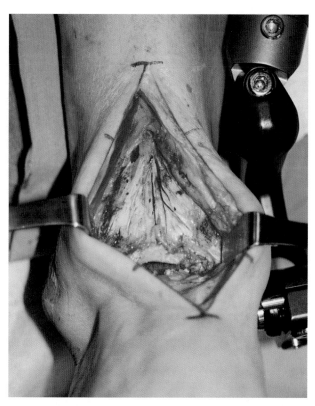

**Figure 39-7.** Subperiosteal dissection of the ankle is used to expose the joint after the deep neurovascular structures are identified and protected laterally.

to the anterolateral edge of the fibula while ensuring that no injury occurs to the branches of the superficial peroneal nerve. Subperiosteal dissection is carried anteriorly to the syndesmosis (Fig. 39-9). The syndesmotic ligaments are excised, and the syndesmosis is mobilized with an osteotome. It is important to ensure that the syndesmosis widens easily by using an osteotome to spring the fibula laterally.

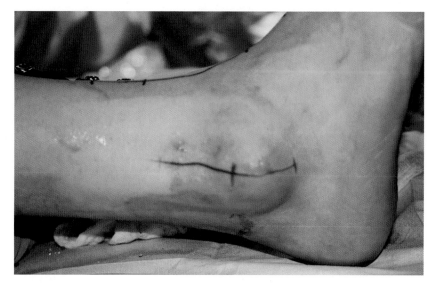

**Figure 39-8.** The lateral incision to expose the syndesmosis is made directly over the distal fibula to keep a healthy skin bridge between it and the anterior incision.

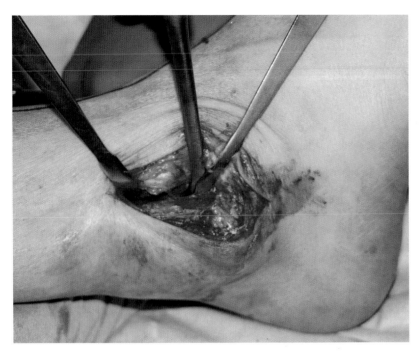

**Figure 39-9.** The syndesmosis is dissected and mobilized so that it is easily opened with a periosteal elevator.

The alignment jig is placed parallel to the tibial axis, with the proximal end centered just distal to the tibial tubercle and the shaft in line with the tibial crest (Fig. 39-10). The alignment jig distal footpads should now rest somewhat above the ankle joint. Only the medial footpad should rest on the surface of the distal tibia (Fig. 39-11). The appropriate size cutting block (as determined preoperatively) is now placed on the distal end of the alignment jig overlying the ankle joint. The footpads of the alignment jig are now secured to the tibia by placing 0.125-inch pins through the jig holes and into the tibia. The use of an image intensifier is strongly recommended to check for proper cutting block alignment. The correct determination of the cutting block's cuts is made when all four cutting slots are completely visualized (Fig. 39-12). By moving the alignment jig's fine tuning screw, the block is centered proximal-distal so that sufficient bone is removed to create bleeding of the trabecular bone on the distal tibia and talus. The cutting block is centered in the medial-lateral direction so that a small portion of the medial malleolus is removed and about one third of the medial fibula is removed. The surgeon drills two 0.125-inch pins into the cutting block to secure it in the appropriate position. If the cutting jig is placed too far medially, fracture of the medial malleolus is more likely. If the cutting jig is placed too far laterally, the tibial prosthesis will displace the talus laterally, causing deltoid overtightening and postoperative varus tilting of the talus.

The bone is resected by using an oscillating saw and reciprocating saw through the cutting block captures (Fig. 39-13). A small osteotome may be placed in the syndesmosis during bone resection to ensure that only a third of the medial fibula is resected. The triangular-shaped cutting slot at the superior end of the cutting block is used to resect a V-shaped bone cut for the tibial component fin (Fig. 39-14). This cut should not reach the posterior cortex of the distal tibia. The cutting block and alignment jig are removed, and all bone resection is completed with a reciprocating saw or osteotome (Fig. 39-15). After resected bone is removed, the tibial trial component is placed to ensure appropriate fit. Holding the trial component with the alignment handle, the surgeon inserts it by spreading the syndesmosis with an osteotome. Using the dorsal fin of the tibial trial as a reference, it is inserted straight, anterior to posterior within the distal tibia (Fig. 39-16). The tibial component articular surface will be positioned obliquely lateral 20° in relation to the trial's dorsal spine. The medial wall of the trial component should be flush with the lateral wall of the

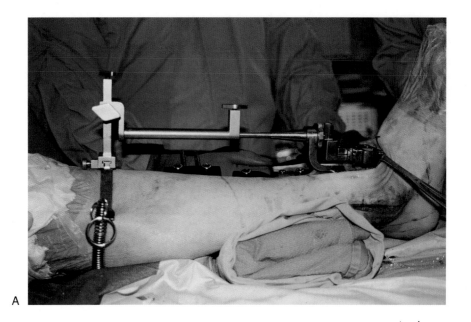

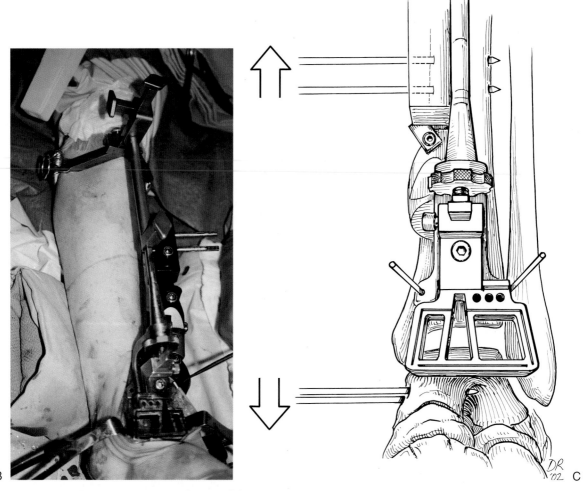

**Figure 39-10.  A:** Lateral view of the alignment jig on the leg. The jig is parallel to the long axis of the tibia. **B:** Anterior view of the jig shows the jig aligned with the crest of the tibia. **C:** The drawing shows the distal alignment foot pegs resting on the crest of the tibia and the proper alignment of the jig and cutting block.

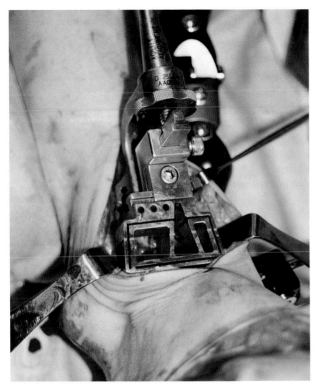

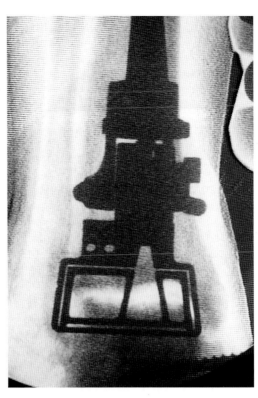

**Figure 39-11.** Close-up anterior view shows the connection of the proper-size cutting block to the alignment jig and the fine-tuning screw used to adjust the block position proximally and distally.

**Figure 39-12.** Fluoroscopic anterior view of the ankle shows proper alignment of the fluoroscopy machine with the cutting block so that all four resection guides are seen in one view.

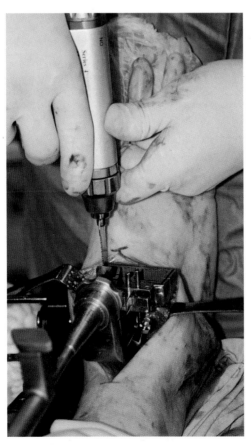

**Figure 39-13.** Bone resection is done with an oscillating and reciprocating saw using the saw captures on the cutting block.

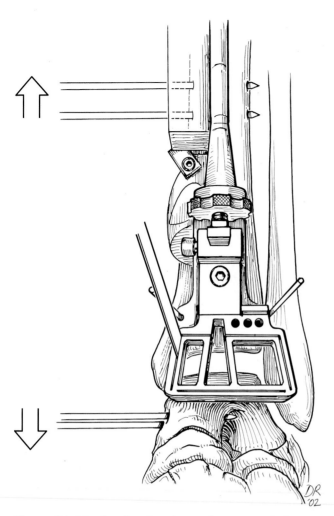

**Figure 39-14.** The drawing shows the cut needed to accommodate the spine on the tibial component.

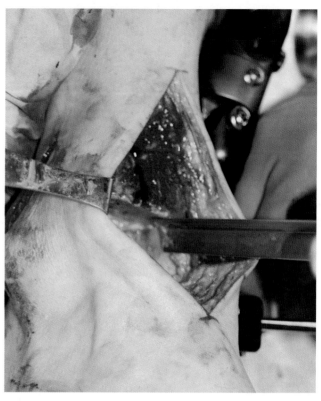

**Figure 39-15.** Use of the angled cutting osteotome ensures that the medial corner of the tibia is prepared without any rough edges or bone, which can prevent proper seating of the tibial component or could result in fracture of the medial malleolus during component seating.

medial malleolus, and the lateral wall of the trial should be flush with the medial wall of the fibula.

The talar cutting guide that corresponds to the same side and size as the tibial component is placed on the cut talar surface, with the handle aligned with the second ray (Fig. 39-17). With a marking pen, the track is marked for bone resection of the talus to allow for the talar component fin. The talar fin track is cut with a reciprocating saw. The cut starts at the junction of the talar neck and the talar body, and the cut is centered in the middle of the talar dome cut surface. The V-shaped cut should be deep enough (about 5 mm) to accommodate the talar component fin but should not extend completely to the posterior cortex of the talus (Fig. 39-18). The talar trial is inserted, making it flush with the cut surface of the talus. The trials should fit loosely because the final components will have a porous coating that adds about 1 mm to the thickness of the final components (Fig. 39-19). If the trial components fit snugly, further bone resection should be completed with the appropriate rasp to allow for an adequate fit of the final components.

At this point, the external fixator is completely removed and the joint is copiously irrigated to remove any debris. The final components are seated in place. To place the talar component, it is often necessary to manually distract the ankle joint and place the foot in a plantarflexed position (Fig. 39-20). After all components are seated, soft tissue balancing

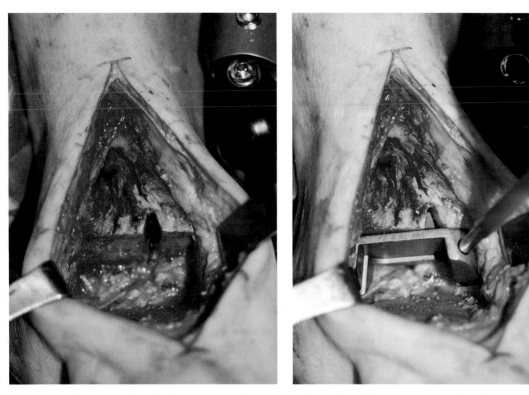

A                                                                      B

**Figure 39-16. A:** Appearance of the distal tibia after all bone is removed. **B:** Using the tibial component trial to ensure adequate fit before final component seating.

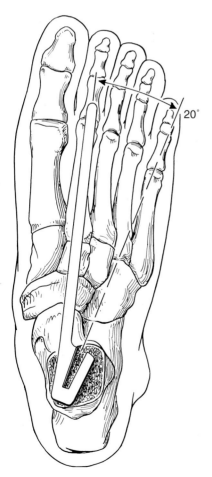

**Figure 39-17.** The drawing shows alignment of the talar cutting jig for proper alignment. The handle of the jig points to the second ray.

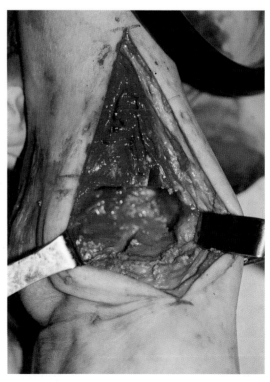

**Figure 39-18.** The V-shaped cut is completed in the talus. Notice that the cut does not go all the way to the posterior cortex of the talus.

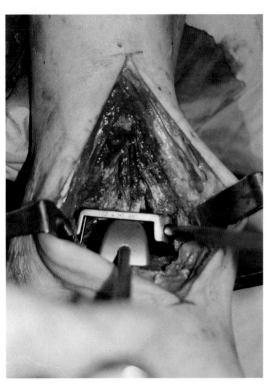

**Figure 39-19.** Final testing of the trial components. Notice that there is an approximately 1-mm gap around the entire trial component. This gap allows for the porous coating of the final components.

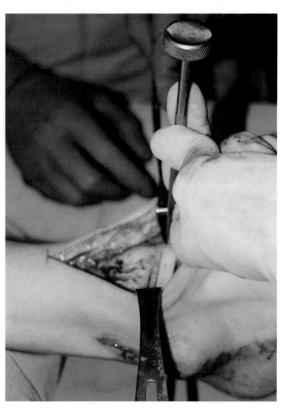

**Figure 39-20.** Seating of the talar component with the tibial component already in place. Notice that the foot is plantarflexed to allow easier seating of the talar component.

can be achieved. Routine release of the posterior half of the deep deltoid ligament is then performed.

The range of motion of the ankle is tested. It should achieve 5° of dorsiflexion with the knee straight. If this degree of dorsiflexion cannot be achieved, a percutaneous heel cord lengthening or gastrocnemius slide may be needed to release contractures. If these fail to allow 5° of dorsiflexion, the talar component should be removed and the posterior portion of the ankle joint assessed for bony spurs or contractures of the soft tissues. Additional bone resection may be needed to obtain adequate motion.

If the ankle tilts into varus after final seating of the components, several factors must be considered. First, the surgeon must ensure that the medial and lateral gutters are cleared of all bony and soft tissue debris. Second, the surgeon ensures that the superficial and deep deltoid ligaments are not contracted. A third incision may be placed at this time from the tip of the medial malleolus for a distance of approximately 3 cm. The superficial deltoid can be released transversely at this time. If the lateral ligaments are incompetent and this is the cause of the varus tilt, a peroneus brevis tenodesis may be needed. If this fails to correct the deformity, a calcaneal osteotomy or plantarflexion first metatarsal osteotomy may be needed to place the heel into valgus.

After the components are in place and all deformities are corrected, attention is again turned to the syndesmosis, where cortical flaps are created and displaced posteriorly. The resected cancellous bone from the distal tibia is fashioned into a single block and placed into the syndesmosis to obtain a solid fusion. Two 3.5-mm, fully threaded cortical lag screws are inserted parallel to each other just above the ankle joint from the fibula to the

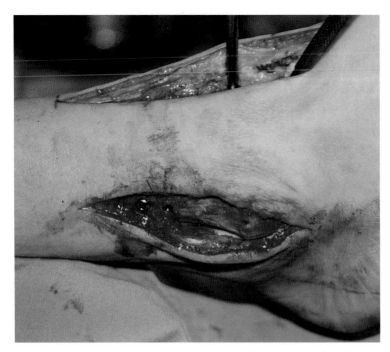

**Figure 39-21.** Two syndesmotic screws are placed across the fibula after bone graft is placed in the syndesmosis. These screws are placed in a lag fashion.

tibia to rigidly fix the syndesmosis (Fig. 39-21). After this step is completed, the edges of the resected talar dome are beveled and coated with bone wax. The wounds are irrigated with pulsed lavage and closed in layers. The anterior wound is closed by first closing the capsule over the components using nonabsorbable suture. The extensor retinaculum is repaired to prevent bow stringing of the extensor tendons. The subcutaneous tissue is repaired with an interrupted absorbable suture, and the skin is reapproximated with staples or interrupted nylon stitches. The lateral wound is closed in a similar fashion.

## POSTOPERATIVE MANAGEMENT

A well-padded posterior splint is placed on the leg, and the patient is allowed to immediately place 40 pounds of weight on the leg at the bedside. The patient is encouraged to elevate the leg above the heart as much as possible for the first 2 weeks. The splint is removed in 2 weeks, and the patient is encouraged to perform active range of motion of the ankle. A removable cam walker boot is given to the patient to allow for daily range of motion. However, weight bearing remains protected with the boot and at 40 pounds of pressure for 6 weeks. At 6 weeks, the patient is advanced to full weight bearing without the cast boot and formal physical therapy begins. Therapy is directed at passive and active range of motion, as well as strengthening the extrinsic and intrinsic muscles of the foot and ankle. Routine radiographs of the ankle are obtained at 6 weeks, 3 months, 6 months, and yearly thereafter if the syndesmotic fusion is solid (Fig. 39-22). Annual radiographs of all ankle replacements are recommended to detect early asymptomatic aseptic loosening and provide early intervention.

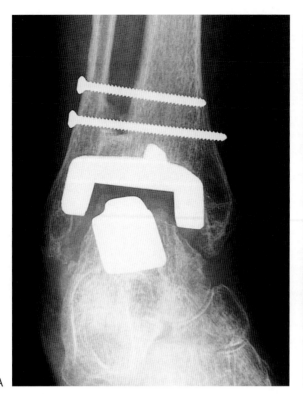

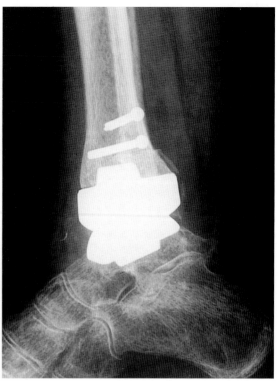

A                                                                                                                      B

**Figure 39-22. A:** Mortise radiograph of a total ankle replacement at 6 months post-operatively. There is good alignment of the components, good bone ingrowth, and solid fusion of the syndesmosis. This patient needs only annual radiographs. **B:** The lateral radiograph shows good alignment and good bone ingrowth.

## COMPLICATIONS

The most common complication with ankle arthroplasty is *fracture* of the medial or lateral malleolus during final component insertion. This occurs because the saw cut beyond the cutting block boundaries or the cuts left too little bone and the force needed to seat the components resulted in a fracture. Placing the fin cut too medially causes the medial shoulder of the prosthesis to displace the malleolus, resulting in fracture. If the medial malleolus fractures, it can be fixed with two parallel, 4.0-mm, cancellous screws directed from the tip of the malleolus to the tibia. Occasionally, Kirschner wires or a tension band wire technique is necessary. If the fibula is fractured, it can be repaired with a low profile plate and screws or a tension band technique with pins and wires.

The posterior tibial tendon runs directly behind the medial malleolus and can be injured during bony resection. It is imperative that this tendon be repaired to avoid a postoperative flatfoot deformity from developing.

*Wound problems* can result from the anterior approach, especially in rheumatoid arthritis patients. Gentle retraction of the skin, limiting of the tourniquet time, and ensuring patient compliance with postoperative leg elevation can help reduce this complication.

*Nonunion* of the syndesmosis fusion sometimes has been encountered. Although many nonunions are asymptomatic, a solid fusion is needed to prevent migration of the component particularly if a substantial portion of the tibial component is positioned lateral to the lateral edge of the distal tibia. In these cases, if external bone stimulation fails to obtain union, reoperation with takedown of the nonunion with subsequent bone grafting and internal fixation may be necessary. If the patient is a smoker, he or she should be strongly encouraged to cease smoking at least until union occurs.

## RECOMMENDED READING

1. Alvine FG: *Agility total ankle system: surgical technique*. Warsaw, Indiana:DePuy Inc., 1999.
2. Alvine FG: Total ankle arthroplasty: new concepts and approach. *Contemp Orthop* 22: 397–403, 1991.
3. Gould JS, Alvine FG, Mann RA, et al.: Total ankle replacement: a surgical discussion. Part I. *Am J Orthop* 29: 604–609, 2000.
4. Gould JS, Alvine FG, Mann RA, et al.: Total ankle replacement: a surgical discussion. Part II. *Am J Orthop* 29:675–682, 2000.
5. Neufeld SK, Lee TJ: Total ankle arthroplasty, indications, results and biomechanical rationale. *Am J Orthop* 29:593–602, 2000.
6. Pyevich MT, Alvine FG, Saltzman CL, et al.: Total ankle arthroplasty: a unique design. *J Bone J Surg Am* 80: 1410–1420, 1998.

# 40

# Bridle Posterior Tibial Tendon Transfer

Richard E. Gellman, Robert B. Anderson, and W. Hodges Davis

## INDICATIONS/CONTRAINDICATIONS

Tendon transfers for the treatment of paralytic foot drop are performed to allow patients to ambulate without the use of ankle-foot orthoses. These transfer procedures were first developed for the flaccid paralyses of polio and leprosy and later expanded to treat spastic paralysis, primarily childhood cerebral palsy. The most commonly performed transfer for spastic and flaccid foot drop is an isolated posterior tibialis tendon, first reported by Watkins in 1954 (7). Results of the isolated posterior tibialis transfer were conflicting, with two large series reporting a significant number of postoperative deformities (5,6).

To correct the problem of varus or valgus malposition, Riordan modified the posterior tibialis transfer by creating a dual insertion through the anterior tibialis and peroneus longus tendons (2). After transferring the posterior tibialis tendon through the interosseous membrane, he formed a tritendon anastomosis of the posterior tibialis tendon to the anterior tibialis and peroneus longus tendons. The peroneus longus tendon is first brought anterior to the lateral malleolus. Riordan coined the term *bridle procedure* to describe the balanced pull of the posterior tibialis transfer through the peroneus longus laterally and the tibialis anterior medially. In theory, the balanced pull of the tibialis anterior and peroneus longus prevent a varus or valgus hindfoot deformity. Riordan and others performed this procedure primarily in pediatric cerebral palsy patients.

In a bridle transfer, the peroneus longus and anterior tibialis tendons function as tendons of the posterior tibialis muscle. The tibialis anterior and peroneus muscles do not have clinically significant motor strength. In this situation, the posterior tibialis muscle serves as the motor function to the transfer and the tritendon anastomosis provides the balance to the foot.

In 1996, Prahinski et al. (3) reported long-term follow-up on 10 adult patients with flaccid paralysis treated with the dual insertion Riordan bridle transfer. They felt that the Rior-

R. E. Gellman, M.D., P.C.: Portland Orthopedic Specialists, Portland, Oregon.

R. B. Anderson, M.D.: Foot and Ankle Service, Department of Orthopaedics and Department of Orthopaedic Surgery, Carolinas Medical Center; and Private Practice, Miller Orthopaedic Clinic, Charlotte, North Carolina.

W. H. Davis, M.D.: Foot and Ankle Service, Department of Orthopaedic Surgery, Carolinas Medical Center; and Private Pactice, Miller Orthopaedic Clinic, Charlotte, North Carolina.

dan transfer works well in the low-demand patient, but they reported four failures from an acute tearing of the transfer or a gradual stretching out of the transfer. Moreover, four of the 10 patients returned to wearing braces.

In 1992, Rodriguez reported on a modification of the Riordan bridle procedure (4). Rodriguez created a triple insertion by passing the posterior tibialis tendon into the middle cuneiform bone after anastomosis with the anterior tibial tendon and the peroneus longus tendon (Fig. 40-1). In theory, the outer tendons maintain a balanced foot, while the central posterior tibialis transfer is strengthened by its direct line of pull from origin to a bone insertion. The procedure eliminates the need for a precise placement of the posterior tibialis insertion

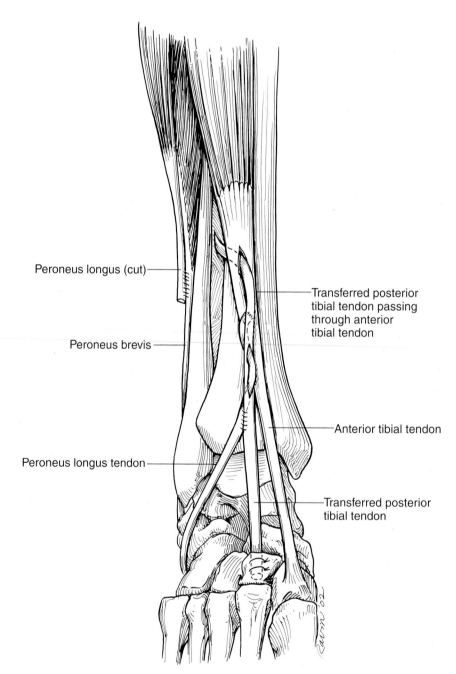

Peroneus longus (cut)

Transferred posterior tibial tendon passing through anterior tibial tendon

Peroneus brevis

Anterior tibial tendon

Peroneus longus tendon

Transferred posterior tibial tendon

**Figure 40-1.** Rodriguez bridle transfer. The posterior tibialis is transferred through the interosseous membrane, and anastomosis is achieved with the peroneus longus and tibialis anterior, as in the Riordan bridle procedure. Rodriguez created a triple insertion by passing the posterior tibialis tendon into the middle cuneiform bone after anastomosis with the anterior tibial tendon and the peroneus longus tendon.

because the balance of the tibialis anterior and peroneus longus tendons prevent varus or valgus malposition. Rodriguez did not have any failures in his group of 10 adult patients.

Since 1993, we have used the bridle procedure described by Rodriguez to treat 23 patients with paralytic foot drop (4). We believe the bridle tendon transfer provides a strong transfer with more reliable balancing to prevent varus or valgus deformity than an isolated posterior tibialis tendon transfer.

After the bridle tendon transfer, all of our patients have been able to ambulate without ankle-foot orthosis braces. Patients have minimal to absent plantarflexion and limited dorsiflexion that functions similar to a tenodesis. The limited range of motion in a bridle tendon transfer compared with the isolated transfer may result from a more limited excursion of the tritendon anastomosis.

The bridle transfer allows reliable, brace-free ambulation, but it does not restore sufficient motion in the ankle and subtalar joints for comfortable running. Walking easily on uneven surfaces may also be difficult. Wearing certain shoes or boots for patients undergoing a bridle procedure will be difficult or impossible because of the limitations of motion.

The bridle procedure is indicated for several causes of flaccid paralysis. Our population comprises mostly patients with traumatic peripheral nerve injuries. The most frequent diagnosis in our series was a common peroneal nerve injury after a knee dislocation. The second most common was an injury to the peroneal division of the sciatic nerve injury, after a femur fracture or total hip arthroplasty. The bridle transfer was also performed for patients with peroneal nerve lacerations or resections.

Contraindications for a bridle transfer include a recent incomplete nerve injury with a likelihood of significant neurologic recovery. If there is return of significant peroneal tendon strength, a symptomatic flatfoot deformity could develop, which has occurred in one of our patients who underwent a sural nerve graft to his peroneal nerve at the time of his bridle procedure. A high potential for recovery of anterior compartment muscle strength would be a contraindication because the foot drop would resolve once the muscle strength returns and overpull of the anterior compartment could result in a calcaneus gait.

Absence of gastrocsoleus muscle strength from a partial injury to the tibial nerve is a relative contraindication, because this patient may still require bracing after correction of the foot drop to provide stability during mid-stance and toe-off phases of gait.

Because the bridle transfer involves transferring tendons at the level of the subcutaneous tissues, a relative contraindication is significant scarring of the skin and soft tissues at the anterior ankle that could create wound healing problems or prevent wound closure over the transfer.

Insufficient vascular status in the limb to allow healing of the seven incisions on the foot and leg necessary for the operation is a contraindication to surgery. The physical exam must include a careful vascular evaluation and possible referral for vascular studies. The surgeon and patient must then weigh the risks and benefits of vascular reconstruction preceding a bridle procedure versus the decision to continue using an ankle-foot orthosis brace.

## PREOPERATIVE PLANNING

### Neurologic and Muscle Strength Examination

Patients suitable for a bridle tendon transfer must have appropriate evaluation of their nerve injury. Referral for neurologic evaluation with electromyography and nerve conduction studies (EMG/NCS) can determine the level of the nerve injury and the potential for recovery. The neurologist or physiatrist completing the study should understand the reason for referral and the plan for possible tendon transfer. The examiner should have experience treating posttraumatic nerve injury and feel comfortable making specific recommendations regarding the likelihood of recovery and the potential success of transferring the posterior tibialis muscle based on the clinical and EMG/NCS findings.

A patient who is more than 1 year from a peripheral nerve injury who has complete motor and sensory loss does not require a preoperative EMG/NCS. The chance of significant recovery after 1 year of paralysis is insignificant as fibrosis progresses and diminishes any potential for reinnervation of the motor end plates (1). If there is a changing motor or sensory examination result, referral is recommended.

The ideal patient for the bridle tendon transfer has normal motor strength in the posterior tibialis muscle, but motor strength of 4/5 is also acceptable and will provide enough power for ambulation out of a brace. Although the transfer does seem to function similar to a tenodesis, there is still a possibility the transfer could stretch out if there is not sufficient strength in the transferred muscle. Gastrocnemius-soleus strength must also be sufficient to allow ambulation out of the brace. A motor strength of 4/5 is recommended to provide enough stability during stance phase of gait. If there is insufficient calf strength, ambulation out of the brace may not be possible despite correction of the foot drop.

### Equinus and Toe Flexion Contractures

Inspection of the lower extremity for sufficient passive ankle dorsiflexion range of motion is critical. If the ankle can be brought to 10° of passive dorsiflexion with the knee extended, Achilles tendon lengthening or gastrocnemius fascia release is unnecessary. However, if motion is more limited, as is usually the case, a lengthening procedure is recommended. For mild to moderate equinus contracture, we prefer the Strayer gastrocnemius slide technique, which heals more rapidly than a percutaneous lengthening of the Achilles tendon with less risk of overcorrection.

Some patients demonstrate toe flexion deformities after correction of their foot drop that makes walking in bare feet difficult. Flexor hallucis longus (FHL) and flexor digitorum longus (FDL) contractures are sometimes addressed at the time of surgery with tendon lengthening or tenotomies. Often, these deformities are not easily determined until the equinus contracture of the heel cord is corrected at surgery.

### Fixed Joint Deformity

As in all tendon transfers, any fixed joint deformities must be corrected to gain a successful result. Patients need careful assessment for rigid deformities in the ankle, hindfoot and midfoot. Any fixed deformities require correction at the time of the transfer. Correction depends on the specific deformity and requires arthrodesis, osteotomy, or soft tissue release.

### Patient Expectations

Patients can expect a high rate of successful brace-free walking. No patient in our study has required a return to an ankle-foot orthosis. The patients studied also demonstrate normal walking speed and stride length after surgery. However, patients must understand that they will not have normal foot and ankle function. They will have little or no plantarflexion motion and only a small degree of ankle dorsiflexion. Running will not be possible, except for short distances, and prolonged work or recreation on uneven surfaces may be difficult unless supportive, above-ankle footwear is worn. Shoes with a heel greater than 0.5 to 1 inch will probably not be comfortable.

## SURGERY

The patient is positioned supine, with placement of a thigh pneumatic tourniquet. Patients are given preoperative intravenous antibiotics. After induction of anesthesia, testing for equinus contracture is performed (Fig. 40-2). If a gastrocnemius slide or Achilles tendon lengthening is required, a bump can be placed under the contralateral hip to allow easier visualization of the posterior mid-distal leg.

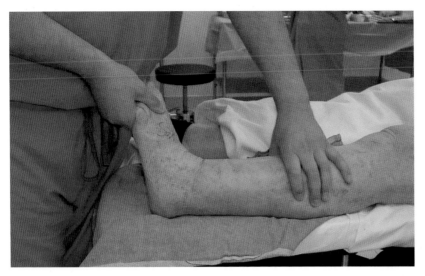

**Figure 40-2.** Evaluation for equinus contracture. The hindfoot is held in a neutral position, and the foot is dorsiflexed with the knee fully extended. If the foot can reach 10° of dorsiflexion, a tendon-lengthening procedure is unnecessary. Most patients require a lengthening procedure.

## Technique: Gastrocnemius Slide

A 4-cm, vertical incision is made on the mid-distal posterior leg, slightly medial to midline. The subcutaneous layer is dissected, taking care to bluntly retract the overlying sural nerve (Fig. 40-3). The medial and lateral margins of the tendon are identified after opening the paratenon and placing deep retractors on either side of the tendon. A transverse incision is made exposing the underlying soleus muscle fascia or soleus muscle. The decision to release both the gastrocnemius and soleus fascia depends on the degree of equinus contracture (Fig. 40-4). The foot is then forcefully dorsiflexed, completing the procedure. The

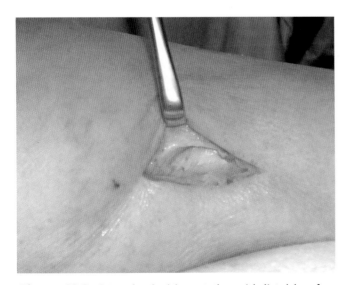

**Figure 40-3.** Posterior incision at the mid-distal leg for gastrocnemius recession shows the sural nerve retracted to reveal the tendon. The incision is made slightly medial to the midline. Left is proximal, right is distal.

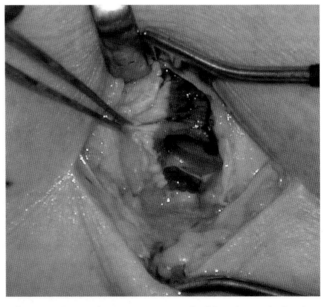

**Figure 40-4.** After a transverse incision is made in the gastrosoleus tendon, dorsiflexion of the foot distracts the proximal (grasped with pickup) and distal ends, exposing underlying soleus muscle belly.

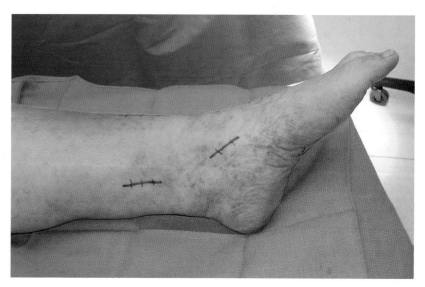

**Figure 40-5.** Medial foot and leg incisions for harvesting the posterior tibialis tendon. Notice the posture of the foot in plantarflexion.

bump is then removed from the contralateral hip and placed under the ipsilateral hip if needed for access to the lateral leg.

### Technique: Tendon Transfer

The medial foot and leg incisions are marked for harvest of the posterior tibialis tendon (Fig. 40-5). The posterior tibialis tendon is harvested through a 4-cm medial foot incision at its insertion on the navicular tuberosity. Extra length can be gained by dissecting tendon and periosteum attached to a thin wedge of bone off the navicular. The end of the tendon is then tagged with nonabsorbable suture, and traction is placed on the tendon to allow freeing of adhesions within the sheath with a blunt scissors (Fig. 40-6). The tendon is retracted proximally through a second 4-cm incision that is made 8 cm above the medial malleolus, along the posterior border of the tibia. After dissecting the subcutaneous and retinacular layers, the first tendon usually encountered is the FDL tendon, which must be retracted for visualization of the posterior tibialis tendon (Figs. 40-7 and 40-8).

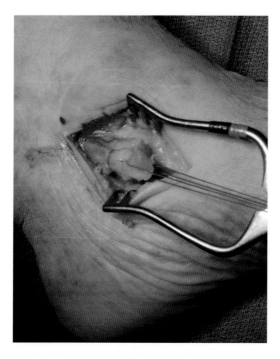

**Figure 40-6.** Through medial foot incisions, the posterior tibialis tendon has been detached from the navicular bone and tagged with nonabsorbable suture. With traction on the tendon, a blunt-tipped scissors can be carefully advanced along the tendon proximally to release adhesions.

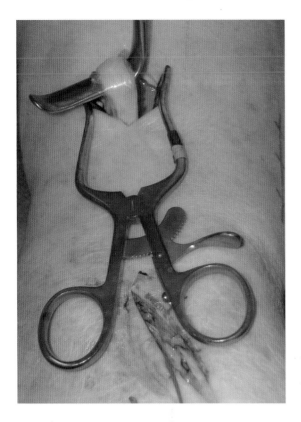

**Figure 40-7.** A large, blunt retractor is placed under the posterior tibialis for safe retrieval of the tendon into the medial leg incision.

A third incision, measuring approximately 6 cm is made over the distal anterior leg. The subcutaneous tissue is dissected and the anterior fascia divided just lateral to the tibialis anterior tendon. The tibialis anterior tendon is then retracted laterally exposing the interosseous membrane (Fig. 40-9). The neurovascular bundle is usually encountered between the tibialis anterior and the extensor hallucis longus tendons and should be mobilized to prevent injury. A large clamp is passed from the medial leg incision along the posterior aspect of the tibia and through the interosseous membrane. A generous opening is made in

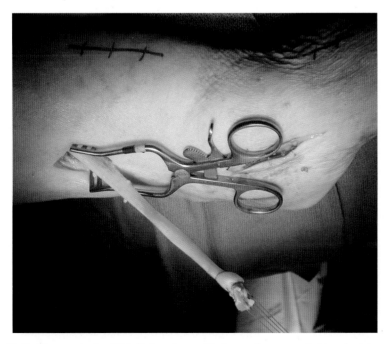

**Figure 40-8.** The posterior tibialis tendon withdrawn from medial leg incisions before transfer. Skin incision is marked for anterior leg incisions.

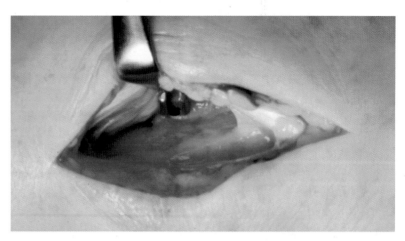

**Figure 40-9.** Through an anterior leg incision, the tibialis anterior is retracted laterally, protecting the neurovascular bundle. Notice the blunt clamp penetrating the interosseous membrane.

the membrane to allow easy excursion of the muscle belly and a direct line of pull for tendon (Fig. 40-10). A narrow opening may prevent excursion of the muscle belly. The tag sutures on the posterior tibialis tendon are now passed with a curved clamp over the posterior border of the tibia through the interosseous membrane and the posterior tibialis tendon is safely pulled into the anterior compartment of the leg (Figs. 40-11 and 40-12). To gain more length and excursion for the transfer, a portion of the posterior tibialis muscle belly may be freed from the fibula with an elevator.

Next, the peroneus longus tendon must be harvested and brought anterior to the lateral malleolus and into the anterior leg incision. A fourth incision is made 10 cm superior along the posterior border of the lateral malleolus. The retinaculum over the peroneal tendons is opened, and the peroneus longus tendon is identified, cut, and tagged with nonabsorbable suture (Fig. 40-13). A fifth incision distal to the inferior peroneal retinaculum is made over the peroneus longus tendon on the lateral border of the foot. This allows retraction of the tendon distally (Fig. 40-14). A large clamp holding the tag sutures on the peroneus longus tendon is then passed subcutaneously to the anterior leg incision (Fig. 40-15). Although the peroneus brevis tendon seems to be a more ideal tendon for transfer because it inserts on the lateral border of the foot, the peroneus brevis tendon is too short to reach the anterior leg incision for anastomosis with the other two tendons.

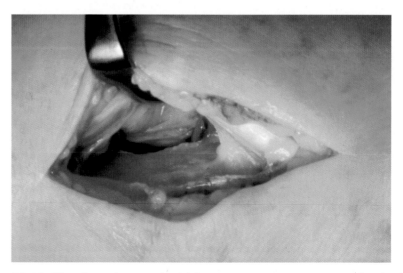

**Figure 40-10.** The clamp is spread widely to create a generous opening in the interosseous membrane.

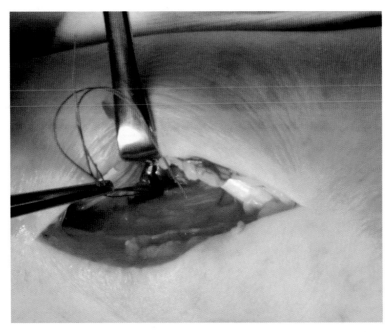

**Figure 40-11.** A clamp holding the tag sutures to the posterior tibialis tendon is passed along the posterior border of the tibia and through the interosseous membrane.

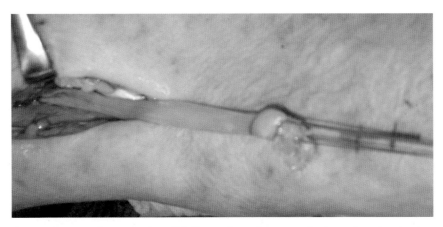

**Figure 40-12.** The posterior tibialis tendon after transfer into the anterior leg.

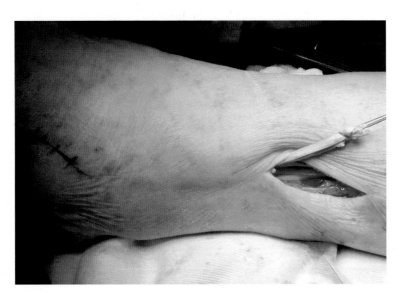

**Figure 40-13.** Lateral view. The peroneus longus tendon is released proximally through a lateral leg incision. Notice the skin incision is marked for the lateral foot incision along the peroneal tendons anterior to the lateral malleolus.

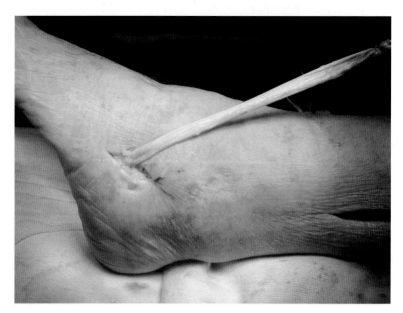

**Figure 40-14.** The peroneus longus tendon previously sectioned proximally is withdrawn from the lateral foot incision. There is sufficient tendon length to reach the anterior leg.

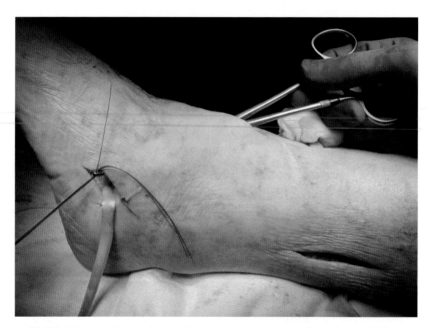

**Figure 40-15.** A large clamp draws the peroneus longus subcutaneously into the anterior leg incision.

### Technique: Tritendon Anastomosis

The tritendon anastomosis of the posterior tibialis, anterior tibialis, and peroneus longus tendons is now performed (Fig. 40-16). The posterior tibialis tendon is passed through a slit in the anterior tibialis tendon just above the ankle joint and sewn with nonabsorbable suture (Fig. 40-17). It is important to hold the foot in dorsiflexion during the anastomosis procedure (Fig. 40-18). The peroneus longus is then woven into the posterior tibialis in a similar fashion through slits or with a Pulvertaft tendon-weaving clamp and then sutured (Fig. 40-19).

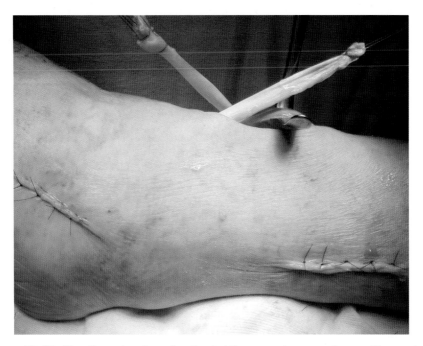

**Figure 40-16.** The three tendons for the bridle procedure are shown. The posterior tibialis tendon is being pulled distally, the peroneus longus proximally, and the tibialis anterior held by a retractor.

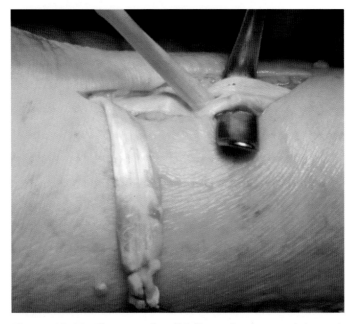

**Figure 40-17.** The posterior tibialis tendon is passed through a slit in the anterior tibialis tendon just proximal to the ankle joint and sewn with nonabsorbable suture.

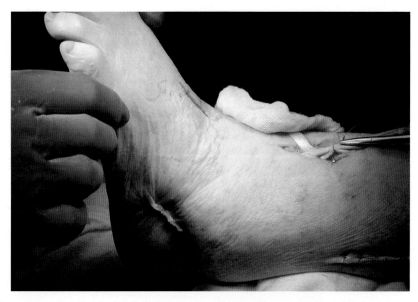

**Figure 40-18.** The foot is held in maximum dorsiflexion during the anastomosis.

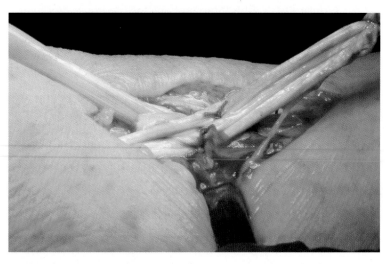

**Figure 40-19.** The peroneus longus tendon is woven through the posterior tibialis tendon and sutured with nonabsorbable suture.

A sixth, 2-cm incision is made on the dorsum of the foot at the middle cuneiform, and the tag sutures of the posterior tibialis tendon are passed with a clamp subcutaneously into the midfoot incision (Fig. 40-20). A bone tunnel large enough to accommodate the posterior tibialis tendon is made from dorsal to plantar in the middle cuneiform with the use of drill bits and curettes (Figs. 40-21 and 40-22). In theory, the bridle transfer can provide varus-valgus balance so that radiography is unnecessary to confirm insertion in the second versus the third cuneiform. A straight Keith needle is used to pass each arm of the tag sutures through the bone tunnel, exiting the sole of the foot (Fig. 40-23). A 2-cm incision is made on the sole of the foot, and dissection is carried to the plantar fascia. The posterior tibialis transfer is then tied over the plantar fascia with the foot held in dorsiflexion. We avoid tying over a button on the sole of the foot because of problems with skin necrosis and patient complaints of pain. After the posterior tibialis tendon insertion is secure, the tibialis anterior and peroneus longus tendons can be tensioned with nonabsorbable suture until the desired balance is achieved. If possible, the anterior leg fascia should be closed over the anastomosis before skin closure (Figs. 40-24 and 40-25).

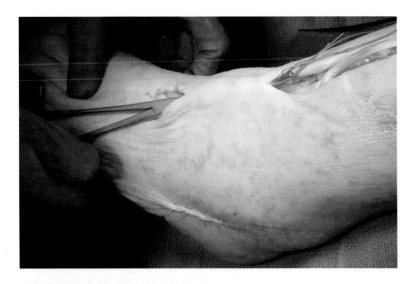

**Figure 40-20.** A 2-cm dorsal foot incision is made over the middle cuneiform, and a clamp is passed proximally subcutaneously to retrieve the posterior tibialis tendon.

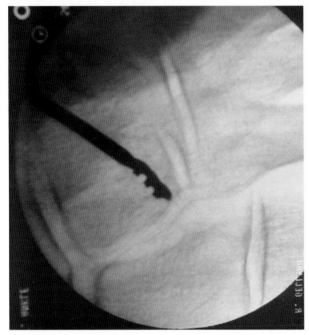

**Figure 40-21.** A fluoroscopic image of the foot confirms the position over the middle cuneiform. Radiographic confirmation is optional.

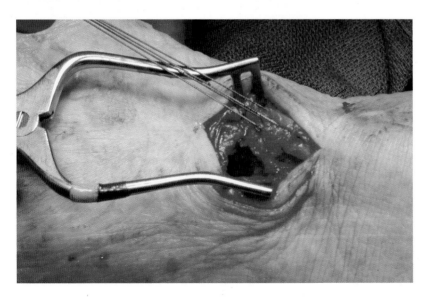

**Figure 40-22.** Through dorsal foot incision, the bone tunnel is widened with drill bits and curettes to accommodate the transfer.

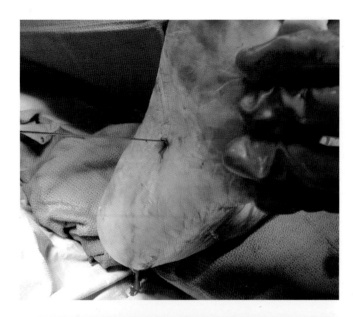

**Figure 40-23.** Sutures exit the plantar foot. The skin is incised so that the knot can be visualized as it is tied over the plantar fascia.

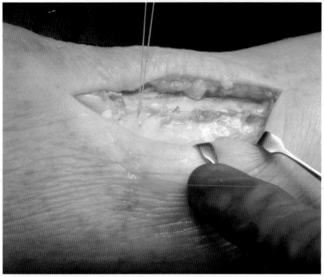

**Figure 40-24.** Anterior leg incision. Closure of the anterior leg fascia over the tritendon anastomosis.

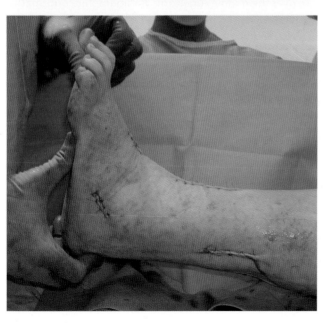

**Figure 40-25.** Final foot position after completion of the transfer.

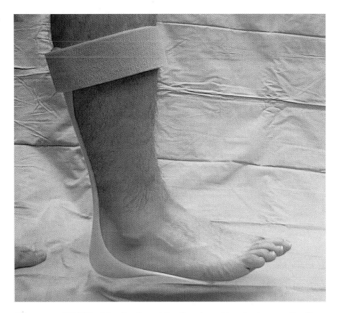

**Figure 40-26.** Typical ankle-foot orthosis is used after cast removal at 6 weeks postoperatively. An ankle-foot orthosis is recommended for an additional 3 to 4 months.

## POSTOPERATIVE MANAGEMENT

Initially, patients are immobilized for 2 weeks in a toe-touch, weight-bearing plaster splint with the foot held in maximum dorsiflexion. Sutures are removed, and a short-leg fiberglass walking cast is applied for 4 weeks with partial or full weight bearing allowed, depending on surgeon preference. At 6 to 8 weeks, casts are removed, and the patient is instructed to ambulate in an ankle-foot orthosis brace or walker boot (Fig. 40-26). Protected ambulation is continued for 3 to 4 months. Compression stockings or socks are often ordered to manage the postsurgical edema common in neurologic patients.

Patients are instructed in active ankle dorsiflexion and warned *not* to perform toe raises or calf muscle strengthening to prevent stretching out the transfer. Clear understanding of the permanent loss of plantarflexion is critical at this point so that an early failure does not result. In our experience, patients are referred to physical therapy for gait training on an as

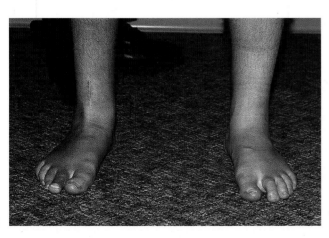
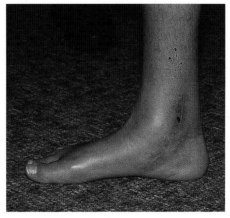

A                                                                                                                B

**Figure 40-27.** Typical appearance of healed incisions after a successful bridle procedure on the right foot. **A:** Anterior view. **B:** Medial view. *(continued)*

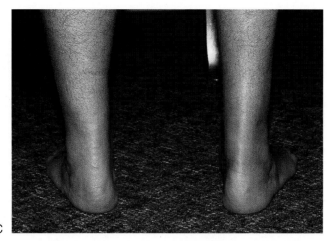

C

**Figure 40-27.** *Continued.* **C:** Posterior view.

needed basis, but electrical stimulation to re-educate muscle transfer is not ordered. Our series demonstrated an average ankle dorsiflexion of 10°, and plantarflexion most commonly measured 0°. Subtalar joint range of motion was significantly reduced to 0% to 25% of the nonoperative side. Walking speed and stride length on a level surface returned to normal in our series of patients tested 1 to 5 years after surgery, with patients reporting maximum improvement by 6 months (Fig. 40-27).

## COMPLICATIONS

No patients in our series developed deep infections. Several complications are specific to the bridle tendon transfer.

*Wound problems* may occur. The skin over the distal anterior leg where the three tendons are sutured together may present an area of delayed healing. Only two patients in our series developed superficial wound problems, which resolved with local care and oral antibiotics.

*Tendon transfer* may produce complications. Patients may be bothered by the presence of a bulky tritendon anastomosis just above the anterior ankle subcutaneously, especially if it is irritated by their shoes. Treatment is education and shoe modification.

*Tendon elongation or failure* may occur. The transferred tendon may stretch if patients do not follow postoperative instructions and attempt early ambulation or plantarflexion motion. Usually, mild to moderate elongation does not require the patient to resume brace wear. This has occurred in only one patient. No patients have resumed brace wear.

A *calcaneus gait* may be caused by insufficient plantarflexion if the transfer is set in too much dorsiflexion or if an Achilles lengthening procedure is performed unnecessarily. Two patients in our series have been effectively managed with shoe modifications.

*Progressive flatfoot* has been seen in one patient who had a sural nerve graft for his common peroneal nerve injury at the same time as the bridle transfer. As peroneal tendon strength returned, the patient developed a progressive, painful flatfoot that required subtalar arthrodesis. In retrospect, it may have been more appropriate to delay tendon transfer surgery until his neurologic status was more stable.

*Toe flexion deformities* may occur. Excessive clawing of the great or lesser toes should be assessed after gastrocsoleus lengthening. Several patients have required tenotomies or flexor tendon lengthening procedures. Three patients in our series that were not corrected noticed a problem postoperatively, but none has elected surgical correction. We recommend preoperative counseling and consent for tenotomy of the lesser toes and lengthening of the FHL as needed to prevent this complication in selected patients.

## RECOMMENDED READING

1. Lee SK, Wolfe SW: Peripheral nerve injury and repair. *J Am Acad Orthop Surg* 8: 243–252, 2000.
2. McCall RE, Frederick HA, McCluskey GM, et al.: The bridle procedure: a new treatment for equinus and equinovarus deformities in children. *J Pediatr Orthop* 11:83–89, 1991.
3. Prahinski JR, McHale KA, Temple HT, et al.: Bridle transfer for paresis of the anterior and lateral compartment musculature. *Foot Ankle* 17:615–619, 1996.
4. Rodriguez RP: The bridle procedure in the treatment of paralysis of the foot. *Foot Ankle* 13:63–69, 1992.
5. Schneider M, Balon K: Deformity of the foot following anterior transfer of the posterior tibial tendon and lengthening of the Achilles tendon for spastic equinovarus. *Clin Orthop* 125:113–118, 1977.
6. Turner JW, Cooper RR: Anterior transfer of the tibialis posterior through the interosseous membrane. *Clin Orthop* 83:241–244, 1972.
7. Watkins MB, Jones JB, Ryder CT, et al.: Transplantation of the posterior tibial tendon. *J Bone Joint Surg Am* 36:1181–1189, 1954.

# 41

# Syme Amputation

James W. Brodsky

## INDICATIONS/CONTRAINDICATIONS

The Syme amputation is indicated for the patient who requires amputation of most of the foot because of loss of viability from infection, gangrene, or trauma. This is the patient for whom a partial foot amputation is no longer possible but still has a viable heel pad. The advantages of the Syme amputation over the next amputation alternative in a patient with a nonviable foot (i.e., below-knee amputation) are enormous. They are manifested in its mechanical, physiologic, and functional superiority. The mechanical advantage of the Syme amputation is the tremendously longer lever given to the function of the quadriceps muscles and to the knee joint. Physiologically, this results in a lower energy expenditure in walking than in patients with a more proximal amputation, an important factor in all patients, but especially in patients with underlying debilitating chronic disease such as diabetes or chronic peripheral vascular disease (5).

Functionally, the patient with a Syme amputation requires only a fraction of the rehabilitation and training to become ambulatory required by a below-knee amputee. Not only is the extensive training in donning and doffing the prosthesis not necessary, but almost none of the Syme amputees requires admission to a rehabilitation facility for gait training. The Syme amputation has the advantage that the distal stump is covered with plantar skin and the pad of the heel, and is therefore thicker and better able to withstand the pressure of weight bearing. The Syme stump is partially end-bearing on this specialized tissue, with the remaining pressure distributed through the proximal tibial metaphysis, where all of the pressure is borne in a below-knee amputation. Some patients (although not advised to do so by their surgeons) nonetheless report weight bearing directly on the stump when getting up in the night to go to the bathroom.

The Syme amputation has also been widely and successfully used in various congenital deformities and deficiencies of the lower limb, including proximal focal femoral defi-

J. W. Brodsky, M.D.: Department of Orthopaedic Surgery, University of Texas Southwestern Medical School; Foot and Ankle Surgery Fellowship, Baylor University Medical Center and University of Texas Southwestern Medical School, Dallas, Texas.

ciency, fibular hemimelia, and congenital pseudarthrosis of the tibia. As in amputations at other levels, the most common underlying disease is diabetes, followed by arteriosclerotic peripheral vascular disease, and trauma.

The primary and absolute contraindication to a Syme ankle disarticulation is the absence of an intact and viable heel pad. This means that the patient needs to have completely intact skin over the posterior, medial and lateral, and plantar aspect of the heel. Posterior skin compromise in particular, especially over the Achilles tendon, will doom the procedure to failure. The only exception would be in the unusual case of a Syme amputation to be performed for trauma in an otherwise healthy individual, in which superficial injury to the heel soft tissue might rapidly heal, particularly with normal vascularity of the limb.

The Syme amputation is likewise contraindicated in patients for whom the procedure is contemplated because of severe infection of the foot but in whom the infection has extended too far proximally and involves the area of the heel itself. Because the primary advantages of this procedure are focused on the enhancement of the patient's walking ability, there is no indication to perform this procedure rather than a below-knee amputation in a wheelchair-bound or otherwise nonambulatory patient. Partial foot amputations are still generally preferable to a Syme procedure whenever a viable outcome is possible, because partial foot amputations can usually be fitted with shoe modifications to ambulate, whereas the Syme amputation is the lowest level amputation that requires a prosthesis. A properly performed Chopart amputation (which must always include Achilles tenotomy) usually requires the use of a polypropylene ankle foot orthosis, which also extends to just below the knee. Although this is also somewhat cumbersome, it is still more cosmetic and lighter than a Syme prosthesis, and it can fit into a limited range of footwear, all of which are preferable to a prosthesis.

## PREOPERATIVE PLANNING

The most important determinant of a successful outcome in the Syme amputation, as in many surgeries, is proper patient selection. The purpose of the preoperative planning is to identify those patients with sufficient vascularity and the appropriate problem that warrant Syme amputation. The lower extremity should be carefully examined to determine the integrity of the skin. The extent of any skin ulcerations needs to be assessed. Involvement of underlying deep soft tissues, bones, and joints needs to be documented. The presence of pulses should be determined, because multiple investigators have demonstrated the relation between palpable posterior pulses and success of Syme amputation. Radiographs should be taken to make certain that there is not osteomyelitis of the distal tibia or fibula. Osteomyelitis of the talus would also be a likely contraindication.

The role of magnetic resonance imaging (MRI) is not as clearly defined. This technique is sensitive but sometimes difficult to interpret. The marrow edema (i.e., change from adipose to water density) of infection is nonspecific, and trauma or even reaction to nearby infection may elicit this indistinct change. On the other hand, if the MRI shows a plantar abscess that extends into the heel pad, this information is clearly most helpful in the decision making.

Most important to the preoperative planning is evaluation of the vascular status of the patient's lower limbs. This is particularly true because most patients who require this procedure are diabetic or dysvascular, or both. The arterial Doppler ultrasound is still the most widely available and most readily applied test of limb perfusion. However, it is to be considered a screening test and not a definitive measure of perfusion. Other technologies, including transcutaneous oxygen measurement and arteriography, are more authoritative with regard to the amount of tissue perfusion (see Chapter 16). A vascular surgery consultation is frequently required before proceeding with this operation. Revascularization procedures may be indicated. The key issue is that there be adequate perfusion of the heel pad, which is supplied by branches of the posterior tibial artery. Although the adipose tissue of the heel pad is a relatively avascular tissue, the absence of sufficient perfusion to this area is the primary cause of failure of the Syme amputation.

## SURGERY

Although there are points of technical finesse to be elucidated in any operative procedure, much amputation surgery is relatively straightforward. However, the Syme amputation is not only the least commonly performed, but unquestionably the most technically difficult of lower extremity amputations. Its functional superiority makes worthwhile the effort expended by the surgeon to obtain a good result with this operation.

Although the two-stage Syme amputation has been much discussed, most Syme amputations are now done at a single sitting (i.e., one-stage). The second stage, which is usually performed 6 or more weeks after the initial procedure, refers to delayed resection of the malleoli. This has been recommended in the past for severely infected cases in which the surgeon does not wish to expose the medullary cavities of the tibia and fibula to likely infection. The number of Syme amputations that are considered to require a second stage are few.

The patient is placed in the supine position. If there is much external rotation of the hip in this position, a pad, made of two to three folded sheets is placed beneath the ipsilateral buttock to compensate by internally rotating the limb. If there is an open, draining wound (Fig. 41-1), it can be covered and sealed off before the prep using an adhesive plastic incise drape. The draped off area is included in the prep, and any drainage is blocked from the area of the incisions. If a tourniquet is used, which is frequently the case, it is a pneumatic cuff placed high on the thigh over several layers of cast padding (Fig. 41-2). If there has been a previous vascular bypass in the thigh, the tourniquet is usually foregone. An Esmarch bandage can still be considered for use as a tourniquet at the ankle level. Preoperative antibiotics are usually given, but can be withheld until the deep wound cultures are taken, so as not to confuse the culture results.

### Technique

First, the skin incisions are marked out (Figs. 41-3 and 41-4). In a two-stage procedure, the anterior incision is along a line that connects two points that are placed 1 to 1.5 cm below and 1 to 1.5 cm anterior to the midpoint of the tip of each malleolus. In the one-stage procedure, especially if done for trauma, the points from which the incisions originate can be more proximal, either on the tips of the malleoli or on the midpoints of the two malleoli. The two malleolar points are then connected by a second incision across the sole, which will delineate the plantar side of the closure.

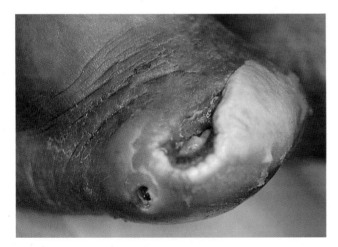

**Figure 41-1.** Infected, failed transmetatarsal amputation with deep plantar abscess that does not extend to the heel pad. A revision to the Syme amputation was elected.

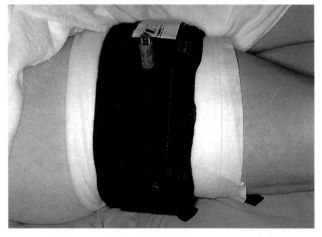

**Figure 41-2.** The pneumatic tourniquet is applied on the proximal thigh over cast padding.

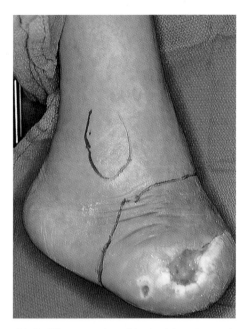

**Figure 41-3.** The anterior skin incision is marked. The line connects two points that are placed about 1 cm distal and anterior to the tips of the malleoli.

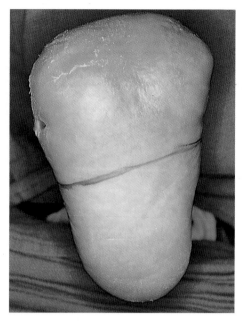

**Figure 41-4.** The plantar incision is marked.

Using a no. 10 scalpel, the dorsal incision is made down to the dome of the talus (Fig. 41-5). The plantar incision is then made all the way down to bone (i.e., down to the calcaneus) (Figs. 41-6 and 41-7). The collateral ligaments of the talus are released, working alternately between lateral and medial sides placing traction on the talus forward and downward (Figs. 41-8 and 41-9). A large bone hook in the talus is extremely helpful, if not

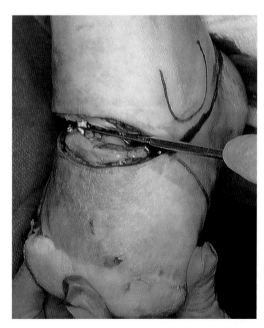

**Figure 41-5.** Using a no. 10 blade scalpel, the dorsal incision is made full thickness down to the dome of the talus.

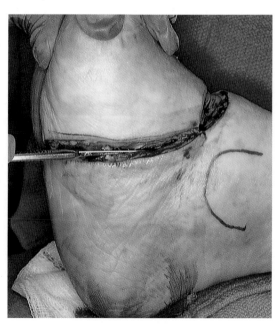

**Figure 41-6.** The plantar incision is then made down to the calcaneus (*side view*).

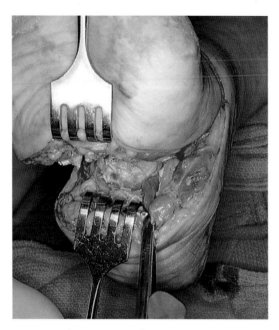

**Figure 41-7.** Plantar view of Figure 41-6, with retraction in place.

essential, to obtain the forward and downward traction to keep the soft tissues under tension to facilitate soft tissue sectioning (Fig. 41-10).

Great care is taken to circumvent the neurovascular bundle (posterior tibial vessels and nerve), one of the two most critical points of the operation, as was described by Syme himself. The neurovascular bundle lies between the flexor hallucis longus and the flexor digitorum longus, and can be accidentally injured if care is not taken (Fig. 41-11). The flexor hallucis longus tendon is the primary landmark, as the bundle lies just behind it. After it is identified, a blunt dissection is done (e.g., with a broad Key elevator) to separate the bone from the entire soft tissue envelope (Fig. 41-12).

The dissection of the calcaneus and its neat separation from the soft tissue constitute the second major critical point in the operation: the subcutaneous attachment of the Achilles tendon. Penetrating or "buttonholing" through the skin at this point often condemns the procedure to failure, because the Syme stump does not heal after this type of injury to the

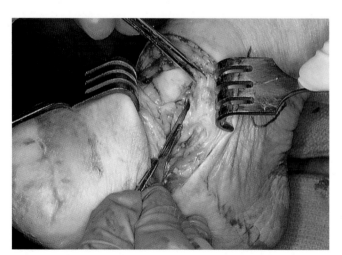
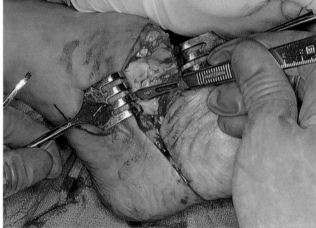

**Figures 41-8 and 41-9.** The collateral ligaments of the talus are released, working alternately on the medial *(left)* and lateral *(right)* sides while placing traction on the talus downward and forward.

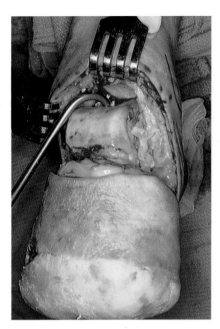

**Figure 41-10.** A large bone hook placed into the dome of the talus is essential to apply the traction needed to keep the dissection under tension. This is essential to "peel" the calcaneus out of its soft tissue envelope.

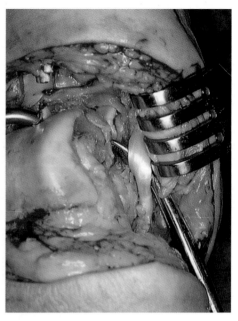

**Figure 41-11.** Care is taken to protect and avoid the neurovascular bundle between the flexor digitorum (on the clamp) and flexor hallucis tendons (at the point of clamp).

heel pad. Figure 41-13 shows how closely the attachment of the Achilles tendon approximates the skin posteriorly. This is the point at which penetration of the skin is most likely.

Alternating use of sharp and blunt dissection with scalpel and periosteal elevator works best to dissect the calcaneus from the adjacent soft tissues (Figs. 41-14 and 41-15). It is this portion of the procedure that is responsible for making the Syme amputation the most technically difficult foot amputation. It is important to work methodically and patiently, exercising vigilance to avoid a penetrating stroke to the posterior soft tissue.

The subperiosteal dissection alternates from above at the Achilles tendon and from the undersurface and sides of the calcaneus until the bone is free from the soft tissue. This

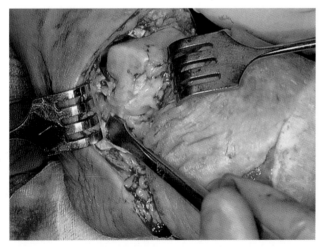

**Figure 41-12.** Blunt dissection with a broad elevator is done to separate the calcaneus from the full-thickness flap of soft tissue.

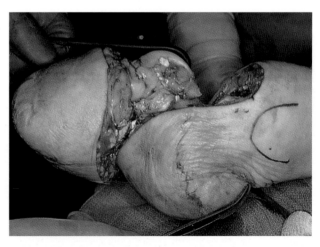

**Figure 41-13.** The clamp points to a dimple in the posterior skin where the attachment of the calcaneus is closest to the surface. This is the point of greatest risk of error in the operation. Penetration of the skin while dissecting out the calcaneus may cause failure.

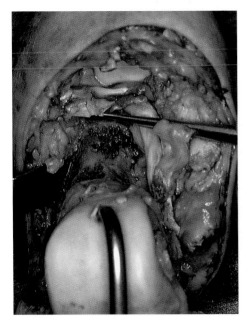
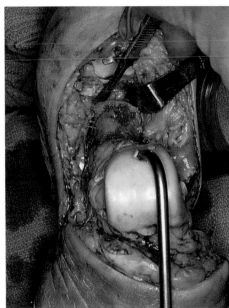

**Figures 41-14 and 41-15.** Alternating sharp and blunt dissection on the calcaneus is preferred for the difficult task of dissecting the bone from the thin layer of soft tissue.

leaves the distal tibial, fibular, and heel pad for final shaping and closure. Notice the appearance of the specimen once the dissection has been completed (Fig. 41-16).

The anterior tibial artery and accompanying veins are then ligated (Fig. 41-17). The extensor and flexor tendons are then pulled distally with a large clamp and divided so that they retract proximally (Fig. 41-18). Avoid the neurovascular bundle within the posterior flap as described to avoid damage to the blood supply to the heel pad.

Before performing the closure, the malleoli are cut off flush with the level of the tibial plafond (Figs. 41-19 and 41-20). Although some surgeons have advised narrowing the medial-lateral flare of the tibial metaphysis, it is desirable to conserve the flare because it gives

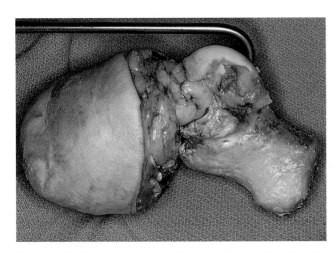

**Figure 41-16.** Appearance of the specimen after the dissection is completed.

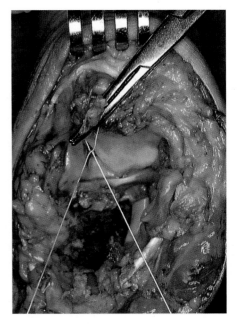

**Figure 41-17.** The anterior vascular bundle is ligated.

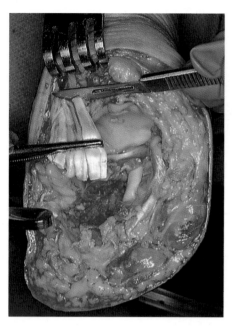

**Figure 41-18.** The extensor tendons are divided under tension.

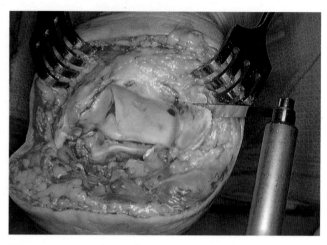

**Figure 41-19.** The malleoli are resected at the level of the tibial plafond using the small oscillating saw.

wider internal support to the bulbous Syme stump. It is specifically important because the tibial flare is the main structure that holds the prosthesis on and keeps it from slipping up and down (Fig. 41-21). It is not necessary to remove the cartilage from the distal tibia.

The heel pad is then gently held up with digital pressure to visualize the appearance of the wound closure (Fig. 41-22). If the pad appears to be too mobile at the time of closure,

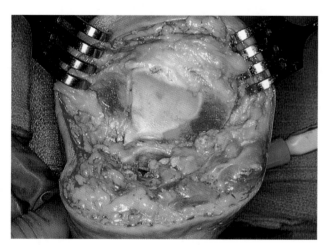

**Figure 41-20.** Appearance after resection of both malleoli.

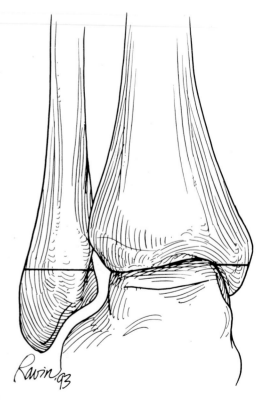

**Figure 41-21.** The level of bone resection of the malleoli.

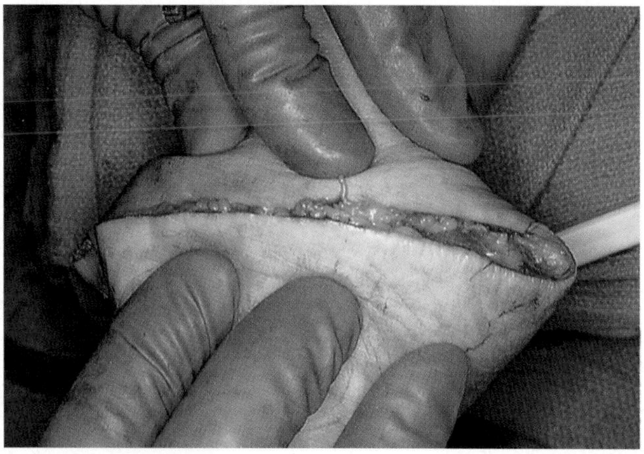

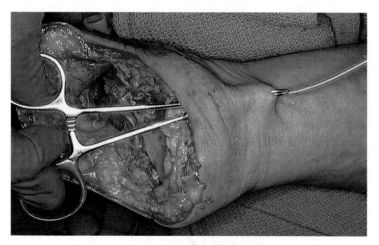

**Figure 41-22.** The final shape of the stump is checked with gentle manual soft tissue approximation to verify the easy apposition of the flaps.

additional tissue should be resected from the distal (plantar) edge of the heel pad, and the pad sutured to the bone. If the soft tissue is too thick to allow easy apposition of the two skin edges, it is usually caused by the thick plantar fat pad on the inferior side. It is often necessary to carefully thin or "plane" down this fat pad so that it does not distract the edges of the wound. Prudence must be applied to prevent excessive thinning and devascularization of the flap. The closure is done over a suction drain that is brought out through a separate tiny stab wound proximally (Figs. 41-23 and 41-24).

Drill holes are made in the anterior lip of the tibial plafond (Fig. 41-25) to anchor the plantar fascia. Alternatively, the plantar fascia can be sutured to the deep fascia anteriorly.

The closure is done in three layers. First, the plantar fascia is sutured either through the drill holes in the distal tibia or to the fascia as described (Figs. 41-26 and 41-27). This is followed by a subcutaneous closure with inverted interrupted absorbable sutures (Fig. 41-28). The skin is closed with nylon sutures or staples (Fig. 41-29). A soft dressing is applied.

In the two-stage Syme procedure done for infected cases, the resection of the malleoli is deferred at the time of the initial operation. At the second stage, the "dog ears" of soft tissue on the medial and lateral sides are excised. The malleoli are then resected through the elliptical openings created on either side before closure. If the pad is excessively mobile at this stage, correction is obtained by removing larger ellipses of skin and subcutaneous tissue.

**Figure 41-23.** Closure is performed over the 0.125-inch suction drain withdrawn through a separate, proximal stab incision.

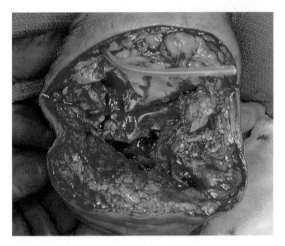

**Figure 41-24.** The drain is placed in the wound.

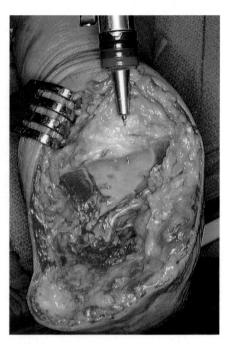

**Figure 41-25.** Drill holes are made in the anterior lip of the distal tibial plafond to anchor sutures to the plantar fascia.

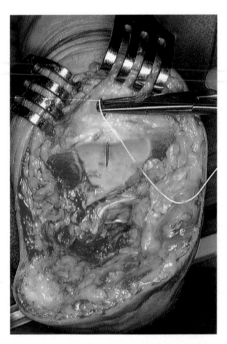

**Figure 41-26.** The suture is placed through the drill holes in the anterior margin of the tibia.

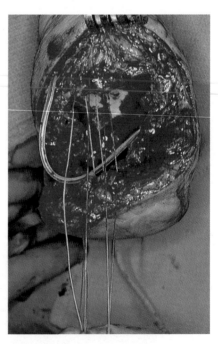

**Figure 41-27.** The sutures are passed through the plantar fascia, taking care to avoid entrapping the drain.

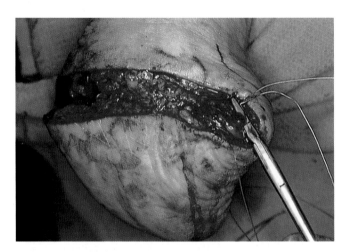

**Figure 41-28.** A subcutaneous closure is done with interrupted, inverted absorbable sutures.

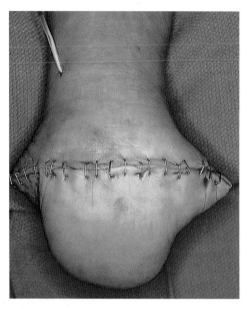

**Figure 41-29.** The skin is closed with staples or interrupted sutures.

## POSTOPERATIVE MANAGEMENT

Initially, a soft dressing or a plaster shell over the dressing can be used. The suction drain is usually removed after 24 hours. The patient is instructed in proper technique for non–weight-bearing gait using crutches or walker. After the first week, a cast is usually applied to protect the stump. If the patient is diabetic or dysvascular, a non–weight-bearing program is maintained for at least 4 to 6 weeks. Earlier ambulation on the cast can sometimes be allowed in cases of amputations done for trauma, depending on the advancement of wound healing.

The removal of the skin sutures or staples may be delayed until 6 to 8 weeks after surgery, or even more. Sutures are generally left in place a minimum of 4 weeks. It is not unusual to see a small amount of serous drainage after closure, as occurs in most foot amputations, but this usually resolves over the first 1 to 2 weeks.

Prosthetic fitting, especially in the diabetic and dysvascular patients is done after complete healing of the stump has occurred. Weight bearing is not permitted if areas of delayed soft tissue healing persist. Most patients with a successful outcome will be able to be fitted with a prosthesis and ambulate at least on a limited basis, within 10 to 12 weeks.

The success rate of Syme amputations varies from 50% to 90%. Most physicians report about a 70% to 75% success rate for healing of Syme amputations in diabetic and dysvascular patients. Weaver et al. (7) described results of 35 patients who underwent Syme amputation preceded by revascularization and 10 (77%) of 13 undergoing amputation alone. Successful rehabilitation was accomplished with 97% of patients with successful primary healing. Laughlin and Chambers (5) studied 52 patients with severe forefoot gangrene from diabetes treated by Syme amputation and found that posterior tibial artery Doppler examination was predictive of healing. Twenty-nine percent had a posterior tibial artery with a triphasic waveform or normal pulse, and 26 (90%) achieved a healed wound. Twenty-three patients had monophasic flow in the posterior tibial artery, and 13 (57%) achieved a healed wound.

Most failures in the diabetic and dysvascular patient population occur early as the result of failure to achieve primary wound healing, usually because of ischemia of the heel pad, which is supplied by branches of the posterior tibial artery.

Late failure of the Syme amputation is usually caused by progressive peripheral vascular occlusion, which results in gangrene through a wider area of the lower limb, rather than complications inherent within the Syme stump.

Good prosthetic fitting of the Syme stump is vital, and usually requires a prosthetist with experience. The difficulty lies in the fact that a secure fit is required but the broad, bulbous end of the stump must pass through a narrow portion of the prosthesis corresponding to the narrow width of the distal tibia just above the metaphysis. This challenge has been handled with a number of different techniques including placing a hinged window in the prosthesis, placing a wraparound filler above the bulb, or using an elastic double-wall construction for the distal part of the prosthesis. Many prostheses are equipped with a solid ankle cushion heel (SACH) that enhances the patient's gait.

A minor and the only significant disadvantage of the Syme amputation compared with a below-knee amputation is that the Syme prosthesis is less cosmetic because of the wide "ankle" portion of the prosthesis, which is required to allow passage of the stump. However, in virtually every other way, the Syme prosthesis is preferable to a below-knee amputation. The Syme stump is a partially end-bearing area, and even diabetic patients have fewer problems with skin breakdown over the proximal leg that would occur with a below-knee amputation. Suprapatellar suspension straps are not needed. The mechanical advantage of a full lower leg segment is immense. Even more important, most patients with Syme amputations need minimal prosthetic training, and require much less extensive physical therapy because the Syme amputation functions like a partial foot amputation. Prosthetic walking is similar to the use of a cast, which most of the patients have used previously. The lower energy cost (i.e., oxygen consumption per meter) of the Syme amputation compared with more proximal amputations was addressed in the introduction to this chapter. The Syme amputee also has a higher velocity of gait and a longer stride length (5).

## COMPLICATIONS

The Syme amputation is an excellent procedure with potentially excellent function for the patient. Because this is often used as a salvage-type procedure, in an attempt to avert performing a below-knee amputation, there will be a certain number of failures and complications, and the numbers will be related to the individual surgeon's threshold criteria for doing this procedure. Although the morbidity of a second, more proximal amputation is not negligible, the ultimate result for the patient is not significantly prejudiced by the need to revise to a below-knee amputation if the Syme amputation fails. There are five major complications of the Syme amputation.

*Early (dysvascular) failure of the wound to heal* is the most common complication of the Syme procedure is primary failure of the soft tissue to heal. Some occurrences of this complication cannot be precluded if the surgeon strives for the goal of maximal limb salvage. However, proper preoperative vascular evaluation is the solution to keep the frequency of this complication to a reasonable level. At the time of surgery, if the wound edges do not demonstrate adequate bleeding once the disarticulation is completed, it is advisable to proceed to a more proximal amputation.

*Hypermobility or migration of the stump* may occur. Some mobility of the stump is normal, and a few patients can even dorsiflex and plantarflex the stump through the action of the residual tendons. Stump mobility becomes problematic when the stump moves or migrates side to side, because this can interfere with or compromise the fitting and function of the prosthesis. If modification of the prosthesis is unsuccessful, it is usually addressed by excision of full-thickness wedges of tissue from the medial and lateral sides of the stump or distally. Suturing the fascia of the distal pad to the tibia through drill holes is sometimes required as well.

*Late ulceration of the stump* occurs infrequently, primarily in diabetics. Although this complication may result from an isolated incident of trauma to the tissue, it is usually caused by pressure from a bony prominence such as the distal margin of the fibula. Stump mobility and shrinkage of the tissue can exacerbate the problem. Initial treatment with local wound care and total contact casts is advisable. If the problem persists, the treatment is excision of the underlying bone causing pressure on the skin. The ulcer can be debrided or excised as well.

*Poor cosmesis* of the prosthesis in the Syme amputee is occasionally a problem, particularly for women who would like to wear dresses instead of pants. It is important to discuss this with the patient preoperatively, and if necessary, even show photos of the prosthesis so that the patient understands what to expect of the final appearance. Most patients choose improved function over image.

*Painful stumps* occur infrequently, usually in Syme amputations that have been done for trauma. The most common cause of pain is neuroma formation in one of the major nerves or anterior superficial sensory nerves near the level of the ankle joint where they have been transected. The treatment is surgical excision or burying the end of the nerve. Accurate diagnosis is aided by selective injection with small amounts of local anesthetic.

Rarely, the entire pad of the stump is persistently painful in a patient who has had the amputation done for a crushing injury to the hindfoot. Most of these are industrial accidents. Treatment is by revision to a long below-knee amputation.

## ILLUSTRATIVE CASE

This patient is a 23-year-old construction worker who sustained a severe crushing injury on the job while working with a paving machine. The forefoot was mangled and the midfoot was contaminated and degloved. The patient underwent initial aggressive debridement, followed by redebridement and a partial foot amputation that was left open (Figs. 41-30 and 41-31). The patient was then treated with appropriate intravenous antibiotics and vigorous

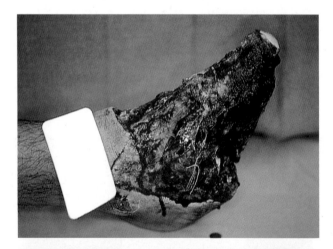

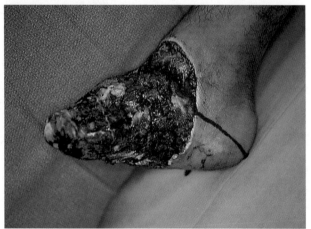

**Figures 41-30 and 41-31.** Appearance of the foot after primary debridements, local wound care, and antibiotics but before performing the Syme procedure.

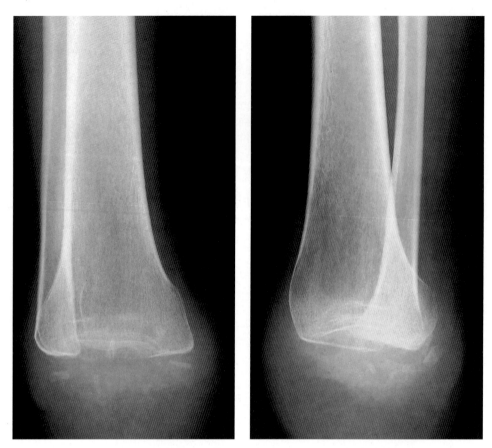

**Figure 41-32.** Radiographs of the Syme stump 6 months postoperatively.

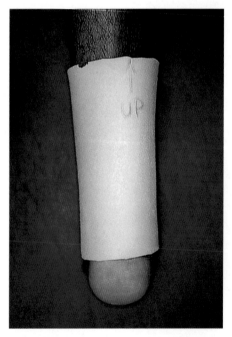

**Figure 41-33.** The Syme limb with a Plastazote molded filler applied just above the bulb. This converts the limb to a cylinder, facilitating early prosthetic fitting.

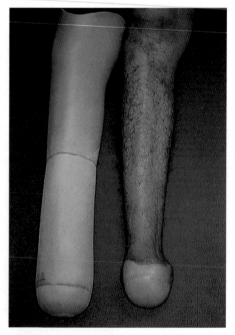

**Figure 41-34.** The appearance of the limb and the liner for the prosthesis 9 months postoperatively.

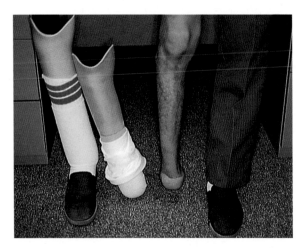

**Figure 41-35.** *Left to right*: the Syme prosthesis, the liner of the prosthesis, the Syme limb, and the normal limb 9 months postoperatively.

local wound care. The open amputation was converted to a Syme amputation 1 week after injury.

Initially, the patient was kept from bearing weight until all the skin sutures were removed. He was then placed in a temporary prosthesis made of synthetic cast material with a rubber heel and started on a vigorous physical therapy program. He was fitted with a Syme prosthesis at about 2.5 months postoperatively. The patient had significant persistent pain for many months, presumably because of the crushing nature of the injury. The patient required another 3 months of physical therapy because of his stump pain and slow progress. There were no problems with healing of the wound, and no specific point tenderness could be found that might indicate neuroma formation. The radiographic appearance of the limb is seen in Figure 41-32. Eventually the patient became independent in his ambulation and virtually pain-free, and returned to a sedentary type of job at about 9 months after injury. The limb and the patient's prosthesis at the time of completion of his treatment are shown in Figures 41-33 through 41-35.

## RECOMMENDED READING

1. Anderson L, Westin GW, Oppenheim WL: Syme amputation in children: indications, results, and long-term follow-up. *J Pediatr Orthop* 4:550–554, 1984.
2. Francis H III, Roberts JR, Clagett GP, et al.: The Syme amputation: success in elderly diabetic patients with palpable ankle pulses. *J Vasc Surg* 12:237–240, 1990.
3. Herring JA, Barnhill B, Gaffney C: Syme amputation. *J Bone Joint Surg Am* 68:573–578, 1986.
4. Jany RS, Burkus JK: Long-term follow-up of Syme amputations for peripheral vascular disease associated with diabetes mellitus. *Foot Ankle* 9:107–110, 1988.
5. Laughlin RT, Chambers RB: Syme amputation in patients with severe diabetes mellitus. *Foot Ankle* 14:65–70, 1993.
6. Waters RL, Perry J, Antonelli D, et al.: Energy cost of walking of amputees: the influence of level of amputation. *J Bone Joint Surg Am* 56:42–46, 1976.
7. Weaver FA, Modrall JG, Back S, et al.: Syme amputations: results in patients with severe forefoot ischemia. *Cardiovasc Surg* 4:81–86, 1996.

# 42

# Tibial Periarticular Fracture Reduction and Fixation

Roy Sanders and Joel D. Stewart

## INDICATIONS/CONTRAINDICATIONS

Fractures of the distal tibia involving the weight-bearing articular surface present a significant treatment challenge for the orthopedic surgeon. These fractures, commonly known as pilon or plafond fractures, represent 1% to 10% of all lower extremity fractures. They occur after low- or high-energy trauma, and they usually result in significant soft tissue and cartilage damage. The most predictable results are obtained when anatomic reconstruction of the joint is obtained and early motion of the ankle can be initiated. Operative treatment in the past focused on obtaining an anatomic reduction at the expense of the soft tissue envelope surrounding the ankle joint. This resulted in significant soft tissue complications, including skin slough, deep infections, and amputation. Because of these complications, techniques using external fixators to protect the soft tissues while minimizing the risk of infection were developed. Unfortunately, anatomic reduction was rarely achieved using these limited techniques. More recent approaches attempt to protect the soft tissues while still obtaining an anatomic reduction of the joint. This technique employs immediate "portable traction" followed by staged reconstruction of the joint and tibia when the soft tissue envelope is not acutely compromised.

R. Sanders, M.D.: Division of Orthopaedic Surgery, University of South Florida; and Department of Orthopaedics, Tampa General Hospital, Tampa, Florida.

J. D. Stewart, M.D.: Department of Surgery, Uniformed Services University of the Health Sciences, Bethesda, Maryland; and Department of Orthopaedics, Naval Medical Center Portsmouth, Portsmouth, Virginia.

Results of nonoperative treatment of displaced pilon fractures were disappointing. Nonoperative treatment should therefore be reserved for nondisplaced fractures or in patients with a poor medical prognosis. Operative indications include distal tibial fractures with articular displacement of more than 2 mm, unacceptable axial alignment, and open fractures. Another indication is adjacent nerve or vascular injury, which require repair and would be protected by bony stabilization of the fracture.

Many classification systems are used to describe pilon fractures. The most commonly used classification is the Rüedi-Ällgower classification, which has been shown to correlate with both complications and outcome (Fig. 42-1A). The AO/OTA classification provides the most detail and is useful for research but is the most complex (Fig. 42-1B). This classification is less useful and reliable beyond distinguishing the fracture type.

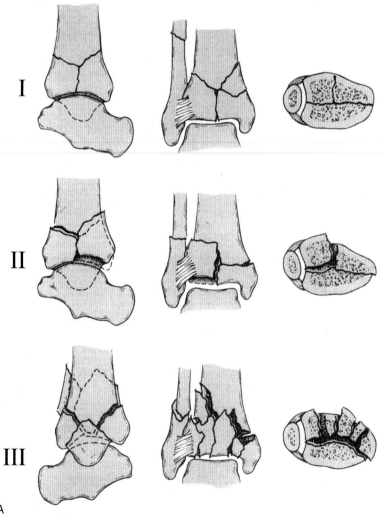

A

**Figure 42-1.  A:** Rüedi and Ällgower classification of pilon fractures. *(continued)*

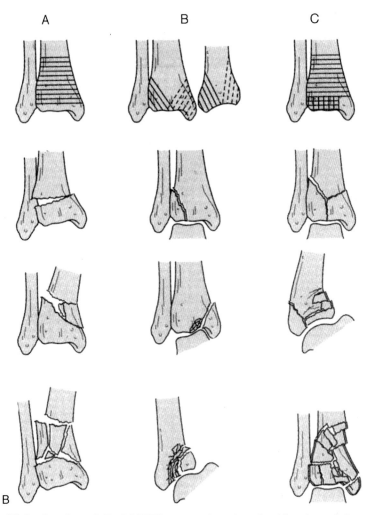

**Figure 42-1.** *Continued.* **B:** AO/OTA comprehensive classification of fractures of the distal tibia. (**A** from Rüedi TP, Ällgower M: Fractures of the lower end of the tibia into the ankle joint: result 9 years after open reduction and internal fixation. *Injury* 5: 120, 1973, with permission; **B** from Muller ME, Schneider R, Ällgower M, et al.: *Manual of internal fixation.* New York: Springer-Verlag, 1991:146–147, 596, with permission.)

## PREOPERATIVE PLANNING

Initial examination includes a standard trauma evaluation of the entire patient. These patients often have other injuries caused by the high-energy mechanism. Evaluation of the injured extremity includes examination of the distal neurovascular structures, evaluation for compartment syndrome, and soft tissue integrity. Evaluation of the soft tissues should assess the severity of damage. Tscherne's classification of soft tissue trauma, grades closed injuries to the limb on a 0 to 3 scoring system (Table 42-1).

Radiographic evaluation includes standard anteroposterior, lateral, and mortise views of the ankle to delineate articular comminution and integrity. Anteroposterior and lateral views of the entire tibial shaft are required to appreciate the metaphyseal and diaphyseal extent of the injury and to evaluate for proximal injuries. Foot radiographs are indicated when foot injuries are suspected, in AP, lateral, and oblique views. Computed tomography

**Table 42.1.** *Tscherne's classification of soft tissue trauma*

| Grade | Diagnosis |
|-------|-----------|
| 0 | Absent |
| 1 | Indirect, contusion from within, superficial abrasion |
| 2 | Direct with deep contaminated abrasion or severe indirect with blistering and edema, impending compartment syndrome |
| 3 | Usually direct, extensive contusion or crush, possibly severe muscle damage, vascular injury, or compartment syndrome |

(CT) is a useful adjunct to plain film radiography. CT scans allow the surgeon to understand the degree of three-dimensional anatomic disruption and to plan surgical incisions and placement of implants.

## SURGERY

The timing of the operative procedure is determined by the technique of stabilization. We prefer a staged protocol with immediate operative intervention once the patient is stabilized (within 12 to 18 hours of injury) with open reduction internal fixation (ORIF) of the fibula and the application of a medial bridging external fixator. Although any external fixation construct can be employed, we have found that using an EBI or Orthofix type of medial frame affords not only axial, but rotational stability and requires a minimum number of pins (Fig. 42-2). When applying this frame, pins should be placed as far as possible from the edges of the proposed incision site. The incision for the fibula ORIF is placed slightly posterolaterally to increase the width of the skin bridge between it and the subsequent anterior incision. It must be emphasized that calcaneal skeletal traction, even with the leg on a Böhler-Braun frame has essentially no place in the treatment of these fractures. This type of traction tends to gradually pull the patient out of bed and to allow the foot to displace posteriorly, causing the distal end of the fractured tibia to impinge and violate the anterior pretibial skin, severely compromising subsequent surgery.

Patients with isolated injuries are typically treated as described earlier and then sent home and kept on a non–weight-bearing program. When the soft tissue edema is no longer present, a safe open reduction with internal fixation of the tibial fracture can be performed (usually 10 to 21 days).

The patient is positioned supine on a radiolucent table or a radiolucent extension. A nonsterile tourniquet is placed on the thigh. The scrub nurse and his or her table are on the ipsilateral side of the patient, while the fluoroscopic C-arm is brought in from the contralateral side of the injured limb (Fig. 42-3). The fixator is removed, but the pins are left in

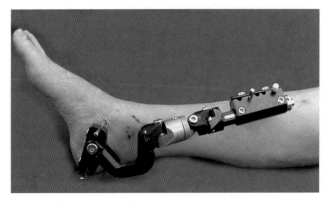

**Figure 42-2.** The medial bridging external fixator should be kept well clear of the planned incision.

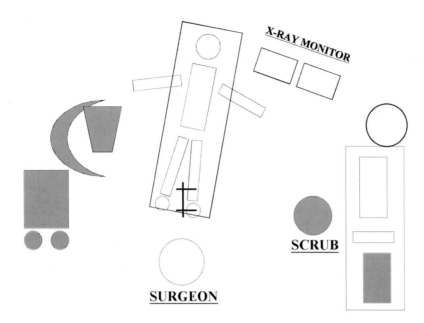

**Figure 42-3.** Operating room setup shows the surgeon at the foot of the table, with the C-arm monitor on the ipsilateral head of the table and the scrub technician on the ipsilateral side of the patient.

place. The limb is prepped. During the prep, the fixator frame is sterilized for 10 minutes so that it can be used intraoperatively as a distractor, if needed. Before exsanguination, the tibial incision is drawn out. The incision must be based on the fracture pattern and fixation techniques to be employed. After the incision is drawn, the limb is exsanguinated and the tourniquet is inflated to 350 mm Hg. This can be left inflated for a maximum of 150 minutes (2.5 hours).

## Technique

**Incisions and Approaches.** If the fracture mostly involves the distal tibial medially, a standard anteromedial approach may be employed. This incision begins just lateral to the medial crest of the tibial shaft, so that the scar does not irritate the patient. The incision is carried distally across the ankle joint, staying just medial to the anterior tibial tendon throughout the entire incision. This is a modification of the "classic" approach described by Schatzker, in which the distal end of the incision curves around and under the medial malleolus. This latter incision is not extensile (i.e., cannot be extended distally if necessary), and tends to prevent access to the middle and lateral portions of the anterior distal tibia. By following the tendon, our modification allows access to the midline and most of the joint surface (Fig. 42-4).

After the skin is incised, the medial skin flap is only developed until the medial aspect of the anterior tibial tendon sheath can be identified. The medial sheath, along with the extensor retinaculum, should be incised and taken down to bone or joint. The incision is carried down to the periosteum, and full-thickness flaps are raised. Periosteal stripping is not performed. Similarly, fat should not be arbitrarily excised. Removing fat for visualization will cause excessive scarring of the joint in the long term. Fracture edges are identified, as are blood clots and periosteal strands. Once completely exposed, fracture reduction may then begin. This approach is ideally suited for the application of a medial pilon plate, especially when shaft extension is present.

A third incision, the anterior midline incision, is a modification of the standard anteromedial exposure that wraps around the medial malleolus, as it is more extensile and less confining. A midline incision is ideally used when the fracture is a pure anterior crush type injury.

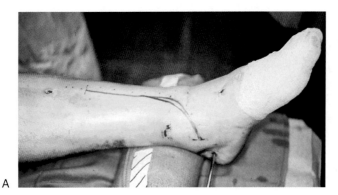
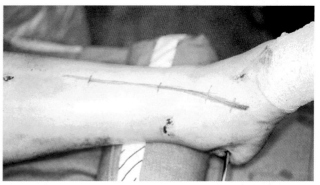

A                                                                                              B

**Figure 42-4.  A:** Standard medial pilon incision wraps around the medial malleolus. **B:** In the modified approach, the incision follows the medial border of the anterior tibial tendon distally. This approach is more extensile and less confining.

In these injuries, this approach will not only permit excellent fracture exposure and reduction, but will easily allow the placement of a low profile anterior tibial plate. This approach may be used if a subsequent total ankle replacement is contemplated. This latter philosophy is very similar to that of midline incisions for tibial plateau fractures, recognizing that some severe injuries may require a total knee replacement. A midline incision will expose the joint between the anterior tibial tendon and the extensor hallucis longus. Care must be taken to identify the superficial peroneal nerve directly under the skin. Once this has been mobilized, the neurovascular bundle lying between the two tendons should be identified and retracted laterally together with the EHL tendon. The joint can then be entered and exposure should be completed with debridement of blood clots and periosteal strands from the fracture fragments.

Finally, the anterolateral, or Böhler, incision should be used when large lateral fragments such as Tillaux-Chaput avulsions are the predominant radiographic finding. This incision must be carefully contemplated as it may jeopardize the skin bridge immediately lateral to it, if the fibula incision is placed too anteriorly. Some judgment must be made at the time of presentation shortly after the injury about what sort of incisions may be needed for addressing the tibial fracture, because this choice will affect the location of the fibula incision. In cases of severe comminution, a small portion of this incision may be needed in addition to an anteromedial one to reduce a lateral fracture fragment. Because of these issues, we typically use a posterolateral incision for fibula fixation. This ultimately affords us the largest skin bridges possible when three incisions are needed.

The Böhler incision starts proximal to the ankle joint and slightly medial to Chaput's tubercle and extends distally in a straight line toward the base of the third and fourth metatarsals (Fig. 42-5). The superficial peroneal nerve is identified and protected while the dissection proceeds through the subcutaneous tissue to expose the superior and inferior extensor retinaculum. After dividing the superior and inferior extensor retinaculum, a medial mobilization of the tendons of the extensor digitorum longus and peroneus tertius, the deep peroneal nerve, and the dorsalis pedis artery is performed. In the distal aspect of the incision, the muscle of the extensor digitorum brevis can be seen. If greater exposure is needed, the muscle can be retracted laterally if possible, divided in the direction of its fibers, or detached from its origin and reflected distally. The lateral branch of the deep peroneal nerve and the lateral tarsal artery should be protected. This approach affords the surgeon a wide exposure of the distal tibia, the middle and lateral ankle joint, and most of the lateral talar body.

**Technical Pearls and Pitfalls.**  For most articular fractures, certain time-tested principles developed by Rüedi, Weber, Heim, and Mast should be followed. The joint surface must be anatomically reconstructed first, as articular malalignment is totally unacceptable, whereas the ankle can tolerate a bit of axial malalignment. Shaft reconstruction is performed secondarily. In some simpler fractures, periarticular and percutaneous reduction and fixation may be possible. If the joint reduction is attempted through the shaft plating, the joint reduction will invariably shift and become suboptimal. As a result, we believe in anatomic joint reduction using isolated lag screws followed by neutralization plating of the metaphyseal-diaphyseal component.

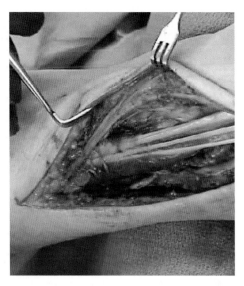

**Figure 42-5.** Böhler incision reveals the tendons of the extensor digitorum longus and peroneus tertius and the superficial peroneal nerve crossing the superior lateral portion of the wound.

The joint surface needs to be reconstructed anatomically. If there are centrally crushed components, the only way they can be mobilized is to carefully retract the perimeter fragments to better visualize and reconstruct the fracture. Typically, the medial malleolus is retracted for most of the operation. If the fibula is stable and out to length and the lateral ligaments are intact, reduction can be performed around the anterolateral corner (i.e., Chaput-Tillaux tubercle). Care must be taken to evaluate for impaction of the anterolateral tibia. Sequential reduction is begun, with the goal of combining fragments until only the medial malleolus is needed to complete the puzzle (Fig. 42-6).

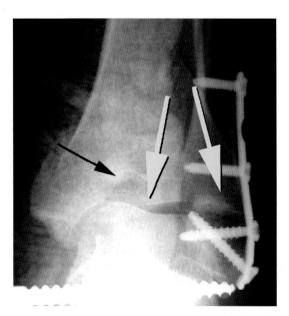

**Figure 42-6.** On the anteroposterior radiograph of a C2 pilon fracture after anatomic reduction of the fibula and bridging external fixation, notice the impacted and displaced Chaput fragment *(green arrows)*. The *black arrow* identifies the centrally impacted articular surface.

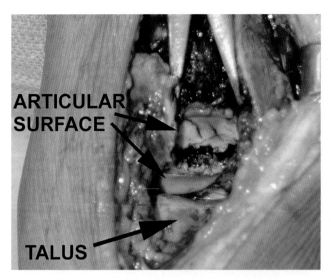

**Figure 42-7.** Pilon fracture after anteromedial exposure. The anterior joint surface is displaced and rotated 90° (Chaput fragment is on the right, medial malleolus is on the left).

The edges of the fragments need to be cleaned of debris and their shapes and imperfections are studied, as these will give the surgeon clues about how they fit together, much like a complicated jigsaw puzzle (Fig. 42-7). Fragments must be connected provisionally, and 1.6-mm Kirschner wires are typically employed. The 2.0-mm wires are too large and can damage the fragments, whereas 1.25-mm wires are too flexible and cannot hold the fragments securely during screw placement. Kirschner wires tend to deviate or deflect within the fragments and may shift the fragments slightly during placement. The wires may have to be passed several times, which may damage the fragments. For these reasons, the authors prefer to use pointed reduction clamps of various sizes to obtain the initial reduction, employing Kirschner wires to maintain the reduction before final fixation. After the fragments are finally secured with Kirschner wires, the clamps are usually left on for stability, and removed only if they interfere with a particular reduction maneuver. Kirschner wires should be placed with deliberation, to ensure they do not interfere with ideal screw placement for final stabilization.

Fragments of the articular surface that are too small to hold screws are stabilized using bioabsorbable pins. These can often be placed through the Kirschner wire holes instead of drilling a separate hole for the pin (Fig. 42-8).

We only rarely use cannulated screws over the wires, though the 1.6-mm wires are employed in case this is necessary. Cannulated lag screws are only partially threaded and have a larger core diameter and therefore a smaller root area of the tapped thread (RATT). This results in an overall inferior purchase as compared with a standard fully threaded cortical or cancellous screw used in a lag mode. Each large fragment is separately lagged to the stable main fragment, usually posterior or posterolaterally, much like the techniques applied to calcaneal (sustentacular fragment) or acetabular (iliosacral fragment) fractures.

Large, centrally depressed fragments can be reduced and fixed with lag screws, without the need for bone graft that could interfere with the reduction. When small, however, these fragments need to be "squeezed" together from the periphery. Lag screws placed though these small fragments will rotate, shift, or cause them to explode. When using the latter technique, cancellous graft must be liberally packed into the defect above the fragments, so that they do not shift during peripheral compression.

After a stable and secure reconstruction of the entire joint has been accomplished, buttress plating using low profile plates is performed to connect the articular surface to the shaft. Rotational and varus-valgus injuries benefit from medial pilon plates, whereas anterior crush injuries should be plated with an anterior pilon plate. Supplemental washer plates

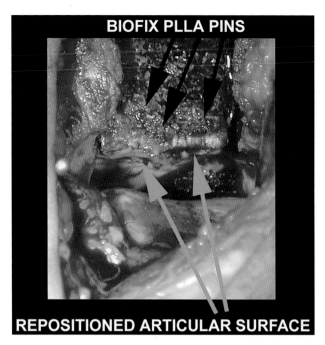

**Figure 42-8.** After reduction of the small articular fragments, they are fixed using bioabsorbable pins (Bionx Implants, Blue Bell, PA).

may be needed depending on the fracture pattern (Figs. 42-9 and 42-10). Stabilization of the articular surface to the shaft can be performed using percutaneous techniques. Stabilization of the construct is achieved by inserting previously contoured plates though small skin incisions onto the bone. The plates are then secured to the bone with screws placed through skin incisions under fluoroscopic guidance. Soft tissue stripping is minimized (Figs. 42-11 through 42-14).

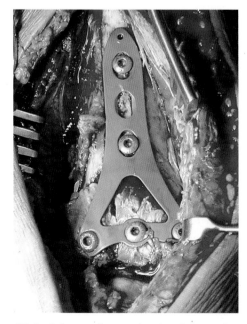

**Figure 42-9.** Joint surface reduction is completed first, and then the metaphyseal fragments are reduced and fixed using a low-profile, contoured titanium periarticular buttress plate (ACE DePuy, Warsaw, IN).

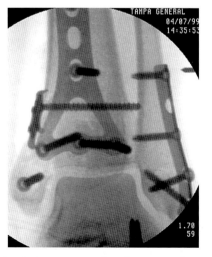

**Figure 42-10.** Intraoperative fluoroscopic images are used to ensure adequate joint reduction. Note spider washer plate medially (ACE DePuy, Warsaw, IN).

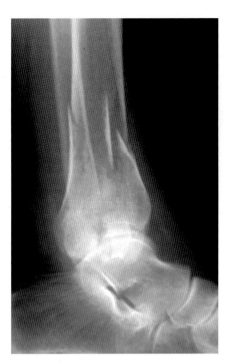

**Figure 42-11.** The C1 fracture is amenable to limited dissection and percutaneous techniques.

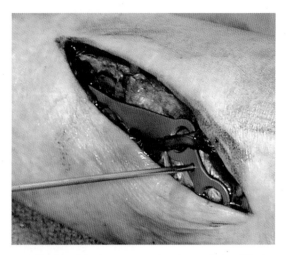

**Figure 42-12.** After open reduction of the fibula and closed reduction of the tibia, the anteromedial surface of the tibia is exposed through a limited incision. The surgeon slides the buttress plate up the tibia extraperiosteally.

Skin closure is performed over a small drain to minimize the development of a postoperative hematoma. The deep layers are closed with interrupted 2-0 absorbable sutures, and the skin is closed with 3-0 nylon with modified Donati or interrupted mattress sutures.

Pitfalls include performing definitive surgery immediately. Fracture patterns are still unclear and soft tissue swelling is too great. Use of an unstable fixator or failure to stabilize

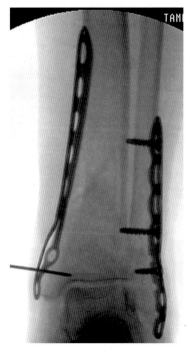

**Figure 42-13.** The reduction and position of the plate are checked using fluoroscopy.

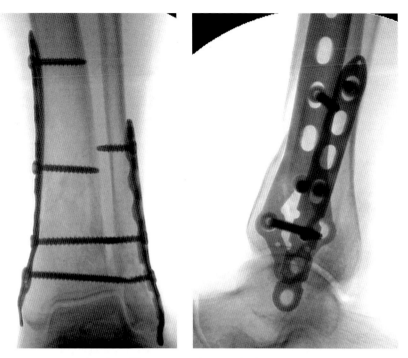

**Figure 42-14.** Postreduction films were obtained after percutaneous plating (ACE DePuy, Warsaw, IN).

the fibula fracture will result in continued motion, resulting in persistent swelling, blistering, and skin breakdown, making subsequent surgery difficult. Use of standard ankle fracture incisions may cause complications. These incisions are not extensile and often prevent appropriate exposure. Attempts to stabilize all fragments at once usually extend the tourniquet time unnecessarily and results in a suboptimal outcome.

### Postoperative Management

The patients are placed in a bulky splint. The drain is removed on the first postoperative day. Patients are maintained on intravenous antibiotics for 48 hours after surgery. The patient is typically discharged when he or she becomes independent on crutches, usually on the second postoperative day. The patient is seen back in the office in 1 week and wounds are examined. At that time the patient is placed in a compression stocking and a removable boot, so that early motion can be initiated. The sutures are removed only when the wound is healed usually at 3 weeks, but sometimes as late as 5 to 6 weeks. Formal physical therapy is started at 4 to 6 weeks, as soon as wound healing is complete. Weight bearing is instituted at 3 months if radiographs indicate complete union of the fracture. The patient must wear the boot at all times, even to sleep; if he or she does not, the patient may develop an equinus contracture.

   Good to excellent results historically are observed in approximately 80% of patients with low energy, minimally displaced fractures. High-energy, OTA grade C2 or C3, or Rüedi and Ällgower type III fractures have significantly higher rates of complications and worse outcomes. Most studies show good to excellent results in 50% to 70% of these high-energy injuries. Outcome is affected by severity of injury (Rüedi classification), quality of articular reduction, and development of postoperative infection. Delayed arthrodesis can be expected in less than 10% of type I or II fractures and approximately 25% of type III fractures.

## COMPLICATIONS

*Wound complications and infection* may occur. Superficial skin necrosis is treated with local wound care, joint immobilization, and oral antibiotics if any evidence of cellulitis is present. Deep infection is more likely to occur in more severe fracture types, open fractures, and those that are associated with postoperative skin slough. Deep infection should be initially treated with debridement and intravenous antibiotics until the fracture has healed. The implants are left in place until the fracture has healed, and then the infection can be treated more effectively by removal of hardware, debridement of all necrotic tissue, and an additional six weeks of culture-specific intravenous antibiotics. If the fracture has not healed, removal of any necrotic fragments, stable fixation of large fragments, antibiotic polymethylmethacrylate beads and culture specific intravenous antibiotics are required. After the infection is cleared, delayed bone grafting or joint fusion can be performed. Wound dehiscence should be treated with free flap coverage if indicated. With close attention to the timing of surgery, and meticulous attention to the handling of soft tissues, these complications can be minimized. In our series, there were no severe wound complications in patients with closed injuries. When significant articular surface loss is coupled with severe soft tissue injury, a below-knee amputation may provide the patient the best outcome.

Anatomic reduction with stable fixation and early motion gives the best opportunity to prevent posttraumatic *arthritis*. Posttraumatic arthritis usually presents within 1 to 2 years. Initial treatment is symptomatic, including physical therapy, anti-inflammatory medications and ambulatory aids. If symptomatic treatment fails, ankle arthrodesis or arthroplasty can be considered.

*Malunions* of the joint surface or shaft can be prevented by adequate initial reduction and stable fixation. The benefit of this "soft tissue friendly" two-stage technique is better access to the joint to allow anatomic reduction at the time of stabilization, because delayed reconstruction (greater than 3 weeks) of the joint is difficult and often results in less favorable outcomes. It is our experience that the use of an external fixator as the sole treatment modality is associated with a high incidence of metaphyseal nonunion, or varus collapse resulting in tibial malunion. Most surgeons who advocate this technique suggest a fibular osteotomy to correct this problem. We do not feel that this is a rational way to treat a fracture. Even if the fracture heals, the leg is subsequently shorter than the other. Similarly, if the metaphyseal area is plated and not grafted or if load bearing begins before complete consolidation, the plate is at risk for failure.

## RECOMMENDED READING

1. Bone L, Stegmann P, McNamara K, et al.: External fixation of severely comminuted and open tibial pilon fractures. *Clin Orthop* 292:101–107, 1993.
2. Brumback RJ, McGarvey WC: Fractures of the tibial plafond: evolving treatment concepts for the pilon fracture. *Orthop Clin North Am* 26:273–285, 1995.
3. Brunner CH, Weber EG: *Special techniques in internal fixation.* New York: Springer-Verlag, 1982.
4. Heim U, Pfeiffer, KM: Internal fixation of small fractures: technique recommended by the AO-ASIF group. New York: Springer-Verlag, 1988.
5. Helfet DL, Koval K, Pappas J, et al.: Intraarticular "pilon" fracture of the tibia. *Clin Orthop* 298:221–228, 1994.
6. Mast JW, Spiegel PG, Pappas JN: Fractures of the tibial pilon. *Clin Orthop* 230:68–82, 1988.
7. McFerran MA, Smith SW, Boulas HJ, et al.: Complications encountered in the treatment of pilon fractures. *J Orthop Trauma* 6:195–200, 1992.
8. Rüedi TP, Állgower M: The operative treatment of intra-articular fractures of the lower end of the tibia. *Clin Orthop* 138:105–110, 1979.
9. Sirkin M, Sanders R, DiPasquale T, et al.: Results of a staged protocol for wound management in complex pilon fractures. *J Orthop Trauma* 13:78–84, 1999.
10. Teeny SM, Wiss DA: Open reduction and internal fixation of tibial plafond fractures; variables contributing to poor results and complications. *Clin Orthop* 292, 108–117, 1991.

# 43

# Mosaicplasty for Osteochondral Lesions of the Talus

Gary Kish

Mosaicplasty represents a surgical technique for the restitution of articular surfaces of weight-bearing diarthrodial joints with multiple small autogenous osteochondral cylindrical grafts. Since 1992, the method has been applied to focal articular lesions of the talar dome, as well as the femoral condyle, patella, and tibial plateau. This chapter focuses on the indications, implementation, and rehabilitation of talar mosaicplasty.

## INDICATIONS/CONTRAINDICATIONS

The major indications for mosaicplasty about the ankle are grade III and IV osteochondral lesions of the talus (OLT) (Fig. 43-1). The cause of these lesions remains elusive, but is related in part to trauma and ischemia. When the lesions have progressed to produce clinical symptoms of pain, locking from loose fragments, and altered biomechanics, operative intervention could be considered. Mosaicplasty addresses the removal of the loose and damaged surface elements, and subsequently restores the surface with contoured autogenous osteochondral plugs obtained from the supracondylar ridge of the ipsilateral femoral condyles.

As experience and success is gained with OLT, there is a tendency to expand the indication to larger traumatic lesions and certain benign tumors such as unicameral and synovial cysts and enchondromas. Under these conditions, the goals and expectations need to be carefully weighed and discussed with the patient.

Contraindications to mosaicplasty include septic lesions, generalized arthritis, large traumatic chondral lesions that have laminated much of the talar surface, and defects related to malignancy. Additionally, avascular necrosis of the talar body cannot support graft ingrowth.

G. Kish, M.D.: Department of Orthopaedics, Portsmouth Regional Hospital, Portsmouth, New Hampshire.

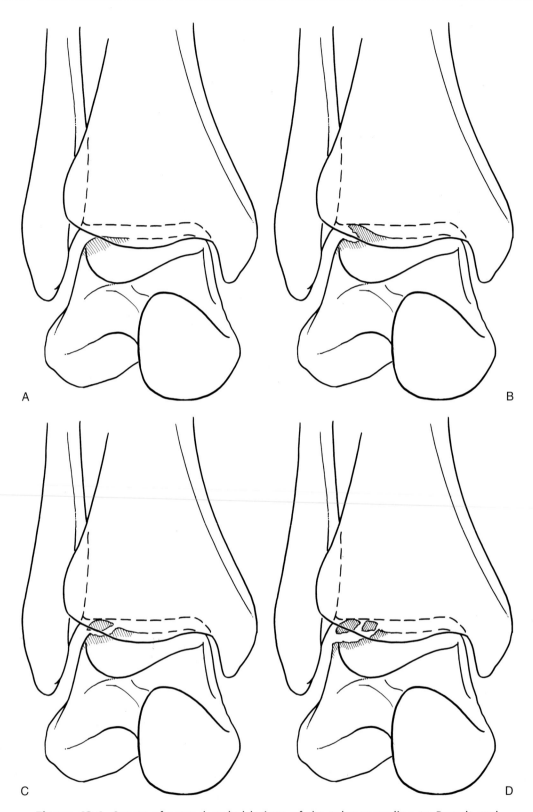

**Figure 43-1.** Stages of osteochondral lesions of the talus according to Berndt and Harty (1959). **A:** Stage I, small area of compression of subchondral bone. **B:** Stage II, osteochondral fragment partially detached. **C:** Stage III, complete detachment from its underlying bed, but fragment remains in anatomic position. **D:** Stage IV, complete detachment with displacement. [From Berndt AL, Harty M: Transchondral fractures (osteochondritis dissecans) of the talus. *J Bone Joint Surg* 41A: 996, 1959.]

## PREOPERATIVE PLANNING

Most patients with symptomatic OLT are in their twenties or thirties, active in sports, and have been treated by a variety of conservative therapies. Many have had previous unsuccessful surgeries, including removal of loose bodies, abrasion arthroplasty, or microfracture. Marginal osteophytes, particularly of the talar neck may be present but do not represent contraindications. As reflected in the literature, lateral talar dome lesions have a clearer link to a single traumatic event, with patients enduring symptoms for a briefer period of time than medial dome OLT. With either type of lesion, the symptoms can be acute, intermittent, or smoldering. Consequently, symptoms include sharp pain, locking, swelling, clicking, catching, giving way, and deep aching in the ankle. Associated ligamentous tears or laxity may also increase episodes of instability.

Plain films can make the diagnosis of the Grade III and IV OLT, while further grading of the lesion can be detailed by MRI, CT scan, and arthroscopy (Fig. 43-2). When radiographs demonstrate an OLT but the symptoms are vague, a bone scan can be helpful in determining if the lesion is actively inflamed.

After an OLT has been defined, graded as a III or IV lesion, and the symptoms are of sufficient magnitude, the option of mosaicplasty is discussed. The patient is counseled about the nature of the problem, the specifics of the surgery, the need to begin early postoperative range of motion of the knee and ankle, and the absolute necessity of adhering to the rule of not bearing weight for a minimum of 4 weeks postoperatively. A concerted and controlled rehabilitation program during the first 6 postoperative months is advised.

Special attention is directed to the use of the ipsilateral knee as the donor site. The supracondylar ridge of the femoral condyle, in the absence of patellar symptoms or arthritis, remains the best source for autogenous osteochondral plugs. The quality of the cartilage

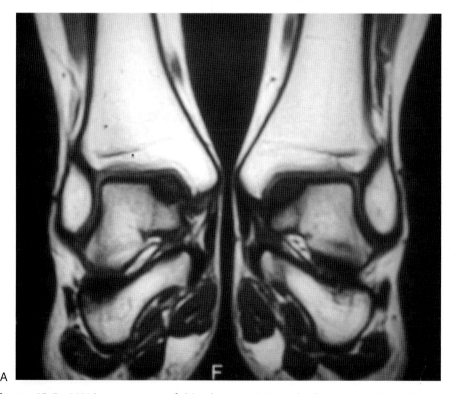

A

**Figure 43-2.** MRI images are useful in characterizing talar lesions. **A:** Coronal view of bilateral, medial lesions. *(continued)*

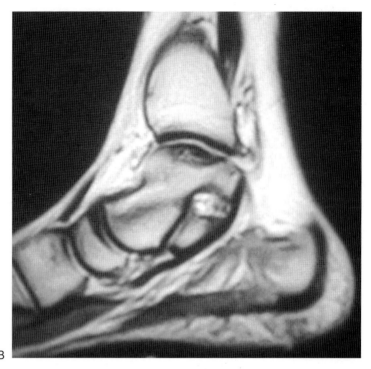

B

**Figure 43-2.** *Continued.* **B:** Sagittal view of a different patient with medial lesions.

closely matches the talar dome articular cartilage; the ridges offer large enough surface areas to obtain enough plugs to cover the talar dome surface; and there has been no long-term morbidity when multiple *small* grafts are taken.

Secondary sources of grafts could be small grafts from the talar head and talar malleolar surfaces. Use of fresh allograft remains an attractive alternative but should be reserved for large defects or when there are absolute contraindications to using the femoral condyles.

Consultation with a physical therapist aids the patient in understanding the need for initial non–weight bearing, range of motion exercises, and use of ambulating aids.

## SURGERY

The procedure is done under general anesthesia, supplemented by local blocks and a postoperative bupivacaine delivery catheter. Proper exposure and freedom to move the lower extremity is facilitated by positioning the patient supine on an adjustable bean bag, and a radiolucent OR table that can be tilted from side to side. Whether it is a medial or lateral lesion (Fig. 43-3), an arthroscopic survey initiates the procedure to confirm the diagnosis and to assess the extent and quality of the articular cartilage in the remainder of the joint.

### Technique: Medial Lesions

When exposure of the medial lesion is sought through an anterior medial capsular incision, only the anterior one fifth of the medial talus can be effectively approached. In most cases, a medial OLT is in a central-medial location, ensconced by the medial malleolus, and exposure through a medial malleolar trap door is required.

If attempting exposure through a medial malleolar osteotomy, the following issues should be kept in mind:

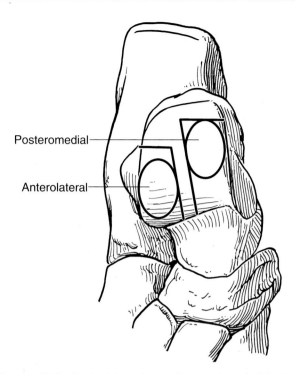

Posteromedial

Anterolateral

**Figure 43-3.** Typical locations of osteochondral lesions of the talus. Areas of access are available through medial malleolar osteotomy *(dotted line)* and anterior lateral approaches *(dashed line)*.

1. Perpendicular instrument access to the lesion will be denied unless the line of the cut is sufficiently vertical, and then enters the joint at the junction of the medial malleolar and tibial plafond.
2. The more oblique the cut, the more eversion and abduction of the talus are needed. The lateral capsule and lateral malleolus will be the limiting factors to these excursions and visualizations.
3. The more vertical the cut, the more vertical shear will be placed on the fixation during active range of motion through the posterior tibial and Achilles tendons.
4. Fixation of the fragment should be initiated by scoring the line with cautery and predrilling the screw holes to avoid loss of orientation and to ensure precise reduction to the "elective fracture."
5. Available hardware should include 4.0-mm malleolar screws ranging up to 50 mm long, 2.7- and 3.5-mm cortical screws, and a small, semitubular plate if apical compression is needed.

To expose the full breadth of the medial ankle, a curvilinear incision is centered over the medial malleolus (Fig. 43-4). By blunt dissection and gentle retraction, thick flaps are developed for preserving and protecting the saphenous vein and nerve. A small anterior incision is made in the anterior capsule at the medial border of the anterior tibial tendon (ATT) to identify the joint line, apex of the medial malleolus, and the lesion (Fig. 43-5). The posterior tibial tendon (PTT) is palpated immediately behind the malleolus. The overlying flexor retinaculum is incised longitudinally, leaving cuffs for later repair. The PTT is retracted off the capsule to expose the capsule to the lateral lip of the PTT groove. A blunt, small, right-angle or Homan retractor is used to protect the PTT and the more posterior lateral flexor digitorum longus tendon, neurovascular bundle, and flexor hallucis longus tendon. A blunt probe is passed through the joint from anterior to posterior. The exposed ends of the probe and the center of the lesion serve as guides for the line of the osteotomy (Fig. 43-5). The surgeon predrills the screw holes and scores the sides of the intended cut (Figs. 43-6 through 43-8). He or she begins and completes the osteotomy with a 1-cm, fine-tooth

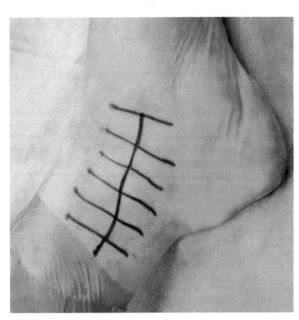

**Figure 43-4.** Surgical approach for medial osteochondral lesions. The medial view shows placement of medial incision over the medial malleolus.

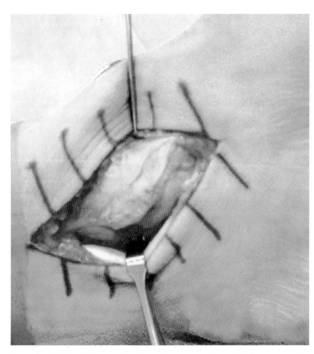

**Figure 43-5.** The malleolus is exposed, and the posterior tibial tendon is retracted posteriorly. A blunt probe is passed through the capsule from anterior to posterior aspects to define the inner margin of the osteotomy.

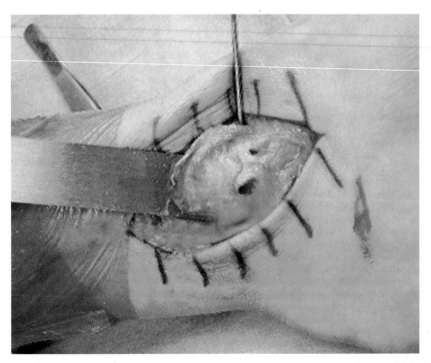

**Figure 43-6.** In the medial malleolar osteotomy, notice the screw holes predrilled for later fixation. A probe is inserted from anterior to posterior aspects to help identify the proper orientation of the osteotomy.

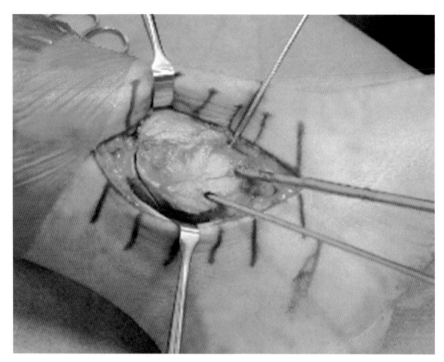

**Figure 43-7.** In the medial malleolar osteotomy, drill bits show the orientation of the predrilled holes. A probe in the ankle from anterior to posterior is shown.

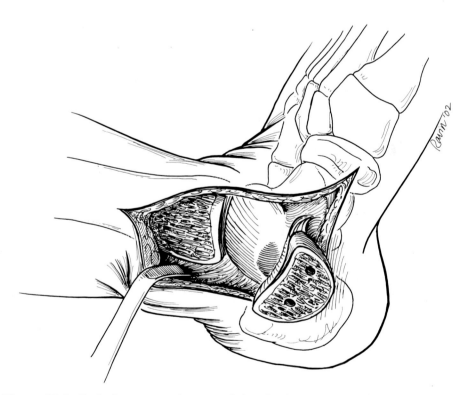

**Figure 43-8.** Typical exposure after a medial malleolus osteotomy shows the ankle everted and foot abducted.

sagittal blade. Performing the osteotomy with care and distraction of the joint can avoid a jagged entry into the joint and scoring of the talus.

A no. 5 suture is passed through the fragment drill holes, the fragment is levered downward, and the capsule is sharply incised anteriorly and posteriorly (Fig. 43-9). The fragment position and blood supply are maintained by the remaining attached deltoid ligament. At this point, the exposure is still limited. To access the talar dome and expose the lesion, the ankle must be everted and drawn forward and the forefoot abducted in a slow, concerted manner. With patience, the dome will come into proper view (Fig. 43-8).

The size and number of grafts will be determined by the dimensions of the OLT, and the contour of the involved portion of the talar dome. The area of the adult talar dome averages 10 cm$^2$, of which 4 cm$^2$ can be approached through the medial exposure and 4 cm$^2$ through the lateral exposure. The dome has a subtle but defined anterior to posterior convexity with a sagittal radius of convexity of 20 mm on the average. A shallow, concave sulcus divides the surface coursing from anterior-medial to posterior-lateral. Osteochondral plugs in the range of 3.5 to 6.5 mm in diameter conform to this undulating surface.

After the lesion has been exposed, the surgeon removes the loose fragments, clears the crater bed of scar tissue and necrotic bone, and trims the edges of the lesion to normal articular cartilage (Figs. 43-9 and 43-10). Have a knowledgeable assistant keep the ankle correctly positioned and stable during the sequence of drilling and dilating the recipient hole, and delivery of the grafts. Release of the tension between steps will provide respite for the soft tissue. Small Homan retractors, 3-tine rakes, and pressure of the delivery tube against the lateral osteotomy wall will keep the field open during the implantation. On occasion, when there is significant subtalar motion, a joystick through the talar neck will help evert and stabilize the talus (Fig. 43-11).

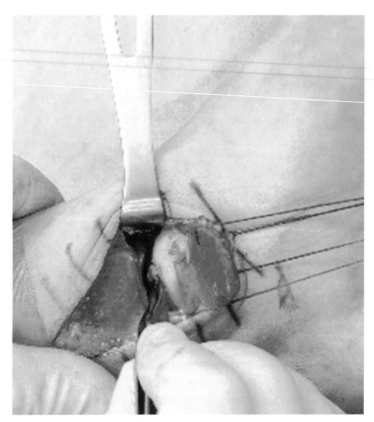

**Figure 43-9.** The surgeon identifies and removes loose osteochondral fragments. Traction is placed on a malleolar fragment with a no. 5 suture.

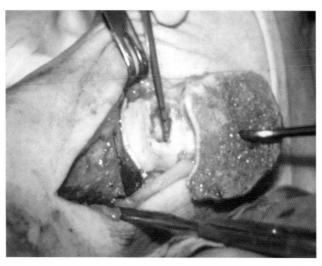

**Figure 43-10.** The lesion is defined down to bleeding, cancellous bone. The edges are trimmed to normal articular cartilage.

The specific instrumentation used is based on availability and the surgeon's preference. The mosaicplasty instruments, Acufex Mosaicplasty Comprehensive System (Smith and Nephew Endoscopy Division, Andover, MA) is described.

Plan and mark the insertion points with the appropriately sized universal guide. Under direct vision, create the recipient sockets with aid of the chisel guide. While keeping the guide perpendicular to the surface, drill the recipient socket to a depth of 18 mm with a sharp-tipped drill (Figs. 43-11 and 43-12). Recently these drills have been converted to

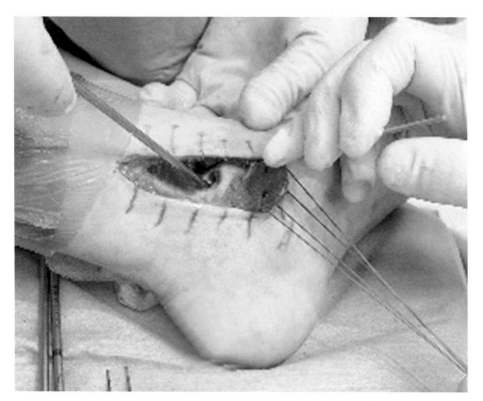

**Figure 43-11.** The lesion is measured carefully to determine the best size and placement of grafts with various sizes of dilators (e.g., 3.5 mm, 4.5 mm, 6.5 mm).

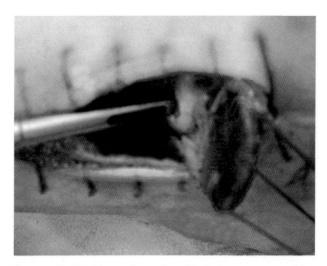

**Figure 43-12.** The universal guide is in proper position for drilling the first hole in the medial talus.

nontapered shanks, which keep the drill bit from "hanging up" in the windows as the drill bit is withdrawn.

The surgeon uses a small Fraser suction to remove the bone fragments from the recipient socket and repeats the process for the remaining sites. The direction of the drill is carefully monitored to ensure there is at least 1 mm of intervening bone between the holes. Because of the undulation of the talus, the direction sometimes needs to be moved off perpendicularly by a few degrees to keep the holes spaced properly (Fig. 43-13). Convergence in the depths of the talar body may occur. In such instances, the cancellous portion of the donor plugs will lock into each other, rather than to the retaining walls. At this point,

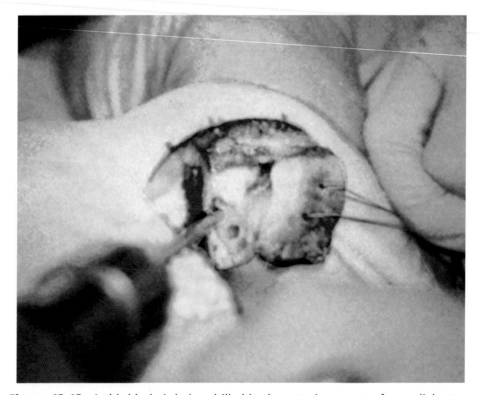

**Figure 43-13.** A third hole is being drilled in the anterior aspect of a medial osteochondral lesion. Drill holes are spaced 1 to 2 mm apart.

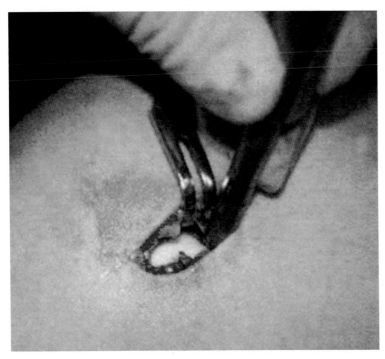

**Figure 43-14.** Grafts are harvested from the knee through a 2-cm incision to expose the medial supracondylar ridge of the medial condyle.

the surgeon removes the instruments, reduces the ankle, and compresses the wound in preparation to obtain the donor grafts from the ipsilateral knee.

The donor grafts can be gained arthroscopically or through a mini-arthrotomy. By direct and controlled access, the mini-arthrotomy allows the surgeon to consistently procure flat, well-spaced grafts. The lateral ridge is the first option because of its flatter surface; the medial ridge is more easily reached arthroscopically (Figs. 43-14 and 43-15). Consider the lat-

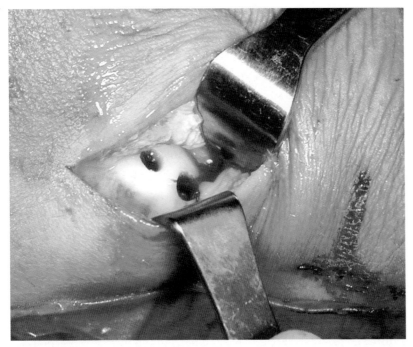

**Figure 43-15.** The donor site after removal of multiple grafts from the lateral supracondylar ridge through a 3-cm incision. The grafts are spaced 2 to 3 mm apart.

ter approach in patients with increased Q angles. When more grafts are needed, both ridges can be used as long as the entrance to the femoral sulcus is not violated. By flexing and extending the knee, up to six 4.5-mm grafts can be obtained through the mini-arthrotomy or an extended arthroscopy portal. The sulcus terminalis serves as the distal end point of available donor articular cartilage.

On selecting a site, the surgeon holds the grafting tool firmly on the cartilage and strikes the tube smartly. The first blow must be of sufficient force to drive through the cartilage and subchondral bone. A tentative first blow allows the tube to drift as it transfers from the cartilage to bone, resulting in a crooked graft with an unstable chondral-bone interface. Complete seating of the chisel to the 15-mm mark is accomplished (Fig. 43-16 left). Using the tamp, the surgeon toggles the chisel from medial to lateral until the cancellous bone at the tip of the chisel is broken as indicated by a palpable "give" (Fig. 43-16 right). Then the chisel is extracted with the captured graft. The tamp is used to push the graft out of the chisel from tip to head, protecting the cutting tip. Subsequent grafts are spaced 1 to 2 mm apart, taking care not to enter the previous cancellous defect. When taking 6.5- and 4.5-mm grafts, the sizes should be alternated to lessen the chances of cancellous confluence and chondral bridge fracture. The grafts should measure 15 mm or less, and the chondral-osseous junction should be stable. The grafts are saved in a dedicated, moist basin on the back table. Typically, these defects fill in with fibrocartilage (Fig. 43-17).

The knee wound may be closed at this point or at the completion of the talar grafting. In either case, the holes are filled with gel-foam, and the knee is drained with a Hemovac. The joint is infused with another bolus of bupivacaine before tourniquet release and opening of the suction drain.

If a thigh tourniquet has been used, it should be deflated after insertion of the drain and

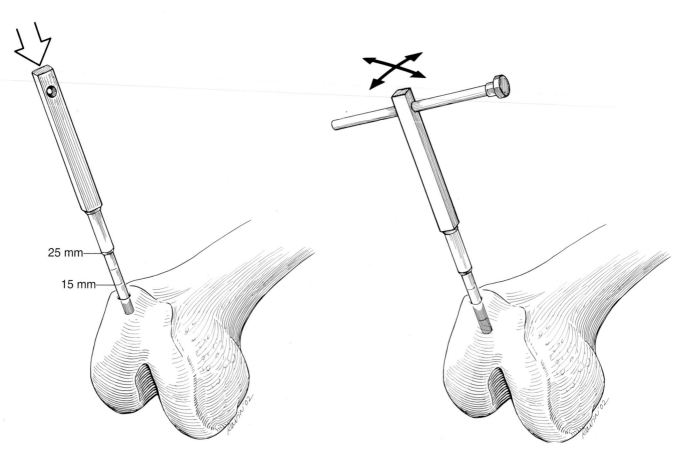

25 mm
15 mm

**Figure 43-16.** The graft is harvested *(left)* in the medial supracondylar ridge with a tubular chisel to a depth of 15 mm. Graft tissue is removed *(right)* by toggling the chisel in multiple directions to free the deep end of the graft. The chisel captures the graft.

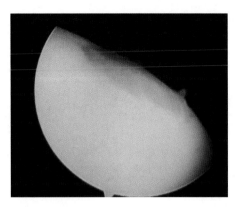

**Figure 43-17.** Example of the appearance of a 4.5-mm donor site in the lateral supracondylar ridge at 1 year of follow-up. The defect was filled with fibrocartilage flush with the articular surface.

knee closure. An above-ankle tourniquet can be used for the insertion of the osteochondral grafts.

The recipient site is exposed as before and the sockets cleared by lavage and Fraser-tip suction. Dilation just before *each* graft insertion is important in this method because the grafts tend to expand by 0.6 to 0.75 mm when removed from the donor site and because the seated grafts can push the common walls, compressing and distorting the adjacent sockets.

The surgeon measures the depth of the holes of the dilator markings, ensuring that each hole is 1 to 3 mm deeper than the length of the intended graft. Press-fit fixation occurs from the sidewalls and adjacent grafts. The 15-mm graft is loaded into the universal tube guide, and the delivery tamp is adjusted to a length flush with the distal shoulder of the guide windows. The graft and plunger are assembled into the guide, and the graft is slowly inserted by pushing, lengthening the plunger (by counterclockwise rotation of the adjustable head), and pushing again until the chondral surface of the plug is slightly proud of the recipient surface (Fig. 43-18). The final sitting of the graft can be done by gently tapping on the plunger head. Care must be exercised in removing the guide from the graft. By lengthening the plunger and putting slight pressure on it, the tube guide can be rotated away from the graft and slid back up the plunger until it clears the graft head, and then removed. Insert each of the subsequent grafts in a similar fashion, preceded by dilating the recipient hole. Strict attention must be paid to the previously inserted grafts as it is possible to push them below the surface with the shoulder of the chisel guide when the grafts are tightly packed (Figs. 43-19 and 43-20). Final seating of the grafts is done with the tamp head (Fig. 43-21). In most medial OCD lesions, the surgeon should expect to use one 6.5- and two 4.5-mm grafts to fill the defect. Once satisfied with the construct, the medial malleolus can be repaired.

Unlike a fractured malleolus, the fragment does not lock with cancellous interdigitization. As such, rotation is controlled with finger pressure, a Kirschner wire, or an awl. The malleolar fragment is restored with two 4.0-mm, partially threaded lag screws. The screws are seated alternately. If the osteotomy line gaps proximally, the surgeon should consider an apical cortical screw or antiglide plate to compress and stabilize the fragment (Fig. 43-22). The ankle is moved though its range of motion from plantarflexion and dorsiflexion positions, checking the fixation, screw position, and reduction with a C-arm.

## Technique: Lateral Lesions

Lateral OLTs invariably are located on the anterior-lateral surface, making their exposure possible through a standard anterior lateral ankle incision (Fig. 43-23). The 5-cm incision is centered at the joint line extending from the upper flare of the anterior tibial tubercle to

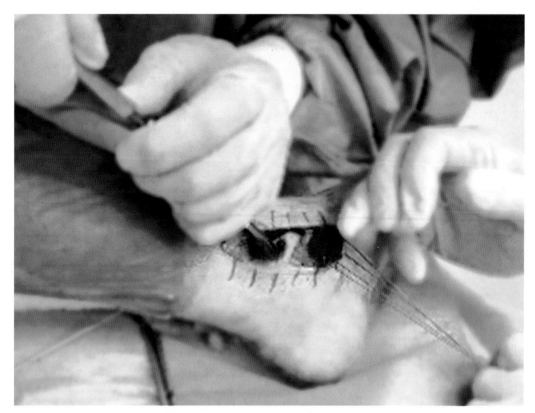

**Figure 43-18.** The selected graft is placed in 4.5-mm universal guide, and the first plug is placed until the cartilage is flush with the talar surface.

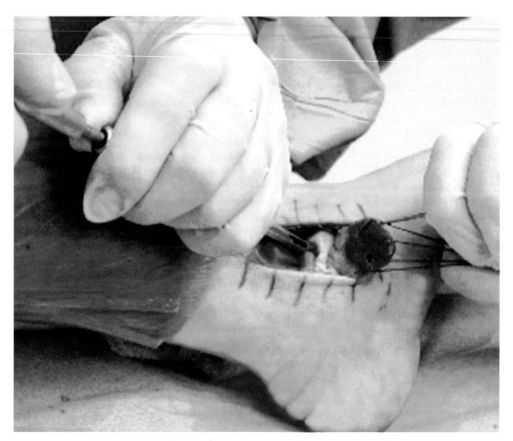

**Figure 43-19.** A third graft is inserted. Each recipient site is dilated before insertion.

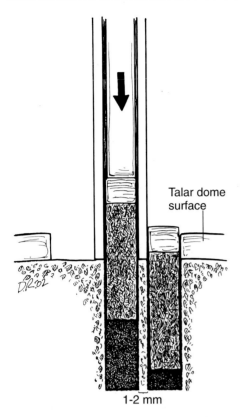

**Figure 43-20.** The second graft is placed 1 to 2 mm from the first graft. The surgeon avoids pushing the graft below the surface of the talus.

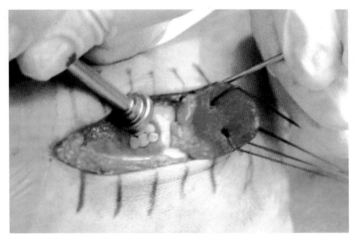

**Figure 43-21.** Multiple grafts are gently impacted for final seating.

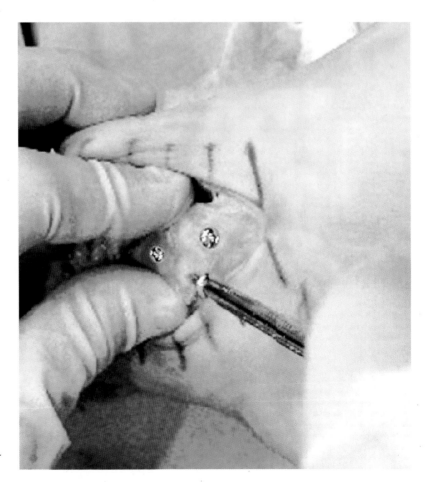

**Figure 43-22.** Fixation of the malleolar osteotomy.

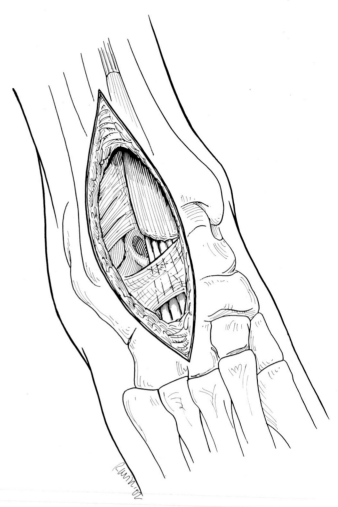

**Figure 43-23.** Anterior lateral lesions are exposed through an anterior lateral skin incision, which permits the lateral two thirds of talus to be exposed.

origin of the extensor digitorum brevis. On entering the ankle joint, the inferior edge of the anterior tibiofibular ligament serves as upper border and the anterior lip of the talar dome as the lower border. Blunt rake retractors are placed on each side of the capsular incision, and the ankle is plantarflexed to see if the lesion can be exposed through this limited arthrotomy. If the lesion extends further posteriorly, the surgeon sequentially releases and tags the anterior talofibular and the calcaneofibular ligaments for later repair. Release of these ligaments allows for anterior translation of the talus, providing perpendicular access to two thirds of the lateral half of the talar dome (Fig. 43-24). Further extensile options include a chevron-shaped osteotomy of the fibula, and posterior capsule release; these options are rarely needed in the cases of lateral OLT.

After perpendicular access has been obtained, the mosaicplasty technique is essentially the same as described for the medial lesions. The lateral lesions usually are wafer-like and reside in the anterior-lateral quadrant of the dome (Fig. 43-24). The surgeon should expect to use two to four 4.5-mm plugs for average-size lesions or one 6.5-mm and two 4.5-mm plugs for larger lesions (Figs. 43-25 through 43-28).

Closure of the ankle incision includes repair of the anterior talofibular and calcaneofibular ligaments if they had been sectioned. Use of bone suture anchors can be helpful particularly if the ATFL has been taken off the talar neck. The knee mini-arthrotomy is closed over a suction drain, which remains in place for 24 hours. With the use of small 3.5- to 6.5-mm grafts, drainage should be less than 100 mL. A well-padded, short-leg posterior splint is applied with the ankle positioned at neutral dorsiflexion.

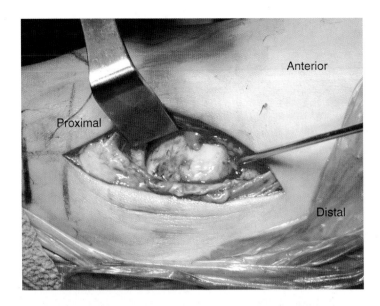

**Figure 43-24.** Anterior lateral exposure. The pin in the talar neck assists in plantarflexing the talus for greater exposure when it is used as a joystick.

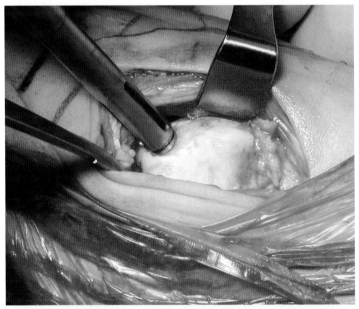

**Figure 43-25.** The universal guide is positioned for drilling the first hole in the lateral talus.

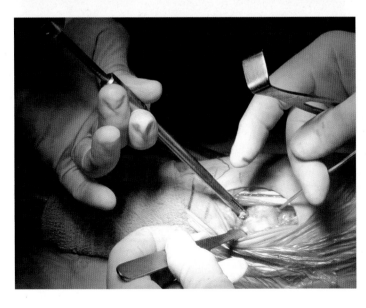

**Figure 43-26.** A second hole is drilled in a lateral talar osteochondral lesion with a 4.5-mm drill.

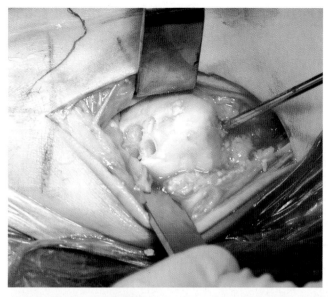

**Figure 43-27.** Completion of four 4.5-mm drill holes in the lateral talus. They are spaced 2 mm apart.

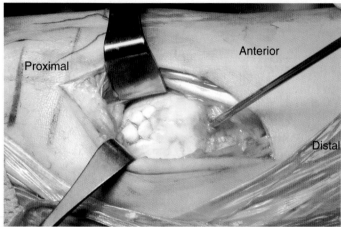

Proximal

Anterior

Distal

**Figure 43-28.** Placement of four grafts in the anterior lateral osteochondral lesion. Notice the traction pin.

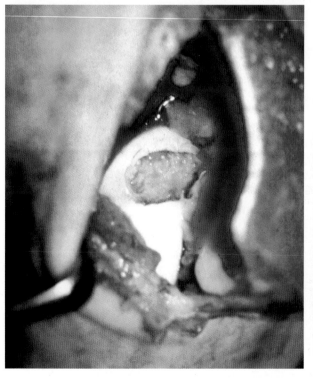

A

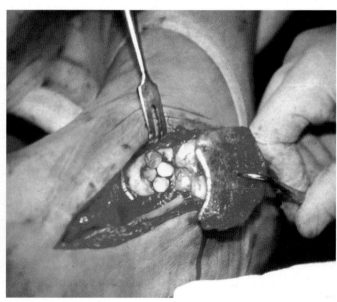

B

**Figure 43-29.  A:** The defect extends over the medial edge of the talar dome and into the medial joint line. **B:** Grafts are inserted with cartilage, following the contour of the adjacent cartilage.

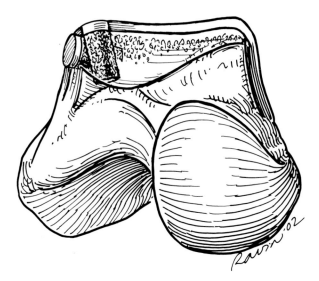

**Figure 43-30.** Grafts are placed along the contour of the medial edge of the talar dome.

Osteochondral lesions can occur in the medial or lateral "edge" of the talar dome (Figs. 43-29 and 43-30). In such cases, the placement and size of the grafts need to be carefully planned and inserted so that a buttress of cancellous bone is created. An absent lip of the talus usually involves 5 mm of articular cartilage and subchondral bone to a depth of 5 mm. By placing one or two 6.5-mm plugs at a slightly oblique inward angle and keeping their length at 15 mm, secure fixation can be gained. The raw cancellous outer surface is then rounded off to conform to the shape of the surrounding outer wall of the talar body. This relatively low-weight-bearing surface can be expected to transform to fibrocartilage. No additional fixation is required (Fig. 43-29).

## POSTOPERATIVE MANAGEMENT

An overnight stay ensures constant elevation of the extremity, allows administration of intravenous prophylactic antibiotics, and provides parenteral pain control. The preemptive marcaine ankle and foot block and intraarticular bupivacaine knee infusion can provide 6 to 12 hours of pain relief. Use of the pain catheter system depends on the surgeon's preference. If inserted in the ankle joint, it should be removed at 48 hours. Some form of deep vein thrombosis prophylaxis could be used.

There are several phases of rehabilitation to full recovery. The better educated the patient, the smoother the postoperative course will be. In phase I (initial 30 days), the patient should not bear weight for 1 month. After the incisions have healed, encourage the patient to actively move the joints. Preoperative counseling, and postoperative re-enforcement makes this critical phase tolerable for the goal-oriented patient. Every part of the patient's activities of daily living can be incorporated into this phase. Crutch walking, in itself is an aerobic exercise, promotes better oxygenation to healing tissues, better overall equilibrium, and may enable the patient to sleep more easily at night. Knee complaints are rare. Any increased pain, swelling, or slow healing of the incision should prompt concerns of problems such as infection or reflex sympathetic dystrophy, and be treated appropriately. For patients needing the unrestrained use of both hands while standing, devices such as a Roll-A-Bout offer a safe standing and ambulatory aid.

In phase II (2 to 3 months), after the wounds have healed, the osteotomy united, and the cancellous portion of the grafts incorporated radiographically, weight bearing can be initiated. A protective, removable walker can limit swelling and bear some of the load as the patient progresses from minimal (one fourth of body weight), to moderate (one half of body weight), and then to full, protected weight bearing incrementally over this 60-day period. The physician prescribes active and active-assisted exercises of the knee, ankle, and foot; aqua therapy; and other modalities during this phase.

Phase III (3 to 6 months) can be called the transition rehabilitation phase for the mosaicplasty patient. The tendency is to remove the harness, rather than to loosen it. With unrestrained activities, the patient will soon return with increased pain, clicking, popping, swelling, and other symptoms reflecting overuse of the soft tissue envelope, which still needs several more months to heal. Preoperative counseling about the expectations during this period helps maintain compliance and alleviate the patient's concerns. If such symptoms arise, reuse of the ankle walker for a short time and antiinflammatory drugs will be helpful.

During phase IV (6 to 12 months), full recovery from talar mosaicplasty for OLT varies considerably. It depends on the size of the lesion, postoperative compliance during the first 6 months, and the patient's habitus and expectations. Full recovery can be measured by full, active weight bearing; full range of motion of the ankle, foot, and knee; 5/5 muscle strength; and criteria as defined by various clinical scales such as the AOFAS ankle and hindfoot scale, Hanover Foot and Ankle Scale, and the Modified Bandi Patellar Femoral Joint scale. The patient can be evaluated on a yearly basis. Experience indicates that, if the ankle condition is good at 24 months, the long-term results will be good.

## COMPLICATIONS

Many of the potential complications and pitfalls have been discussed in the above sections. In general, the major complications of infection, thrombophlebitis, and articular incongruity can be minimized by good patient care and attention to detail at surgery. Some of the problems associated with graft placement may be lessened by proper exposure, including a correctly oriented malleolar osteotomy (Figs. 43-31 through 43-34).

A specific concern about the mosaicplasty involves *late pain and ankle dysfunction* after 6 months. Late knee pain after the procedure may be related to scarring in the patellar-femoral joint or exuberant prominent fibrocartilage ingrowth at the donor sites. If the pain is associated with clicking and catching after 6 months, an arthroscopic evaluation should

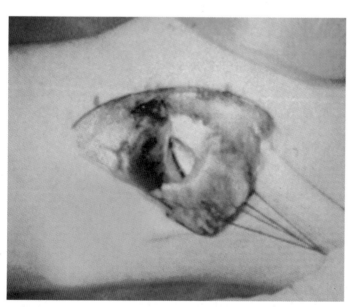

**Figure 43-31.** A common pitfall of medial malleolar osteotomy is orientation that is too horizontal, which limits exposure.

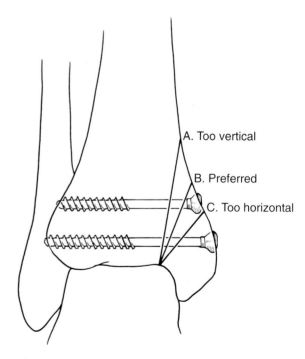

**Figure 43-32.** Medial osteotomy. Too vertical *(A)*. Preferred position *(B)*. Too horizontal *(C)*.

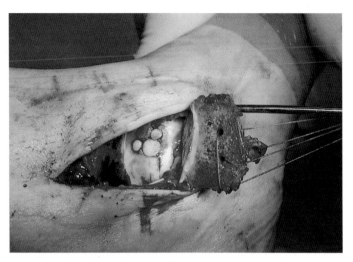

**Figure 43-33.** Medial view of the ankle shows a common pitfall of medial malleolar osteotomy. The osteotomy entered the joint too medially (medial to apex). Adequate visualization is accomplished with more torque on the foot by placing a pin in the talus to evert the talus.

be considered. Otherwise, persistent physical therapy for strengthening and stretching should be continued.

Late ankle pain associated with similar physical signs of catching, intermittent locking or giving-way of the joint may indicate a loosened donor fragment or nonincorporation of a graft. Radiographs may give evidence of a loose osseous fragment, whereas MRI is needed to determine whether a defect in the articular surface has reappeared. If either of these imaging modalities is positive, an arthroscopic examination can be considered. At the time of the arthroscopy, the entire construct can be evaluated, debridement performed as necessary, and physical therapy reinstituted.

*Loss of motion* not associated with intrarticular problems can be associated with gait dysfunction. The most troublesome restriction will be loss of ankle dorsiflexion. Most com-

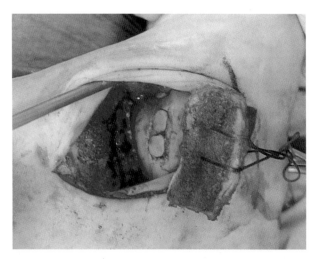

**Figure 43-34.** Medial view of the ankle after malleolar osteotomy. The osteotomy entered the joint slightly lateral to the apex. Notice the excellent exposure that does not require excessive torque on the foot or a talar pin. Angling the osteotomy to enter the joint lateral to the apex is useful if the lesion is large or more centrally located or if the ankle is stiff.

monly, the cause is contracture of the soleus or gastrocnemius-soleus complex, which can be addressed by stretching exercises and rocker-bottom soles. The other cause could be accumulation of scar at the talar neck. In such cases, if dorsiflexion cannot be improved at least to neutral, and is associated with pain and dysfunction, then arthroscopic debridement at the talar neck and lengthening of the soleus or gastrocnemius can be considered.

## ACKNOWLEDGMENTS

The author appeciates the contributions of László Hangody, M.D., Ph.D., D.Sc., Department of Orthopaedics and Trauma, Uzsoki Hospital, Budapest, Hungary, and of Robert E. Eberhart, M.D., Sports Medicine Atlantic Orthopaedics, Portsmouth, New Hampshire.

## RECOMMENDED READING

1. Ferkel RD: *Arthroscopic surgery: the foot and ankle.* Philadelphia: Lippincott-Raven, 1996:145–184.
2. Hangody L, Kish G, Kárpáti Z, et al.: Treatment of osteochondritis dissecans of the talus: use of the mosaic-plasty technique—a preliminary report. *Foot Ankle Int* 18:628–634, 1997.
3. Hangody L, Kish G: Osteochondritis dissecans of the talus. *Surg Tech Orthop Traumatol Paris* 55:630, 2000.
4. Hoppenfeld S, de Boer P: *Surgical exposures in orthopaedics.* New York: J.B. Lippincott, 1983.
5. Jackson DW, Scheer MJ, Simon TM: Cartilage substitutes: overview of basic science and treatment options. *J Am Acad Orthop Surg* 9:37–52, 2001.
6. Kitaoka HB, Alexander IJ, Adelaar RS, et al.: Clinical rating systems for the ankle, hindfoot, midfoot, hallux and lesser toes. *Foot Ankle Int* 15:349–353, 1994.

# Subject Index

Page numbers followed by f indicate figures; those followed by t indicate tables.